AF324156

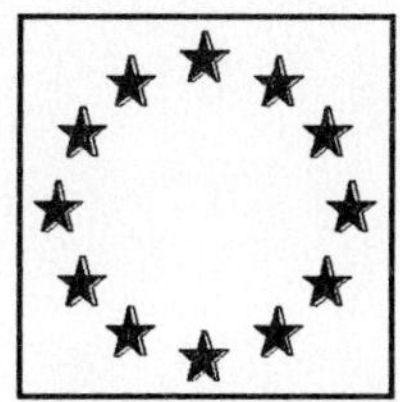

Published on behalf of

Commission of the European Communities

VETERINARY DRUG RESIDUES

Residues in food producing animals and their products: Reference Materials and Methods.

Second Edition

Edited by
R.J.Heitzman
1, Churn Road
Compton
Newbury
Berkshire RG16 0PP
United Kingdom

Contract Numbers 5464/1/5/272/91/04-BCR-UK(10) & 5326/1/5/272/90/3-BCR-UK(10)

Final Report

Measurements and Testing Programme (BCR)
Directorate General for Science, Research and Development

Directorate for Agriculture.

OXFORD

BLACKWELL SCIENTIFIC PUBLICATIONS

LONDON EDINBURGH BOSTON

MELBOURNE PARIS BERLIN VIENNA

1994   EUR 15127-EN

Published on behalf of the
COMMISSION OF THE EUROPEAN COMMUNITIES
Directorate General
Telecommunications, Information Industries and Innovation
L-2920 Luxembourg
by
Blackwell Scientific Publications
Osney Mead, Oxford OX2 0EL

Publication no. EUR 15127-EN of the
Commission of the European Communities,
Dissemination of Scientific and Technical Knowledge Unit
Directorate-General Information Technologies and Industries
and Telecommunications,
Luxembourg

First edition published 1992
Second edition published 1994

Luxembourg: Office for Official Publications of the European Communities 1994
ISBN 0-632-03786-5

ECSC-EEC-EAEC, Brussels – Luxembourg, 1994

Printed in Great Britain by
the University Press, Cambridge

PREFACE

Food quality, especially public concern about residues in meat, is one of
the important issues in Europe. This is the first revision of a book whose
purpose is to bring together and update the activities in residues of
veterinary drugs within the Community. The increasing vigilance and
control of residues of veterinary drugs in farm animals and their primary
products relies on effective control of residues. This is only made
possible by having adequate technical resources to carry out relevant
legislation. The analytical methodology used must have an acceptable
quality assurance supported by good quality control criteria, sufficient
reference materials and technical data.

This book addresses each of these needs in detail. There is a summary of
relevant EEC legislation including a section on Maximum Residue Limits
(MRLs). The methods used in each Member State for the examination of
residues of a large number of drugs is summarised and a selection of the
methods are described in detail. There is supporting information on
residues and chemical/physical data of the most important veterinary drugs.
Also one section of the book covers quality assurance and gives the
criteria for the methods to be used in routine analysis of residues.

The project to produce this book was supported by funds from the
Directorate General for Science, Research and Development (Measurements and
Testing Programme, BCR) and from the Directorate General for Agriculture
(Division of Veterinary and Animal Husbandry Legislation and the Division
for the Coordination of Agricultural Research).

The Commission wishes to thank all those who contributed to the successful
completion of this book and in particular the editor, Doctor R.J.Heitzman.

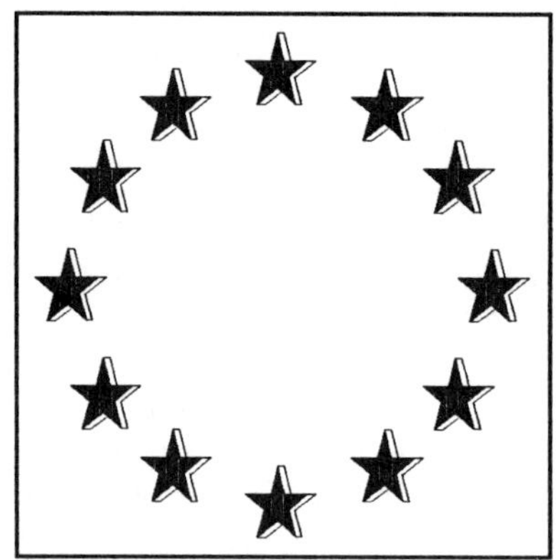

RESIDUES IN FOOD-PRODUCING ANIMALS AND THEIR PRODUCTS: REFERENCE MATERIALS AND METHODS.

CONTENTS.

1. Introduction

2. Residue groups requiring analytical methods. Maximum Residue Limits

3. Community and National Reference Laboratories

4. Summary of routine screening methods used by EC Member States

5. Criteria for routine methods and quality assurance guidelines.

6. Methods. Techniques; Screening methods; Confirmatory methods.

7. Levels of residues and naturally occurring substances.

8. Reference materials and sources of reference compounds and reagents.

9. Chemical and physical data for residue substances.

10. EEC Directives and Decisions concerning residues.

11. Literature references.

12. Annexes

13. Index.

[Note: The pages are numbered separately for each section, e.g. section 3 page 5 is 3/5. The analytical methods in section 6 are numbered separately for each method, e.g. page 3 of routine method Cy 1.2 is Cy 1.2/3.]

SECTION 6.   ROUTINE METHODS FOR DETECTING RESIDUES.

THE METHODS CHOSEN FOR INCLUSION IN THIS MANUAL ARE A SELECTION OF METHODS
USED IN VARIOUS MEMBER STATES.   THEY DO <u>NOT</u> HAVE OFFICIAL STATUS FROM THE
EUROPEAN COMMISSION AND AT THIS STAGE <u>CANNOT</u> BE TREATED AS OFFICIAL
COMMUNITY REFERENCE METHODS.

SCREENING METHODS (Sg)

Sg 1.0   **METHODS FOR ANABOLICS**

Sg 1.1   Anabolics - A routine method for the determination of residues of anabolics in perirenal fat using HPLC-HPTLC. *[Origin, Belgium]*

Sg 1.2   Anabolics - a routine method for the detection of residues of anabolics in bovine urine using GC-MS in the electron impact mode. *[Origin, France]*

Sg 1.3   Diethylstilboestrol - method for the detection of residues of diethylstilboestrol in bovine urine using radioimmunoassay (RIA). *[Origin, Ireland]*

Sg 1.4   Thyreostats - method for the measurement of residues of thyreostatic substances in animals and animal tissues on the basis of high performance thin layer chromatography (HPTLC). *[Origin, Belgium]*

Sg 2.0   **METHODS FOR ß-AGONISTS**

Sg 2.1   ß-agonists - a screening method for the detection of ß-agonists in bovine urine by GC-MS in the electron impact mode for the trimethylsilyl derivatives. *[Origin, France]*

Sg 2.2   ß-agonists - An ELISA screening method using a commercially available kit for the detection of ß-agonists in bovine urine. *[Origin, Italy]*

Sg 2.3   ß-agonists - an EIA screening method for the detection of ß-agonists in bovine urine. *[Origin Belgium]*

Sg 2.4.   ß-agonists - a screening method for the detection of ß-agonists in bovine liver, kidney and meat by GC-MS in the electron impact mode for the trimethylsilyl derivatives. *[Origin, France]*

Sg 3.0   **METHODS FOR ANTIBIOTICS**

Sg 3.1.   Antibacterial substances. A screening method for the detection of antibacterial substances in fresh meat using a modified four plate test. *[Origin, France]*

Sg 3.2.   Sulphonamides - Screening method using HPTLC for the detection of sulphonamides and dapsone in the meat of farm animals. *[Origin - the Netherlands]*

Sg 3.3.   Chloramphenicol - RIA screening method for the detection of chloramphenicol in meat, milk and eggs. *[Origin, Germany]*

Sg 3.4.   Nitroimidazoles and Nitrofurans - Analysis with dialysis and on-line HPLC for determining residues of nitroimidazoles and nitrofurans in poultry (chickens, ducks and turkeys) meat. *[Origin, The Netherlands]*

Sg 3.5.   Ciprofloxacin and Enrofloxacin - Routine screening method for the determination by HPLC after cation-exchange column chromatography in pig muscle, bacon and bovine muscle. *[Origin, UK]*

Sg 3.6.   Gentamicin and Neomycin - routine screening method for the determination by HPLC in muscle of cattle, sheep and pigs and in muscle, liver, kidney and fat of veal calves. *[Origin, France]*

Sg 4.0   **METHODS FOR OTHER SUBSTANCES.**
Sg 4.1.   Tranquillizers - An HPLC method with on-line UV spectrum identification by diode-array for residues in pig kidneys. *[Origin, The Netherlands]*
Sg 4.2.   Carbadox as QCA - routine screening method for the determination by HPLC of quinoxaline carboxylic acid (QCA) in pig kidney tissue. *[Origin, UK]*
Sg 4.3   Carbadox as Desoxycarbadox - routine screening method for the determination by HPLC of Carbadox and Desoxycarbadox in pig meat, liver and kidney tissue. *[Origin, The Netherlands]*
Sg 4.4   Ionophores - a routine method for the determination of residues of ionophores in chicken meat, liver and kidney using HPTLC. *[Origin, The Netherlands]*
Sg 4.5   Levamisole - a routine method for the determination of residues of levamisole in liver tissue by GC-MS. *[Origin, UK]*

CONFIRMING METHODS (Cy)

Cy 1.0   **METHODS FOR ANABOLIC AGENTS.**
Cy 1.1.   Anabolic Agents - A modular method for the analysis of biological materials for residues of anabolic agents. *[Origin; The Netherlands and Italy]*
Cy 1.2.   Anabolic Agents - A multi-residue method for determining residues of anabolic agents in animal tissues. *[Origin; Germany]*
Cy 1.3.   Stilbenes - Confirmation of stilbenes in bile by gas chromatography-mass spectrometry. *[Origin; UK]*
Cy 1.4.   Trenbolone - Confirmation of trenbolone in bile by gas chromatography-mass spectrometry *[Origin; UK]*
Cy 1.5.   Zeranol - Confirmation of zeranol in bile by gas chromatography-mass spectrometry. *[Origin; UK]*
Cy 1.6[*]   Zeranol - Method for measurement of residues of zeranol in animals and animal tissues using HPLC/radioimmunoassay (RIA). *[Origin; The Netherlands and UK]*
Cy 1.7[*]   Stilbenes - Method for the measurement of residues of the stilbenes, diethylstilboestrol, hexoestrol and dienoestrol in animals and animal tissues on the basis of HPLC/RIA. *[Origin; The Netherlands and UK]*
Cy 1.8.   Ethinyloestradiol - Method for the measurement of residues of ethinyloestradiol in cattle urine by GC-MS *[Origin; Belgium]*
Cy 1.9.   Thyreostats - method for the measurement of residues of thyreostatic substances in animals and animal tissues on the basis of high performance thin layer chromatography and gas chromatography - mass spectrometry (GC-MS). *[Origin, Belgium]*

Cy 2.0   **METHODS FOR ß-AGONISTS**
Cy 2.1   ß-agonists - a method for the detection and identification of ß-agonists in biological samples and animal feed.*[Origin; The Netherlands]*
Cy 2.2.   Clenbuterol - Determination of clenbuterol at residue levels in bovine plasma and tissues by GC-MS. *[Origin; France]*
Cy 2.3.   ß-Agonists - a method for confirming the detection of ß-agonists in bovine urine by GC-MS in the positive chemical ionisation mode for the trimethylsilyl derivatives. *[Origin, France]*
[*][Note; The use of spectroscopic methods for the confirmation of the stilbenes and zeranol is preferred].

Cy 3.0   **METHODS FOR ANTIBIOTICS**
Cy 3.1.   Sulphonamides - Confirmation of sulphonamides by GC-MS.
             [Origin; UK]
Cy 3.2   Sulphadimidine. Determination of sulphadimidine in pig kidney
             and diaphragm muscle tissue by high performance liquid
             chromatography. *[Origin UK-NI]*
Cy 3.3.   Sulphadimidine - HPLC analysis of sulphadimidine in porcine
             kidney. *[Origin; UK]*
Cy 3.4.   Sulphadimidine. Determination of sulphadimidine in reference
             material and fresh tissues by high performance liquid
             chromatography. *[Origin UK-NI]*
Cy 3.5.   Chloramphenicol - Confirmation of chloramphenicol in meat,
             eggs, milk and urine by GC-MS. *[Origin; The Netherlands]*
Cy 3.6.   Chloramphenicol - Confirmation of chloramphenicol in meat by
             GC-MS *[Origin; Germany]*
Cy 3.7.   Chloramphenicol - HPLC analysis of chloramphenicol in milk.
             [Origin; France]
Cy 3.8.   Tetracyclines - Determination by HPLC of tetracyclines at
             residue levels in animal tissues. *[Origin; UK]*
Cy 3.9.   Nitrofurans - HPLC combined with dialysis for determining
             residues of nitrofurans in eggs, milk and meat. *[Origin; The
             Netherlands]*

Cy 4.0   **METHODS FOR OTHER SUBSTANCES.**
Cy 4.1.   Benzimidazoles - Determination by HPLC of Benzimidazole type
             anthelmintics at residue levels in animal tissues and milk.
             [Origin; UK]
Cy 4.2.   Lasalocid - Determination by HPLC of Lasalocid at residue
             levels in poultry muscle and eggs. *[Origin; UK]*
Cy 4.3.   Carbadox - Determination by GC-MS of quinoxaline carboxylic
             acid (QCA) at residue levels in kidney tissue. *[Origin; UK]*
Cy 4.4.   Ivermectin - Determination by HPLC of Ivermectin at residue
             levels in animal tissues.*[Origin; UK]*
Cy 4.5.   Tranquillizers and carazolol - an HPLC method with on-line UV
             spectrum identification and off-line TLC confirmation for
             residues in pig kidneys. *[Origin; The Netherlands]*
Cy 4.6.   Tranquillizers - Identification using GC-MS confirmation for
             residues of tranquillizers in pig kidneys. *[Origin; The
             Netherlands]*

1.INTRODUCTION

The Council Directive (86/469/EEC) concerning the examination of animals
and fresh meat for the presence of residues requires that samples are
analyzed "in accordance with methods which are applied by Member States and
have been submitted to the Commission under their inspection plans". These
methods are routine methods of analysis for screening and confirmation
purposes. All positive findings must, if challenged, be confirmed by a
laboratory officially approved for that purpose by the competent
authorities, using the reference methods established pursuant to Article
4(1)(b) of Directive 64/433/EEC.

This manual brings together those parts of EEC legislation concerned with
residues, the National Surveillance programmes for residues, and the latest
progress and developments in routine methods and Reference Materials (RMs).

More specifically the purpose of the manual is to provide a reference
manual describing the methods and materials (standards and reference
materials) for use in the identification, measurement and confirmation of
residues in food of animal origin.

Analytical technology is continually changing and progressing. Thus in the
first edition in 1991 methods were reported at various advanced stages of
development and with special emphasis on multi-residue and modular methods.
In this edition there are more methods, including a new section describing
a selection of routine <u>screening</u> methods used by Member States. The
routine methods used throughout the Community are summarised in table form
for each analyte. Where possible the routine methods are differentiated as
screening or confirmatory methods.

For many analytes there are excellent confirmatory methods used by one or
more Member States which for a variety of reasons have not yet been raised
to the status of Reference Methods. Until such time as a reference method
is available a selection of these routine confirming methods is detailed.
Many of these methods are probable candidates for Reference Methods.

This edition includes a section on quality assurance which complements the
criteria for methods set out in EEC Decision 93/256 and reproduced in
section 5.

The book is aimed primarily for use in reference laboratories or other
laboratories performing residue analysis. Many international and national
authorities may also find the book helpful as a reference work for problems
associated with residues.

REFERENCE METHODS AND ROUTINE CONFIRMING METHODS.

The routine confirming methods as defined in EEC 93/256 and used by Member
States may in the future be approved by the Commission and given the status
of Community Reference Methods. Reference methods could be used to settle
disputes (e.g between Member States) by providing an approved analytical
tool for the means of controlling residues in food through the specific and
accurate determination of the residue content in food. The routine
confirming methods when fully developed meet the criteria in EEC 93/256
(see section 5) and are suitable for
(i)   being performed in EEC reference laboratories.
(ii)   identifying unambiguously an analyte (residue)
(iii)   measuring the concentration of analytes accurately.

REFERENCE MATERIALS (RMs).

The purpose of the RMs is the quality control of analytical methods by;-
(i)   use in development of a method
(ii)   determination of accuracy and precision
(iii)   quality assurance
(iv)   providing RMs with concentrations of analytes at or near the
        tolerance limits (MRL) set by the EEC or when MRL are zero at or
        close to the lower limit of detection of the method.
(v)   a standard for traceability

The RMs will be available commercially through the Measurement and Testing
Programme of DG12. Certified RMs are now available for the stilbenes in
bovine urine.
RMs are stable materials of animal origin containing residues at known
concentrations. They are prepared by collecting samples (muscle, liver,
kidney, fat, bile, urine, blood or faeces) from animals administered
veterinary drugs or other substances. The samples are prepared as
lyophilised material which are stable and have stated residue
concentrations.

2. RESIDUE GROUPS; TESTS AND MRLs.

2.1 ANNEX I, DIRECTIVE 86/469/EEC, lists the groups of residues which will require tests.

The list is:-

A. GROUPS COMMON TO ALL MEMBER STATES.

Group I.
       (a) Stilbenes, stilbene derivatives, their salts and esters.
       (b) Thyreostatic substances.
       (c) Other substances with oestrogenic, androgenic or gestagenic
           action.

Group II   Authorised Substances
            Natural (endogenous) hormones.

Group III
       (a) Inhibitors: Antibiotics, sulphonamides and similar antimicrobial
           substances.
       (b) Chloramphenicol.

B. SPECIFIC GROUPS.

Group I: Other medicines.
       (a) Endo- and ectoparasitic substances.
       (b) Tranquillizers and beta-blockers.
       (c) Beta-agonists
       (d) Other veterinary medicines.

Group II: Other residues.
       (a) Contaminants present in feeding stuffs.
       (b) Contaminants present in the environment.
       (c) Other substances

2.2. MAXIMUM RESIDUE LIMITS, (MRL)

A summary of the MRLs allocated by the Committee on Veterinary Medicinal Products (CVMP) of DG3/EEC and the WHO/FAO Joint Expert Committee on Feed Additives (JECFA) is given for compounds of interest in table 1. More detailed information on the MRLs allocated by the CVMP and published as Commission Regulation (EEC) №675/92 is given in table 2.

Table 1; MRLs allocated by CVMP and JECFA.

MRL in µg per kg tissue or fluid

Group and Compound	EEC	JECFA
Group A I;		
Dienoestrol (DEN),	0^1	0
Diethylstilboestrol (DES),	0^1	0
Hexoestrol (HEX),	0^1	0
Medroxyprogesterone acetate	0	
Methyltestosterone (MT),	0	
19-Nortestosterone (NT),	0	
Tapazole (TAP),	0^1	
Trenbolone (TB),	0^1	$2 (\beta TB, M)^C,$ $10 (\alpha TB, L)^C$
2-Thiouracil (2-TU),	0^1	
Zeranol (Z),	0^1	$2(M)^C, 10(L)^C$
Group A II;		
17ß-Oestradiol (ßE$_2$),	0.04^3	unnecessary
Progesterone (P),	?	unnecessary
Testosterone (T),	$10 \& 30^3$	unnecessary
Group A III		
Ampicillin,	$4 \& 50^2$	
Amoxicillin	$4 \& 50^2$	
Benzylpenicillin,	$4 \& 50^2$	50(M,L,K), 4(Mk)
Chloramphenicol (CAP),	10^2	not allocated
Chlortetracycline,	$100 \text{ to } 600^2$	
Cloxacillin	$30 \& 300^2$	
Dicloxacillin	$30 \& 300^2$	
Dihydrostreptomycin,		1000 (M), 200 (Mk), 500 (Eg)
Furazolidone	5^2	not allocated
Nitrofurans	5^2	
Nitrofurazone	5^2	not allocated
Oxacillin	$30 \& 300^2$	
Oxytetracyline,	$100 \text{ to } 600^2$	100 (M,Mk), 300 (L) 600(K),10(F),200 (Eg)
Sulphadimidine,	100^2	300 as total (M,L,K,F) 100 as parent (M,L,K,F) 50 as total (Mk) 25 as parent (Mk)

Group and compound	MRL in µg per kg tissue or fluid	
	EEC	JECFA
Sulphaquinoxaline,	100^2	
Sulphathiazole	100^2	not allocated
Tetracycline	100 to 600^2	
Trimethoprim	50^2	

Group and compound	EEC	JECFA
Group B		
Albendazole,	under evaluation	100 (M,F,Mk) as sulphone 5000(L,K)
Azaperone	50 & 100^2	not allocated
Carazolol,	5 & 30^2	5(F), 30(L,K)^{C,P}
Carbadox,	$	30 as QCA(L)^P 5 as QCA(M)^P
Chlorpromazine,		not allocated
Clenbuterol,		
Closantel		1500(M,L),5000(K), 2000(F)^S 1000(M,L), 3000(K,F)^C
Cimaterol,		
Dapsone	25^2	
Dimetridazole,	10^2	not allocated
Diminazene		not allocated
Febantel,	10 or 1000^2	100(M,F,K), 500(L)^{C,P,S} 100(Mk)^C N.B.^{4}
Fenbendazole,	10 or 1000^2	as Febantel
Flubendazole		10(M,L)^P 200(M), 500(L)^{Py} 400 (Eggs)
Isometamidium		100 (M,F,Mk), 500(L)^C, 1000(K)^C
Ivermectin,	15 & 20^2	100(L), 40(F)^C, 15(L), 20(F) other species
Ipronidazole,		not allocated
Lasalocid,	$	
Levamisole,	10^2	10 (all) Temporary
Metronidazole,		not allocated
Monensin,		
Narasin,		
Olaquindox	$	not allocated
Oxfendazole	10 or 1000^2	as febantel ^{4}
Propionylpromazine,		not allocated
Ractopamine		not allocated
Ronidazole,	2^2	not allocated
Salbutamol,		
Salinomycin,		
Spiramycin	50(M), 300(L)^{C,P} 200(K),^{C,P} 100(Mk)^C	50(M), 300(L)^{C,P} 200(K),^{C,P} 100(Mk)^C
Thiabendazole,		100 (M,L,K,F)^{C,P,S,G,5} 100(Mk)^{C,G,5}
Triclabendazole		200(M), 300(L,K), 100(F)^{C,6} 100(M,L,K,F)^{S,6}
Tylosin		not allocated

Specific species are indicated by superscripts, C is cattle, P is Pig. S
is sheep, G is goats.
Superscript 1 indicates that these compounds are prohibited from use in EC
Member States.
Superscripts 2 and 3 refer to data in tables 2 and 3 respectively.
Superscript 4 refers to three benzimidazoles which have a group MRL. The
MRL is the sum of the concentrations of fenbendazole, oxfendazole, and
oxfendazole sulphone, calculated as oxfendazole sulphone equivalents.
Superscipt 5, the MRL is the sum of thiabendazole and 5-
hydroxythiabendazole.
Superscript 6, the MRL is expressed as the marker residue, 5-chloro-6-
(2',3'-dichlorophenoxy)-benzimidazole-2-one.
$ indicates that these compounds are classed as feed additives and as such
are not covered by EEC Directives 81/851 and 81/852. They are covered by
EC Directive 70/524.
Note; The JECFA values are those recommended to the Codex Alimentarius
Commission, they may not yet be officially adopted by Codex. "Not
allocated" means there was insufficient information to allocate an MRL.
A full list of the status of ADI and MRL evaluated by JECFA (32nd-40th
meetings) may be found in the FAO Monograph, Food and Nutrition Paper 41/5,
Residues of some veterinary drugs in animals and foods. (1993).

Table 2. MRLs recommended by the Committee for Veterinary Medicinal Products for residues of certain active substances used in veterinary medicine. The MRLs are published in the Commission Regulation № 675/92 "amending Annexes I and III of Council Regulation (EEC) № 2377/90 laying down a Community procedure for the establishment of maximum residue limits of veterinary medicinal products in foodstuffs of animal origin."

Compound	Species	MRL(s) µg/kg	Marker Residue	Target food Commodity	Status
GROUP A III					
ß-LACTAMS.					
Ampicillin	All	50	parent drug	meat, all tissues	Final
		4		milk	Final
Amoxicillin	All	50	parent drug	meat, all tissues	Final
		4		milk	Final
Benzylpenicillin	All	50	parent drug	meat, all tissues	Final
		4		milk	Final
Cloxacillin	All	300	parent drug	meat, all tissues	Final
		30		milk	Final
Dicloxacillin	All	300	parent drug	meat, all tissues	Final
		30		milk	Final
Oxacillin	All	300	parent drug	meat, all tissues	Final
		30		milk	Final
Chloramphenicol[m]	All	10	parent drug	meat, all tissues	1.1.94[P]
Spiramycin	C,P	300	parent drug	liver	1.7.95[P]
	C,P	200	parent drug	kidney	1.7.95[P]
	C,P	50	parent drug	muscle	1.7.95[P]
	C	150	parent drug	milk	1.7.95[P]
Sulphonamides	All	100	parent drug	meat, all tissues	Final
	C,S,G	100	parent drug	milk	1.1.94[P]
Tetracyclines	All	600	parent drug	kidney	1.1.94[P]
		300		liver	1.1.94[P]
		200		eggs	1.1.94[P]
		100		muscle, milk	1.1.94[P]
Trimethoprim	All	50	parent drug	meat, all tissues milk	1.1.96[P]

<u>B GROUP</u>

Substance	Species	MRL (µg/kg)	Marker residue	Tissue	Date
Azaperone	All	100	azaperol	kidney	1.1.96[p]
		50	azaperol	muscle, liver kidney	1.1.96[p]
Carazolol	All	30	parent drug	liver, kidney	1.7.95[p]
		5		muscle, fat	1.7.95[p]
Dapsone	All	25	parent drug	meat, all tissues, milk	1.1.94[p]
Dimetridazole	All	10	all residues with intact nitro-imidazole structure	meat, all tissues	1.1.94[p]
Febantel[a]	All	1000	oxfendazole +	liver	1.7.95[p]
		10	oxfendazole-sulphone + fenbendazole	muscle, kidney, fat, milk	1.7.95[p]
Fenbendazole[a]	All	1000	oxfendazole +	liver	1.7.95[p]
		10	oxfendazole-sulphone + fenbendazole	muscle, kidney, fat, milk	1.7.95[p]
Ivermectin	C,P,S,H	15	H_2B_1a	Liver	Final
		20	metabolite	fat	Final
Levamisole	All	10	parent drug	meat, all tissues milk	1.1.95[p]
Nitrofurans group	All	5	all residues with intact 5-nitro structure	meat, all tissues, eggs	1.7.93[p]
Oxfendazole	All	1000	oxfendazole +	liver	1.7.95[p]
		10	oxfendazole-sulphone + fenbendazole	muscle, kidney, fat, milk	1.7.95[p]
Ronidazole	All	2	all residues with intact nitro-imidazole structure	meat, all tissues	1.1.94[p]

Superscripts; a; The CVMP was agreed that there is no need to establish separate ADIs for febantel and fenbendazole because these are metabolised into oxfendazole which is the more toxic metabolite.
p; provisional date.
m; no MRLs are allocated for residues in milk or eggs because the CVMP specifically recommends that chloramphenicol not be authorised for use in lactating animals or laying birds.

Species are C, cattle; P, pigs; S, sheep; G, goats, H, horses.

2.3. Amendments to Directive 86/469/EEC

There are some amendments to the National Plans for examinations for
residues provided for in Article 4 of Directive 86/469/EEC.   They include;

2.3.1. Naturally Occurring Steroid Residues.

- Until the Scientific Veterinary Committee makes its report on the
  physiological levels of "natural" sex hormones in plasma the
  following provisional procedures for dealing with the illegal use of
  "natural" sex hormones for fattening purposes in bovine animals for
  the year 1991 shall be adopted.

  If, in the course of testing for "natural" sex hormones in accordance
  with Directive 86/469/EEC (live bovine animals at the farm or at the
  slaughterhouse) or in the course of any other testing, levels of
  oestradiol or testosterone exceeding the level given in the table
  below, are found in the blood plasma of at least one bovine animal,
  the investigations and measures foreseen in Article 6, paragraphs 1
  ,2 and 3 of Directive 85/358/EEC should immediately be carried out.

	AGE (months)	Maximum Plasma Concentrations	
		Male Bovine (μg per L)	Non-pregnant female bovine (μg per L)
free oestradiol-17ß	$\leq$ 6		0.04
	$\leq$ 18	0.04	
free testosterone-17ß	<6	10	
	6 - 18	30	
	$\leq$ 18		0.5

2.3.2. Xenobiotic Anabolic Agents with Hormonal Activity.

- In order to detect the presence of residues of stilbenes, trenbolone
  or zeranol in urine, bile or faeces, a routine method with a decision
  limit less than or equal to 2 ppb (μg per kg or L) shall be used.

- Testing shall include the substances, 19-nortestosterone,
  melengestrol acetate, chlormadinone acetate and megestrol acetate.

3. REFERENCE LABORATORIES.

The Community has two levels of Reference Laboratories. There are four
<u>Community</u> Reference laboratories (CRL) and thirty six <u>National</u> Reference
Laboratories (NRL).

(a) COMMUNITY Reference Laboratories.

The role of the Community Reference Laboratories is delineated in Articles 1
and 2 of the Council Decision, 89/187/EEC, "determining the powers and
conditions of operation of the Community Reference Laboratories provided for
by Directive 86/469/EEC concerning the examination of animals and fresh meat
for the presence of residues".

The Community Reference Laboratories are;-

Robert Von Osterag Institut des Bundesgesundheitsamt   (BGA)
Diederdorfer Weg 1
D-1000 Berlin 48, Germany

Istituto Superiore di Sanita   (ISS)
Viale Regina Elena 299
00161 Roma, Italy

Rijksinstitut voor Volksgezondheid en Milieuhygiëne   (RIVM)
Antonie van Leeuwenhoeklaan 9
NL-3720 BA Bilthoven, The Netherlands

Laboratoire des Medicaments Veterinaires   (LMV)-(CNEVA)
La Haute Marche
Javene
F-35133 Fougeres, France

(b) NATIONAL Reference Laboratories

The list of National Reference Laboratories is given in Annex II in the
Commission Decision 93/257/EEC   "laying down the reference methods and the
list of National Reference Laboratories for detecting residues" and revoking
Decision 89/610/EEC" (see list below). A major difference from the first
edition of this book is that laboratories in Germany are regrouped because of
the unification of Germany. Each Reference Laboratory is responsible for
certain groups of compounds as described in section 2.

Member State. Reference Laboratories and Residue groups measured (in italics)

Belgium   Institut d'Hygiène et d'Épidémiologie
             Rue J. Wijtsman, 14
             1050-Brussels   *ALL*

Denmark   Veterinaerdirektoratets Laboratorium
             Odinsvej 4
             Postboke 93
             DK 4100-Ringsted   *ALL*

             Levnedsmiddelstyrelsens Centrallabatorium
             Morkhoj Bygade 19
             DK-2860 Soborg   *B*

Germany   Robert Von Osterag Institüt des Bundesgesundheitsamt
            Diederdorfer Weg 1
            D-1000 Berlin 48   *ß-agonists, CAP, Sulphonamides*

            Landesuntersuchungsamt für das Gesundheits- und Veterinärwesen
            Institüt Chemnitz
            Hohe Straße 27/29
            D-9005 Chemnitz   *Stilbenes*

            Staaliches Medizinal-, Lebens- Mittel- und Veterinärsuchungs-
            Druselteistraße 63
            D-3500 Kassel   *Trenbolone, 19-Nortestosterone*

            Staaliches Medizinal-, Lebens- Mittel- und Veterinärsuchungs-
            Amt Mittelmessen
            Marburger Staß3 54
            D-6300 Gießen   *Gestagogenic substances*

            Chemisches Landesuntersuchungsamstalt Freiburg
            Bifflerstraße 5
            D-7800 Freiburg 1   *Organochlorine PCBs*

            Landesuntersuchungsamt für das Gesundheitswesen
            Südbayern
            Veterinärstraße 2
            D-8042 Oberschleißheim   *Natural Hormones*

            Staatliches Veterinärsuchungsamt Arnsberg
            Zur Traubeneiche 10/12
            D-5760 Arnsberg 2   *Zeranol, Ethynyloestradiol, Thyreostats*

            Chemische Landesuntersuchungsanstalt Stuttgart
            Breidscheidstraße 4
            D-7000 Stuttgart 1   *Nitrofurans*

            Chemische Landesuntersuchungsanstalt - Karlsruhe
            Hoffstraße 3
            D-7500 Karlsruhe   *Avermectin*

            Chemische Landesuntersuchungsanstalt - Nordrhein-Westphalien
            Sperlichstraße 19
            D-4400 Münster   *Tranquillizers & ß-blockers*

            Staatliches Veterinär- und Lebelsmitteluntersuchungsamt - Potsdam
            Pappelallee 2
            D-1572 Potsdam   *Heavy metals*

            Staatliches Veterinärsuchungsamt - Hannover
            Eintrechtweg 17
            D-3000 Hannover 1   *Penicillins, Tetracyclines, Quinolone*

Greece   Institute of Biochemistry, Toxicology and Nourishment of Animals
            25, Neapoleos Street
            GR-153 10 Aghia Paraskevi Athens   *AI,a,c; AII; AIII,b; BII,a,b*

Institute of Food Hygiene
Dept. Residue Analysis   *Thyreostats, Antimocrobials*
75, Iera Idos, Botanikos   *Parasiticides, Tranquillizers,*
GR-118 55 Athens   *ß-blockers, ß-agonists, PCBs, BII,c.*

Spain   Centro Nacional de Alimentacion Y Nutrition
            c/Pozuelo-Majadahonda Km 6.2
            28023 - Majadahonda (Madrid)   *AI,a,c; AII; AIII,a,b; ß-agonists*

            Laboratorio de Sanidad y Produccion Animal
            18320 Santa Fe (Granada)   *AI,b; BI,a,b,c*

            Laboratorio de Sanidad y Produccion Animal
            28806 Algete (Madrid)   *AI,b; BI,b*

            Laboratorio Arbitral del Ministerio de Agricultura, Pesca y
            Alimentacion
            Ctra. de la Coruno, Km 10.7
            28032 Madrid   *Pesticides, Heavy metals*

France   Laboratoire Central d'Hygiene Alimentaire
            43, rue de Dantzig
            75015 Paris   *BI,a; BII,a,b,c*

            Laboratoire des Medicaments Veterinaires (LMV)
            La Haute Marche
            Javene
            F-35133 Fougeres,   *BI,b,c; AIII,a,b*

            Laboratoire de dosages hormonaux École nationale vétérinaire de
            Nantes
            CP 3028
            F-44087 Nantes Cedex 03   *AI; AII*

Ireland   Central Meat Control Laboratory
            Abbotstown
            Castleknock
            Dublin 15   *AI, AII, AIII, BI, BII (not pesticides)*

            State Laboratory
            Abbotstown
            Castleknock
            Dublin 15   *AI, AII, AIII, BI, BII*

Italy   Istituto Superiore di Sanita
            Viale Regina Elena 299
            I-00161 Roma   *ALL*

Luxembourg
            RIVM Bilthoven   *ALL*

            Institut d'hygiène et d'épidémiologie
            Rue J. Wijtsman, 14
            1050-Brussels   *ALL*

Netherlands
          Rijksinstitut voor Volksgezondheid
                    en Milieuhygiëne (RIVM)
          Antonie van Leeuwenhoeklaan 9
          NL-3720 Bilthoven   *ALL*

          Rijkskwaliteitsinstituut voor Land- en Tuinbouwprodukten (RIKILT)
          Bornesteeg 45
          NL-6708 Wageningen   *ALL*

Portugal Laboratorio Nacional de Investigacao
          Veterinaria
          Estrada de Benfica 701
          1500 Lisboa   *ALL*

United
 Kingdom Central Veterinary Laboratory (CVL)
          New Haw
          Addlestone
          Surrey KT15 3NB   *AI, AII, AIII, BI*

          Food Science Laboratory
          Colney Lane
          Norwich NR4 7UA   *AIII, BI, BII*

          Veterinary Research Laboratories (VRL-NI)
          Stormont
          Belfast BT4 3SD   *AI,a,c; AII, AIII, BI, BII*

          Food and Agric. Chem. Res. Division
          Dept. Agriculture for N.I.
          Newforge Lane,
          Belfast BT9 5PX   *AI,b; AIII, BI, BII*

4.0. ROUTINE METHODS

4.1. The purpose of this section is to summarise the <u>routine</u> methods used
by the Member States of the European Community for the control of residues
in food-producing animals and their products in accordance with the
Directive 86/469.

The definitions and criteria for ROUTINE methods are given in Section 5 and
are in the Commission Decision 93/256/EEC. Routine methods are used for
surveillance or regulatory purposes and are divided into two types.

 1. SCREENING METHODS.

Methods used to detect the presence of an analyte (residue) or class of
analytes at the level of interest. They have a high sample throughput
capacity and are used to sift large numbers of samples for potential
positives and aim to reduce the number of false negative results.

 2. CONFIRMATORY METHODS.

These methods are applied to positive samples identified in the screening
methods. They are methods which provide unequivocal identification of the
analyte at the level of interest. They are aimed to prevent false positive
results and an acceptable probability of false negative results.

4.2. A selection of screening and confirmatory methods are described in
ISO format in this edition (see section 6).

4.3. For the first edition, a survey of routine methods used throughout
the Member States was carried out by the Commission (DGVI) in the period
May-July 1990 and updated during the period April-June, 1991. In this
edition the survey covers the period April-August, 1993. Responses were
received from the National Reference Laboratories in Belgium, Denmark,
France, Germany, Greece, Ireland, Netherlands and UK.

The results are summarised below giving the methods used for each analyte
or group of analytes. LLD in the tables is either the limit of detection
or the limit of determination and is that claimed by the member nation and
is not necessarily as defined in EEC Directive 89/610. The methods may not
have been validated by another laboratory.

The procedures for some of the methods are published in Section 6 following
selection by the editor in consultation with the CRL.

STILBENES

Method	Type Sg,Cy	Ext.	Purif.	Det.	Type	Size mL or g	LLD µg/kg or/L	Member State
TLC	Sg,Cy	Sv	CC	UV	U,M	50	1-5	P
HPTLC	Sg	no	C18,HPLC	Fl	U	15	2	S
	Sg	Sv	C-Si	UV	U,M(i.s)	2	5	F
	Sg,Cy	Sv	C18,HPLC	UV	U,F	20(U),25(F)	2	B
	Sg	Sv	C18,HPLC	UV	Fc	30	2	B
HPLC	Sg	Sv	C18	ECD	M	10	1	S
	Cy	Sv	C18,HPLC	RIA	U	0.05-1	0.02-0.05	Gr
RIA	Sg	Sv	C18	RIA	Bi	0.05	2	UK
	Sg	Sv	C18	RIA	Fc	1.0	2	UK
	Sg	Sv	C18	RIA	U	0.1	2	B
	Sg	Sv	C18	RIA	U	0.05	0.5-1	Gr
	Sg	Sv	C18	RIA	M	1	0.02-0.05	Gr
	Sg	Sv	C18	RIA	U	0.1	2	P
	Sg	Sv	C18/HPLC	RIA	Fc	1	2	B
	Sg	Sv	no	RIA	Se	0.5	0.05	UK
	Sg	Sv	no	RIA	U	0.1	2	UK
	Sg	Sv	no	RIA	Fc	1.0	2	D
	Sg	Sv	no	RIA	U	0.05	2	It
	Sg	Sv	no	RIA	U	0.2	0.5	Ir
	Sg	Sv	no	RIA	U	0.5	1	F
	Sg	Sv	no	RIA	U	0.5	0.4	UK-NI
	Sg	Sv	no	RIA	M	1	0.2	UK-NI
	Sg	Sv	Sv	RIA	M	1.0	0.3	It
EIA	Sg	no	C18	EIA	U	0.5	0.2	G
GC-MS	Sg,Cy	Sv	C18,HPLC	MS	U	10	1	S
	Cy	Sv	C18	MS	U	10	1	G
	Sg	Sv	C18,HPLC	MS	Fc	30	2	B
	Sg	Sv	C18,HPLC	MS	U	10	1	It
	Cy	IAC	HPLC	MS	U	10	0.1	NL*
	Cy	Sv	IAC	MS	M	5	0.1	NL*
	Sg,Cy	no	C18,C-Si	MS	U,L,K	20	0.5	F
	Cy	Sv	CC	MS	M	30	0.3	It
	Cy	Sv	SPE	MS	Bi	5	5	UK-NI
	Sg,Cy	Sv	CC	MS	U,Bi	25(U),	0.5-1	NL
	Cy	Sv	HPLC	MS	Bi,Fc	5(Bi), 2(Fc)	5	UK
	Cy	Sv	HPLC	MS	U	3	2	UK

Abbreviations are at the end of this section.

19-NORTESTOSTERONE

Method	Type Sg,Cy	Ext.	Purif.	Det.	Type	Size mL or g	LLD µg/kg or/L	Member State
TLC	Sg,Cy	Sv	CC	UV	U,M	50	0.5-2	P
HPTLC	Sg	Sv	C-Si	UV	U,M(i.s.)	2	5	F
	Sg,Cy	Sv	C18,HPLC	UV	U,F	20(U),25(F)	2	B
	Sg	Sv	C18,HPLC	UV	Fc	30	2	B
HPLC	Cy	Sv	C18	UV	U	5	2	Ir
EIA	Sg	Sv	no	EIA	U	0.5	1.5	D
	Sg	Sv	IAC	EIA	Se,Pl,U,Bi	0.25-0.5	0.2-1	UK-NI
	Sg	Sv	IAC	EIA	U	0.5	1	G
RIA	Sg	Sv	C18	RIA	U	0.1	5	It
	Sg	Sv	C18	RIA	U	0.1	2	B
		Sv	C18	RIA	M	1	0.5	It
	Sg	Sv	C18	RIA	U	0.2	1	P
	Sg	Sv	IAC	RIA	M	4	0.5	G
	Sg	Sv	C18/HPLC	RIA	Fc	1	2	B
	Sg	no	C18	RIA	U	0.5	1	F
	Sg	Sv	no	RIA	Se	0.5	2	UK
	Sg	Sv	no	RIA	U	0.2	0.5	Ir
	Sg	Sv	no	RIA	U	0.1	2	UK
	Sg	Sv	HPLC	RIA	U	1	0.2	NL*
	Sg	Sv	IAC	RIA	Bi	0.25	0.2	NL*
	Sg,Cy	Sv	IAC	RIA	U	0.1	0.2	Gr
GC-MS	Cy	Sv	CC	MS	U	20	2	G
	Sg,Cy	Sv	CC	MS	U	25	0.5-1	NL
	Cy	Sv	CC	MS	M	30	0.5	It
	Sg	Sv	C18,HPLC	MS	Fc	30	2	B
	Cy	Sv	C18,HPLC	MS	U	10	1	It
	Cy	Sv	HPLC	MS	U	3	5	UK
	Cy	Sv	IAC	MS	U,M	5	0.2	NL*
	Cy	Sv	IAC	MS	Bi	1	0.2	NL*
	Sg,Cy	no	C18,C-Si	MS	U,L,K	20	0.5	F
	Sg,Cy	no	C18,HPLC	MS	U	10	1.2	S
	Cy	Sv	IAC	MS	Bi	5	0.2	UK-NI

Abbreviations are at the end of this section.

TRENBOLONE

Method	Type Sg,Cy	Ext.	Purif.	Det.	Type	Size mL or g	LLD µg/kg or/L	Member State
TLC	Sg,Cy	Sv	CC	UV	U,M	50	0.5	P
HPTLC		Sv	C18	UV	U	10	0.5	It
	Sg	no	C18,HPLC	Fl	U	15	1	S
	Sg	Sv	C-Si	UV	U,M(i.s.)	2	5	F
	Sg,Cy	Sv	C18,HPLC	UV	U,F	20(U),25(F)	2	B
	Sg	Sv	C18,HPLC	UV	Fc	30	2	B
	Cy	no	IAC	Fl	U	5	2	S
HPLC		Sv	C18,CC	UV	U	9	2	It
	Cy	Sv	C18	UV	U	5	2	Ir
HPLC/EIA	Sg	Sv	HPLC	EIA	Bi	1	1	UK-NI
EIA	Sg	Sv	no	EIA	Pl	0.5	0.43	D
	Sg	Sv	no	EIA	U	0.5	2.4	D
	Sg	Sv	IAC	EIA	Se	0.5	0.1	UK-NI
	Sg	Sv	no	EIA	Bi	0.04	2	UK
	Sg	Sv	no	EIA	U	0.08	2	UK
	Sg	Sv	IAC	EIA	M	5	0.2	UK-NI
	Sg	Sv	IAC	EIA	Fc	3	0.4	UK-NI
	Sg,Cy	Sv	IAC	EIA	U	0.1	0.1	Gr
	Sg	Sv	C18	EIA	U	0.5	1	G
	Sg	Sv	C18	EIA	M	10	1	G
RIA	Sg	Sv	C18	RIA	U	0.1	2	B
	Sg	Sv	C18	RIA	U	0.1	0.2	P
	Sg	Sv	C18	RIA	Fc	1	2	UK
	Sg	Sv	C18/HPLC	RIA	Fc	1	2	B
	Sg	Sv	no	RIA	Se	0.5	0.02	UK
	Sg	Sv	no	RIA	U	0.2	0.5	Ir
GC-MS	Sg,Cy	Sv	CC	MS	U	25	1-2	NL
	Cy	Sv	IAC	MS	U,M	5	0.5(M),0.3	NL*
	Cy	Sv	IAC	MS	Bi?	5	1	NL
	Sg,Cy	no	C18,C-Si	MS	U,K,L	20	2	F
	Sg	Sv	C18,HPLC	MS	Fc	30	2	B
	Cy	Sv	C18,HPLC	MS	Bi,Fc,U	5(Bi),2(Fc),3(U)	1	UK
	Cy	no	C18,HPLC	MS	U	5	2	S

Abbreviations are at the end of this section.

ZERANOL

Method	Type Sg,Cy	Ext.	Purif.	Det.	Type	Size mL or g	LLD µg/kg or/L	Member State
TLC	Sg,Cy	Sv	CC	UV	U	50	5	P
HPTLC	Sg,Cy	Sv	C18,HPLC	UV	U,F	20(U),25(F)	2	B
	Sg	Sv	C18,HPLC	UV	Fc	30	2	B
EIA	Sg	Sv	no	EIA	Bi,U	0.08	2	UK
	Sg	Sv	IAC	EIA	U	0.25	0.5	Gr
	Sg	Sv	C18	EIA	U	0.5	0.125	G
HPLC/RIA	Sg	Sv	no	RIA	Bi	1	2	UK-NI
RIA	Sg	no	C18	RIA	U	0.5	2	D
	Sg	Sv	no	RIA	U	0.2	2	Ir
	Sg	Sv	C18	RIA	U	0.1	2	It,B
	Sg	Sv	C18	RIA	U	0.1	2	P
	Sg	Sv	C18	RIA	F	1	5	P
	Sg,Cy	Sv	IAC	RIA	U	0.1	0.5	Gr
	Sg	Sv	C18/HPLC	RIA	Fc	1	2	B
	Sg	Sv	no	RIA	U,Fc	0.5(U),1(Fc)	1	G
	Sg	Sv	no	RIA	Pl,Se	0.5	0.2	UK-NI
	Sg	Sv	no	RIA	U	0.5	1	UK-NI
	Sg	Sv	no	RIA	M	3	0.5	UK-NI
GC-MS	Cy	Sv	no	MS	U	3	0.2	G
	Sg,Cy	Sv	CC	MS	U	25	0.5-1	NL
	Sg	Sv	C18,HPLC	MS	Fc	30	2	B
	Cy	Sv	HPLC	MS	Bi,Fc,U	5(Bi),2(Fc),3(U)	2	UK
	Cy	Sv	IAC	MS	U,M	5	0.3	NL*
	Sg,Cy	no	C18,C-Si	MS	U,K,L	20	2	F
	Sg,Cy	no	C18,HPLC	MS	U	10	2	S

Abrreviations are at the end of this section.

ETHINYLOESTRADIOL

| Method | Type Sg,Cy | ----Procedures-------- | | | ---Sample---- | | | Member |
		Ext.	Purif.	Det.	Type	Size mL or g	LLD µg/kg or/L	State
EIA	Sg	Sv	C18	EIA	U	0.5	0.2	G
GC-MS	Cy	Sv	C18,CC	MS	U,Fc	10(U), 2(Fc)	1	G
	Sg,Cy	C18	C-Si	MS	U	20	2	F

ACETYL-GESTAGENS

| Substance. | Method Sg,Cy | ------Procedures------ | | | | --Sample-- | | | Member |
		Type	Ext.	Purif.	Det.	Type	size mL or g	LLD µg/L or/kg	State
MPA,MGA	RIA	Sg	no	C18	RIA	Pl	2	1	D
CMA	RIA	Sg	no	C18	RIA	Pl	2	1.5	D
MLA	RIA	Sg	no	C18	RIA	Pl	4	2.5	D
Various	EIA	Sg	Sv	C18	EIA	Fat	2	0.1	G
Various	HPLC/EIA	Sg	Sv	C18	EIA	I.S	actual	various	UK-NI
Various	HPLC	Sg	Sv	HPLC	UV	Fat	50	5	UK-NI
Various	GC-MS	Cy	Sv	CC	MS	I.S.	actual	various	UK-NI

MPA is medroxyprogesterone acetate, MGA is megestrol acetate, CMA is
chlormadinone acetate and MLA is melengestrol acetate.

Other abbreviations are at the end of this section.

NATURAL STEROIDS

Method	Type Sg,Cy	Ext.	Purif.	Det.	Type	Size mL or g	LLD μg/kg or/L	Member State
			Procedures		**Sample**			
TLC	Sg	Sv	CC	UV	U,M	50	<2	P
HPTLC	Sg	no	C18,HPLC	Fl	U	15	2	S
	Sg	Sv	C-Si	UV	U	20	2	F
EIA	Sg	Sv	no	EIA	Pl,Se	0.5	0.1(T)	UK-NI
RIA	Sg	Sv	C18	RIA	Pl	1	0.04-	B
	Sg	Sv	no	RIA	Pl	0.5	0.2(P,T)	D
		Sv	no	RIA	Pl	0.5	0.002($E_2\beta$)	D
	Sg	Sv	no	RIA	Pl	0.1	0.01	Gr
	Sg	Sv	no	RIA	Se	0.5-1	0.008-0.1	G
	Sg	Sv	no	RIA	Se	0.15-0.5	0.01-0.5	UK
	Sg	Sv	no	RIA	Pl,Se	0.05-0.1	0.02-0.2	It
	Sg	Sv	no	RIA	Pl	1-2	0.02-0.09	F
	Sg	Sv	CC	RIA	Pl,	0.1-1	0.01-0.1	Ir
	Sg	no	no	RIA	Pl	0.05-0.2	0.008-0.05	P
	Sg	Sv	no	RIA	Se	0.05-0.1	0.02-0.2	NL
	Sg	Sv	no	RIA	Pl,Se	0.5	0.01($E_2\beta$)	UK-NI
							0.1(P)	UK-NI
GC-MS	Sg,Cy	Sv	CC	MS	U	25	0.5-1	NL
	Cy	Sv	IAC	MS	U,M	5	0.2	NL*
	Cy	Sv	IAC	MS	Pl,Se	10	0.01	NL*
	Cy	Sv	HPLC	MS	Imp.	all	10μg total	UK
	Sg,Cy	no	C18,HPLC	MS	U	10	1-2	S

Abbreviations are at the end of this section.

THYREOSTATS

Method	Type Sg,Cy	Ext.	Purif.	Det.	Type	Size mL or g	LLD µg/kg or/L	Member State
Grav	Sg	no	no	Grav	Th	whole	>55g	UK, UK-NI
Grav	Sg	no	no	Grav	Th	whole	>50g	B
HPTLC	Cy	Sv	C-Si	Fl	Th	2	200	UK,
	Sg	Sv	CC	Fl	Th	2-5	100-200	S
	Sg	Sv	C-Si	Fl	M	2	100	D
	Sg,Cy	Sv	CC	Fl	M,U	2	50-100	Gr
	Sg	Sv	no	Fl	Pl	2	100	D
	Sg,Cy	Sv	CC	Fl	U	2	50-100	NL
	Sg,Cy	Sv	CC	UV	U	2	50-100	It
	Sg,Cy	Sv	CC	UV	U	2	100	P
	Sg,Cy	Sv	CC	UV	Th,M	2	100	P
	Sg,Cy	Sv	CC	UV	Th,U	2	10-50	B
	Sg	Sv	CC	UV	M	2	25-100	Ir
	Sg,Cy	Sv	C18	UV	M,Th	2	50-100	It
TLC	Sg	Sv	no	UV	M,Th	5	20	G
	Sg	Sv	no	UV	Se	1	100	G
	Cy	Sv	CC	Fl	Th	2	25	UK-NI
HPLC	Cy	Sv	CC	Di.A	Th	2-5	100-200	S
	Sg	Sv	CC	UV	Th	5	50-100	F
GC-MS	Cy	Sv	no	MS	M,Th	5	50-100	G

Abbreviations are at the end of this section.

B-AGONISTS

Member Substance.	Method	Type Sg,Cy	Ext.	Purif.	Det.	Type	size mL or g	LLD µg/kg or µg/L	State
Cl	TLC	Sg,Cy	Sv	C18	Vis	U	20	1	P
Cl,Ci	HPTLC	Sg	no	C18	Vis	U	10	1	S
Cl,Ci	HPTLC	Sg	no	C18	Vis	L	5	2	S
Unspec.		Sg,Cy	Sv	CC	Vis	U	16	1	Gr
Cl,Sa,T		Cy	Sv	C18	UV	U	22.5	2	Ir
Cl, Mab		Sg	Sv	C-Si	ECD,UV	U	20	1	F
Sa, T		Sg	Sv	C8	ECD,UV	U	20	1	F
Cl		Sg	acid	CC	UV	U	10	<5	Ir
Cl,Ci		Cy	no	C18	Di.A	U	20	1-2	S
Cl.Ci		Cy	Sv	C18	Di.A	L	10	2	S
Cl	HPLC	Sg	Sv	C18	UV	L	5	1	Ir
Cl,Ci,Mab		Sg,Cy	Sv	C18	Di.A	U,L	10	1-2	B
Sa		Sg,Cy	Sv	IAC	Fl	U,L	5	1-2	B
Unspec	GC	Cy	Sv	CC	ECD	M	5	2	Ir
Cl,Sa,T	RIA	Sg	Sv	no	RIA	U	1	0.05	Ir
Cl		Sg	Sv	no	RIA	L	1.25	0.5	Ir
Cl		Sg	Sv	no	RIA	U	0.1	0.8	Gr
Cl		Sg	Sv	no	RIA	U	0.5	1	P
Various (>8)	EIA	Sg	no	no	EIA	U	10	1-2	NL
Mab,Ci,Sa		Sg	Sv	C18	EIA	L	1	1-5	D
Cl		Sg	Sv	C18	EIA	L	1	0.25	D
Cl,Ci,Sa,Mab,Terb,Carb		Sg	no	C18	EIA	U	1	0.1-2.6	G
Cl		Sg	Sv	-	EIA	M,L,K,U	5	0.25	UK
Sa		Sg	Sv	C18	EIA	L	10	1	UK
Cl,Mab		Sg	Sv	no	EIA	Bi,U,R	0.5	0.5-2	UK-NI
Cl,Mab		Sg	Sv	no	EIA	K,M,L	5	0.2-4	UK-NI
Cl,Ci,Sa		Sg	Sv	no	EIA	U	0.5	0.1-1	Gr
Unspec.	GC-MS	Cy	Sv	IAC	MS	U	10	0.5	NL*
Various (>8)		Sg,Cy	C18	IAC	MS	U,L	5	0.5-1	NL
Various (9)		Sg,Cy	Sv	C8/CSO$_3$H	MS	U,L,K	10	0.2-1	G
Cl		Cy	CC	C18	MS	U	10	1	Ir
Unspec		Sg,Cy	Sv	CC	MS	U,L,K	20	0.5-2	F
Cl		Cy	Sv	HPLC	MS	L	5	0.5	UK
Sa		Cy	Sv	HPLC	MS	L	5	0.5	UK
Cl,Mab		Cy	Sv	Sv	MS	U,Bi,L,K,M	10	0.2-4	UK-NI
Cl,Mab		Cy	Sv	Sv	MS	R	0.5	0.5	UK-NI

Cl is Clenbuterol, Ci, Cimaterol; Sa, Salbutamol; T is Terbutaline, Mab is Marbuterol
Unspec. is unspecified. Other abbreviations are at the end of this section.

CHLORAMPHENICOL

Method	Type Sg,Cy	Procedures Ext.	Purif.	Det.	Sample Type	Size mL or g	LLD µg/kg or/L	Member State
HPLC	Cy	Sv	Sv	Di.A	U	25	2	B
	Cy	Sv	Sv	Di.A	M,Eg,Fish	10	2	B
	Cy	Sv	Sv	Di.A	K, Mk	10	2	B
		Sv	Sv	UV	M,L,K,Mk	5	2,1(Mk)	F
	Sg	Sv	C18	UV	M,Mk	5	10	UK-NI
		Sv	CC,C18	UV	M,Eg	5	2	It
	Sg	H_2O	CC	UV	M	10	1	NL
	Sg	Sv	C-Si	UV	Eg	20	0.5	NL
	Sg	no	CC	UV	Mk	15	0.5	NL
	Cy	Sv	CC	Di.A	M	10	10	S
	Cy	Sv	C-Si	Di.A	M	50	10	NL
GC	Cy	Sv	C18	ECD	M,Mk,Eg	3,Mk(5)	0.5	G
		Sv	IAC	ECD	K,U	3(K0,1(U)	2(K),0.5(U)	G
	Cy	Sv	CC-Si	ECD	M	5	2	Ir
	Sg	Sv	CC-Ion	ECD	L	5	10	Ir
	Sg,Cy	Sv	Sv	ECD	M,K	5	1	Ir
EIA	Sg	H_2O	no	EIA	M	20	5	NL
	Sg	no	no	EIA	U	0.1	50	NL
	Sg	Sv	no	EIA	M,K,Mk	10	7	B
	Sg	Sv	no	EIA	U	0.05	5	P
	Sg	Sv	no	EIA	M	10	20	P
	Sg	Sv	no	EIA	M,K	10	20	UK-NI
	Sg	Sv	no	EIA	M	3	1	D
	Sg	Sv	no	EIA	M	0.5	0.1	Gr
	Sg	no	no	EIA	K	1	1.0	UK
	Sg	Sv	C18	RIA	Fc	1	2	UK
	Sg	no	no	EIA	U	1	5	NL*
RIA	Sg	Sv	no	RIA	Mk	1	0.2	G
	Sg	Sv	Sv	RIA	M,Eg	3	0.2	G
	Sg,Cv	Sv	C18	RIA	M	1	0.2	Gr
		Sv	no	RIA	M	3	10	P
	Cy	Sv	HPLC	RIA	U	1	0.5	NL*
	Sg	Sv	no	RIA	M	3	0.5	Ir
GC-MS	Cy	H_2O	CC	MS	M	10	0.5	NL
	Cy	no	CC	MS	Mk	10	0.5	NL
	Cy	Sv	Sv		M	10	2	B
	Cy	CC	HPLC	MS	U,M,Eg	10	0.1	NL*
	Cy	Sv	CC-Ion	MS	L	5	10	Ir
	Cy	Sv	C18	MS	M,Mk	M(3),Mk(5)	0.1,0.2	G
LC-MS	Cy	Sv	C18	MS	L	10	1	UK-NI

Abbreviations are at the end of this section.

TRANQUILLIZERS

Substance.	Method	Type Sg,Cy	Ext.	Purif.	Det.	Type	size mL or g	LLD µg/kg µg/L	Member State
Various (6)	TLC	Sg,Cy	Sv	Sv	Vis	K	20	1.2-3	P
Various(3)	HPLC	Sg,Cy	Sv	C18	Di.A	M	5	50	B
Various (5)		Sg,Cy	Sv	C18	UV	M	5	1-10	Gr
Various (4)		Sg	Sv	no	UV	K	2	50	D
Various(6)			Sv	C-DIOL	UV	K	20	1-10	F
Various		Sg	Sv	C18	UV	K	5	1-5	Ir
Various (6)		Sg	Sv	C18	UV	M,K	5	1-6	NL
Various (6)		Cy	Sv	C-DIOL	UV	K	20	1-10	NL*
Various (5)		Sg,Cy	Sv	HPLC	UV	Pl,Se	2	6	UK-NI
Various (5)		Sg	Sv	C18	UV	K	5	0.1	UK
Various (5)	GC-MS	Cy	Sv	C18	MS	K	10	50	NL
Various (3)		Cy	Sv	C18	MS	M	5	25	B
Various (5)		Sg,Cy	Sv	CC	MS	K,M,U	10	10-30	G

BETA-BLOCKERS

Substance.	Method	Type Sg,Cy	Ext.	Purif.	Det.	Type	size g or mL	LLD µg/kg or µg/L	Member State
Carazolol	TLC	Sg,Cy	Sv	no	Vis	K	20	1.5	P
Carazolol	HPLC	Sg,Cy	Sv	C18	Fl	M	5	50	B
Carazolol			Sv	C-DIOL	UV	K	20	1	F
Carazolol		Cy	Sv	C-DIOL	UV	K	20	20	NL*
Carazolol		Sg	Sv	Sv	Fl	K	10	2	G
Carazolol		Sg	Sv	C18	Fl	M,K	5	0.3	NL
Carazolol		Cy	Sv	C18	Di.A	K	5	50	NL
Carazolol		Sg	Sv	no	UV	K	2	25	D
Carazolol		Sg,Cy	Sv	C18	UV	M	5	1	Gr
Carazolol		Sg,Cy	Sv	C18	UV	K	5	0.3	UK
Carazolol		Sg	Sv	no	UV	Pl,Se	10	10	UK-NI

Unspec. is unspecified. Other abbreviations are at the end of this section.

SULPHONAMIDES

Substance.	Method	Type Sg,Cy	Ext.	Purif.	Det.	Sample Type	size mL or g	LLD µg/kg or µg/L	Member State
Unspec.	TLC	Sg	Sv	no	Fl	M	1	25	F
Unspec.			Sv	C-Si	Fl	K	10	20	NL*
Various(4)	HPTLC	Sg	Sv	C-SO$_3$H	Fl	M,K	10	5	B
Unspec		Sg	Sv	C-Si	UV	M,K,Mk	5(Mk),10	5-10	NL
Various(11)		Sg	Sv	NH$_2$,CSX	Fl	K	2.5	20	UK
Various		Sg	Sv		Fl	K	2.5	50	UK-NI
SMZ		Cy	Sv	no	Fl	M	2.5	<50	D
Various		Sg	Sv	C-Si	Fl	M	10	50	S
Various(11)	HPLC	Cy	Sv	C-SO$_3$H	Di.A	M,K	10	5	B
Unspec.			Sv	Sv	UV	Eg,Mk	5	2-5	F
Unspec.		Sg,Cy	Sv	Sv	Di.A	M,L,K,Eg,Mk	10	2	G
Unspec.		Cy	Sv	C18	Di.A	M	10	20	NL*
Unspec.		Sg	H$_2$0	dial.	Vis	M,Mk,Eg	10	25	NL
Various (3)		Sg	Sv	no	UV	Se	4	100	D
Various		Cy	Sv	CSX	Di.A	M	10	50	S
Various (3)			Sv	CC,C18	UV	M,K	10	25	It
Various (5)		Cy	Sv	C-Si	UV	M	5	10	F
Unspec.		Cy	Sv	C18	UV	M	10	20	Ir
Unspec.		Cy	Sv	C-Si	Di.A	M	10	25	NL
Various(4)		Cy	Sv	NH$_2$CSx	UV	K	2.5	20	UK
SMZ		Cy	Sv	no	UV/Vis	K,M,L	5	50	UK-NI
SMZ	EIA	Sg	no	no	EIA	Se	0.01	13	D
SMZ		Sg	no	card	EIA	U	5	0.5	P
SMZ		Sg	no	no	EIA	U	0.02	100	UK-NI
SMZ		Sg	no	no	EIA	K,M	2.5	20	UK-NI
SMZ		Sg	no	no	EIA	U	0.01	100	Gr
Unspec.		Sg	Sv	no	EIA	K	2.5	3	UK
Unspec.		Sg	Sv	no	EIA	U	0.01	100	Ir
SMZ		Sg	Sv	no	EIA	K	2.5	80	Gr
Various	HPLC/MS	Cy	Sv	C-Si	MS	M	5	30-80	G
Various(11)		Cy	Sv	HPLC	MS	K	5	100	UK
SMZ	GC-MS	Cy	Sv	SCX	MS	K,M,L	5	20	UK-NI

Abbreviations are at the end of this section.

NITROFURANS

Substance.	Method	Type Sg,Cy	Ext.	Purif.	Det.	Sample Type	size mL or g	LLD µg/kg or µg/L	Member State
Various (4)	TLC	Sg,Cy	Sv	C-Si	Fl	M	5	1	F
Furazolidone & Furaltadone	HPLC	Sg,Cy	Sv	Sv	Di.A	M,Fish,Eg	10	5	B
Unspec.		Sg	Sv	C18	UV	U	22.5	2	Ir
Various (3)			Sv	C18	UV	M,L,Eg	5	2	It
Unspec.		Sg	Sv	Sv	UV	M,L,K,Eg Mk,Fish	50	5	G
Furazolidone		Sg	Sv	Sv	UV	Eg	50	5	NL
Furazolidone		Sg	Sv	Sv	UV	L	1	1	UK
Furazolidone		Sg	Sv	Sv	Vis	Meal	1	10	UK-NI
Various (4)		Sg	H_2O	Dial.	UV	M,Mk,Eg	10	1-10	NL
Various (4)		Sg,Cy	Sv	no	UV	M	10	5	D
Furazolidone		Cy	Sv	Sv	Di.A	M	20	5	NL
Furazolidone		Cy	Sv	Sv	Di.A	Eg	50	15	NL
Furazolidone		Cy	Sv	Sv	Di.A	Eg	50	15	NL
Furazolidone	LC-MS	Cy	Sv	C-NH_2	MS	M,L,K	2	1	UK-NI

Unspec. is unspecified. Other abbreviations are at the end of this section.

CARBADOX

Method	Type Sg,Cy	Ext.	Purif.	Det.	Type	Size mL or g	LLD µg/kg or/L	Member State
HPLC	Sg	Sv	CC(Al)	Vis	M,L,K,Eg	10	2, (Eg,1)	NL
	Cy	Sv	CC(Al)	Di.A	K	10	10	NL
GC		Sv	CC	ECD	L	5	30	Ir
GC-MS	Cy	Sv	HPLC	GC-MS	K	20	<1	NL*
	Cy	Sv	CC(I-Ex)	MS	Meal	5	2	UK-NI

Residues of carbadox are normally monitored by measuring a metabolite.

ANTHELMINTICS

Substance.	Method	Type Sg/Cy	Ext.	Purif.	Det.	Type	size mL or g	LLD µg/kg or µg/L	Member State
Levamisole	HPLC	Sg,Cy	Sv	Sv	UV	M	10	50	B
Levamisole	HPLC	Sg	Sv	Sv	UV	L	10	20	NL
Levamisole		Sg			UV	L	10	5	UK
Fenbendazole		Sg	Sv	Sv	UV	Pl	1	20	UK-NI
Thiabendazole		Sg	Sv	Sv	Fl/UV	M,L	10	10	B,NL
Benzimidazoles (5)		Sg	no	Dial.	UV	Mk	10	10-50	NL
Benzimidazoles (5)		Sg,Cy	Sv	C2	UV	L	5	250	UK
Ivermectin		Sg	Sv	C18,C-Si	Fl	L	2.5	2.5	D
Ivermectin		Sg	Sv	C8	Fl	M	10	10	NL
Ivermectin		Sg,Cy	Sv	C-Si	Fl	M	5	50	B
Ivermectin		Sg,Cy	Sv	C8,C-Si	Fl	M,l,Mk	5	0.4	G
Ivermectin		Cy	Sv	C8	Fl	M	5	1	UK-NI
Oxfendazole	HPLC-MS	Cy	Sv	HPLC	MS	M	3	100	UK-NI
Fenbendazole		Cy	Sv	Sv	UV	M	3	50	UK-NI
Rafoxanide		Cy	Sv	no	MS	L,M	3	20	UK-NI
Nitroxynil		Cy	Sv	no	MS	L,M	2	20	UK-NI
Levamisole	GC/MS	Cy	Sv	Sv	MS	L	10	5	UK

Abbreviations are at the end of this section

ABBREVIATIONS for Section 4.

TECHNICAL / METHODS
Procedures,
Ext., extraction; Purif., purification/clean-up; Det, detection system

Immunoassay,
IA, immunoassay; RIA, radioimmunoassay; EIA, enzymeimmunoassay;

Chromatography (C);
CC, column chromatography;
GC, gas chromatography;
HPLC, high performance liquid chromatography;
IAC, immunoaffinity chromatography;
TLC, thin-layer chromatography;

SPE; solid phase extraction; C8, SPE on C8 cartridges; C18, SPE on C18
cartridges;
C-Si, SPE on silica cartridges; $C-SO_3H$, SPE on sulphated cartridges
C-DIOL, SPE on hydroxylated silica cartridges, CSX is ion-exchange column,
$C-NH_2$ is aminated cartridge.

Spectrometry;
MS, mass spectrometry; UV, ultra-violet spectrometry;
IR, infra-red spectrometry,

Dens, densimetric;
Dial, dialysis;
Di.A, diode array;
ECD, electro-chemical detector;
Fl, fluorescence;
FPT, four-plate test;
GIB, growth inhibition of bacteria; Grav, gravimetric;
H_2O, aqueous extraction
Sv, solvent extraction;
Vis, visible

b) SAMPLES;- M, muscle; L, liver; K, kidney; F, fat; U, urine; Fc,
faeces; Mk, milk; Eg, eggs; Bi, bile; Th, Thyroid; Pl, plasma; Se, Serum;
I.S., injection site - normally muscle; Imp, implant; Meal, animal meal.

c) Hyphenated techniques are on-line, / are off-line.'

d) LLD is lower limit of detection (sometimes limit of determination).

e) Member States. P, Portugal; S, Spain; F, France; G, Germany (several
Federal labs); It, Italy; Ir, Ireland; UK, United Kingdom; UK-NI, UK-
Northern Ireland; D, Denmark; B, Belgium; L, Luxembourg; Gr, Greece; NL,
Netherlands (Holland)

f) NL* are methods from RIVM submitted direct to manual and are not
officially used in the initial screening part of the National Programme on
hormones and other substances by the National Inspection Service (RVV).
The methods are used to confirm positives where confirmation is required
from a second laboratory.
g) Type of method;- Cy is confirmatory, Sg is screening

5.0.   CRITERIA FOR ROUTINE METHODS AND QUALITY ASSURANCE GUIDELINES.
5.1.   CRITERIA FOR ROUTINE METHODS

These criteria were formulated by a group of experts forming an Ad Hoc
Committee brought together by DGVI. The members of the committee were;

A. Sanabria, DGVI, C. Gaudot (Chairmen);
C. Ring, (Rapporteur to Sc. Vet. Committee, EEC)
F. André, LDH, École Nat. Vet., Nantes
D. Arnold, BGA, Berlin,
N.F. Cunningham, CVL, Weybridge;
N. De Ruig, RIKILT, Wageningen;
H. Durbeck, Kernforschungsanlage Institut, Jülich;
R.J.Heitzman, Private consultant.
H. Meyer, Institute for Physiology, Weihenstephan-Freising;
G. Moretti, Instituto Superiore di Sanita, Rome;
R.W. Stephany, RIVM, Bilthoven.

The full text is published in Commission Decision 93/256 laying down the
methods to be used for detecting residues of substances having a hormonal
or thyrostatic action. *[Editors comment; Note that the title of the
Decision relates to hormonal and thyrostatic substances. In practice the
criteria can and should be applied to residues of all veterinary drugs].*

Article 1 states that the routine analytical procedures for detecting
residues of substances having a hormonal action and of substances having a
thyrostatic action shall be ;- immunoassay; thin-layer chromatography;
liquid chromatography; gas chromatography; mass spectrometry; spectrometry
: or any other method which fulfils comparable criteria to those laid down
for related methods in the Annex of this Decision.

The Annex is a revision of the guidelines published in the first edition of
this manual. The criteria now cover methods for both screening and
confirmatory purposes.

<u>ANNEX OF 93/256/EEC</u>

1.   DEFINITIONS AND GENERAL REQUIREMENTS

1.1.   DEFINITIONS

1.1.1.   **Routine Methods of analysis**

          These are methods of analysis used by Member States to
          implement National Plans for the control of residues in food-
          producing animals and their products in compliance with
          Directive 86/469/EEC. Routine methods must have been validated
          by operational laboratories, and must fulfil the relevant
          criteria set out in this Annex. They may be used for screening
          and/or confirmatory purposes:

          - Methods used for <u>screening</u> purposes (screening methods) are
          methods which are used to detect the presence of an analyte or
          class of analytes at the level of interest. These methods
          have a high sample throughput capacity and are used to sift
          large numbers of samples for potential positives. They are
          aimed at avoiding false negative results.

5/1

- Methods used for <u>confirmatory</u> purposes (confirmatory methods) are methods which provide full or complementary information enabling the analyte to be identified unequivocally at the level of interest. These methods are aimed at preventing false positive results as well as having an acceptable low probability of false negative results.

1.1.2. **Analyte**

This is a component of a test sample which has to be detected, identified and/or quantified. The term "analyte" includes, where appropriate, derivatives formed from the analyte during the analysis.

A quantitative measure of an analyte has to be reported as:

- an <u>amount</u>, expressed as a mass quantity (e.g. μg, ng)
- a <u>content</u>, expressed as a mass fraction (e.g. μg/kg, ng/kg), a mass concentration (e.g. μg/L) or a concentration (e.g. mol/L).

1.1.3. **Samples**

1.1.3.1. Laboratory sample

This is a sample as prepared for sending to the laboratory and intended for inspection or testing.

1.1.3.2. Test sample

This is a sample prepared from the laboratory sample and from which test portions will be taken.

1.1.3.3. Test portion

This is the quantity of material drawn from the test sample (or, if both are the same, from the laboratory sample) and on which the test or observation is actually carried out.

1.1.4. **Standard analyte**

This is a well-defined substance in its highest available purity to be used as a reference in the analysis.

1.1.5. **Reference material**

This is a material of which one, or several, properties have been confirmed by a validated method, so that it can be used to calibrate an apparatus or to verify a method of measurement.

1.1.6. **Blank determinations**

1.1.6.1. Sample blank determination

This is the complete analytical procedure applied to a test portion taken from a sample from which the analyte is absent.

1.1.6.2.   Reagent blank determination

This is the complete analytical procedure applied with omission
of the test portion or using an equivalent amount of suitable
solvent in place of the test portion.

1.1.7.   **Specificity**

Specificity is the ability of a method to distinguish between
the analyte being measured and other substances. This
characteristic is predominantly a function of the measuring
principle used, but can vary according to class of compound or
matrix.

Details concerning specificity must relate at least to any
substances which might be expected to give rise to a signal
when the measuring principle described is used, e.g.
homologues, analogues, metabolic products of the residue of
interest. From the details concerning specificity it must be
possible to derive quantitatively the extent to which the
method can distinguish between the analyte and the other
substances under the experimental conditions.

1.1.8.   **Accuracy**

In this Decision this refers to accuracy of the mean. The
definition which shall be used is laid down in ISO 3534-1977
under 2.83 (Accuracy of the mean: the closeness of agreement
between the true value and the mean result which would be
obtained by applying the experimental procedure a very large
number of times).

The principal limitations on accuracy are:

     (a) random errors;
     (b) systematic errors.

For a very large number of experiments, the accuracy of the
mean approaches the systematic error. For desk review of a
method, the number of experiments must be specified.

The measure of accuracy is the difference between the mean
value measured for a reference material and its true value,
expressed as a percentage of the true value. If no reference
material is available, relevant parameters may be evaluated by
analyzing fortified sample material.

In cases where neither absolute defining methods nor certified
reference materials are available, the analyte content of a
sample may be defined by the results obtained with the aid of a
method which exhibits the highest degree of specificity,
accuracy and precision for the analyte.

1.1.9.   **Precision**

This is the closeness of agreement between the results obtained
by applying the experimental procedure several times under

prescribed conditions (ISO 3534-1977, 2.84), and covers
repeatability and reproducibility.

Repeatability: The closeness of agreement between mutually
independent test results obtained under repeatability
conditions, i.e. with the same method on identical test
material in the same laboratory by the same operator using the
same equipment within short intervals of time.

Reproducibility: The closeness of agreement between mutually
independent test results obtained under reproducibility
conditions, i.e. with the same method on identical test
material in different laboratories with different operators
using different equipment.

According to the Annex to Directive 85/591/EEC the precision
values for methods of analysis which are to be considered for
adoption under the provisions of that Directive shall be
obtained from a collaborative trial which has preferably been
conducted in accordance with ISO 5725-1986. For this purpose,
the terms repeatability and reproducibility are defined in ISO
5725-1986. For conducting such trials sample materials of
known analyte content ranging around the maximum residue limit
to be enforced shall be used.

Until such time as the reproducibility of a method has been
established by a collaborative trial, then for the purpose of
preselection of candidate methods by desk review, it is
sufficient that data on repeatability are available.

The measure of repeatability and reproducibility to be used is
the coefficient of variation as defined in ISO 3534-1977, 2.35
(Coefficient of variation: the ratio of the standard deviation
to the absolute value of the arithmetic mean).

1.1.10.   **Limit of detection**

The smallest measured content from which it is possible to
deduce the presence of the analyte with reasonable statistical
certainty (at least 95% for unauthorized substances - see
1.2.6.1).
The limit of detection can be calculated using different
approaches:

(a)   One way is to carry out sample blank determinations on at
       least 20 representative blank samples. The limit of
       detection is calculated as the apparent content
       corresponding to the value of the mean plus three times
       the standard deviation for the blank determinations.
       Note 1: The amount of test portion typically used in the
       analysis should be specified.
       Note 2: If it is to be expected that factors such as
       species, sex, age, feeding or other environmental factors
       may influence the characteristics of a method, then a set
       of at least 20 blank samples is required for each
       individual homogeneous population to which the method is
       to be applied.

(b)   Alternatively, in the case of spectrometric
        determinations in which blank determinations give white
        noise only, the limit of detection is calculated as the
        apparent content corresponding to three times the peak-
        to-peak noise.

1.1.11.   Limit of determination

This is the smallest analyte content for which the method has
been validated with specified accuracy and precision.

1.1.12.   Sensitivity

This is a measure of the ability of a method to discriminate
between differences in analyte content. In this Decision,
sensitivity is calculated as the slope of the calibration curve
at the level of interest.

1.1.13.   Practicability

This is a characteristic of an analytical procedure which is
dependent on the scope of the method and is determined by
requirements such as sample throughput and costs.

1.1.14.   Applicability

This is a list of the sample materials and/or analytes to which
the method can be applied as presented or with specified minor
modifications.

1.1.15.   Interpretation of results

1.1.15.1.   Positive result

The presence of the analyte in the sample is proved, according
to the analytical procedure, when the general criteria, and the
criteria specified for the individual detection method, are
fulfilled.

(a)   For substances with a zero tolerance, the result of the
        analysis is "positive" if the identity of the analyte in
        the sample is proved unambiguously.

(b)   For substances with an established maximum residue limit,
        the result of the analysis is "positive" if the
        experimentally determined content of the analyte in the
        sample (after applying any correction factor) is greater
        than that established maximum residue limit, which takes
        into account the acceptable probability of obtaining
        false positive or false negative results.

1.1.15.2.   Negative result

The result of the analysis is regarded as "negative" according
to the analytical procedure, when the general criteria and the
criteria specified for the individual detection method are

fulfilled in the case of appropriate reference materials and blank determination and:

(a)   in the case of substances for which there is a zero tolerance, the identity of the analyte has not been proved unambiguously, or

(b)   in the case of substances with an established maximum residue limit, the measured content of the analyte in the sample is below the level specified in 1.1.15.1 (b) above.

Note: A negative result does not prove in case (a) that the analyte is absent from the sample, or in case (b) that the true content of the analyte is below the maximum residue limit.

1.1.16.   **Co-chromatography**

This is a procedure in which the purified test solution prior to the chromatographic step(s) is divided into two parts and:

(a)   one part is chromatographed as such;

(b)   the standard analyte that is to be identified is added to the other part, and this mixed solution of test solution and standard analyte is chromatographed. The amount of added standard analyte has to be similar to the estimated amount of the analyte in the test solution.

1.1.17   **Immunogram**

In this Decision an immunogram is defined as a graphical plot of immunochemical response versus retention time or elution volume as obtained from chromatographic separation with (in general off-line) immunochemical detection of the components of the sample extract.

1.2.   GENERAL REQUIREMENTS

1.2.1.   **Criteria**

In accordance with the Annex to Council Directive 85/591/EEC, the criteria set out below shall apply to the examination of methods of analysis.

1.2.2.   **Screening methods**

Fixed requirements cannot be set for screening methods. The most important aspect of performance is that the incidence of false negatives at the level of interest must be minimal.

1.2.2.1.   <u>Specificity</u> must be defined.

1.2.2.2.   <u>Accuracy and precision</u>: Quantification may not be necessary. Depending on whether the use of a substance is prohibited or authorised, a screening method may be qualitative or

quantitative. False positives are acceptable but false
negatives at the level of interest should be minimal.

1.2.2.3. Limit of detection: This should be appropriate for the purpose.
For substances with an established maximum residue limit, it
must be sufficiently low to detect residues at this level. For
substances which are not authorised for use in food-producing
animals, the limit of detection should be as low as possible.

1.2.2.4. Practicability: A high sample throughput capability is required
and costs should be low.

1.2.3. **Confirmatory methods**

1.2.3.1. Specificity: As far as possible, confirmatory methods must
provide unambiguous information on the chemical structure of
the analyte. When more than one compound gives the same
response, then the method cannot discriminate between these
compounds.

Methods based only on chromatographic analysis without the use
of molecular spectroscopic detection are not suitable for use
as confirmatory methods.

If a single technique lacks sufficient specificity, the desired
specificity may be achieved by analytical procedures consisting
of suitable combinations of clean-up, chromatographic
separation(s) and spectrometric or immunochemical detection,
e.g. GC-MS, LC-MS, IAC/GC-MS, GC-IR LC-IR, LC-Img.

1.2.3.2. Accuracy: In the case of repeated analysis of a reference
material, the guideline ranges for the deviation of the mean
experimentally determined content (after applying any
correction for recovery) from the true value are as follows:

True content (mass fraction)	Range
$\leq$ 1 µg/kg	-50% to +20%
> 1 µg/kg to 10 µg/kg	-30% to +10%
> 10 µg/kg	-20% to +10%.

1.2.3.3. Precision: In the case of repeated analysis of a reference
material under reproducibility conditions, typical values for
the inter-laboratory coefficient of variation (CV) calculated
according to the Horwitz equation [CV(%) = $2^{(1-0.5\ \log C)}$, where
C is the content as a power of 10] are as follows:

Content (mass fraction)	CV (%)
1 µg/kg	45
10 µg/kg	32
100 µg/kg	23
1 mg/kg[a]	16

[Editors Note; [a] this is a correction of µg/kg in official text]

For analyses carried out under repeatability conditions, the
intra-laboratory CV would typically be one-half to two-thirds
of the above values.

1.2.3.4.   <u>Limit of detection</u>: Adequate for the purpose (see 1.2.6.1).

1.2.3.5.   <u>Limit of determination</u>: Adequate for the purpose (see 1.2.6.2).

1.2.3.6.   <u>Sensitivity</u>: Adequate for the purpose.

1.2.3.7.   <u>Practicability</u>: Speed and cost are of lesser importance
compared with screening methods.

For confirmatory methods, most aspects of practicability are of
minor significance compared with the other criteria defined in
this Decision. It is usually sufficient that the required
reagents and equipment are available.

1.2.4.   Calibration curves

If the method depends on a calibration curve then the following
information must be given:

- the mathematical formula which describes the calibration
curve
- acceptable ranges within which the parameters of the
calibration curve may vary from day to day
- the working range of the calibration curve

Whenever possible, suitable internal standards and reference
materials should be used for the quality control of calibration
curves of confirmatory methods, and details of the variance of
the variables which is valid at least for the working range of
the calibration curve should be given.

1.2.5.   Susceptibility to interference

1.2.5.1.   For all experimental conditions which could in practice be
subject to fluctuation (e.g. stability of reagents, composition
of the sample, pH, temperature) any variations which could
affect the analytical result should be indicated. The method
description shall include means of overcoming any foreseeable
interference. If necessary, alternative detection principles
suited for confirmation shall be described.

1.2.5.2   If co-chromatography is carried out, then only one peak should
be obtained, the enhanced peak height (or area) being
equivalent to the amount of added analyte. With GC or LC, the
peak width at half maximum height should be within the range
90-110% of the original width, and the retention times should
be identical within a margin of 5%. For TLC methods, the spot
presumed to be due to the analyte should be intensified only; a
new spot should not appear, and the visual appearance should
not change.

1.2.5.3   It is of prime importance that interference which might arise
            from matrix components should be investigated.

1.2.6.   **Relationship between permitted residue levels and analytical
            limits**

1.2.6.1.   For substances which are not authorised for use in
            food-producing animals, the limit of detection of the
            analytical method must be sufficiently low that residue levels
            which would be expected after illegal use will be detected with
            at least 95% probability.

1.2.6.2.   For substances with an established maximum residue limit, the
            limit of determination of the method plus three times the
            standard deviation which the method produces for a sample at
            the maximum residue limit shall not exceed the established
            maximum residue limit.

1.2.6.3.   For substances with an established maximum residue limit, the
            method should be validated at that limit and at one-half and
            twice the limit.

2.   <u>CRITERIA FOR THE IDENTIFICATION AND QUANTIFICATION OF RESIDUES.</u>

2.1.   GENERAL REQUIREMENT

            Laboratories carrying out analyses for the final confirmation
            of the presence of residues of low molecular weight organic
            substances shall ensure that the criteria for the
            interpretation of results are fulfilled in accordance with the
            requirements of this section. The criteria are designed for
            the identification of the analyte and aim to prevent false
            positive results. For a positive conclusion, the analytical
            results have to fulfil the criteria laid down for the
            particular analytical method.

2.2.   GENERAL CONSIDERATIONS FOR THE WHOLE ANALYTICAL METHOD

2.2.1.   **Preparation of the sample**

            The sample should be obtained, handled and processed in such a
            way that there is a maximum chance of detecting the analyte, if
            present.

2.2.2.   **Susceptibility to interference**

            Information as detailed under 1.2.5 (Susceptibility to
            interference) should be submitted.

2.2.3.   **General criteria for the whole procedure**

2.2.3.1.   The specificity (1.1.7) and the limit of detection (1.1.10) of
            the method for the analyte in the matrix under investigation
            have to be known.

5/9

Note: this information can be obtained from experimental data and/or theoretical considerations.

2.2.3.2.   For a positive result, the physical and chemical behaviour of the analyte during the analysis should be indistinguishable from those of the corresponding standard analyte in the appropriate sample material.

2.2.3.3.   The positive or negative result of the analysis will hold only within the borders of specificity and limit of detection of the procedure for the analyte and sample material under investigation.

2.2.3.4.   Reference material containing known amounts of analyte should preferably be carried through the entire procedure simultaneously with each batch of test samples analyzed. Alternatively, an internal standard may be added to test samples.

2.2.4.   **Criteria for off-line physical and/or chemical preconcentration, purification, and separation**

2.2.4.1.   The analyte should be in the fraction which is typical for the corresponding standard analyte in the appropriate sample material under the same experimental conditions.

2.2.4.2.   Retention data for standards, control samples and test portions should be submitted together with the final result: positive or negative.

2.2.5.   **Criteria for quantitative measurements**

2.2.5.1.   The recovery must be controlled and specified for all quantitative measurements.

2.2.5.2.   Intra-laboratory variability in recovery should be as low as possible.

2.2.5.3.   It must be clearly stated whether or not final results have been corrected for recovery using a correction factor. If they have then the method used for correction must be described.

2.3.   CRITERIA FOR METHODS OF ANALYSIS WHICH MAY BE USED FOR CONFIRMATORY PURPOSES ONLY IN COMBINATION WITH OTHER METHODS.

The methods considered in this Section may only be used for confirmatory purposes in combination with other methods.

2.3.1.   **Quality requirements for the determination of an analyte by IA**

2.3.1.1.   The working range of the calibration curve has to be specified and has in general to cover a concentration range of at least one decade.

2.3.1.2.   A minimum of six calibration points is required, adequately distributed along the calibration curve.

2.3.1.3.   Adequate quality control parameters have to be in line with those of preceding assays, e.g. NSB and parameters of the calibration curve.

2.3.1.4.   Control samples have to be included in each assay. Concentration levels: zero and at lower, middle and upper parts of the working range. Results for these have to be in line with those of previous assays.

            All raw data for the control samples and for the test portion should be submitted together with the final result: positive or negative.

2.3.2.   **Criteria for the determination of an analyte by GC or LC using non-specific detection.**

2.3.2.1.   The analyte should elute at the retention time which is typical for the corresponding standard analyte under the same experimental conditions.

2.3.2.2.   The nearest peak maximum in the chromatogram should be separated from the designated analyte peak by at least one full width at 10% of the maximum height.

2.3.2.3.   For additional information, co-chromatography may be used and chromatography using at least two columns of different polarity.

2.3.3.   **Criteria for the determination of an analyte by TLC.**

2.3.3.1.   The R_f value(s) of the analyte should agree with the R_f value(s) typical for the standard analyte. This requirement is fulfilled when the R_f value(s) of the analyte is (are) within ± 3% of the R_f value(s) of the standard analyte under the same experimental conditions.

2.3.3.2.   The visual appearance of the analyte should be indistinguishable from that of the standard analyte.

2.3.3.3.   The centre of the spot nearest to that due to the analyte should be separated from it by at least half the sum of the spot diameters.

2.3.3.4.   For additional information, co-chromatography and/or two-dimensional TLC may be used.

2.4   CRITERIA FOR METHODS OF ANALYSIS WHICH MAY BE USED FOR CONFIRMATORY PURPOSES

2.4.1.   **Criteria for the determination of an analyte by LC/IA or LC/Img**

2.4.1.1.   For LC/Img, the analyte peak in the Img should be constructed from at least 5 LC fractions.

2.4.1.2.   Criteria 2.2.4.1 and 2.2.4.2 must be fulfilled.

2.4.1.3.   **Reagents**

The source and characteristics of the antibody and other reagents should be specified.

2.4.1.4.   **Calibration curve**

As the method depends on calibration curves, the information itemised under 1.2.4 (Calibration curves) must be given. The quality requirements specified for IA (2.3.1.1 to 2.3.1.4) must be fulfilled.

2.4.1.5.   For confirmatory purposes, if the method is not used in combination with other methods, then two different LC or two immunograms using antibodies with different specificities must be carried out.

2.4.2.   **Criteria for the determination of an analyte by LC-SP.**

2.4.2.1.   The absorption maxima in the spectrum of the analyte should be at the same wavelengths as those of the standard analyte within a margin determined by the resolution of the detection system. For diode array detection this is typically within ± 2 nm.

2.4.2.2.   The spectrum of the analyte above 220 nm should not be visually different from the spectrum of the standard analyte for those parts of the two spectra with a relative absorbance ≥10%. This criterion is met when the same maxima are present and at no observed point is the difference between the two spectra more than 10% of the absorbance of the standard analyte.

2.4.2.3.   For confirmatory purposes, if the method is not used in combination with other methods, then co-chromatography in the LC step is mandatory. See 1.2.5.2 for the requirements to be fulfilled by co-chromatography.

2.4.3.   **Criteria for the determination of an analyte by TLC-SP**

2.4.3.1.   The method must fulfil the criteria specified for TLC (2.3.3.1 to 2.3.3.3).

2.4.3.2.   The absorption maxima in the spectrum of the analyte should be at the same wavelengths as those of the standard analyte, within a margin determined by the resolution of the detection system.

2.4.3.3.   The spectrum of the analyte should not be visually different from the spectrum of the standard analyte.

2.4.3.4.   For confirmatory purposes, if the method is not used in combination with other methods, then co-chromatography in the TLC step is mandatory. See 1.2.5.2 for the requirements to be fulfilled by co-chromatography.

2.4.4.   **Criteria for the determination of an analyte by GC-MS**

2.4.4.1.   GC criteria

2.4.4.1.1. Criteria 2.3.2.1 and 2.3.2.2 must be fulfilled

2.4.4.1.2. An internal standard should be used if a material suitable for
this purpose is available. It should preferably be a stable
isotope labelled form of the analyte or, if this is not
available, a related standard with a retention time close to
that of the analyte.

2.4.4.1.3. The ratio of the retention time of the analyte on GC to that of
the internal standard, i.e. the relative retention time of the
analyte, should be the same as that of the standard analyte in
the appropriate matrix, within a margin of ± 0.5%.

2.4.4.1.4. For use as a confirmatory method: if no internal
standard is used, then identification of the analyte must be
supported by using co-chromatography.

2.4.4.2.   **Criteria for LRMS**

2.4.4.2.1. For use as a screening method, at least the intensity of the
most abundant diagnostic ion must be measured.

2.4.4.2.2. For use as a confirmatory method, the intensities of at least
four diagnostic ions should be measured. If the compound does
not yield four diagnostic ions with the method used, then
identification of the analyte should be based on the results of
at least two independent GC-LRMS methods with different
derivatives and/or ionization techniques, each producing two or
three diagnostic ions.
The molecular ion should preferably be one of the four
diagnostic ions selected.

2.4.4.2.3. The relative abundances of all diagnostic ions monitored from
the analyte should match those of the standard analyte,
preferably within a margin of ± 10% (EI mode) or ± 20% (CI
mode).

2.4.5.   **Criteria for the identification of an analyte by IR.**

2.4.5.1.   **Definition of adequate peaks**

            Adequate peaks are absorption maxima in the IR spectrum of a
            standard analyte, fulfilling the following requirements:

2.4.5.1.1. The absorption maximum is in the wavenumber range 1800-500cm^{-1}.

2.4.5.1.2. The intensity of the absorption is not less than:
            (a) A specific molar absorbance of 40 with respect to zero
            absorbance and 20 with respect to peak base line, or

            (b) A relative absorbance of 12.5% of the absorbance of the
            most intense peak in the region 1800-500 cm^{-1} when both are

measured with respect to zero absorbance, and 5% of the absorbance of the most intense peak in the region 1800-500 cm^{-1} when both are measured with respect to their peak base line. Note: Although adequate peaks according to (a) may be preferred from a theoretical point of view, those according to (b) are easier to determine in practice.

2.4.5.2.   The number of peaks in the IR spectrum of the analyte whose frequencies correspond with an adequate peak in the IR spectrum of the standard analyte, within a margin of $\pm$ 1 cm^{-1} is determined.

2.4.5.3.   **IR criteria**

2.4.5.4.1   Absorption must be present in all regions of the analyte spectrum which correspond with an adequate peak in the reference spectrum of the standard analyte.

2.4.5.3.2.   A minimum of 6 adequate peaks is required in the IR spectrum of the standard analyte. If there are less than 6 adequate peaks, then the IR spectrum at issue cannot be used as a reference spectrum.

2.4.5.4.3.   The "score", i.e. the percentage of the adequate peaks found in the IR spectrum of the analyte, shall be at least 50.

2.4.5.4.4.   Where there is no exact match for an adequate peak, the relevant region of the analyte spectrum must be consistent with the presence of a matching peak.

2.4.5.4.5.   The procedure is only applicable to absorption peaks in the sample spectrum with an intensity of at least 3 times the peak-to-peak noise.

2.5.   **OTHER METHODS OF ANALYSIS**

Analytical methods or combinations of methods other than those considered in Sections 2.3 and 2.4 (e.g. LC-MS, MS-MS, GC-IR) may be used for screening or confirmatory purposes provided they fulfil comparable criteria which permit unambiguous identification of the analyte at the level of interest.

LIST OF ABBREVIATIONS AND SYMBOLS

CI	=	chemical ionization
EI	=	electron impact ionization
GC	=	gas chromatography
IA	=	immunoassay
IAC	=	immunoaffinity chromatography
IMG	=	immunogram
IR	=	infrared spectroscopy
LC	=	liquid chromatography
LRMS	=	low resolution mass spectrometry
MS	=	mass spectrometry
NSB	=	non-specific binding
R_f	=	distance moved relative to the solvent front
SP	=	spectrometry, e.g. diode array
TLC	=	thin-layer chromatography
/	=	off-line hyphenated techniques
-	=	on-line hyphenated techniques

e.g. LC/GC-MS = LC off-line followed by GC with on-line MS

5.2. QUALITY ASSURANCE

5.2.1. Introduction.

Clients of laboratories need to know that measurements, tests or analyses carried out for them are accurate and reliable. Laboratories often provide this level of quality assurance (QA) by working to internationally or nationally accepted standards. The main standards are set out in the documents, EN 29000, ISO 9000, ISO Guide 25 and EN 45001.

There is an International Laboratory Accreditation Conference (ILAC) which aims to harmonise criteria and procedures for laboratory accreditation as a means of dismantling technical barriers to trade, as required by the General Agreement of Tariffs and Trade (GATT), and to facilitate international acceptance of calibration measurements, test data and certificates from accredited laboratories. The results of this technical work are published as ISO/ICE Guides.

Several countries have mutual recognition agreements recognising the equivalence of services and mutual recognition of calibration and test results of accredited laboratories.
In Western Europe laboratory accreditation in EC and EFTA is coordinated by two organisations whose members are national accreditation bodies. These organisations are;
- Western European Calibration Cooperation (WECC) for calibaration laboratories and
- Western European Laboratory Accreditation Cooperation (WELAC) for testing laboratories.

The criteria used by these bodies for Accreditation are based on the EN 45000 series and ISO/IEC Guide 25.

Two Multilateral Agreements, one for WECC and one for WELAC have been signed. The signatories are;
WECC; Denmark, Finland, France, Germany, Italy, the Netherlands, Norway, Sweden, Switzterland and the United Kingdom.

WELAC; Denmark, France the Neterlands, Spain, Sweden and the United Kingdom.
It is expected that the number of signatories will very soon be increased.

Many laboratories and especially those carrying out contract work find that they are only able to obtain and undertake work if they can show that they are working to accepted standards. In the field of veterinary drugs and their residues, the standards required are either working under "Good Laboratory Practice" (GLP) or through a recognised analytical accreditation scheme. GLP is found more useful for drug development and assessment, particulary toxicology, where animal studies are required. On the other hand, analytical measurement accreditation is probably more appropriate for the measurement of residues.

This section summarises the general requirements of QA and makes suggestions as to how QA can be achieved and improved for the measurement of residues.

5.2.2. Definitions

<u>Quality</u> is fitness for purpose.

The USDA, FSIS, "Chemistry Quality Assurance Handbook, (1982) states that
quality assurance (QA) and quality control (QC) have been defined in
several different ways. QC may be understood as "internal quality
control", namely, routine checks included in normal internal procedures,
periodic calibrations, duplicate checks, split samples and spiked samples.
QA may also be viewed as "external quality control", those activities that
are performed on a more occasional basis, usually by a person outside of
the normal routine operations, e.g. laboratory inspections, independent
performance audits, interlaboratory comparisons, and periodic evaluation of
internal QC data.

As in the FSIS handbook the term <u>Quality Assurance</u> is used in this section
to include the above meanings of QA and QC.

Analytical Quality Assurance covers "All activities and functions
concerned with the attainment of accurate and precise information of the
<u>required</u> quality".

<u>Accreditation</u> of a Laboratory is achieved through a third party (competent
authority) providing an independent assurance of the competence of a
laboratory and the validity of the test data or calibration it produces.
Accreditation should not be carried out in-house or by the customer.

<u>Interlaboratory Comparison Tests</u>. These tests are carried out by a
recognised authority (e.g. CRL) using reference samples and formalised
protocols. The results are appraised by the competent authority using
approved statistical methods. ISO/IUPAC/AOAC have recently published "The
international harmonised protocol for the proficiency testing of (chemical)
analytical laboratories" and is recommended for further information on this
type of QA testing (ISO/REMCO N280 report paper by Thompson & Wood, 1993).

5.2.3. Role of Community Reference Laboratories (CRLs).

The Council Decision, 89/187/EEC, lists in Article 1 the functions of the
CRL. Many of these refer to providing a QA programme for the measurement
of residues by the National Reference Laboratories (NRLs). In particular
the following summarised clauses are relevant;-

The CRLs will;-
     a) coordinate the application, within the various NRL, of GLP, in
     accordance with Directives 87/18/EEC and 88/320/EEC.
     b) distribute blank samples and control samples containing known
     amounts of analyte to be analyzed blind in comparative tests to be
     carried out by NRLs.
     c) organize comparative tests between NRLs...
     d) conduct training courses for the analysts in the NRLs.

5.2.4. Role of Management

The management of an organisation/laboratory are responsible for setting up
and managing a QA system. The QA system will address the resources,
processes and procedures by which measurements of the required standard are
achieved.

5/17

The management should have a written quality policy.

The management should identify responsibility and authority for managing the QA system. This may entail the appointment of a "Quality Manager", the choice of inspectors, auditors and testers.

The management are responsible for achieving, allocating and maintaining the necessary resources for the QA system. The key resources are accommodation, staff and equipment. A laboratory will not get accreditation if any of these do not meet the required standards set by the accreditation bodies.

The management should review the QA system periodically and consider all audits and complaints.

Equipment should be adequate for the required measurements and should be calibrated and maintained on a systematic basis (see below).

5.2.5. The QA System

The system which should be set out in the QA manual, will have to take into account most of the components listed below.

1.   Management and Organisation.
2.   Sampling and Sample Handling.
3.   Staff standards.
4.   Equipment Maintenance and Calibration.
5.   Methods and Procedures.
6.   Records
7.   Certificates and Reports.
8.   Audit and Review.
9.   Calibrants, reagents and supplies.
10. Handling of complaints and anomalies.

5.2.5.1. Management and Organisation.

A QA manager should be appointed who will have the responsibility of managing and organising the QA system preferably on an independent basis as described in the EN 45000 series.

He (or she) would report directly to senior management and work very closely with the head/manager of the laboratory.

He is responsible for checking and assuring that all the activities in the laboratory are set up and performed to the required standard.

He will have a major input into the assessment and training of staff.

He must ensure that the documentation for methods, procedures, records and reports meet the accreditation requirement (e.g EN 45000
series)

He will be responsible for internal auditing, checking and calibration of the performance of procedures and equipment.

He will liaise with any external auditors and have a major role in inter-laboratory comparison studies.

5.2.5.2.   QA System Procedures

These procedures cover the whole of the QA system. All procedures must be
documented, controlled and made available to the staff concerned. There
should be a "Quality Manual" giving a general guide to the QA system. This
should be produced by the laboratory staff and will describe the quality
policy objective and the system to achieve it. It will include, detail of
the scope of the laboratory's accreditation, an organization chart of the
laboratory and the staff together with their job descriptions and
authorities. There should be a list of approved signatories.

There should be easily accessible written procedures to cover,
administration, documentation, sampling, calibration and standardisation,
analytical methods, testing protocols, QC and QA analytical procedures,
verdicts, certificates, reports and records. Some of these procedures are
expanded below.

5.2.5.3.   Document Control

The control of documents covers approval and issue and also any changes and
alterations. There should be a set of master documents which are properly
identified. Copies are issued to those that need them and a record of
their distribution kept. Alterations and changes of documents should be
done at the master copy level and then new copies and identities issued and
recorded. Previous master copies should be kept and marked "SUPERSEDED".
All obsolete copies should be collected and destroyed.

5.2.5.4.   Staff

Staff should have the required skills, always where complex techniques and
equipment are used. Training and continuous education is essential and
within the Community attendance at EC workshops should be encouraged.

5.2.5.5.   Equipment.

All measuring equipment that can influence quality must be controlled,
calibrated and maintained.

The choice of equipment is important. The equipment must be capable of
measuring to the required sensitivity and tolerance. An established design
from a reputable company is preferred. Consideration should be given to
the availability of good and reliable service, maintenance, spares and
repairs. In third world countries this is of vital importance.

The replacement of equipment should be planned in collaboration with the
management.

The equipment should be uniquely identified.

The documentation for the equipment should be properly filed. It will
consist of the manufacturers instructions/manuals and an in-house file.
This file should contain;
        List of equipment
        Equipment requiring calibration and maintenance.
        Dates or intervals for calibration and maintenance.
        Calibration procedures to be performed by authorised staff.
        Records of calibration and maintenance.

Maintenance and Calibration of Equipment;-
The regular maintenance and calibration of important measuring equipment is
essential for achieving accuracy an precision of results. For residue
analysis at least the following items should be checked and /or calibrated.
>   Balances,
>   pipettes (especially the automatic type, check the automatic pipette
>   stations including those for HPLC or GC),
>   pH meters,
>   spectrophotometers, Mass spectrometers
>   HPLC and GC;
>   Radioisotope counters
>   Temperature of fridges, freezers and cold rooms,
>   Thermometers

5.2.5.6.   Sampling and Sample Handling.

The sample should be representative and its history documented and
transferred to the analyst. It must arrive at the laboratory in a
condition which does not alter the content of the analyte from that at the
immediate time of sampling. The procedures for proper sampling of animals
and food products are described in section 6 (6.3.1). Even with the best
analytical methods and QA, inaccurate results are guaranteed if the
original sample is wrongly taken or has deteriorated and the content of the
analyte been affected .

There should be detailed written procedures of how to handle, store and
record samples on arrival at the laboratory. The procedure should preserve
best approximation of the true content of the analyte in the sample to be
analyzed and in replicate samples and contra-samples. Special attention
has to be paid to those analytes, e.g. the nitrofurans, which degrade very
quickly in biological tissues.

5.2.5.7.   Analytical Methods

Analytical methods may be from different sources;-
>   Official Standard Methods (e.g. ISO methods)
>   Standard Operating Procedures which have been accredited by a
>   recognised authority or scheme.
>   In-house methods which are validated but not accredited.
Several of the methods in section 6 are Standard Operating Procedures (SOP)
which have received accreditation.

Methods should include the following,
>   Sampling, sample handling and storage.
>   Safety precautions.
>   Scope, field of application, references, definitions, principle of
>   method.
>   Details of Materials; reagents, standards and calibrants.
>   Details of equipment.
>   Details of calibration
>   Test sample preparation.
>   Testing procedure.
>   Data handling; Calculation of results, checking results, data
>   transfer, estimation of uncertainty.
>   Quality control procedure which include using CRMs and/or in-house
>   reference materials.
>   Flow diagrams.

The methods require planned quality control and there should be records of all QA measurement. It is vital that what is written in the procedure is carried out, any variation should be recorded.

5.2.5.8.   QC Procedures for analytical methods for residues.

The criteria for the methods are set out in the "Criteria Document", EC 93/256, given in this section. How these are controlled varies between laboratories. This is evident from the different QC procedures detailed in section 6. However some of the most important and common features for QC are listed below.
1.   Method is accredited or fully validated (some of the texts in section 6 are similar to the official SOP).
2.   The analysis, testing, calibrating, calculations and recording of results are done by authorised staff and exactly as in the written procedures.
3.   QC samples are used. These ideally should be in-house reference materials preferably standardised against EC certified reference materials (CRM) or other internationally approved standards if available. The QC samples recommended are;-
     i). a blank with no analyte present,
     ii). an incurred sample either with the analyte concentration equal to the MRL for the analyte or in the case of prohibited substances at a concentration at or just above the limit of detection and/or determination of the method.
     iii). an incurred sample above the MRL or limit of detection but approximating to a concentration which might be found in practice.
4.   QC samples are measured in every assay. The use of <u>blind</u> check samples might be used for both internal and external performance assessment.
5.   Spiked samples (with analyte and/or internal standard) are used to check recoveries, linearity of response and to produce calibration curves.
6.   Major equipment, which must be suitable for the measurements, is calibrated and maintained.
7.   The method for the calculation of results is detailed and the quality of the results is tested using approved statistical procedures such as laid down in ISO REMCO N263 (1992) (Thompson & Wood, 1993) and see also Heydorn (1991).

5.2.5.9.   Tools for checking data.

The statistical control of data is recommended and reviewed by Heydorn (1991). Some good examples of the use of charts is given in volume I of the USDA, FSIS, Chemistry Quality Assurance Handbook, 1987 and also Griepink (1990a, 1990b).

Charts are a useful approach to reviewing measurement. Their construction is used to detect trends, biases and performance of an analytical method. Eaasy to use and construct are either Cusum or Shewhart charts.

<u>Cusum Charts.</u>   A Cusum (Cumulative sum) control chart is useful in a laboratory carrying out the same analyses many times over a long period of time. It is a graphic plot of the running summation of process deviation from a control value. Its underlying mathematical concepts are highly involved, but its construction is simple. An example which might be appropriate to residue analysis is shown below. In this example the recovery of an internal standard is measured; the normal expected recovery is 60% and values between 50% and 65% are acceptable. During the first six months the analysis is functioning properly but by September there is a clear warning that the analysis may be out of control. By November the analysis is out of control. Remedial action had clearly cured the problem by December and into the new year.

Date of Analyses.	Recovery (%)	Cusum (%)
Jan	61	1
Feb	63	4
March	61	5
April	63	8
May	60	8
June	61	9
July	56	5
August	58	3
Sept	55	-2
Oct	53	-9
Nov	50	-19
Dec	59	-20
Jan	60	-20
Feb	58	-22
March	62	-20

<u>Cusum Chart</u>

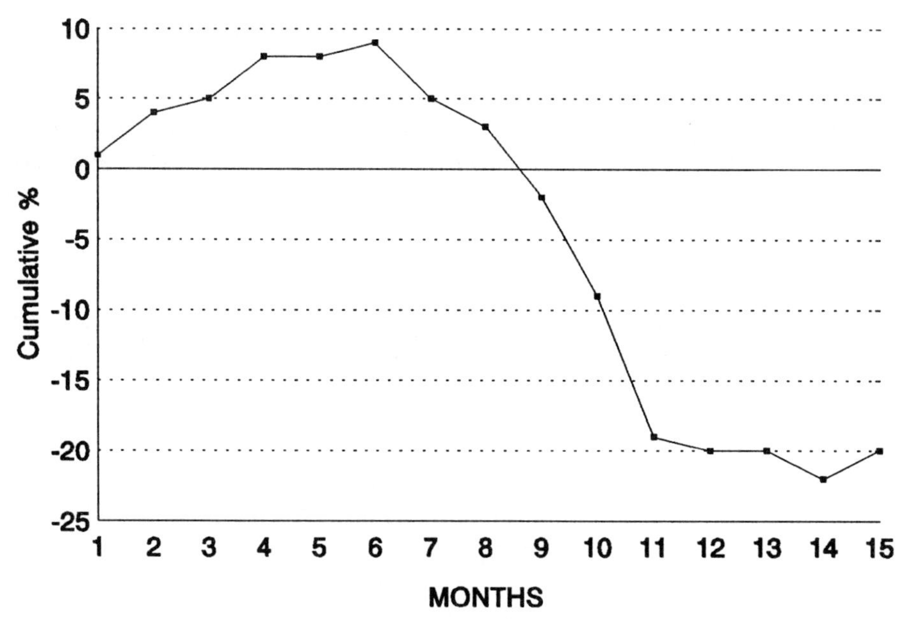

<u>Shewhart Control Charts.</u>   These charts are a graphical representation of
control limits for the average mean and range of results for a set of
analyses. The determination of the appropriate control limits (upper and
lower confidence limits and the upper and lower warning limits) can be
based on the capability of the procedure itself as known from past
experience or on the specified requirements of the measurement procedure
(e.g. a function of the standard deviation as set out in the Criteria
Decision, 93/256/EEC, see above).

An example (hypothetical) of a Shewhart graph is shown below. A reference
sample was measured in duplicate as a QC control in each of a series of
analyses. The results of the mean values and the range for the QC samples
are plotted. The mean values are all within the confidence limits although
one value (analysis 9) is suspiciously high especially since the range was
low probably caused by a systematic error. One of the values (analysis 6)
for the range is unacceptable. Checking the raw data for this analysis may
well indicate that one or both of the results is a "rogue" or "outlier".
This may be caused by a random error.

Figure 2. Shewhart Control Graphs for means and ranges.

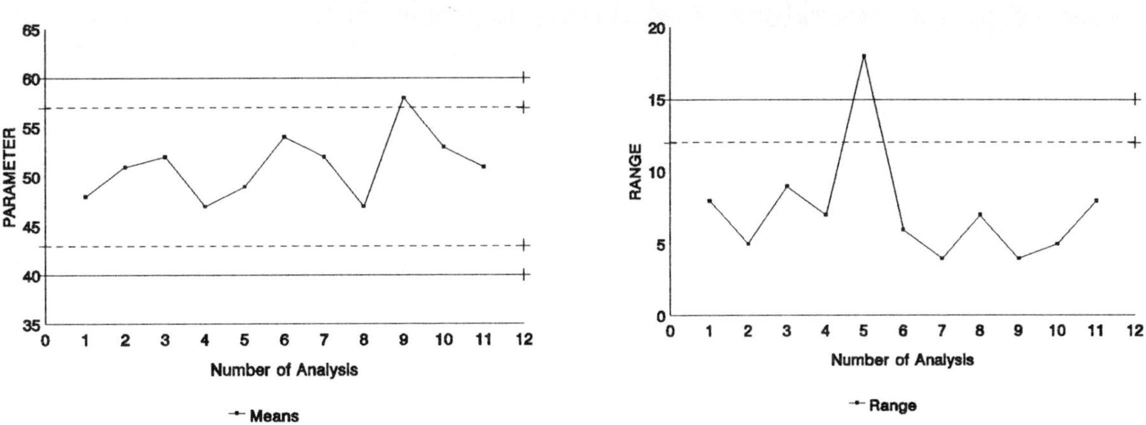

The upper and lower confidence limits are shown as solid lines; the dotted
lines are the upper and lower warning limits which are sometimes set at
twice the SD. Further information can be found in volume I of the USDA,
FSIS, Chemistry Quality Assurance Handbook, 1987.

5.2.5.10.   Audit and Review.

Audit; The laboratory should always carry out regular internal audits of
the QA system and pay particular attention to the procedures and methods
for analysis. With both GLP and accreditation of methods, audits are
compulsory. Under GLP all procedures are audited on a regular basis by
personnel who are independent of the laboratory staff carrying out a
particular study. Under most accreditation schemes, there is third party
examination of the analytical methods. Failure to meet the required
standards after being allowed a short period for corrective action can lead
to loss of accreditation. Under the NAMAS scheme in the UK the
laboratories may be required to measure audit samples.   Similarly under EC
Directive 86/469 the CRLs could make use of RMs to check the performance of
the NRLs in their measurement of residues.

Review; Reviews of the QA system should be done on a regular basis by
senior management in consultation with the QA management. The results of
the review should be communicated to the relevant staff.

5.2.5.11.   Reports and Records.

The laboratory will keep all raw data and copies of results, reports and
records. The QA manager will be responsible for checking and auditing that
the data is calculated, recorded and reported according to the agreed
procedures. Good quality reports and records are of great benefit in the
event of problems with the analyses, queries by customers and for external
audit. The retention time of the reports and records is decided and
written into the procedures. For GLP they must be kept for 10 years, for
an accreditation scheme e.g. NAMAS, UK, for 6 years.

5.2.5.12.   Corrective Actions.

The QA system should have a documented procedure to investigate anomalies,
complaints and serious non-compliancies. All corrective actions and their
effectiveness is recorded. All non-compliancies reported through the
audits must be subject to corrective action. If doubt arises about the
data reported by the laboratory, the clients must be notified in writing.

References.
Griepink, B.(1990a). Quality and Certified Reference Materials. In
"Element concentration cadasters in ecosytems." Ed. H. Leith & B. Markert.
Publ. VCH, Weinheim, Germany, pp 181-205.

Griepink, B. (1990b). The role of CRM's in measurement systems. Fres. J.
Anal. Chem. 338, 360-362.

Heydorn, K. (1991), Quality Assurance and Statistical Control.
Mikrochimica Acta. III, 1-10.

Thompson, M. and Wood, R. (1993), The international harmonised protocol for
the proficiency testing of (chemical) anlytical laboratories. Pure &
Applied Chem., 65, 2123-2144 also as ISO/REMCO N280.

6. ROUTINE METHODS FOR DETECTING RESIDUES.

THE METHODS CHOSEN FOR INCLUSION IN THIS MANUAL ARE A SELECTION OF METHODS USED IN VARIOUS MEMBER STATES. THEY DO <u>NOT</u> HAVE OFFICIAL STATUS FROM THE EUROPEAN COMMISSION AND AT THIS STAGE <u>CANNOT</u> BE TREATED AS OFFICIAL COMMUNITY REFERENCE METHODS.

The definitions of routine methods for screening and confirmatory purposes is given in section 5.1.1. All of the methods covered in this section should meet the criteria laid down in section 5 and published as EC Decision 93/256/EEC. The routine screening and some of the confirmatory tests used by Member States as of August 1993 are tabled in section 4.

The Council Decision 91/664 designating the Community reference laboratories (CRL) for testing certain substances for residues and the Council Decision 89/187 determining the powers and conditions of operation of CRL provided for by directive 86/469 EEC concerning the examination of animals and fresh meat for the presence of residues have established a major role for the four CRL in the development, testing, quality assurance, advice and training for analytical methodology. This manual serves as an adjunct to their role.

6.1. ROUTINE SCREENING METHODS.

Routine screening methods should be rapid with high throughputs, rugged, inexpensive and be sensitive enough to monitor the levels of interest (e.g. MRLs) with the minimum of false negatives.

The wide variety of drugs and their residues requires that several different procedures are needed to monitor all the possibilities. The ideal would be to analyze a sample for all possible residues using one procedure. The complete separation of residues by chromatography coupled with a sensitive end-point detection system has been attempted with limited success (e.g. Verbeke, 1979, Malisch, 1986). In general the most promising results are where procedures have been limited to residues of substances within classes of drugs. Multiresidue screening methods are available for;

1.   Antibiotic substances using the Four Plate Test
2.   Sulphonamides by TLC or IA.
3.   Anabolics by IA or GC-MS
4.   Benzimidazoles by HPLC
5.   ß-agonists by GC-MS or IA.
6.   Sedatives and tranquillisers by HPLC.

6.1.1 Assay Kits for screening for Residues.

Screening procedures are well suited for the application of commercially available assay kits. The kits must be rugged and transportable on an international basis. A list of commercial suppliers and their assay kits is given in section 8.4 and a summary is shown in table 1 below. Some important antibodies and other reagents for assays are also listed in Section 8.

Table 1. Assay Kits for Veterinary Drug Residues.

Group	Drug Residue	Assay	Supplier
AI Anabolics	19-Nortestosterone 19-Norandrostenedione	EIA	Euro-diagnost ica, NL
	Stilbenes, Zeranol, Trenbolone.	RIA	Genego, Italy
	Zeranol, DES, 19-Nortestosterone,	ELISA	Genego, Italy
	19-Nortestosterone, Trenbolone,	ELISA	Randox, UK-NI
	19-Nortestosterone, Ethinyloestradiol, Trenbolone, DES, Zeranol.	ELISA	R-BIOPHARM GmbH Germany
	DES, 19-Nortestosterone Zeranol, Taleranol, Trenbolone, Oestradiol, Ethinyloestradiol, Testosterone, Acetylgestagenes	ELISA	RIEDEL-DE-HAEN Germany
AII Natural Steroids	Progesterone	ELISA	Genego, Italy
	Testosterone	ELISA	Randox, UK-NI
	Oestradiol-17β Testosterone	ELISA	R-BIOPHARM GmbH Germany
	Progesterone	ELISA	RIEDEL-DE-HAEN Germany
AII Antibiotics	Chloramphenicol	EIA	Euro-diagnost-ica, NL
	Chloramphenicol, Sulphadimidine, Penicillin-G	ELISA	Genego, Italy
	Sulphonamides	ELISA	Randox, UK-NI
	Chloramphenicol, Sulphadimidine, Sulphamethoxine, Gentamicin	EIA Card	Rhone-Poulenc, France
	Chloramphenicol, Sulphadimidine, Streptomycin, Tetracycline.	ELISA	R-BIOPHARM GmbH Germany

Table 1 continued.

Group	Drug Residue	Assay	Supplier
ß-agonists	Clenbuterol, salbutamol, mabuterol & mapenterol	EIA	Euro-diagnostica, NL
	Clenbuterol, salbutamol, mabuterol, mapenterol and terbutaline	ELISA	Genego, Italy
	Clenbuterol, salbutamol mabuterol, terbutaline,	ELISA	R-BIOPHARM GmbH, Germany
	Clenbuterol, mabuterol, salbutamol, mapenterol and terbutaline	ELISA	RIEDEL-DE-HAEN Germany
	Clenbuterol, mabuterol, salbutamol, terbutaline, cimaterol	ELISA	MARLOIE, Belgium

6.1.2 Residues in Milk.

This manual does not give detailed methods for residues in milk as the methods are suitably described in the <u>Bulletin of the International Dairy Federation</u> №258/1991. The methods are divided into two sections;-
1. Methods for the detection of inhibitors.
   - Microbial inhibition tests, screening and confirmatory
   - Other tests not based on microbial inhibition.
2. Special Methods for the detection of the antibiotics, ß-lactams, chloramphenicol, tetracyclines, macrolides, aminoglycosides and sulphonamides in milk and milk products.
   - Many of these methods are similar to those used for testing animals and other animal products but are specially adapted for use with milk and milk products. They include IA, HPLC, TLC, electrophoresis and GC.

6.1.3 Screening for residues of antimicrobial substances.

6.1.3.1. Introduction.
Antimicrobial substances are widely used in farm animals. There is both therapeutic and prophylactic use. The drugs are administered either parentally or added to the drinking water or feed. The unique property of antimicrobial substances is that they can be assayed for their antimicrobial activity. Vast numbers of meat (and milk) samples are assayed for the determination of the antimicrobial activity of any residues present. Because there is such a large variety of antimicrobial compounds with very different chemical structures and molecular weights it is not easy to identify the nature of the chemical substance causing the antimicrobial activity in the tests. Also the microbiological methods are less sensitive for some drugs than others and many antibiotics (e.g. chloramphenicol, sulphonamides, nitrofurans) are not successfully detected in the standard tests such as the "Frontier Post Test". Many antimicrobials and especially those insensitive to the "Frontier Post Test" are regulated as individual substances using chemical methods. These methods are sensitive enough to regulate MRLs (see section 2).

6.1.3.2. General scheme for testing for antibiotics.

Routine Screening tests; These are carried out using one of the following
procedures for testing meat;-

1. The official EC "Frontier Post Test" (Bogaerts and Wolf, 1980) which
    is sometimes called the Four Plate Test, or a modified version of
    this test. In 1993 the CRL at Fougeres recommends a modified version
    (see method Sg 3.1) for general use by Member States.
2. An enzyme immunoassay test. (e.g. for sulphonamides, chloramphenicol
    gentamicin)
3. Chromatographic methods using TLC, HPLC or occasionally GC.

Numerous sensitive and well developed methods for testing for antibiotics
in milk are available (see 6.1.2).

Routine Confirmatory Tests; Methods based on GC-MS, LC-MS or HPLC, are
well developed for confirming the presence of individual substances which
have been tentatively identified in the screening tests. Examples of
methods are given in section 6 for the confirmation of residues of the
sulphonamides, chloramphenicol, tetracyclines and nitrofurans. It is
difficult to identify the nature of residues which are positive with
respect to their antimicrobial activity. A method combining the separation
of antibiotics into groups by using High Voltage Electrophoresis and
identifying the separated groups with a microbial inhibition test has had
some success (Smither and Vaughan, 1978).

Tests based on Antimicrobial Activity.

Frontier Post Test.

This test is carried out as an agar diffusion test, and the meat samples
are applied to four plates of agar medium inoculated with Bacillus subtilis
spores (at pH 6.0, 7.2 and 8.0) and Micrococcus luteus (at pH 8.0).
Trimethoprim is incorporated into the pH 7.2 medium to enhance the test's
sensitivity toward sulphonamide residues. Diffusion of an antibacterial
substance is shown by the formation of zones of inhibition of one or both
microorganisms. The test is an official EC method based on the method of
Bogaerts and Wolf, (1980).

The detection of an antimicrobial agent by this test depends on the lower
limit of sensitivity for that agent using the most sensitive combination of
test organism and growth conditions applied to the target tissue.   The
data shows that the test is sensitive for ß-lactam antibiotics, all tested
aminoglycosides, macrolides and tetracyclines, novobiocin, and the one
tested polypeptide antibiotic, bacitracin. The test is relatively
insensitive for chloramphenicol, furazolidone and trimethoprim. Many other
groups of antibiotics have only been partially tested. The CRL at
Fougeres, have modified the method by reducing the volume of agar in the
Petri dishes. This modified method which is replacing the official method
in France is given in full detail in Method number Sg 3.1.

It is suggested that for all agents which cannot be measured by this test
at a sensitivity of 1 mg per kg muscle, alternative assay procedures are
developed in order to reach this level of sensitivity. Agents of special
interest in this class are chloramphenicol, sulphonamides and nitrofurans.

High Voltage Electrophoresis (HVE) Method.

Since "false positive" results must be eliminated from the Frontier Post
Test results by further analysis, it makes sense to determine at the same
time which antimicrobial agent is present in the "true positive" results.
This may be achieved in a method combining HVE with microbial inhibition
(Smither and Vaughan, 1978). The antimicrobial substances are separated on
an agar coated plate into groups which are then positionally identified
with a microbial inhibition test.

The test is both difficult to perform and sometimes lacks precision.
Nevertheless fifty antimicrobial substances have been identified by this
test including chloramphenicol and furazolidone.

[Editor; There is probably scope for improvement in this type of test
because of the rapid development in techniques for separation by
electrophoresis.].

Chemical Methods.

The methods used for the measurement and detection of antimicrobials with a
molecular weight less than 1000 daltons (e.g. tetracyclines, sulphonamides,
ß-lactams and chloramphenicol) are no different from those for other
veterinary drugs of similar molecular weights.

Some antimicrobials are very big molecules with high molecular weights and
these drugs are among the most difficult to measure and identify. These
substances are not ideal for GC-MS or immunoassay methods. Immunoassay is
sometimes a problem because of the difficulty of making a suitable
immunogen without disturbing the quaternary structure of the large parent
molecule. These drugs can often be best measured using HPLC, where mild
solvents and low temperatures are less damaging. A good example is the
measurement of Ciprofloxacin and Enrofloxacin (see Method number Sg 3.5.
The combination of HPLC with MS (LC-MS) is new technology which is being
successfully applied to the analysis of high molecular weight veterinary
drugs and proteins.

6.2 ROUTINE CONFIRMATORY METHODS.

The purpose of the confirmatory methods is to determine the presence or
absence of a residue in a sample found positive in a routine screening
analysis. In the future some of the confirmatory methods may be approved
by the Community and be designated Community Reference methods.

The selection of a method depends on a combination of resources and the
selectivity of the method. The selectivity index (see Van Ginkel and
Stephany, 1989; Stephany and Van Ginkel, 1990) is based on the summation of
the partial indices for each stage of the method. Not surprisingly methods
with several stages have a high selectivity index and those methods which
combine chromatographic clean up (particulary IAC, HPLC and GC) with end-
point spectrometry score best.

Confirmatory methods should preferably be based on molecular spectrometry
to provide direct information about the molecular structure of the residue
(see Criteria, section 5). The application of spectrometry to residue
determination is progressing rapidly but the measurement of residues at
concentrations <1 µg per kg is difficult, especially in the transfer of

methods to other laboratories. In the interim period until spectroscopic methods are further developed, validated methods, or a battery of methods, providing indirect information on the molecular structure may be used.

An earlier problem with detection and determination of anabolics at concentrations in the sub ppb level was the sensitivity of the end-point detection system. Until recently routine confirmatory methods were limited to the use of immunoassay at this level whereas spectroscopic methods were applied at higher levels. The sensitivity and availability of MS and IR has improved and although the HPLC/RIA methods have been shown to give the same results as MS methods (Jansen et al, 1986) the spectroscopic methods are the recommended methods of choice (see Criteria, Section 5).

The approximate applicability limits for various molecular "full spectrum" detectors as such or on-line with chromatographic separation techniques can be estimated by considering the sensitivity of the detectors as shown below.

Spectrum Detector	Minimum mass for full spectrum (ng)	Lowest content for 1 g sample[R] (ug per kg)	Mass of sample to find 1 μg per kg[R] (g)
IR	100	100	100
GC-IR	100	100	100
HPLC-UV	100	100	100
TLC-UV	100	100	100
*GC-FTIR (cryotrapping)	1	1	1
GC-MSD	0.1	0.1	0.1
[e]LC-MS	0.02	0.02	0.02
GC-MS	0.01	0.01	0.01
MS-MS	0.001	0.001	0.001

Data presented by R. Schothorst at EEC Workshop, RIVM - RIKILT, 28th Nov. 1988; * at EEC Workshop, RIVM, 22-26 April, 1991; [e] at Euroresidues II, Veldhoven, The Netherlands, May,1993.
[R] assuming 100% recovery of analyte.

The rapid emergence of spectroscopic methods has a drawback for this manual in that the technology is continually developing and methods are either not published or are published as single methods used in only one or two laboratories. Many of these methods and the other types of confirmatory methods have not been validated by ring tests between the Member States nor have they been approved as Community Reference Methods.

6.2.1 EEC WORKSHOPS.

There is a programme organised through DGVI to hold EEC workshops where scientists from the Member States receive training in residue method technology. To date the following workshops have been held;

DATE	PLACE	TITLE
1981	BGA, Berlin	RIA methods for the stilbenes.
1985	Brussels	TLC methods for thyreostats

1986	BGA, Berlin	RIA method for chloramphenicol
1987	Weihenstephan	IA methods for anabolic agents
1988	RIVM, Bilthoven	HPLC and IAC/GC-MS for anabolic agents
1990	Brussels	TLC methods for ß-agonists
1991	RIVM, Bilthoven	MS methods for ß-agonists
1994 also	RIVM, Bilthoven	GLP for NRLs
1993	Univ. Liege - EC-Flair Workshop , MS for residue analysis	

6.2.2. Multiresidue and Modular Methods.

Traditional analytical strategies are gradually being replaced by multiresidue techniques of a modular nature. Van Ginkel and Stephany (1990) conclude that these alternative strategies are more flexible with respect to changes in matrix and analyte.

More than thirty of the most probable residues which could occur in animal products can be determined using just three multi-residue GC-MS methods. Special attention is also given to making these multi-residue methods into modular methods. The purpose of these methods is to reduce the number of methods which a laboratory needs to establish. The methods contain options which could fulfil the Criteria in Section 5. The methods contain three key elements, an initial extraction, a clean-up and purification by chromatography and an end point determination using either GC or HPLC coupled to MS. Future development will almost certainly include GC-FTIR using a cryotrapping technique (Visser et 1993). For some large molecules the application of capillary gel electrophoresis coupled to MS is an exciting prospect.

6.2.3 Availability of reagents and standards.

The choice of method is also governed by the availability of reagents and standards. In some cases there is difficulty obtaining immunoaffinity chromatography (IAC) columns or the antibodies for IAC, also the availability of pure standards and especially deuterated standards is a problem. The Measurement and Testing Programme (BCR) is funding programmes and encouraging the production of many of these reference compounds and RMs so that they are available throughout the Community (see section 8). For the validation of these methods certified reference materials are of great importance. Many reagents and reference compounds are available commercially but in an industry where the market is small the supply of the materials may change very quickly. A list of suppliers of immunochemicals and reagents is given in section 8.4.

6.3. GENERAL PROCEDURE FOR ROUTINE METHODS TO DETERMINE RESIDUES OF ORGANIC ANALYTES.

All the methods follow a similar sequence of procedures shown in the flow chart. In some of the methods the extraction and chromatographic purifications steps may overlap or be merged and for some screening methods a simple extraction procedure followed by a rapid end-point determination is often sufficient.

FLOW CHART OF PROCEDURES.

        (i) Representative sample or RM.
       (ii) Add internal standard
      (iii) Homogenise tissues / dilute fluids
       (iv) Hydrolyse
        (v) Initial extraction
       (vi) Clean up extraction by solvent/solvent partition
      (vii) Clean up and/or resolution by chromatography
     (viii) End point determination
       (ix) Quality assurance procedures.
        (x) Calculation of results.
       (xi) Reporting of results

GENERAL COMMENTS ON PROCEDURES.

6.3.1 (i) Representative sample;
6.3.1.1 Legal Basis (EC legislation).
The sampling for the National Surveillance Schemes is regulated under

- The Council Directive 86/469 concerning the examination of animals
  and fresh meat for the presence of residues. This Directive is
  undergoing modification.
- Commission Decision 83/153 concerning the correlation of samples
  taken for residue examination with animals and their farm of origin.

6.3.2. Technical and Administrative Procedures.
6.3.2.1. Which Samples?
The choice of matrix shall depend on :

- the analyte and its route of excretion.
- the analytical method of detection

The biological fluid sample is either urine, bile, blood (as plasma or
serum) or milk.
The tissue samples are either muscle, liver, kidney, fat or eggs. In rare
cases other organs may have to be examined (e.g. residues of ß-agonists may
investigated using the eyes of cattle).

Also the difficulty/ease of collecting the sample should be considered: It
is easier to collect blood or faeces than urine from live bovine animals at
the farm. In this case the laboratory has to develop specific clearing
procedures if faecal materials are the only matrix at its disposal.

6.3.2.2. Quantity (How much?)
This must be divided into several parts (see 6.3.2.4.) and each part
sufficient for the analysis. Large volumes of fluids are recommended
although the use of a diuretic to increase the volume of urine is not
recommended as this may have a dilution effect on the concentration of the
residue.

6.3.2.4. Division of the Samples.
According to the different national laws it can be compulsory to divide the
sample into two or three parts as aliquots into suitable containers (e.g
bottles, tubes or bags). These samples are used
        1. for the routine analyses.

2. as contra-samples for use by the owner of the animal or meat.
3. put at the disposal of a Court of Justice.

The sample may be divided at the point of collection i.e. farm or
slaughterhouse. More usual and to be recommended is the division of the
sample on reception at the laboratory. This latter procedure is preferred
especially where some pretreatment of the sample is essential before
storage.

6.3.2.5. Identification.
The identification on the container should be;

- indelible
- marked on the main part of the container (not just the removable top)
- linked with the complete information written on the official sampling
  form.
The following information must be recorded;-
- the name and address of the owner or person in charge of the animal;
- the name and address of the premises where the sample was taken;
- the species, sex and age of the animal;
- the type, amount and method of collection;
- the identification of the animal or a reference permitting the farm
  of origin of the animal to be identified;
- the name, position and signature of the official agent collecting the
  sample
- the date of sampling and the date of expedition to the laboratory.

6.3.2.6. Sealing.
The package shall be sealed (e.g. wax or lead seal) in order to prevent any
change in the matrix during storage or transport.

6.3.2.7. Storage.
If the sample cannot go immediately to the laboratory, it must be stored as
soon as possible, in a chilling room or freezing room, on the condition
that the freezing procedure does not destroy the molecules of the residue.

6.3.2.8. Transport.
Transport to the laboratory must be carried out under such conditions that
the sample is kept at its temperature of conservation.

Expedition before a week-end or a holiday period shall be avoided. Too
often the laboratories receive samples impossible to use because of bad
conditions of transport, e.g. broken package, matrix at the ambient
temperature or the sampling form lost.

6.3.2.9 Summary.
These general recommendations have to be adapted to each situation, but it
is clear that the reliability of the result is very dependant on the
quality of the sampling procedure.

The samples are usually stored deep frozen and only thawed immediately
before analysis.

6.3.3 (ii) Addition of internal standard (ISTD).
Internal standards are used a) to monitor and measure recovery
b) as calibrants for retention times or reference values in chromatography
systems.

For RIA end point measurements the ISTD is a radiolabelled form of the
analyte in question.

For methods with chromatographic end points a substance with similar
chemical and physical properties to the analyte is used but it must be
clearly separated from the analyte and other major residues in the final
chromatographic analysis.

For MS methods an isotope labelled form of the analyte is used which must
be distinguishable from the analyte in the MS and have a similar ionisation
mechanism compared to the analyte.   If the isotope is deuterium then the
possibility of hydrogen - deuterium exchange between the ISTD and the
analyte should be checked.

6.3.4 (iii) Homogenisation;
Fluids do not normally require homogenisation and bile, urine, plasma or
serum are thawed and an aliquot diluted in buffer. Milk which has separate
fat and aqueous phases will require special treatment depending whether
whole milk or one of the phases is to be tested.

Tissues except fat are thawed and a representative sample is added to a
buffer and the sample homogenised at 0°C using a blade homogeniser or in
some cases a stomacher. Losses can occur due to inadequate transfer of
materials during this procedure.

Fat is often cut into small pieces and either melted or dissolved into an
organic lipophilic solvent from whence it is treated as a fluid.

6.3.5 (iv) Hydrolysis;
Many analytes form conjugates e.g. as sulphates or glucuronides. The
conjugates are normally soluble in buffer solutions and may be hydrolysed
to liberate the free analyte.
Hydrolysis is best achieved using suitable enzyme preparations and mild
conditions. Hydrolysis using acids or alkalis should only be used when it
is certain no degradation of the analyte occurs.

6.3.6 (v) Initial Extraction;
Solvent/solvent partition has formed the basis of extraction and clean up
procedures for most of this century. It still plays an important role and
is the primary extraction step in most assays measuring organic molecules.
The purpose of the extraction is to remove as much of the interfering
cellular material and organic compounds as possible while retaining the
majority of the analyte.

The solvents used depend on the properties of the analyte as determined by
polarity, pH and solubility in different solvents.
The commonly used systems include;-

-    Homogenate or solution in aqueous buffer / immiscible organic solvent
-    Organic solvent / aqueous phase various pH
-    Polar phase (e.g. methanol/water) / Non-polar solvent
                                         (e.g. petroleum ether)

Matrix Solid-phase Dispersion (MSPD).
The method involves the mechanical blending of the sample with bulk
sorbent. The initial studies were performed using a C-18 sorbent, a
silicate based bonded phase that can solubilize samples rich in lipid

material. The silicate particles act as a strong abrasive and also provide
a structurally stable support for the C-18 molecule. As the sample becomes
disrupted it is dispersed over the surface of the support by
hydrophobic/hydrophillic interactions. The mixture is semidry and is
readily packed into columns. The analyte can be eluted using selected
solvents. This technique coupled with SPE (see below) has provided a
successful method for measuring residues of Ivermectin at the 1-2 µg per kg
levels (Schenk, Barker and Long, 1989)

6.3.7 (vi) Chromatographic clean up;
Chromatography is perhaps the most important technique in the methods, not
only is it used to give highly purified fractions containing the analyte
prior to the end point determination but it is also a key step in
hyphenated end point determinations.

Simple clean up procedures;- Two types of chromatography are widely used;
solid phase column chromatography (SPE) and immunoaffinity chromatography
(IAC).

SPE is used to extract groups or classes of residues from the initial
extract. The columns are characterised by low affinity, high capacity and
low specificity. Either very small columns e.g. Sep-Pak C18 cartridges,
are used with small volumes of eluting fluids or larger columns are used
with much larger solvent volumes, e.g. XAD-2 columns for cleaning up
anabolic agents. The small columns are disposable and cost little.

IAC is a relatively new procedure and the system uses a small column packed
with one or more specific antibodies immobilised onto a solid matrix. The
antibodies are specific for one or more analytes. The columns are
characterised by high affinity, low capacity and high specificity. However
attention should be paid to the possibility of interference from unknown
metabolites which may cross-react with the antibodies. The use of IAC in
the determination of steroids and ß-agonists is increasing and examples are
given in methods M 1.1. and M 1.3.

Chromatography as part of end point determination;- HPLC and GC are
powerful techniques used for obtaining highly purified extracts containing
specific analytes. Methods using the resolving power of HPLC and GC in
combination with specific IA or MS can meet all the Criteria of EC Decision
93/256/EEC (see section 5) necessary for the unambiguous identification of
a residue.

HPLC and GC procedures must be carried out using equipment that is suitable
to achieve the minimum Criteria as detailed in section 5 (2.6 and 2.7).
Many of the machines now on the market allow the fulfilment of these
criteria and examples are to found in the specific methods. The ability
of the system to resolve the analyte(s) in question from similar molecules
and separate the analyte from a major proportion of the interfering
substances is very important.

6.3.8 (viii) End point Determination;- The techniques include;-
   - Spectrometry: IR, MS, UV, AA
   - Immunoassay: RIA, EIA
   - Chromatography: TLC
   - Hyphenated techniques: i.e. a combination of two or more
     procedures: TLC & IA; HPLC & IA; HPLC & MS; GC & MS; MS & MS;
     GC & MS & MS; GC & FTIR (see 6.3.1.).

A technical description of the equipment, materials and reagents is
included with each assay method. The quality of the equipment must be
good enough to allow the method to fulfil the Criteria for the
identification and quantification of an analyte as laid down in section 5.

6.3.9 (ix) Quality assurance is covered in section 5.

6.3.10 (x) Calculation of results;- Each method contains instructions on
the calculation of results. The calculation takes into account the
recovery of an internal standard and the quality control of the method
using RMs or other suitable standards.

6.3.11 (xi) Results should be reported in the agreed format. All data
should be properly recorded which together with all raw data must be filed
for future reference. See also section on Quality Assurance in section 5.

6.3.12. Note on GC-FTIR.
IR is an alternative spectroscopic method to MS for the identification of
known analytes. For unknown analytes MS and FTIR are complimentary
techniques, MS yielding information on the molecular masses of the analyte
and of the different fragment ions, FTIR on the functional groups and their
chemical surroundings. The development of very sensitive cryotrapping GC-
FTIR spectrometry with limits of detection in the sub ng range makes this
technique suitable for residue analysis.

The technique of cryotrapping GC-eluates at 77°K on an IR transparent
window has recently bee incorporated into a commercially available GC-FTIR
instrument. The eluates are crystallised onto a window of zinc selenide at
77°K immediately after leaving a small deposition tip at the end of the GC.
The window is slow moving in such a way that each component passes an IR
light beam a few seconds after deposition and can be scanned immediately.
An advantage of the technique is that as a result of movement of the window
the complete chromatogram is "frozen" onto the widow as a trace. It
remains stored for as long as cryogenic conditions are maintained. This
offers the opportunity to perform post-run scanning of the cryotrapped
components and to improve the signal-to-noise ratio of the spectra.

The data processing is carried out on a computer which must have the
capability of handling and storing large numbers of IR spectra.

The technique is successfully used at RIVM, Bilthoven, for the confirmation
of ß-agonists in urine at the 2.5 µg per kg or L level (Visser et al
1993).

6.4. TYPE OF METHODS

The methods are allocated into sections covering either screening or
confirmatory methods. They are sub-divided into modular multi-residue
methods, multi-residue methods, and methods for specific veterinary drug
residues. At this stage the well tried and tested multiresidue methods for
pesticide analysis and the EC documented methods for heavy metals are not
included. A full list of the methods is given in the contents.

REFERENCES

Bogaerts, R. and Wolf, F., (1980), A standardised method for the detection of residues of anti-bacterial substances in fresh meat. Fleischwirtschaft, 60, 672-673

Commission Decision, 93/256/EEC, laying down the methods for detecting residues of substances having a hormonal or thyrostatic action. OJ. № 118, pp 64-74, 14.4.93.

Jansen, E.H.J.M., Den Berg, van R.H., Blitterswijk, van H., Both-Miedema, R. and Stephany, R.W. (1985). A highly specific detection method for diethylstilbestrol in bovine urine by radioimmunoassay following high performance liquid chromatography. Food Addit. Contam. 2, 271-281

Ginkel, van L.A. and Stephany, R.W., (1989) Experimental chemometrics - an alternative approach for estimating the overall reliability of an analytical procedure. Presented at 103rd AOAC annual international meeting and exposition. St. Louis, Missouri, USA, 25-28 September.

Ginkel, van L.A. and Stephany, R.W., (1991), New trends in strategies for residue analysis of growth promoting agents. Microbiologie-Aliments-Nutrition, 9, 89-?

Malisch, R. (1986), Multimethode zur Bestimmung der Rückstände von Chemotherapeutica, Antiparasitica und Wachstumförderern in Lebensmittel tierischer Herkunft. Z. :Lebenm. Unters Forrsch., 182, 385-399

Schenk, F.J., Barker, S.A. and Long, A.R. (1989), Lab. Inform. Bull. (DHSS) 5, 3381-?

Stephany, R.W. and Ginkel, van L.A., (1990) Quality criteria for residue analysis and reference materials. Relationship between legal procedures and materials. Fresenius J. Anal. Chem. 338, 370-377

Verbeke, R. (1979), Sensitive multi-residue method for the detection of anabolics in urine and in tissues of slaughtered animals. J.Chrom. 177, 69-84

Visser, T., Vredenbregt, M.J., De Jong, A.P.J.M, Van Ginkel, L.A., Van Possum, H.J. and Stephany, R.W. (1993), Cryotrapping gas-chromatography-fourier transform infrared spectrometry: a new technique to confirm the presence of ß-agonists in animal material. Anal. Chim. Acta. 275, 205-214

Sg. 1.1 ANABOLICS - A ROUTINE METHOD FOR THE DETERMINATION OF RESIDUES OF ANABOLICS IN PERIRENAL FAT USING HPLC-HPTLC.

WARNING AND SAFETY PRECAUTIONS

0.   INTRODUCTION

Throughout the EEC the use of xenobiotic anabolic agents is prohibited in food-producing animals and no residues of these anabolics should be present in animal products imported into or produced within the Community. Preparations of natural steroids or their esters may be used in farm animals under strictly controlled conditions (see EEC Directive 88/146/EEC) and the maximum concentrations of natural steroids allowed in plasma are set (see section 2) but the levels permitted in edible tissues have not yet been defined (August 1993).

1.   SCOPE

This method of analysis describes the determination of the presence of individual analytes for a large number of Anabolic Agents in samples of perirenal fat. This work is carried out in compliance with the Residues Directive (86/469/EEC) and the method is used in several Member States.

2.   FIELD OF APPLICATION.

The method is used to perform routine screening and confirmatory analyses in bovine perirenal fat samples.
The method can be adapted for muscle and urine. This modular method is suitable for testosterone[*], trenbolone[*], oestradiol[*], oestrone, zeranol, diethylstilboestrol, hexoestrol, dienoestrol, 19-nortestosterone[*], methyltestosterone, ethinyloestradiol, medroxyprogesterone acetate, chlormadinone acetate, melengestrol acetate and megestrol acetate,

[*] either the 17α- or the 17ß- hydroxy compounds.

The limit of detection is about 1 µg per kg for most of the compounds.

3.   REFERENCES.

Commission Decision, 93/256/EEC, laying down the methods for detecting residues of substances having a hormonal or thyrostatic action. [OJ. Nº L.118, 14.4.93. pp 64-74]

ISO Standard 78/2-1982 Layout for standards - Part 2: Standard for Chemical Analysis

Verbeke, R (1979). Sensitive multi-residue method for detection of anabolics in urine and in tissues of slaughtered animals. J.Chromatog. <u>177</u>, 69-84

Smets, F., (1988), Méthode Analytique pour le determination des résidus d'anabolisants dans l'urine à l'aide de la HPLC-HPTLC. Union economique Benelux, SP/LAB/h (88), 33

Smets, F. and Vandewalle, M., (1984), HPLC column switching technique for the clean-up of steroid samples. Z.Lebensm. Unters. Forsch. <u>178</u>, 38-40

De Brabander, H.F., Smets, F. and Pottie, G. (1988), Faster and cheaper
two-dimensional HPTLC. J.Planar Chromat. <u>1</u>, 369-371

4.   DEFINITIONS.

Anabolic substance content is taken to mean the amount of anabolic
substance in perirenal fat determined according to the described method and
expressed as µg anabolic substance per kg of test sample.

5.   PRINCIPLE

The methods comprises 5 stages;-

- Homogenisation of fat samples in acetate buffer.
- Extraction using methanol.(Remove fat with n-hexane)
- Extraction using ether and washing with carbonate buffer
- Purification of concentrated extract by HPLC fractionation.
- Detection and identification by fluorescence and visible light on TLC

6.   MATERIALS

Note: The reagents for which examples of their source are quoted are
known to be satisfactory, nevertheless reagents of comparable purity from
other sources may be equally suitable.

6.1.   Reference Compounds and Standard Solutions.

Testosterone[*], trenbolone[*], oestradiol[*], oestrone, zeranol,
diethylstilboestrol, hexoestrol, dienoestrol, 19-nortestosterone[*],
methyltestosterone, ethinyloestradiol, medroxyprogesterone acetate,
chlormadinone acetate, melengestrol acetate and megestrol acetate,

[*] either the 17α- or the 17ß- hydroxy compounds.

17α-Trenbolone and epi-19-nortestosterone were obtained from the ANAREF
collection (Benelux), all the other compounds were from Steraloids Inc.

6.2   Chemicals
6.2.1   Methanol
6.2.2   Water (HPLC grade)
6.2.3   n-hexane
6.2.4   diethylether
6.2.5   dichloromethane
6.2.6   chloroform
6.2.7   acetone
6.2.8   cyclohexane
6.2.9   ethyl acetate
6.2.10   ethanol
6.2.11   tetrahydrofuran
6.2.12   sulphuric acid

6.3   Solvents and Solutions
6.3.1   HPLC conditioning solvent; Methanol:Water, (75:25 (v/v))
6.3.2   HPLC eluent - mixtures of methanol and water (see procedure 9.16.1)

6.3.3   HPTLC eluents
6.3.3.1   Eluent 1; n-hexane - diethylether - dichloromethane (25/45/30)
6.3.3.2   Eluent 2; chloroform - acetone (90/10)
6.3.3.3   Eluent 3; cyclohexane - ethyl acetate - ethanol (60/40/2.5)
6.3.3.4   Eluent 4; chloroform - n-hexane - acetone (50/40/10)
6.3.3.5   Eluent 5; tetrahydrofuran - n-hexane (35/65)
6.3.4   HPTLC detecting reagent; 5% solution of sulphuric acid in
           ethanol.
6.3.5   0.04M Sodium acetate buffer, pH 5.2
6.3.6   10% Sodium Carbonate buffer, pH ≤10.25

7   EQUIPMENT

7.1   Ultra Turrax homogeniser
7.2   Rotary evaporator
7.3   Vortex mixer(s)
7.4   HPTLC equipment for running HPTLC plates.
7.4.1   HPTLC silica gel plates, (Merck № 5631)
7.5   UV lamp at 366 nm
7.6   Drying cabinet
7.7   Cabinet at 95°C for heating HPTLC plates
7.8   Centrifuge tubes, 300 mL capacity
7.9   Water bath at 80°C
7.10   Centrifuge
7.11   Erlenmeyer flasks, 300 mL capacity
7.12   Cotton wool
7.13   Vortex evaporator (Büchler)
7.14   HPLC
7.14.1   Basic instrument with pump, (Perkin Elmer, Series 4)
7.14.2   Automatic injector (Perkin Elmer, ISS-100)
7.14.3   Automatic switching valve (VICI) (Valco)
7.14.4   UV detector (model 440 - Waters)
7.14.5   Fraction Collector (model 202 - Gilson)
7.14.6   Column - C-18 semi-preparative: ODS (5 μm) 25 cm x 10 mm i.d.
           (Altex part № 235328)
7.14.7   Guard column: pellicular ODS (C18); 37 - 53 μm; 3 cm x 4.6 mm
           i.d. (Whatman № 4102-010)
7.14.8   Precolumn: Cartridge MCH-10 C18 10μ; 3 cm x 4.6 mm i.d. (Varian
           № 00-996750-00)

8.   SAMPLES AND SAMPLING PROCEDURE.

N.B. Attention is drawn to section 6.3.1 and to ISO document 78/2-1982 and
also the following notes derived from Annex II of 2052/VI/84-EN.

8.1.   Nature of the Sample; Samples shall be such as to enable the
           detection of residues in fat as defined in Directive 64/433/EEC.
8.2.   Size of Sample; The size of the sample must be large enough to
           allow the method to be carried out and to allow repeat analysis
           where required. Each analysis needs a 50 g sample.
8.3.   The samples must be taken and packed in such a way as to allow
           proper identification in the laboratory.
8.4.   The method of packing, preservation and transport must maintain
           the integrity of the sample and not prejudice the result of the
           examination.
           Samples for the analysis of anabolics must be stored at
           temperatures below -18°C.

9	PROCEDURE

9   PROCEDURE

9.1   Cut 50 g perirenal fat into small pieces and weigh into a 300 mL centrifuge tube (7.8).

9.2   Add 70 mL sodium acetate buffer (6.3.5) and warm up the mixture in a water bath at 80°C for 10 min.

9.3   Homogenise with an Ultra Turrax

9.4   Extract with 180 mL methanol utilising the Ultra turrax for mixing.

9.5   Centrifuge at 5000 g for 20 min.

9.6   Filter the supernatant through a cotton wool plug into a 300 mL Erlenmeyer flask (7.11).

9.7   Transfer two fifths of the supernatant (equivalent to 20 g fat) into a 250 mL separating funnel.

9.8   Extract with 2 x 20 mL n-hexane and discard the n-hexane phase.

9.9   Add 40 mL water and extract with 2 x 100 mL of diethylether.

9.10   Wash the combined ether phases with 10 mL of carbonate buffer (9.3.6) and 2 x 15 mL water. Discard the aqueous phases.

9.11   Evaporate the ether phase to dryness on a rotary evaporator at 40°C.

9.12   Transfer the contents into a vial with 3 x 1 mL methanol

9.13   Evaporate the mixture to dryness using a Vortex evaporator.

9.14   Dissolve the residue with vortex mixing into 100 µL methanol.

9.15   Inject 100 µL into the HPLC.

9.16   HPLC

9.16.1 Elution Programme

Step	Time (min)	Flow mL/min	Water %	MeOH %	Curve
a. Injection	0	3	25	75	
b. Front cut	1.2	3	25	75	
c. Backflush guard and precolumn	1.3 5	3 3	0 25	100 75	0 0
d. Elution Fn. 1-3 Fn. 4&5	10 5 5	3 3 3	25 0 0	75 100 100	1
e. Reconditioning	15	3	25	25	0

9.16.2 Collection of fractions.

Five fractions are collected over the time period 14 to 22 min. Fractions 1 to 3 are collected during the elution with 25% water and 75% methanol. Fractions 4 and 5 are collected during the gradient period, 17.5 to 22.5 min. The exact time windows should be determined using pure standards.

The five fractions are collected with windows which will allow the collection of the following anabolics.

Fraction 1: DES/HEX/DEN; zeranol; α/ß-trenbolone

Fraction 2: ß-19-nortestosterone; α/ß-oestradiol; oestrone

Fraction 3: α-19-nortestosterone; ß-testosterone

Fraction 4: α-testosterone; methyltestosterone

Fraction 5: medroxyprogesterone acetate; chlormadinone acetate; melengestrol acetate; megestrol acetate.

9.17   HPTLC

9.17.1   Evaporate to dryness the fractions 1 to 5 obtained from the HPLC.
          Dissolve the fractions in either 20 μL acetone or ethanol. Use
          1/4 of the volume (equivalent to 5 g fat) to apply to the HPTLC
          plate (7.4.1). Apply 10 ng of the appropriate standards at a
          separate spot.
9.17.2   Run the plates using eluents 1 (6.3.3.1) and then 2 (6.3.3.2) for
          fractions 1 to 4 from the HPLC.
9.17.3   Run the plates using eluents 3 (6.3.3.3) and then 4 (6.3.3.4) or
          using eluents 4 (6.3.3.4) and then 5 (6.3.3.5) for fraction 5
          containing the gestagens from the HPLC.
9.17.4   Detection of spots; Induction of fluorescence is obtained by
          plunging the plates in a solution of 5% sulphuric acid in ethanol
          (6.3.4) and drying the plates at 95°C for 10 min.
9.17.5   The spots can be detected under UV light at 366 nm and in visible
          light. The spots for the gestagens for instance, have
          characteristic colours in visible light being;-
          Blue - megestrol acetate and chlormadinone acetate
          Pale brown - melengestrol acetate
          Greenish - medroxyprogesterone acetate.

10   INTERPRETATION OF RESULTS
10.1   Identification of the analytes on the TLC is obtained when the
          spots have the same R_f and colours as the standards. The
          analytes must elute in the correct fraction from the HPLC.

11.   SPECIAL CASES

12.   NOTES ON PROCEDURE.

13.   QUALITY CONTROLS

See section 8 of manual detailing the RMs for the anabolics.

14.   TEST REPORT

15.   LIST OF ABBREVIATIONS

A full list of abbreviations is given in Annex I, Section 12

16.   FLOW DIAGRAM

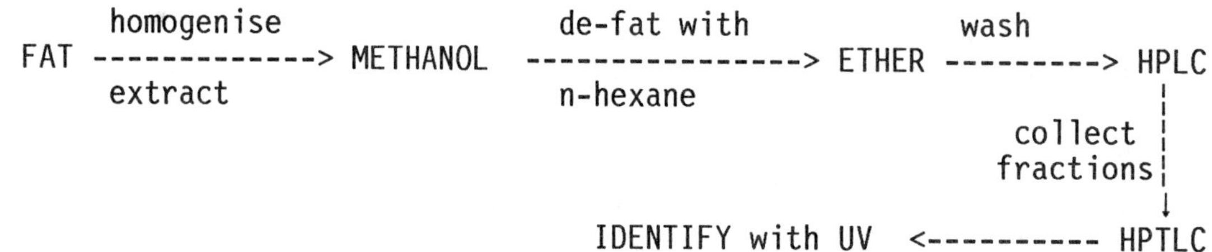

Sg. 1.2 ANABOLICS - A ROUTINE METHOD FOR THE DETECTION OF RESIDUES OF ANABOLICS IN BOVINE URINE USING GC-MS IN THE ELECTRON IMPACT MODE.
[Note; Method can be extended to a confirming method].

WARNING AND SAFETY PRECAUTIONS
Wear gloves for handling acids, bases and organic solvents. Handle solvents in a fume cupboard.

0.   INTRODUCTION

Throughout the EEC the use of xenobiotic anabolic agents is prohibited in food-producing animals and no residues of these anabolics should be present in animal products imported into or produced within the Community. Preparations of natural steroids or their esters may be used in farm animals under strictly controlled conditions (see EEC Directive 86/469/EEC) and the maximum concentrations of natural steroids permitted in edible tissues have not yet been defined (August 1993).

1.   SCOPE

This method of analysis describes the detection of the presence of individual analytes for a large number of Anabolic Agents in samples of bovine urine. This work is carried out in compliance with the Residues Directive (86/469/EEC) and the method is used in France.

2.   FIELD OF APPLICATION.

The method is used to perform routine screening in urine samples. This modular method is suitable for testosterone*, trenbolone*, oestradiol*, oestrone, zeranol, *cis-* and *trans-* diethylstilboestrol, hexoestrol, dienoestrol, 19-nortestosterone*, methyltestosterone, ethinyltestosterone, boldenone, stanolone, norethandrone, dianabol, bolasterone, α-chlorotestosterone, chloromethandienone, vinyloestradiol, ethinyloestradiol, medroxyprogesterone, chlormadinone and megestrol,

*   either the 17α- or the 17ß- hydroxy compounds.

The limit of detection is about 1 µg per L for most of the compounds.

3.   REFERENCES.

Commission Decision, 93/256/EEC, laying down the methods for detecting residues of substances having a hormonal or thyrostatic action. [OJ. № L.118, 14.4.93. pp 64-74]

ISO Standard 78/2-1982 Layout for standards - Part 2: Standard for Chemical Analysis

LeBizec, B., Montrade, M.-P., Monteau, F. and André, F. (1993), Detection and identification of anabolic steroids in bovine urine by gas chromatography-mass spectrometry. Anal. Chim. Acta., 275, 123-133

LeBizec, B., Montrade, M.P. and André, F. (1993), Method of detection and identification of anabolic steroid agents in urine by gas chromatography-mass spectrometry in the electron impact mode. Document. LDH/93/02. Lab. Dosages Hormonaux, Nantes, France.

4.   DEFINITIONS.

Anabolic substance content is taken to mean the amount of anabolic
substance in bovine urine determined according to the described method and
expressed as μg anabolic substance per L of test sample.

5.   PRINCIPLE

The methods comprises 6 stages;-

  - Hydrolysis of urine samples in acetate buffer.
  - Extraction on a C-18 cartridge
  - Wash with carbonate buffer
  - Fractionation of anabolic groups on a Si-gel 60 column.
  - Derivatization
  - Detection on GC-MS in EI mode.

6.   MATERIALS

Note: The reagents for which examples of their source are quoted are
known to be satisfactory, nevertheless reagents from other sources may be
equally suitable.

6.1.   Reference Compounds and Standard Solutions.

6.1.1.   The steroids;- testosterone*, trenbolone*, oestradiol*, oestrone,
zeranol, *cis-* and *trans-* diethylstilboestrol, hexoestrol, dienoestrol, 19-
nortestosterone*, methyltestosterone, boldenone, stanolone, norethandrone,
dianabol, bolasterone, chlorotestosterone, ethinyltestosterone,
chloromethandienone, ethinyloestradiol, vinyloestradiol, norethandrolone,
medroxyprogesterone, chlormadinone and megestrol,
were obtained from Steraloids (Wilton, USA), Sigma (St. Louis, USA) and
Research Plus (Bayonne, USA),
     * either the 17α- or the 17ß- hydroxy compounds.

6.1.2   Internal standards
          Deuterated (d$_3$) methyl-testosterone (Sigma)
          Deuterated (d$_2$) 17ß-oestradiol (Sigma)

6.1.3   External standard
          Dichlorophene (Aldrich)
          Norgestrel (Sigma)

6.2   Chemicals
6.2.1   Methanol (Merck-6009)
6.2.2   Ultra-pure water (>18 MΩ.cm)
6.2.3   n-hexane (Merck-4367)
6.2.4   *Helix pomatia* juice (ß-glucuronidase-arylsulfatase, Merck-4114)
6.2.5   Sodium carbonate (Merck-6392)
6.2.6   Sodium hydroxide (Merck-9137)
6.2.7   Sodium acetate (Merck-6268)
6.2.8   Glacial acetic acid (Merck-55)
6.2.9   Ethyl acetate (Merck-9623)
6.2.10   Absolute ethanol (Merck-693)
6.2.11   Silica gel 60 (Merck-7734)
6.2.12   Nitrogen (dry over Silica gel)

6.2.13   1,1,1-Trichloroethane (Merck-8749)
6.2.14   N-methyl-N-trimethylsilyl-trifluoroacetamide : MSTFA (Fluka-
          69482)
6.2.15   Trimethyliodosilane : TMIS (Fluka-58118)
6.2.16   Dithiothreitol : DTE (Aldrich-15046-0)
6.2.17   N-methyl-N-(tertbutylmethylsilyl)trifluoracetamide : MTBSTFA
          (Pierce-48920)
6.2.18   T.H.P Helium (Carboxyque)

6.3   Solutions
6.3.1   2*M* Acetate buffer, pH 5.2 ± 0.2, for hydrolysis of conjugates.
          Dissolve 164 g sodium acetate (6.2.7) in 900 mL water (6.2.3) and
          adjust the pH to 5.2 ± 0.2 with glacial acetic acid (6.2.8). Make
          up to 1 L with water and store at +4°C. Use for up to 1 month.
6.3.2   10% Sodium carbonate solution; Dissolve 100 g sodium carbonate in
          1 L water.
6.3.3   Eluents
6.3.3.1   Eluent 1; methanol/ethyl acetate 30/70
6.3.3.2   Eluent 2; 1,1,1-trichloroethane/ethyl acetate 80/20
6.3.3.3   Eluent 3; 1,1,1-trichloroethane/ethyl acetate 20/80
6.3.4   Derivatization solution. Prepare under anhydrous conditions IN A
          FUME CUPBOARD a solution of MSTFA (6.2.14) / TMIS (6.2.15) / DTE
          (6.2.16), 100/5/5 (v/v/w). Keep in the freezer excluding light
          and moisture.

7   EQUIPMENT

7.1   Hamilton syringes, 5 μL, 50 μL, 1000 μL
7.2   Automatic pipettes, 20 μL, 200 μL, 1000 μL, 5000 μL
7.3   Vortex mixer(s)
7.4   Ultrasonic bath
7.5   Heating block with nitrogen evaporation system,
7.6   Heating block for derivatization (Pierce-18780)
7.7   Heating block for 6 mL and 12 mL haemolysis tubes with nitrogen
          evaporation system.
7.8   Plastic bottles with screw tops, 30 mL capacity.
7.9   Centrifuge
7.11   Oven for hydrolysis
7.12   Derivatization vials suited for either manual or automatic
          injection into the GC.
7.13   Vacuum suction system for SPE columns (Vac Elut, Prolabo -
          07485001)
7.14   Glass haemolysis tubes, 6 mL and 12 mL, with stoppers use only
          once.
7.15   pH paper
7.16   Pasteur pipettes.
7.17   Parafilm
7.18   Mega Bondelut C-18 columns (Varian-AI 122560-15).
          Contain 2 g grafted resin in a 10 mL container.
          Conditioning; Wash with 10 mL methanol and then 10 mL of
          ultrapure water. Do not allow the column to dry.
7.19   G60 silica column; Use a glass column (15 cm x 10 mm i.d.)
          equipped with a 10 mL reservoir and a manual flow regulator
          (L.N.R.).
          Preparation; Put the gel into a beaker containing Eluent 2;
          1,1,1-trichloroethane/ethyl acetate 80/20 (6.3.3.2) and stir.
          Pour the resin into the column up to 8 cm. Rinse with 6.3.3.2

and tamp the gel. Rinse with a further 10 mL 6.3.3.2. Do not run
to dryness. The column is now ready.

7.20   GC-MS;
7.20.1   GC. (Hewlett Packard HP-5890)
          Injection;   Splitless, open valve at 1 min.
          Volume injected; 2 μL
          Column;   Fused silica capillary type, 30 m x 0.25 mm i.d. with
                     25 μm film of SE-30
          Temperatures; Injector, 280°C, Transfer line, 280°C;

                         15°C / min   *5°C / min*
Oven 120°C for 1 min. -------------> 250°C ---------------> 300°C for 4 min
                                                            then to 120°C

          Carrier gas; T.H.P Helium
          Flow rate; 1 mL per min.
          Pressure at head of column; 5 psi.
7.20.2   MS. (Hewlett Packard HP-5971A)
          EI mode at 70 eV.
          Dwell time (msec) is selected so that the number of cycles per
          sec is close to 2.
          Source temp.; 190°C
          The electromultiplier, ion focus and entrance lens values will be
          calculated by the autotune.

8.   SAMPLES AND SAMPLING PROCEDURE.

N.B. Attention is drawn to section 6.3.1 and to ISO document 78/2-1982 and
also the following notes derived from Annex II of 2052/VI/84-EN.

8.1. Nature of the Sample; Samples shall be such as to enable the
detection of residues in meat as defined in Directive 64/433/EEC. Failing
this biological fluids (here urine) or faeces may constitute the samples
for the detection of residues.

8.2. Size of Sample; The size of the sample must be large enough to allow
the method to be carried out and to allow repeat analysis where required.

8.3. The samples must be taken and packed in such a way as to allow proper
identification in the laboratory.

8.4. The method of packing, preservation and transport must maintain the
integrity of the sample and not prejudice the result of the examination.
Samples for the analysis of anabolics must be stored and transported at
temperatures below -18°C.

9   PROCEDURE
9.1   Thaw the urine sample.
9.2.   Centrifuge >20 mL at 3000 rpm and transfer 20 mL of the
          supernatant to a plastic container (7.8).
9.3   Add 2 mL acetate buffer (6.3.1) and adjust the pH to 5.2 ± 0.2
          with glacial acetic acid (6.2.8). Add 200 ng of d_3-
          methyltestosterone.
9.4   Repeat 9.1 to 9.3 for two blank urines. To one of the blanks add
          anabolic standards.
9.5   Add 100 μL *Helix Pomatia* (6.2.4) to all the urines. Incubate for

	15 h at 52°C in an oven.
9.6	SPE Clean up;
9.6.1	Transfer the hydrolysed urines to a conditioned Mega Bond Elut column (7.18). Allow the column to dry for 30 sec. Wash with 10 mL ultrapure water under vacuum suction until drained. Wash with 10 mL n-hexane.
9.6.2	Elute all the steroids with 5 mL eluent 1 (6.3.3.1) into a 12 mL tube (7.14).
9.7	Add 2 mL carbonate solution (6.3.2) to the eluate and vortex for 10 sec. Centrifuge at 10,000 rpm for 1 min. Transfer the upper organic phase to a clean tube.
9.8	Add 2 mL carbonate solution (6.3.2) to the organic phase and vortex for 10 sec. Centrifuge at 10,000 rpm for 1 min. Transfer the upper organic phase to a clean tube.
9.9	Evaporate the organic phase to near dryness using nitrogen on a 50°C heating block. Avoid thermolysis of the residue.
9.10	Purification on Silica gel 60 column.
9.10.1	Add 1 mL eluting solution 2 (6.3.3.2) to the residue. Vortex and place in an ultrasonic bath for a few seconds.
9.10.2	Transfer the solution to the bed of a prepared Si gel 60 column (7.19) with a Pasteur pipette. Allow to drain into the column. Repeat once 9.10.1 with 0.5 mL of eluent 2 (6.3.3.2).
9.10.3	Wash with 4 mL eluent 2 (6.3.3.2).
9.10.4	Elute oestrogenic substances with 13 mL eluent 2 (6.3.3.2). Collect as fraction I. Add 100 ng dichlorophene as external standard.
9.10.5	Elute the androgens and gestagens with 12 mL eluent 3 (6.3.3.3) and collect as fraction II. Add 100 ng norgestrel as external standard.
9.11	Reduce the volumes of both fractions I and II to ca. 500 µL under a nitrogen stream at 50°C.
9.12	Vortex the tubes to wet the walls and then centrifuge at 1000 rpm for 1 min to bring the liquid to the bottom of the tubes.
9.13	Transfer the contents of the tubes to reactivials (7.12) and evaporate just to dryness using nitrogen on a 50°C heating block. Avoid thermolysis of the residue.
9.14	Derivatization;

[Must be done under anhydrous conditions]

9.14.1	Add 20 µL of derivatising solution 6.3.4 and close vial immediately. Vortex and ultrasonicate. Heat at 60°C for 30 min.
9.14.2	The derivatives are ready for injection but may be stored in sealed vials for up to 48 h at 4°C.

[Note; It is possible to derivatize the stilbenes in Fraction I with N-methyl-N-(tertbutylmethylsilyl)trifluoracetamide : MTBSTFA (6.2.17) to increase the retention times and the mass of the ions, therefore their specificity.]

9.15	Inject 2 µL into the GC-MS equipment using the conditions described in 7.20.

10	INTERPRETATION OF RESULTS
10.1	The approximate retention times of the anabolics are shown in table 1. They will vary and should be studied systematically in relationship to the retention time of the internal standard.
10.2	The ions selected for monitoring should be determined beforehand. As a rule they will be; high mass, high intensity; free of interference with ions from the column and background.
10.3	If 2 or 3 ions have a signal to noise ratio > 3 then the sample

10.4   is suspected "positive".
The criteria in EEC 93/256 (see section 5) must be met for the GC parameters.

10.5 The blank urine must be clear of all evidence of ions attributable to xenobiotic anabolics.

10.6 The ions for the external and internal standards must be present.

11.   SPECIAL CASES

12.   NOTES ON PROCEDURE.

13.   QUALITY CONTROLS

See section 8 of manual detailing the RMs for the anabolics.

14.   TEST REPORT

15.   LIST OF ABBREVIATIONS

A full list of abbreviations is given in Annex I, Section 12

16.   FLOW DIAGRAM

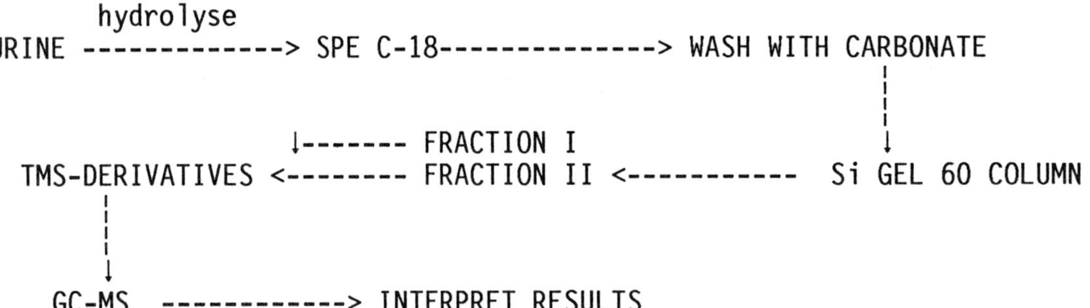

Table 1. List of steroids and their respective ions and retention times.

Substances in Fraction I

Analyte	Retention time (min)	Diagnostic ions m/z	Other ions m/z
cis-DES	11.63	412, 383	397, 368
Dichlorophene (E.S.)	12.07	414, 412, 377	
Hexoestrol	12.33	399, 207,	414
Dienoestrol	12.38	410, 395	381, 217, 193
trans-DES	12.46	412, 383	397, 368
Ethinyloestradiol	16.67	440, 425	300, 285
Vinyl oestradiol	17.00	442, 352	427, 300, 285

Steroids in Fraction II

Analyte	Retention time (min)	Diagnostic ions m/z	Other ions m/z
17α-Nortestosterone	14.75	418, 194	403, 287, 182
17β-Nortestosterone	15.20	418, 194	403, 287, 182
17α-Trenbolone	15.37	414, 283	399, 324
Stanolone	15.39	434, 405	419, 202
Boldenone	15.49	430, 206	415, 325, 299
17β-oestradiol-d_2 (I.S.)	15.50	418, 287	
17β-oestradiol	15.52	416, 285	401, 326
17β-Testosterone	15.63	432, 209	417,301
17β-Trenbolone	15.82	414, 283	399, 324
Norethandrone	16.21	432, 287	417, 342
Dianabol	16.50	444, 206	339, 299, 283
Methyltestosterone-d_3 (I.S)	16.63	449, 301	
Methyltestosterone	16.66	446, 301	431, 356
Bolasterone	16.72	460, 445	355, 315
Ethinyltestosterone	16.82	456, 301	441, 316
Zeranol	16.97	538, 433	523, 379, 307
Norgestrel (E.S.)	17.43	456, 316	
α-chlorotestosterone	17.50	466, 431	468, 451
Norethandrolone	17.57	446, 287	431, 356
β-chlorotestosterone	18.25	466, 431	468, 451
Fluoxymesterone	18.43	552, 462	407, 319
Bromoestradiol	18.90	496, 365	494, 481, 406
Chloromethandienone*	19.20	480, 335	482, 465, 390, 375
Medroxyprogesterone*	19.41	560, 330	545, 455, 315
Megestrol*	19.14	558, 453	543, 353, 231
Chlormadinone*	20.76	578, 488	563, 473, 231

* measured as di-TMS.
The "other ions" may be used as supplementary ions for confirmation purposes.
Data from Lab. des Dosages Hormonaux, Nantes, France.

Sg 1.3. DIETHYLSTILBOESTROL - METHOD FOR THE DETECTION OF RESIDUES OF DIETHYLSTILBOESTROL IN BOVINE URINE USING RADIOIMMUNOASSAY (RIA).

WARNING AND SAFETY PRECAUTIONS.

1.   INTRODUCTION.

Throughout the EEC the use of stilbenes is prohibited in food producing animals.

2.   SCOPE AND FIELD OF APPLICATION

This method of analysis describes the detection of diethylstilboestrol (DES) in bovine urine. The detection limit, defined as three times the standard deviation of the blank determination, is 0.23 µg per litre of urine for the stilbene. The limit of determination defined as six times the standard deviation of the blank determination for 20 samples, is 0.38 µg per litre.

3.   REFERENCES.

ISO Standard 78/2-1982 Layout for standards - Part 2: Standard for Chemical Analysis

Commission Decision, 93/256/EEC, laying down the methods for detecting residues of substances having a hormonal or thyrostatic action. [OJ. № L.118, 14.4.93. pp 64-74]

Standard Operating Procedure for the estimation of diethylstilboestrol in urine from the Central Meat Control Laboratory, Dublin, Ireland.

Other references.
Bates, M.L., Warwick, M.J. and Shearer, G. (1985), Determination of synthetic growth promoters in bile. Food Additives & Contaminants. _2_, 37-46

Gaspar, P. and Maghuin-Rogister, G., (1985), Rapid extraction and purification of diethylstilboestrol in bovine urine hydrolysates using reversed phase C 18 columns before determination by radioimmunoassay. J. Chromat. _328_, 413-416

Harwood, D.J., Heitzman, R.J. and Jouquey, A., (1980), A radioimmunoassay method for the measurement of residues of the anabolic agent hexoestrol in tissues of cattle and sheep. J.Vet. Pharmacol. & Therapeutics, _3_, 245-254

Heitzman, R.J. and Harwood, D.J. (1983), Radioimmunoassay of hexoestrol residues in faeces, tissues and body fluids of bulls and steers. Vet. Rec. _112_, 120-123

Jansen, E.H.J.M., (1985), A highly specific detection method for diethylstilboestrol in bovine urine by radioimmunoassay following high performance liquid chromatography. Food Additives & Contaminants. _2_, 271-281

Vogt, von K., (1985), Vereinfachte Absicherung des radioimmunologischen Nachweises von Diethylstilbestrol in Fleischhaltigen Konserven und tierischen Ausscheidungen. Arch. fur Lebensm.hygiene. _36_, 1-24

4.   DEFINITIONS.

DES content is taken to mean the amount of DES in the substance in
question, regardless of the chemical form, determined according to the
described method and expressed as µg DES per litre of test sample.

5.   PRINCIPLE

The method comprises 5 stages;-

- Diluting urine in buffer
- Hydrolysis of conjugates in buffer/homogenate with enzyme
- Extraction of DES with diethylether
- End point determination with RIA
- The amount of DES is calculated by interpolation from a standard
  curve and taking into account the recovery.

6.   REAGENTS FOR EXTRACTION OF TISSUES.

Note: The reagents for which examples of their source are quoted are
known to be satisfactory, nevertheless reagents from other sources may be
equally suitable.

6.1.   Chemicals
6.1.1.   Acetone
6.1.2.   Dry ice
6.1.3.   Diethyl-ether (peroxide free and very high purity)
6.1.4   Sodium dihydrogen phosphate, anhydrous
6.1.5   Disodium hydrogen phosphate, anhydrous
6.1.6   Sodium chloride
6.1.7   Thiomersal
6.1.8   Gelatin
6.1.9   Methanol
6.1.10   Purified water - by reverse osmosis followed by deionisation,
          absorption and filtration.
6.1.11   Tritiated DES (Amersham, UK. Monoethyl-^{3}H-DES. S.A. 91 Ci/mmol.
          1 mCi per mL). Store at -20°C.
6.1.12   Charcoal (Sigma C-5260)
6.1.13   Dextran (Pharmacia T70)
6.1.14   Scintillation fluid (Optiphase Hisafe 11 - LKB)
6.1.15   Antiserum against stilbenes stored at -20°C. (Marloie, Belgium)
          Cross-reactivities. *Trans*-DES, 100%; *trans*-DES dipropionate,
          9.7%; Hexoestrol, 3.3%; Dienoestrol, 1%; Other stilbenes <0.4%;
          Other anabolics and steroids <0.1%.
6.1.16   Nitrogen

6.2   Standards
6.2.1   DES (Sigma D-4628)

6.3   Solutions
6.3.1   Stock Solution; (100 ng per mL) Dissolve 100 mg DES in methanol
          and make up to 100 mL. Dilute with methanol to give a
          concentration of 100 ng per mL. Store at -20°C.
6.3.2   Working solutions; Prepare working standards from the stock
          solution to give concentrations of DES in methanol of 5, 10, 20,
          50, 100, 200 and 500 pg per mL. Store at +4°C.

6.3.3   Phosphate-gelatin buffer - 4.68 g sodium dihydrogen phosphate
          anhyd. (e.g. Analar BDH). 8.66 g disodium hydrogen phosphate
          anhyd. (e.g. Analar BDH). 9.0 g sodium chloride (e.g. Analar
          BDH). 0.1 g thiomersal (e.g. BDH). 1.0 g gelatin (e.g. BDH).
          Made up to 1 litre (pH 7.0) with purified water, stored at +4°C.
6.3.4   B-glucuronidase (e.g. Sigma G-0876) diluted with ten volumes
          double distilled water.
6.3.5   Charcoal suspension - 5 g charcoal (6.1.12). 0.5 g dextran
          (6.1.13). Made up in 1 litre with phosphate buffer (6.3.3)
6.3.6   Tritiated stilbenes; Dilute 50 µL stock solution 6.1.11 with 10
          mL methanol to give a radioactive concentration of ca. 2µCi per
          mL. Store at -20°C.
6.3.7   Tritiated stilbene assay solution, prepared from stock solution
          6.3.6. by evaporation and redissolving in buffer (6.5.4.) to give
          10,000 cpm/0.1 mL. Prepared on day of use.
[Note; The non-specific binding (NSB) of the 3H-stilbene must be determined
and if it exceeds 10% of the total count (SA) of 3H-stilbene should be
repurified or replaced.]
6.3.8   Prepare solution of antibody in buffer (6.3.3). It will be
          necessary to follow the instructions pertaining to the individual
          antibody preparations. The concentration of antibody in buffer
          should be 8x greater than the concentration needed in the final
          RIA incubation mixture.

7.   EQUIPMENT.

Reference to a company and/or product is for purposes of information and
identification only. Equivalent types or products also may be suitable.

7.1   Liquid scintillation Counter, with automatic sample changer.
7.2   Scintillation vials.
7.3   Cold storage space.
7.4   Cold room/refrigerator space.
7.5   Deep freeze -20°C.
7.6   Fume cupboards.
7.7   Centrifuges.
7.8   Refrigerated centrifuge with large capacity for small tubes.
7.9   Bench centrifuge.
7.10   Heating units.
7.11   37°C water bath/incubator.
7.12   40/45°C water bath.
7.13   Magnetic stirrer.
7.14   Glassware.
7.15   Glass tubes 75 mm x 12 mm.
7.16   Glass stoppered tubes 125 mm x 16 mm.
7.17   Glass universal bottles, approx 25 mL with plastic screw tops.
7.18   Vortex mixer.
7.19   Pipettes and dispensers.
7.20   Semi-automatic pipettes with disposable tips.
7.21   Pasteur pipettes.
7.22   Tilt measures (5 mL for diethyl ether).
7.23   Dispenser for scintillator.
7.24   Apparatus suitable for evaporation of solvents. e.g. Compressed
          nitrogen supply and evaporation manifold or rotary film
          evaporator.
[Note; Solvent should be evaporated at temperatures not exceeding 50°C
using e.g. either a stream of nitrogen or a rotary film evaporator.]

8.   SAMPLES AND SAMPLING PROCEDURE.

N.B. Attention is drawn to section 6.3.1 and ISO document 78/2-1982 and
the following notes derived from Annex II of 2052/VI/84-EN.

8.1. Nature of the Sample; Samples shall be such as to enable the
detection of residues in meat as defined in Directive 64/433/EEC.

8.2. Size of Sample; The size of the sample must be large enough to allow
the reference method to be carried out and to allow repeat analysis where
required.

8.3. The samples must be taken and packed in such a way as to allow proper
identification in the laboratory.

8.4. The method of packing, preservation and transport must maintain the
integrity of the sample and not prejudice the result of the examination.

Samples for the analysis of stilbenes must be stored and transported at
temperatures below -18°C.

9.   PROCEDURE.
9.1.1   Into four test tubes (7.16) or universal bottles (7.17) add 0.5
          mL blank urine.
9.1.2   Into four test tubes (7.16) or universal bottles (7.17) add 0.5
          mL blank urine and 100 pg DES for recovery.
9.1.3.   Into four test tubes (7.16) or universal bottles (7.17) add 0.5
          mL blank urine and 90 pg DES for QC check.
9.1.4   Add 0.2 mL urine sample in duplicate to test tubes or universals.
          Normal equipment would allow 30 samples to be used.
9.2   Add to universals/tubes 9.1.1 - 9.1.4. 50 µL enzyme (6.3.4) and
          incubate for 2 h at 37°C.
9.3   Allow to cool and add 5 mL diethyl-ether (6.1.3.), vortex mix for
          15 seconds.
9.4   Centrifuge at 2000 rpm for 5 min.
9.5   Freeze samples in dry ice/acetone bath and decant ether phase
          into glass tubes (7.15).
9.6   Evaporate to dryness under nitrogen. (7.24).

9.7   Radioimmunoassay.
The method chosen for separation of antibody-bound and free ligand uses
charcoal.
9.7.1.   Into 7 RIA tubes (7.15) pipette 0.1 mL methanol (3 tubes for Non-
          specific binding {NSB} and 4 tubes as zero standard tubes). Into
          RIA tubes, pipette in triplicate 0.1 mL of stilbene standard
          solutions (6.3.2) to give range 5 - 500 pg per tube. Evaporate
          methanol to dryness e.g.under nitrogen (7.24).
9.7.2.1   Add 60 µL methanol to all tubes (9.7.1 and 9.6). Add 640 µL
          gelatin-phosphate buffer (6.3.4) to the 3 tubes for NSBs. and 540
          µL buffer to all the other tubes.
9.7.2.2   Add 0.1 mL tritiated stilbene solution (6.3.7) to all tubes and
          to two scintillation vials (for total counts).
9.7.2.3   Add 0.1 mL antibody (6.3.8) to all tubes except the 3 zero
          standard tubes designated for NSB, to these 3 tubes add 0.1 mL
          buffer (6.3.4).
9.7.3   Vortex mix for a few seconds.
9.7.4   Place all tubes in a water bath at 37°C for 15 minutes and then

incubate overnight at +4°C.
9.7.5   Add 0.5 mL charcoal suspension (6.3.5) at 4°C.
9.7.6   Shake all tubes gently by hand for 1 minute and stand at 4°C for
           10 min.
9.7.7   Centrifuge at 2000-3000 rpm at 4°C for 20 minutes.
9.7.8   Decant supernatant into scintillation vials (7.2).
9.7.9   Add 10 mL scintillator (6.5.2.) to all vials including 2 vials
           containing 0.1 mL tritiated stilbene solution (9.7.2.2) and also
           two vials containing 0.1 mL gelatin-phosphate buffer (Background
           counts)
9.7.10.   Place samples in liquid scintillation counter (7.1) and count
           (preset time or counts) e.g. 10000 counts or 10 minutes.

10.   CALCULATION OF RESULTS.

10.1   Prepare calibration curve by plotting cpm ^{3}H-DES bound (cpm
           bound) to antibody for vials containing standards 0 - 500 pg
           against pg standard.

10.2   Read off calibration curve pg DES against cpm for test samples
           and solvent blanks.

10.4.   Calculate the concentration of DES in sample -

           pg stilbene = (curve pg - blank pg) x 5 x recovery factor.

           curve pg = pg obtained in step 10.2.
           blank pg = pg for solvent blanks obtained in step 10.2.
           recovery factor is determined by the recovery of the 100 pg in tubes
                                                                      (9.1.2)
10.5.   Alternative calculations.

 B = cpm bound to antibody - cpm for NSB (NSB tubes 9.7.2.3.).
 Bo = cpm bound to antibody in zero standard tubes - cpm for NSB.
 Bo should be between 40-60% of total cpm (cpm 3H-DES(SA))

 Prepare calibration curve by plotting B/Bo against pg standard.

 If a microcomputer programme is possible then a best line plot of log pg
standard against Ln Z/(1-Z) where
           Z = B/Bo (LOGIT plot) can be used to interpolate results.

 Calculate B/Bo for test sample and for the solvent blank using cpm - NSB
and estimate pg DES from calibration curve. Proceed as 10.3.

The original counting data should be included with the final results.

10.6   Recovery and Precision Data for fortified blank urines.

           Conc (ng per mL)   Recovery (%)   Within lab. CV (%)
                0.5   85   15
                5   90   12
                10   92   8

Data from Meat Control Lab. Dublin, Ireland.

11.   SPECIAL CASES

12.   NOTES ON PROCEDURE

  - Better results were observed if the RIA tubes were not siliconised.
  - The addition of methanol into the RIA tubes (9.7.2.1) aids the
    reconstitution of the DES into solution.

13.   ANTIBODIES

Antibodies to DES are commercially available but recommend up to date
information is obtained from the Community Reference Laboratories.

14.   QUALITY CONTROLS

See section 8 of manual detailing the RMs available for the stilbenes.

15.   LIST OF ABBREVIATIONS

NSB, non-specific binding; SA, standard addition.
A full list of abbreviations is given in Annex I, Section 12

16.   FLOW DIAGRAM

```
              URINE ------------> Hydrolyse
                                      |
                                      ↓
      Calculate <----- RIA <----- ether extraction
      results
```

Sg. 1.4. THYREOSTATS - METHOD FOR THE MEASUREMENT OF RESIDUES OF THYREOSTATIC SUBSTANCES IN ANIMALS AND ANIMAL TISSUES ON THE BASIS OF HIGH PERFORMANCE THIN LAYER CHROMATOGRAPHY (HPTLC).

WARNING AND SAFETY PRECAUTIONS.

1.   INTRODUCTION.

Throughout the EEC the use of thyreostatic (anti-thyroid) substances is prohibited in food producing animals. Also the MRL for residues of thyreostatics in animal products imported into or produced within the Community is zero.

2.   SCOPE AND FIELD OF APPLICATION

This method of analysis describes the determination of the presence of thyreostatic substances in foodstuffs and samples of animal origin. The method can be used for meat and also for biological material such as animal organs, biological fluids and excreta. The limit of detection for 2-thiouracil (TU); 4(6)-Methyl-2-thiouracil (MTU) and 4(6)-n-propyl-2-thiouracil (PTU) is about 25 μg per kg or L.   Because the recovery of 4(6)-phenyl-2-thiouracil (PhTU) and 1-methyl-2-mercaptoimidazole (tapazole, TAP) from the mercurated column is less efficient the limit of detection for these two compounds is about 100 μg per kg or L.

For confirmation of the thyreostats the spots can be scraped from the HPTLC plate, derivatised and identified by GC-MS in the CI mode (De Brabander et al, 1992). See Method Cy 1.9.

3.   REFERENCES.

Commission Decision, 93/256/EEC, laying down the methods for detecting residues of substances having a hormonal or thyrostatic action. [OJ. № L.118, 14.4.93. pp 64-74]

ISO Standard 78/2-1982 Layout for standards - Part 2: Standard for Chemical Analysis

EEC Working paper VI/3186/84-EN, File 6.21 II-4. Method of analysis for detecting anti-thyroid substances in fresh muscle tissue using a selective mercurated column.

De Brabander, H.F. and Verbeke, R. (1984), Determination of methylthiouracil and analogous thyreostatic drugs. Proc. 30th Eur. Meat Res. Workers, Bristol, 387-388.

De Brabander, H.F., Batjoens, P. and Van Hoof, J. (1992), Determination of thyreostatic drugs by HPTLC with confirmation by GC-MS. J. Planar Chrom. 5, 124-130

4.   DEFINITIONS.

Thyreostatic substances detected in this assay are;

    2-thiouracil (TU);   4(6)-Methyl-2-thiouracil (MTU);
    4(6)-n-propyl-2-thiouracil (PTU);   4(6)-phenyl-2-thiouracil (PhTU);
    1-methyl-2-mercaptoimidazole (tapazole, TAP);

5.   PRINCIPLE

The method comprises 4 stages;
- Homogenisation of tissue samples or diluting fluids in methanol
- Percolation of supernatant through mercurated ion-exchange resin
    chromatographic column
- Derivatization
- Separation and identification by two dimensional HPTLC

Note; See confirmatory method Cy 1.9.

6. CHEMICALS

Note: The reagents for which examples of their source are quoted are
known to be satisfactory, nevertheless reagents from other sources may be
equally suitable. All the reagents must be of analytical grade.

6.1.   Methanol
6.2.   Absolute ethanol
6.3.   Hydrochloric acid, use HCl fumans (min 37% HCl) and dilute with
          water accordingly.
6.4.   KOH
6.5.   Diethyl-ether (peroxide free and very high purity)
6.6.   Anhydrous sodium sulphate
6.7.   Eluting Solution for resin. 0.5M NaCl, 0.1M HCl, pH = 1.
6.8.   NBD-Cl solution. Dissolve 5 mg NBD-Cl (7-chloro-4-nitrobenzo-2-
          oxa-1,3-diazole) in 1 mL methanol. Prepare this solution fresh
          daily and keep in a cool dark place.
6.9.   NaOH
6.10.   NaCl
6.11.   Spray solutions;
6.11.1.   Solution I - mix 50 mL denatured alcohol with 50 mL propan-2-ol.
          Add 2 mL 25% ammonia.
6.11.2.   Solution II - dissolve 0.6 g cysteine hydrochloride (or 2-
          mercaptoethylamine) in 20 mL water. Keep in refrigerator at
          about +4°C. Make fresh daily.
6.11.3.   Spray reagent - Immediately before use, mix 2 mL solution II with
          100 mL solution I.
6.12.   Standards
6.12.1.   The thyreostats, TU, MTU, PTU, PhTU and TAP are prepared as stock
          solutions of 20 mg thyreostat in 100 mL methanol. For MTU,
          distilled water and a trace of HCl must be added to dissolve the
          substance. PhTU is dissolved in a mixture of benzene and
          methanol (8:92 v/v). The working solutions are made by diluting
          aliquots of the stock solution 100 times with buffer (6.12.4)
6.12.2.   The internal standard is 4 (5,6)-dimethyl-2-thiouracil (DMTU).
          20 mg DMTU is dissolved in 100 mL methanol (stock solution) and a
          working solution is made immediately before use by diluting 0.5
          mL stock solution to 100 mL with methanol.
6.12.3.   Spiked tissues. 2.0 g minced meat (or other tissue) is spiked by
          the addition of 100 μL methanol solutions containing 0.05 μg TU,
          MTU, PTU, 0.2 μg TAP and 0.05 μg DMTU as the internal standard.
6.12.4.   Phosphate buffer; 94.5 mL of 0.2M Na_2HPO_4 is mixed with 5.5 mL
          of 0.2m KH_2PO_4. The pH is adjusted to pH 8.8.

7.   EQUIPMENT.

7.1.   Air- and water-tight reaction tubes, 10 mL and 20 mL.
7.2.   Homogeniser (Ultra-Turrax type).
7.3.   Extraction tubes with ground glass neck, 50 mL
7.4.   Refrigerator +4°C
7.5.   Deep freeze -20°C.
7.6.   Centrifuge.
7.7.   TLC ancillary equipment, e.g. solvent tanks
7.8.   UV lamp, 366 nm, with contrast filter or protective
          chromatography spectacles.
7.9.   Glass columns about 300 mm long, 4 mm i.d. and 6 mm o.d.,
7.10.   200 mL glass flasks with B 14 glass joint.
7.11.   Micro-litre syringes with end of needle cut at 90°. Capacity 1
          µL, 10 µL and 100 µL.
7.12.   Preparation of the Mercurated resin.
          20 mL Dowex 1 x 2 (50-100 mesh, Analytical grade) is washed
          successively with 10 bed volumes of distilled water, 0.5M NaOH,
          distilled water, 0.5M acetic acid and distilled water. The wet
          resin (20 mL) is then shaken with 200 mL aqueous solution of 2,7-
          dibromo-4-hydroxymercrifluorescein (500 mg dissolved in 200 mL
          water) for 24 hours. The mercurated resin is then washed with
          water until the eluate is colourless. The resin is treated with
          100 mL 0.1M HCl and 0.5M NaCl, washed with 500 mL distilled
          water, treated with 100 mL 0.1M NaOH and washed with 500 mL
          distilled water. The resin is stored in the dark.
7.13.   Preparation of Micro-Column for clean-up stage.

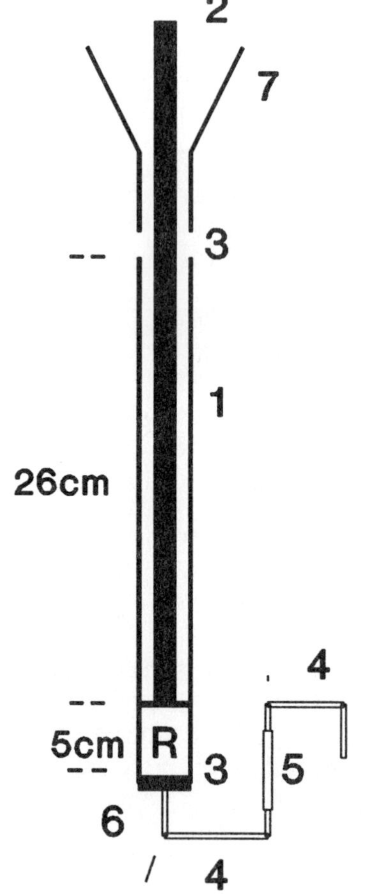

1. glass column 4 mm i.d., 6 mm o.d.
2. glass rod 3 mm i.d.
3. connected with silicone tubing
4. silicone tubing 0.3 mm i.d. 0.7 mm o.d.
5. silicone tubing 0.5 mm i.d. 1 mm o.d.
6. silicone tubing 0.5 mm i.d. 4 mm o.d.
7. glass funnel

R is resin

The column is filled with water and the glass rod removed. Approximately 0.6 mL mercurated resin is suspended in water and added via the funnel. When the resin sediments to a height of 5 cm, the excess resin is removed and the glass rod replaced to rest on top of the resin bed. The column is ready for use.

7.14.   HPTLC
7.14.1.   Plates; Silicagel 60 aluminium sheets without fluorescent
          indicator (e.g. Merck No. 5613 or 5547). The plates are
          activated at 110°C overnight before use.
7.14.2   Solvents. Use either system a or system b.

System a
7.14.2.1a First direction solvent; chloroform : ethanol 95:5 v/v
7.14.2.2a Second direction solvent; chloroform : propionic acid 95:5 v/v.

System b
7.14.2.1b First direction solvent; methylene chloride : methanol 98:2 v/v
7.14.2.2b Second direction solvent; methylene chloride : propionic acid
          98:2 v/v.
7.14.3.   Spray solutions, see 6.11.

Reference to a company and/or product is for purposes of information and
identification only. Equivalent types or products also may be suitable.

8.   SAMPLES AND SAMPLING PROCEDURE.

N.B. Attention is drawn to section 6.3.1 and to ISO document 78/2-1982 and
also the following notes derived from Annex II of 2052/VI/84-EN.

8.1. Nature of the Sample; Samples shall be such as to enable the
detection of residues in meat as defined in Directive 64/433/EEC. Failing
this biological fluids or faeces may constitute the samples for the
detection of residues.

8.2. Size of Sample; The size of the sample must be large enough to allow
the method to be carried out and to allow repeat analysis where required.

8.3. The samples must be taken and packed in such a way as to allow proper
identification in the laboratory.

8.4. The method of packing, preservation and transport must maintain the
integrity of the sample and not prejudice the result of the examination.
Samples for the analysis of thyreostatic substances must be stored and
transported at temperatures below -18°C.

9.   PROCEDURE.

9.1   2 g tissue, 2 mL urine, plasma or skim milk, are homogenised in
          10 mL methanol using an Ultra-Turrax homogeniser (7.2).
9.2.   100 µL internal standard solution, containing 0.2 µg DMTU,
          (6.12.2) is added and the homogenate centrifuged at 10,000 rpm
          (12,000 g) for 10 minutes.
9.3.   The supernatant is decanted and then percolated through the
          mercury column (7.13). Air is removed by moving the glass rod
          carefully up and down.
9.4.   The column is washed with 10 mL water and the thyreostats are
          eluted with 5 mL elution solution (6.7).
9.5.   The eluate is neutralised with 100 µL 4M NaOH and 1 mL buffer
          (6.12.4) and adjusted to pH = 8.
9.6.   0.1 mL NBD-Cl solution (6.8) is added and the reaction allowed to
          proceed in the dark at 40°C for one hour. The optimum reaction
          time may vary between 1 - 2 hours depending on the quality of the

NBD-Cl. The time should be checked in advance.

9.7.   The pH of the reaction mixture is adjusted to pH 3-4 by adding 0.2 mL 6M HCl.

9.8.   The NBD derivatives are extracted with 3 mL, 2 mL and 2 mL diethyl-ether and the combined ether extracts are dried over anhydrous sodium sulphate (0.5 -1 g). No water must be present.

9.9.   The ether is evaporated under a stream of nitrogen to yield, according to the concentration range of interest, a volume between 0.2 mL and 1 mL.

9.10.   Standards are prepared for derivatisation by mixing 0.1 mL stock solution in 5 mL buffer (6.12.4). The mixture is derivatised by carrying out steps 9.6 to 9.9 and evaporating the ether to a volume of 2 mL.

9.11.   50-100 µL of the extracts (9.9) are analyzed by bi-dimensional HPTLC.

9.12.   The plate is run first with solvent 7.14.2.1.(a or b), dried carefully in a stream of air and then run in the other direction using solvent 7.14.2.2.(a or b).

9.13.   Standards which are derivatised at the same time may be run parallel with the extracts during the second solvent step for accurate identification of the individual thyreostats.

9.14.   The plates are sprayed with the cysteine based spray (6.11) and the spots identified. The spots, which are not visible before spraying, should appear as yellow fluorescent spots on a blue background. The relative intensities of the fluorescence at 366 nm of the suspected thyreostats are compared with the intensity of the spot due to the internal standard.

Note; Interferences on the plate may be reduced by allowing the plate to stand overnight.

10.   CALCULATION OF RESULTS.

10.1.   IDENTIFICATION.

The spots are yellow fluorescent spots and must have the same R_f values as the standards.   In the system using the solvents 7.14.2.1a and 7.14.2.2a the R_f values relative to the internal standard DMTU should be similar to those in table 1.

Table 1. RR_f of thyreostats relative to DMTU on HPTLC plates.

Thyreostat	RR_f in 1st solvent	RR_f in 2nd solvent
DMTU	1.0	1.0
TU	0.34	0.22
MTU	0.59	0.43
PTU	0.73	0.77
PhTU	0.94	0.89
TAP	1.09	0.53

Data from EEC Working paper VI/3186/84-EN, File 6.21 II-4.

10.1.   RECOVERIES.

The recoveries of the thyreostats from the mercurated column is >78% for TU, MTU, PTU and DMTU but only about 17% for PhTU and 60% for TAP.

The recoveries of the internal standard, DMTU, from meat, plasma and milk are shown in table 2;

Table 2; Recoveries of 100 µg per kg spike of DMTU.

Sample.   Concentration found ± SD
                               (µg per kg)
                 PTU   MTU   TU

Meat   106 ± 5.5   102 ± 13.7   97 ± 21.8
Plasma   84 ± 6.2   98 ± 5.0   76 ± 5.7
Milk   88 ± 6.9   105 ± 3.6   85 ± 8.0

10.2.   PRECISION
10.2.1. Reproducibility; The reproducibility of the analysis of meat
spiked at the 100 µg per kg level was recorded for each step of the assay.
The results obtained by De Brabander and Verbeke (1984), Ghent, are shown
in table 3;
Table 3;

Step   n   recovery   CV
                                mean ± SD (µg/kg)   %

Column elution   26   81 ± 3.9   4.8
Derivatisation   26   76 ± 5.0   6.6
HPTLC   22   88 ± 4.7   5.4

Total procedure   22   55 ± 6.9   12.6

11.   SPECIAL CASES

12.   NOTES ON PROCEDURE

13.   QUALITY CONTROLS

See section 8 of manual detailing the RMs available for the thyreostatics.

14.   TEST REPORT

15.   LIST OF ABBREVIATIONS

A full list of abbreviations is given in Annex I, Section 12

16.   FLOW DIAGRAM
    Tissue --> add methanol and internal standard ---> Homogenise
                                                           ¦
                                                           ¦
                                                           ↓
      HPTLC <------- Derivatise <------- percolate through Hg column
        ¦
        ↓
      Measure fluorescence at 366 nm -------> Calculate results.

Sg 2.1. ß-AGONISTS - A SCREENING METHOD FOR THE DETECTION OF ß-AGONISTS IN BOVINE URINE BY GC-MS IN THE ELECTRON IMPACT MODE FOR THE TRIMETHYLSILYL DERIVATIVES.

1.   SCOPE

This method of analysis describes the detection of the presence of individual β-agonists in samples of urine of veal calves and adult cattle. The method is used officially in France and is carried out in compliance with the Residues Directive (86/469/EEC).

2.   FIELD OF APPLICATION

The method is used to perform routine screening in urine from veal calves and adult cattle. The method is used to test for the presence of residues of clenbuterol, clenpenterol, hydroxymethyl-clenbuterol, salbutamol, terbutaline, cimaterol, cimbuterol, mabuterol, mapenterol, tulobuterol, fenoterol and ractopamine.
The detection limit, defined as a signal noise ratio >3 is below 1 µg per L

3.   REFERENCES

Montrade, M-P., Le Bizec, B., Monteau, F., Siliart, B. and André, F. (1993), Multi-residue analysis for ß-agonistic drugs in urine of meat-producing animals by gas chromatography - mass spectrometry. Anal. Chim. Acta. <u>275</u>, 253-268

Montrade, M-P., Le Bizec, B. and André, F. (1992), Methode de recherche urinaire (screening) d'agonistes ß-adrenergiques par chromatographie gazeuse couplee à la spectrometie de masse (GC-MS) en mode impact electronique. Document LDH/92/01 Lab. Dosage Hormonaux, Nantes. DGAL/SDHA/№92.8066
[Note; This method is available in French, Spanish or Portuguese]

4.   DEFINITIONS

ß-agonists content is taken to be the amount of β-agonists in the substance in question determined according to the described method and expressed as µg β-agonists per L of test sample.

5.   PRINCIPLE

The method comprises 6 stages;
1. hydrolysis of conjugates
2. methanol precipitation (optional), particulary for "dirty" urine of adult cattle
3. extract purification and concentration using mixed solid-phase extraction (SPE) chromatography
4. derivatisation
5. detection by GC-MS in electron impact mode
6. calculation and evaluation of results

6.   MATERIALS

Note: The reagents (and equipment) for which examples of their source are quoted are known to be satisfactory, nevertheless reagents and equipment from other sources may be equally suitable. All the reagents should be of analytical grade or better.

6.1   Reference compounds and Standards.

Clenbuterol hydrochloride (Interchim, Montlucon, France)
Salbutamol hemisulphate, Terbutaline hemisulphate and metoprolol tartrate
(Sigma).
Cimaterol, clenpenterol (NAB 760), mabuterol, fenoterol hydrobromide and
hydroxymethyl clenbuterol (NA1141) (Boehringer Ingleheim)
Tulobuterol hydrochloride (Abbott)
Ractopamine hydrochloride (Eli Lilly)
Cimbuterol and marpenterol were synthesised by Chem Dept, University of
Rennes, France

6.2   Chemicals
6.2.1   *Helix pomatia* juice (ß-glucuronidase-arylsulfatase, Merck-4114)
6.2.2   Glacial acetic acid   (Panreac - 131008 or Merck.62)
6.2.3   Ultra-pure water (>14 M Ω.cm)
6.2.4   Methanol (Carlo-Erba RS CLHP-412002 or Merck.6009)
6.2.5   Ethyl acetate (Merck ZA-9623)
6.2.6   32% Ammonium hydroxide (Merck 5426)
6.2.7   1*M* Potassium hydroxide (Merck ZA-9018920)
6.2.8   1*M* Acetic acid
6.2.9   N-O-bis(trimethylsilyl)trifluoracetamide (BSTFA) (Regisil-270111
           or FLUKA -15244)
6.2.10   Toluene (FLUKA - 89677) by molecular sieving.
6.2.11   Sodium acetate (Merck ZA-6268)
6.2.12   Potassium dihydrogen phosphate (Merck ZA-4873)
6.2.13   Nitrogen (dried over silica gel)
6.2.14   Helium (very high purity, N55, Carboxyque)

6.3   Solutions
6.3.1   ß-agonists. Prepare stock solutions of the standards (6.1.1) in
           methanol (1 g per L and 100 mg per L) and store at -18°C.
6.3.2   ß-agonists. Prepare working solutions by dilution of stock
           solutions (6.3.1) with methanol to final concentrations of 10 µg
           and 1µg per mL. Store at -18°C in the dark.
6.3.3   2*M* Acetate buffer, pH 5.2, for hydrolysis of conjugates.
           Dissolve 164 g sodium acetate (6.2.11) in 900 mL water (6.2.3)
           and adjust the pH to 5.2 ± 0.1 with glacial acetic acid (6.2.2).
           Make up to 1 L with water and store at +4°C. Use for up to 1
           month.
6.3.4   0.1*M* Phosphate buffer, pH 6.0. Dissolve 13.6 + 0.1 g potassium
           dihydrogen phosphate (6.2.12) in 900 mL water (6.2.3) and adjust
           the pH to 6.0 ± 0.1 with 1*M* potassium hydroxide (6.2.7). Make up
           to 1 L with water and store at +4°C. Use for up to 1 month.
6.3.5   Mix ethyl acetate and 32% ammonium hydroxide 97:3 (v/v). 100 mL
           does 16 samples. Stir/agitate the mixture prior to use and then
           place into an ultra-sonic bath during step 9.13.3.

7.0   EQUIPMENT
7.1.   Centrifuge
7.2   Rotary evaporator
7.3   Vortex mixer
7.4   pH meter
7.5   Pipettes
7.6   Balance

7.7   Vacuum filtration system (Vac-Elut from Analytichem
          International)
7.8   Ultra-sonic bath
7.9   Magnetic stirrer/agitator
7.10   Conical reaction vials for derivatisation
7.11   Heating block for reaction vials 7.10
7.12   Heating block with evaporation system
7.13   SPE-Columns; CLEAN SCREEN DAU (Worldwide monitoring - Horsham,
          PA, USA and sold by Technicol, Stockport, Cheshire, UK). These
          columns of 6 mL volume contain 500 mg of a mixed phase support
          which has hydrophobic and ion-exchange properties.

7.14   GC-MS
7.14.1   GC; GC Hewlett Packard 5890.
          Capillary column, 30 m X 0.25 mm i.d. with SE-30 stationary phase
          of 0.25 μm thickness.
          Injection mode; splitless over 1 minute
          Injection volume; 2 μL
          Injector temp. 250°C; Transfer temp. 280°C

          Temp. programme;

                      18°C/min   *5°C/min*
          70°C (2 min) ------------> 200°C (0 min) ----------> 245°C (0 min)

              25°C/min
          ------------> 300°C (12 min)

          Gas; Helium at 1 mL per min and 5 psi.

7.14.2   MS; Hewlett Packard 5971 with UNIX station.
          Electron Impact ionisation mode (70 eV)
          Source temp. 190°C $\pm$ 5°C
          Pressure, 30-40 mm Torr

8.   SAMPLES AND SAMPLING PROCEDURE.

N.B. Attention is drawn to section 6.3.1 and to ISO document 78/2-1982 and
also the following notes derived from Annex II of 2052/VI/84-EN.

8.1.   Nature of the Sample; Samples shall be such as to enable the
          detection of residues in urine as defined in Directive
          64/433/EEC.
8.2.   Size of Sample; The size of the sample must be large enough to
          allow the method to be carried out and to allow repeat analysis
          where required. Each analysis needs a 10 mL sample.

8.3.   The samples must be taken and packed in such a way as to allow
          proper identification in the laboratory.

8.4.   The method of packing, preservation and transport must maintain
          the integrity of the sample and not prejudice the result of the
          examination.
          Samples for the analysis of ß-agonists must be stored at
          temperatures below -18°C.

Sg 2.1/3

9.0.   PROCEDURE
9.1   Thaw the primary samples and transfer more than 10 mL to a
           centrifuge tube. Centrifuge at 3000 rpm for 15 min. Pipette 10
           mL to a screw-topped tube (e.g. scintillation counting vial).
9.2   Add 60 ng metoprolol as internal standard to all urines including
           two blank urines.
9.3   To one of the blank urines (9.2) add 40 ng (equiv. 4 ppb)
           tulobuterol, fenoterol and ractopamine and 20 ng (equiv. 2 ppb)
           of the other ß-agonist standards (6.3.2).
9.4   Add 1 mL acetate buffer (6.3.3) and check the pH is about 5.2 ±
           0.3. Adjust the pH to about 5.2 with acetic acid if necessary.
9.5   Add 50 µL *Helix pomatia* juice (6.2.1) and incubate overnight at
           50°C in a water bath or oven.
Steps 9.6 to 9.11 are optional and can be used for urines from adult
cattle.
9.6   Transfer the hydrolysed urines to rotary evaporation flasks.
9.7   Add 25 mL methanol. Evaporate the methanol using a rotary
           evaporator and a water bath at about 45°C.
9.8   Concentrate the aqueous phase to about 3 mL.
9.9   Transfer the aqueous phase to a test tube with a pasteur pipette
           and rinse out the flask twice with 5 mL phosphate buffer (6.3.4).
9.10   Centrifuge at 3500 rpm for about 10 min. A precipitate should
           form on the tube.
9.11   Check and adjust the pH to 6.0 ± 0.3 if necessary. Use all the
           clear aqueous phase for step 9.13.
9.12   If steps 9.6 to 9.11 were not carried out add 4 mL phosphate
           buffer (6.3.4) to the hydrolysate, adjust the pH to 6.0 (final
           volume to 15 mL).
9.13   Column extraction;
9.13.1   Place the columns on the Vac-Elut system and successively rinse
           with; 2 mL methanol; 2 mL water (6.2.3); 2 mL phosphate buffer
           (6.3.4).
9.13.2   Transfer the clear extracts (9.11 or 9.12) with a pasteur pipette
           to the top of the column and allow to drain slowly using slight
           negative (ca.12 cm Hg) pressure.
9.13.3   Rinse the columns using negative pressure of about 40 cm Hg with
           1 mL 1*M* acetic acid (6.2.8) and allow to dry before rinsing with
           6 mL methanol by applying a strong vacuum.
9.13.4   Place the ethyl acetate / ammonium hydroxide solution (6.3.5) in
           an ultra-sonic bath to agitate the mixture during step 9.13.3.
9.13.5   Elute the analytes with 6 mL the ethyl acetate / ammonium
           hydroxide solution (6.3.5)
9.14   Evaporate the eluate with nitrogen using an evaporation system
           and a heating block at 40 ± 5°C.
9.15   Dissolve the residue in 200 µL methanol with vigorous vortexing.
9.16   Transfer the solution to a reaction vial.
9.17   Dissolve and transfer to the reaction vial any remaining residue
           with a further 100 µL methanol and vortexing.
9.18   Evaporate the methanol to dryness on a heating block at 40°± 5°C.
9.19   Derivatisation
9.19.1   Add 50 µL BSTFA (6.2.9) and vortex.
9.19.2   Place vials in heating block at 75°C ± 5°C for 90 min.
9.19.3   Transfer the vials to a heating block at 40° ± 5°C. Allow the
           vials and block to cool to room temperature (25°C) evaporate to
           dryness with nitrogen.

9.19.4   Add 25 µL toluene (6.2.10) and vortex vigorously.
9.19.5   The vials may be stored in a refrigerator at +4°C.
9.20   Inject 2 µL of 9.19.5 into the GC-MS.

9.21   The GC-MS is run in the selected ion monitoring mode. The ions
          and the retention times of the derivatives of the ß-agonists are
          shown in table 1.

Table 1.

ß-agonist	N	RT (min)	Selected ions	Mol. Ion
Tulobuterol	1	9.34	86, 194, 284	299
Mabuterol	1	10.36	86, 277, 296	382
Mapenterol	1	11.04	100, 277, 296	396
Terbutaline	3	11.67	86, 356	441
Clenbuterol	1	12.02	86, 243, 262 (264)	348
Cimaterol	1	12.14	72, 219	291
Salbutamol	3	12.27	86, 369	455
Cimbuterol	1	12.36	86, 219	305
Cimaterol	2	12.62	72, 291	363
Metoprolol (I.S)	1	12.7	72, 223	339
Cimbuterol	2	12.8	86, 291	377
Clenpenterol	1	12.86	100, 243, 262 (264)	362
Hydroxymethyl-clenbuterol (NA 1141)	2	14.05	174, 243, 262	436
Fenoterol	4	18.39	322, 356, 412	591
Ractopamine	3	18.63	250, 267	517

N is the number of TMS groups. RT are the retention times recorded in an
analysis at LDH, Nantes.

10.0   INTERPRETATION OF RESULTS

10.1   Validity of Analysis; The criteria set out in EC Decision 256
          must be fulfilled especially the following;-

10.1.1   The relative retention times for the TMS derivatives of the
          standard analytes in the appropriate matrix and the suspected ß-
          agonist must be the same.
10.1.2   The relative intensities of the selected ions to the base peak
          must be same as in the assay of spiked blank urines and of
          standards.
10.1.3   The ions for the internal standard (metoprolol-monoTMS) **must** be
          present at the correct retention time.

10.1.4   The analysis of the blank urine containing the internal standard
          must show NO evidence of carry-over of ß-agonists from the GC-MS
          system. This is a check for contamination of the system.

11.   SPECIAL CASES
12.   NOTES ON PROCEDURE.

13.   QUALITY CONTROLS
See section 8 of manual detailing the RMs for the ß-agonists.

14.   TEST REPORT

15.   LIST OF ABBREVIATIONS
A full list of abbreviations is given in Annex I, Section 12

16. FLOW DIAGRAM

```
              hydrolysis
    URINE ------------> METHANOL PRECIPITATION--------> EXTRACT by SPE
                            (Optional)                 |       Chrom.
                                                       |
                                                       |
                                                       |
      INTERPRET RESULTS <----- GC-MS <------------ TMS DERIVATIVES
                          (EI-mode)
```

Sg 2.2. ß-AGONISTS - AN ELISA SCREENING METHOD USING A COMMERCIALLY AVAILABLE KIT FOR THE DETECTION OF ß-AGONISTS IN BOVINE URINE.

WARNING; The stop solution (6.1.1.9) contains sodium fluoride, handle with care and in case of contact wash thoroughly with tap water.

1.   SCOPE

This method of analysis describes the detection of the presence of β-agonists in urine samples of cattle using a commercially available kit. The method has been mainly tested for residues of clenbuterol, salbutamol, mabuterol, mapenterol and terbutaline. The kit manufacturer claim that the kit may be used for bovine liver and milk and also milk replacer powder. This work is carried out in compliance with the Residues Directive (86/469/EEC).

2.   FIELD OF APPLICATION

This ELISA method is used to perform routine screening in bovine urine for the presence of residues of clenbuterol, salbutamol, terbutaline, mapenterol and mabuterol.
The lower limits of detection for urine (and liver, milk and milk powder) in μg per L or kg calculated (see EEC 93/256) as mean of blanks ± 3 S.D. are;- Clenbuterol and mabuterol, 1; salbutamol and mapenterol, 3.5; terbutaline 4.5.
EIA kits for measuring ß-agonists in urine and serum and using different antibodies are marketed by several manufacturers (see Section 8.4.2). The lower limits of detection and the specificities are different from those in the method reported here.

3.   REFERENCES

Commission Decision, 93/256/EEC, laying down the methods for detecting residues of substances having a hormonal or thyrostatic action. [OJ. Nº L.118, 14.4.93. pp 64-74]

Angeletti, R., Paleologo Oriundi, M., Piro, R. and Bagnati, R. (1993), Application of an enzyme-linked immunosorbent assay kit for ß-agonist screening of bovine tissues in north-eastern Italy. Anal. Chim. Acta.<u>275</u>, 215-219.

Quantitative ß-agonists ELISA kit. Enzyme immunoassay for in vitro diagnostic use. Cat.Nº AG310. Genego S.P.A., 34170 Gorizia, Italy.

4.   DEFINITIONS

ß-agonists content is taken to be the amount of β-agonists in the substance in question determined according to the described method and expressed as μg β-agonists per litre of urine.

5.   PRINCIPLE

The method comprises 3 stages.

1.   Dilution of primary urine sample
2.   ELISA using kit
5.   Calculation and evaluation of results

6.	MATERIALS

Note:	The reagents (and equipment) for which examples of their source are
quoted are known to be satisfactory, nevertheless reagents and equipment
from other sources may be equally suitable.

6.1	Chemicals
6.1.1	ELISA kit (Cat.№ AG310. Genego S.P.A., 34170 Gorizia, Italy.)
		containing;-
6.1.1.1	Clenbuterol standard solutions, 0.3, 0.6, 1.25, 2.5, 5.0, 10 ng
		per mL - ready to use
6.1.1.2	Enzyme conjugate; salbutamol peroxidase - ready to use
6.1.1.3	Anti ß-agonists antibody
6.1.1.4	Wash buffer; Dilute 10x with distilled water.
6.1.1.5	Diluent solution; Dilute 20x with distilled water.
6.1.1.6	Chromogen
6.1.1.7	Citrate buffer
6.1.1.8	Developing solution; Dilute the chromogen (6.1.1.6) 25x with
		citrate buffer (6.1.1.7).
6.1.1.9	Stop solution - ready to use
6.2	Distilled water

7.	EQUIPMENT

7.1	Micropipettes, 50, 100 and 200 µL.
7.2	Multichannel micropipette, 50-200 µL
7.3	Plate washing equipment, manual or automatic
7.4	Microplate reader with 414 or 405 nm filter with optional EIA/RIA
		data processing.
7.5	Normal laboratory glassware.
7.6	Centrifuge (optional)

8. SAMPLES AND SAMPLING PROCEDURE.

N.B. Attention is drawn to section 6.3.1 and to ISO document 78/2-1982 and
also the following notes derived from Annex II of 2052/VI/84-EN.

8.1. Nature of the Sample; Samples shall be such as to enable the
detection of residues in meat as defined in Directive 64/433/EEC. Failing
this biological fluids (here urine) or liver may constitute the samples for
the detection of residues.

8.2. Size of Sample; The size of the sample must be large enough to allow
the method to be carried out and to allow repeat analysis where required.

8.3. The samples must be taken and packed in such a way as to allow proper
identification in the laboratory.

8.4. The method of packing, preservation and transport must maintain the
integrity of the sample and not prejudice the result of the examination.
Samples for the analysis of ß-agonists must be stored at temperatures below
-18°C.

9.	PROCEDURE

9.1	Clarify the urine sample (0.5-2 mL) by centrifugation at 1000 g
		for 5 min or filtration.

9.2   Dilute 0.5 mL urine with 0.5 mL dilution buffer (6.1.1.5)

9.3   ELISA - follow the kit instructions using 50 µL of sample (9.2) or standards (6.1.1.1) in duplicate. The incubation time is 35 min. at room temperature and development time for the chromogen is 30 min. at room temperature.

9.4   Measure the absorbance at 405 or 414 nm of the test samples, the standards and the assay blanks after the addition of the stop solution (6.1.1.9).

10.   INTERPRETATION OF RESULTS

10.1   Precision; The intra-assay and inter assay variation was measured using the 1.25, 2.5 and 5.0 ng per mL standards. The values were

Intra-assay CV (%) was < 6% n=6
Inter-assay CV (%) was < 9% n=5   (Angeletti et al., 1993)

Accuracy was measured by spiking blank urines with 1 ng clenbuterol per mL or 2 ng salbutamol per mL gave a small overestimation of the analyte concentration (10-15% in the low ng per mL range).

10.2   The action limit was estimated for field samples by comparing the number of positives detected above either 0.6 or 1.0 ng per mL with the number of confirmed positives for clenbuterol and salbutamol <u>only</u>. Samples were examined from 815 cattle and the results are shown in the table of the data reported by Angeletti et al., (1993)..

Animals or Herds	Nº +ve >0.6 ng/mL	Nº +ve >1 ng/mL	Nº Confirmed +ve
815 cattle	141	89	59
180 herds	35	25	18

11.   SPECIAL CASES

12.   NOTES ON PROCEDURE.

The kit can be used for testing residues in bovine liver, milk and milk replacer powders (see Genego instructions for the kit).

13.   QUALITY CONTROLS
See section 8 of manual detailing the RMs for the ß-agonists.

14.   TEST REPORT

15.   LIST OF ABBREVIATIONS

A full list of abbreviations is given in Annex I, Section 12

16.   FLOW DIAGRAM

```
                dilute
URINE -----------> ELISA -------------> RESULTS
```

**Sg.2.3.   ß-AGONISTS - AN EIA SCREENING METHOD FOR THE DETECTION OF
ß-AGONISTS IN BOVINE URINE.**

1.   SCOPE

This method of analysis describes the detection of the presence of β-agonists in urine samples of cattle. The method has been mainly tested for residues of clenbuterol and salbutamol. This work is carried out in compliance with the Residues Directive (86/469/EEC).

2.   FIELD OF APPLICATION

This EIA method is used to perform routine screening in bovine urine for the presence of residues of clenbuterol, salbutamol, terbutaline, cimaterol and mabuterol. In principle it is also suitable for the detection and confirmation of other t-butyl or isopropyl-β-agonists.
The lower limit of detection is 0.14 µg per L urine and the limit of determination is 0.18 µg per L. The method was developed at the University of Liege and Laboratoire d'Hormonologie, Marloie, Belgium (Degand et al, 1993)

Note; There is also an RIA kit for the same ß-agonists and using the same antiserum also available from Laboratoire d'Hormonologie, Rue de Carmel 1, 6900-Marloie, Belgium.

An EIA kit for measuring ß-agonists in urine and serum and using a different antibody is marketed by Riedel-de Haen (see Section 8.4.2). The lower limits of detection are higher than those in the method reported here.

3.   REFERENCES

Commission Decision, 93/256/EEC, laying down the methods for detecting residues of substances having a hormonal or thyrostatic action. [OJ. Nº L.118, 14.4.93. pp 64-74]

Degand, G., Bernes-Duyckaerts, A. and Maghuin-Rogister, G. (1992), Determination of clenbuterol in bovine tissues and urine by enzyme immunoassay. J. Agric. Food Chem. <u>40</u>, 70-75

Degand, G., Bernes-Duyckaerts, A., Delahaut, Ph. and Maghuin-Rogister, G. (1993), Determination of ß-agonists in urine by an enzyme immunoassay based on the use of an anti-salbutamol antiserum. Anal. Chim. Acta. <u>275</u>, 241-248

Yamamoto I and Iwalak, 1982 Enzyme immunoassay for clenbuterol, a β-2-adrenergic stimulant. Journal of Immunoassay, 3:15

4.   DEFINITIONS

ß-agonists content is taken to be the amount of β-agonists in the substance in question determined according to the described method and expressed as µg β-agonists per litre of urine.

5. PRINCIPLE

The method comprises 5 stages; the first two are optional.
1.   Preparation of enzyme conjugate.

2.   Coating EIA plates
3.   Dilution of primary urine sample
4.   EIA
5.   Calculation and evaluation of results

6.   MATERIALS

Note: The reagents (and equipment) for which examples of their source are
quoted are known to be satisfactory, nevertheless reagents and equipment
from other sources may be equally suitable. All the reagents must be of
analytical grade.

6.1.   Chemicals and reagents. All chemicals were analytical grade or
          better.

6.1.1.   Reference compounds.

The following standard compounds are used.

Compound	CAS-No	mol formula	Mol. Wt.	
clenbuterol	37148-27-9	$C_{12}H_{18}C_{12}N_2O$	277.18	(Boehringer
cimaterol	54239-37-1	$C_{12}H_{17}N_3O$	219.29	Ingleheim)
salbutamol	18559-94-9	$C_{13}H_{21}NO_3$	239.31	Sigma
terbutaline	23031-25-6	$C_{12}H_{19}NO_3$	235.29	Sigma
mabuterol	56341-08-3	$C_{13}H_{18}ClF_3N_2O$	310.75	Sigma
isoproteronol				Sigma
pirbuterol				Sigma

and additional β-agonists if desired.

6.1.2.   Tween-20 (Merck)
6.1.3.   Thiomersal (Merck)
6.1.4.   Bovine Serum albumin (BSA) (Sigma)
6.1.5.   Antiserum from Marloie. Cat. as anti-salbutamol serum.
          Cross reactivities;
          Salbutamol, 100%; clenbuterol, 115%;
          Mabuterol, 65%; terbutaline, 31%; Cimaterol, 13%
          Pirbuterol, 0.02%; isoproterenol, 0.02%;
          Adrenaline 0.01%, noradrenaline, <0.01%
6.1.6.   Deionised water (Milli Q, Millipore)
6.1.7.   Sodium carbonate
6.1.8   Sodium bicarbonate
6.1.9   6M sulphuric acid
6.1.10   Sodium dihydrogen phosphate (Merck).
6.1.11   Sodium chloride
6.1.12.   Disodium hydrogen phosphate (Merck).

6.2.   Solutions
6.2.1.   Stock solutions of standards containing 1 g/L in ethanol, stored
          at -20°C in the dark.
6.2.1.   Working solutions of standards containing 0.01 g/L in ethanol,
          stored at +4°C for a maximum period of 2 weeks.
          Smallest volume pipetted out of the stock solution is 0.1 mL.
6.2.3.   Phosphate-saline-BSA buffer, 0.01 mol/L, pH = 7.4
          Dissolve in 800 mL water 1.6 g disodium hydrogen phosphate
          (6.1.12.), 0.14 g sodium dihydrogen phosphate (6.1.10), 8.6 g
          sodium chloride (6.1.11), 1 g BSA (6.1.4) and 0.1 g thiomersal
          (6.1.3). Adjust the pH at 7.4 ± 0,1 and add water to a final

volume of 1000 mL.
6.2.4.   Coating Solution.
6.2.4.1   Coating Buffer, 50 mmol per L, pH 9.6
           Dissolve 1.59 g sodium carbonate and 2.93 g sodium bicarbonate in
           1 L distilled water.
6.2.4.2   1 volume of Antiserum (6.1.5) from Marloie is diluted with 9
           volumes PBS buffer (6.2.3) and 10 volumes glycerol. 7 μL of
           diluted antiserum are added to 7 mL coating buffer (6.2.4.1) to
           give a 1 in 20,000 dilution. 100 μL are added to a well.
6.2.5   Washing solution.
           Dissolve 8.76 g sodium chloride and 0.5 mL Tween-20 in 1 L water
           (6.1.6).
6.2.6.   TMB Microwell peroxidase substrate system. KPL Cat. № 50.76.00
6.2.7   Mix equal volumes of TMB chromogen with hydrogen peroxide
           solution. Add 150 μL to a well.
6.2.8   Stopping Solution - use 6M sulphuric acid
6.2.9   Phosphate buffer, 0.01M, pH 7.5. Dissolve 1.49 g Na_2PO_4. $2H_2O$
           and 0.22 g $NaH_2PO_4.H_2O$ in 1 L water (6.1.6).
6.3   Reagents for Preparation of Enzyme Conjugate.
6.3.1   Horse radish peroxidase (Boehringer [Mannheim])
6.3.2   Methanol
6.3.3   Succinic anhydride
6.3.4   Dimethylformamide
6.3.5   N-methylmorpholine
6.3.6   Isobutyl chloroformate
6.3.7   Sephadex G-25

7.   EQUIPMENT

7.1   Dispensing pipettes
7.2   ELISA plates (NUNC-Immuno plate Maxisorb F96-, Roskilde,
           Denmark.
7.3.   Microplate reader, (Multiscan MCC/340, Flow Labs)
7.4.   Oven at 37°C
7.5.   ELISA plate sealer, (plastic film from TechGen, Zellik,
           Belgium)
7.6.   Optional microcomputer with EXCEL (Microsoft) for data
           calculations.
7.7.   For preparation of Enzyme conjugate.
7.7.1   TLC system
7.7.2   Column chromatographic system for purifying conjugate.
7.7.3   Cryostatic bath at -15°C
7.7.4   Dialysis tubing and 3 L vessel.
7.7.5   Ultrasonic bath (Branson 1200 VEL Belgium)
7.7.5   Stirrer (magnetic)

8. SAMPLES AND SAMPLING PROCEDURE.

N.B. Attention is drawn to section 6.3.1 and to ISO document 78/2-1982 and
also the following notes derived from Annex II of 2052/VI/84-EN.

8.1. Nature of the Sample; Samples shall be such as to enable the
detection of residues in meat as defined in Directive 64/433/EEC. Failing
this biological fluids (here urine) or faeces may constitute the samples
for the detection of residues.

8.2. Size of Sample; The size of the sample must be large enough to allow the method to be carried out and to allow repeat analysis where required.

8.3. The samples must be taken and packed in such a way as to allow proper identification in the laboratory.

8.4. The method of packing, preservation and transport must maintain the integrity of the sample and not prejudice the result of the examination. Samples for the analysis of ß-agonists must be stored and transported at temperatures below -18°C.

9.   PROCEDURE.

Note; This method is given with two options.
1. The 96-well plates coated with either anti-clenbuterol or anti-salbutamol antiserum and both the salbutamol-HRP conjugate and the clenbuterol-HRP conjugate may be purchased from Marloie (see Section 8.4.2).

2. In the form of a "do it yourself" EIA, in which all the reagents except the salbutamol-enzyme conjugate can be purchased and the 96-well plates have to be coated and all the solutions prepared.

9.1   Optional Coating of the EIA plates and preparation of enzyme conjugate.
9.1.1   Coating the plates. Add 100 μL of the diluted antiserum (6.2.4.2) to each of the inner 60 wells of a 96-well plate (the values for well to well variation are greatly reduced in certain plates if only the inner wells are used). Cover the plate with the plastic film and store at 4°C for 16 h or at 37°C for 2 h. Wash the plate with four rinses of 6.2.5. before use.
9.1.2   Preparation of enzyme conjugate. Suspend 12.5 mg salbutamol succinate (37.5 μmol) in 2 mL dimethylformamide and 30 μL triethylamine. Place the flask in an ultrasonic bath for 15 min and then add 2 x 200 μL distilled water. Cool the solution at -15°C and add 4 μL N-Methylmorpholine. followed by 37.5 μmol isobutylchloroformate. Stir the mixture for 5 min. Add the cold mixture to horse radish peroxidase (6.3.1) solution in 500 μL 0.1M phosphate buffer, pH 7.5, to yield a molar ratio of 25:1 salbutamol to HRP. Stir for one h at -15°C and 2 h at 0°C. Add 10 mg sodium bicarbonate and dialyse against 3 L of 0.01M phosphate buffer, pH 7.4 Unreacted material can be easily separated by gel filtration on Sephadex G-25.
9.2   Pretreatment of urine samples. It is recommended that the urine is centrifuged gently to remove any solid material. Dilute the clear urine sample 10 times with in the PBS-BSA buffer (6.2.3).
9.3   EIA.
9.3.1   Add 50 μL of diluted urine (9.1.4) in duplicate to the inner wells.
9.3.2   Add 50 μL standards (6.2.1) in duplicate to give six values over the range 0.04-10 μg per L.
9.3.3   Add 100 μL enzyme-conjugate solution which contains a final concentration of 70 ng per mL of HRP. This will require approximately an 8000 fold dilution in PBS-BSA buffer (6.2.3) or follow manufacturers instructions.
9.3.4   Cover the plate with plastic film, shake and incubate overnight

9.3.5   Wash the wells four times with solution 6.2.5.

9.3.6   Add the substrate solution (6.2.7) and incubate for 30 min at 18-20°C in the dark.

9.3.7   Stop the reaction by adding the stopping solution of sulphuric acid (6.2.8) to each well. Do this in the same order and at the same rate as the substrate was added to keep the reaction time near constant. Shake the plate gently and measure the absorbance at 450 nm on a plate reader.

10.0   CALCULATION OF RESULTS.

10.1 The results can be calculated using a logit transformation. The interpolation from the calibration curve using the standards where the bound enzyme activity, expressed as the logit of the ratio (in percent) between absorbance increase per 30 min, at each concentration of salbutamol (B) and the bound activity in the absence of unlabelled salbutamol (B_o) was plotted versus the log of the salbutamol concentration. A suitable EIA data handling package can be adapted to perform this calculation.

10.2. Validation. (Degand et al, 1993). The inter-assay variation was determined using data from 10 separate days. The mean slope ± SD of the curve was -(0.82 ± 0.01), CV = 1%. The mean mid-point of the curve for salbutamol was 16.8 ± 2.2 pg, CV = 6.7%.

The reproducibility of measuring incurred urines containing approximately 2 and 5 µg Salbutamol per L were;

Conc. Salbutamol µg per L	intra-assay CV(%) (n = 8)	inter-assay CV(%) (n = 8)
2	5.9	8.8
5	7.2	9.7

The blank value was determined as the mean + 3 SD using 20 blank urines from untreated veal calves was 0.14 µg. The limit of determination was 0.18 µg as required by EC Decision 89/610.

Recoveries were measured by spiking blank urines and were

Added spike (µg per L)	Measured (µg per L)	Recovery (%)
1	1.1 ± 0.2	112
2	2.2 ± 0.3	113
5	4.8 ± 0.4	97

11.   SPECIAL CASES

12.   NOTES ON PROCEDURE.

The preparation of the enzyme conjugate and coating the plates can be performed as a batch process and stored for use in subsequent assays.

13.   QUALITY CONTROLS

See section 8 of manual detailing the RMs for the ß-agonists.

14.   TEST REPORT

15.   LIST OF ABBREVIATIONS

A full list of abbreviations is given in Annex I, Section 12

16.   FLOW DIAGRAM

```
        COAT EIA PLATES---->-<--------- PREPARE ENZYME CONJUGATE
           (optional)        |                 (optional)
                             |
                             |
                             ↓
        dilute 10 x
  URINE ---------------->  EIA ------------> CALCULATE RESULTS
```

Sg 2.4.   ß-AGONISTS - A SCREENING METHOD FOR THE DETECTION OF ß-AGONISTS IN BOVINE LIVER, KIDNEY AND MEAT BY GC-MS IN THE ELECTRON IMPACT MODE FOR THE TRIMETHYLSILYL DERIVATIVES.

1.   SCOPE

This multi-residue method of analysis describes the detection of the presence of twelve individual β-agonists in samples of liver, kidney and meat of veal calves and adult cattle. The method is used officially in France and is carried out in compliance with the Residues Directive (86/469/EEC).

2.   FIELD OF APPLICATION

The method is used to perform routine screening in liver, kidney and meat from veal calves and adult cattle. The method is used to test for the presence of residues of clenbuterol, clenpenterol, hydroxymethyl-clenbuterol, salbutamol, terbutaline, cimaterol, cimbuterol, mabuterol, mapenterol, tulobuterol, fenoterol and ractopamine.
The detection limit, defined as a signal noise ratio >3 is below 2 µg per kg for most compounds.

3.   REFERENCES

Montrade, M-P., Le Bizec, B., Monteau, F., Siliart, B. and André, F. (1993), Multi-residue analysis for ß-agonistic drugs in urine of meat-producing animals by gas chromatography - mass spectrometry. Anal. Chim. Acta. <u>275</u>, 253-268

Montrade, M-P., Le Bizec, B. and André, F. (1992), Methode de recherche urinaire (screening) d'agonistes ß-adrenergiques par chromatographie gazeuse couplee à la spectrometie de masse (GC-MS) en mode impact electronique. Document LDH/92/01 Lab. Dosage Hormonaux, Nantes. DGAL/SDHA/№92.8066
[Note; This method is available in French]

Montrade, M-P., Le Bizec, B. and André, F. (1993), Methode de depistage (screening) d'agonistes ß-adrenergiques par chromatographie gazeuse couplee à la spectrometie de masse (GC-MS) en mode impact electronique. 2. Analyse de prevevements de foie, rein, viande. Document LDH/93/07 Lab. Dosage Hormonaux, Nantes.

4.   DEFINITIONS

ß-agonists content is taken to be the amount of β-agonists in the substance in question determined according to the described method and expressed as µg β-agonists per litre of test sample (liver, kidney and meat).

5.   PRINCIPLE

The method comprises 8 stages;
1. Homogenisation of sample with Stomacher and ultrasonication.
2. hydrolysis of conjugates
3. acid precipitation
4. solvent/solvent partition.
5. extract purification and concentration using mixed solid-phase extraction (SPE) chromatography
6. derivatisation

7. detection by GC-MS in electron impact mode
8. calculation and evaluation of results

6.   MATERIALS

Note: The reagents (and equipment) for which examples of their source are
quoted are known to be satisfactory, nevertheless reagents and equipment
from other sources may be equally suitable. All the reagents should be of
analytical grade or better.

6.1   Reference compounds and Standards.

Clenbuterol hydrochloride (Interchim, Montlucon, France)
Salbutamol hemisulphate, Terbutaline hemisulphate and metoprolol tartrate
(Sigma).
Cimaterol, clenpenterol (NAB 760), mabuterol, fenoterol hydrobromide and
hydroxymethyl clenbuterol (NA1141) (Boehringer Ingleheim)
Tulobuterol hydrochloride (Abbott)
Ractopamine hydrochloride (Eli Lilly)
Cimbuterol and mapenterol were synthesised by Chem Dept, University of
Rennes, France

6.2   Chemicals
6.2.1   *Helix pomatia* juice (ß-glucuronidase-arylsulfatase, Merck-4114)
6.2.2   Glacial acetic acid   (Panreac - 131008 or Merck.62)
6.2.3   Ultra-pure water (>14 M Ω.cm)
6.2.4   Methanol (Carlo-Erba RS CLHP-412002 or Merck.6009)
6.2.5   Ethyl acetate (Merck ZA-9623)
6.2.6   32% Ammonium hydroxide (Merck 5426)
6.2.7   1*M* Potassium hydroxide (Merck ZA-9018920)
6.2.8   1*M* Acetic acid
6.2.9   N-0-bis(trimethylsilyl)trifluoracetamide (BSTFA) (Regisil-270111
            or FLUKA -15244)
6.2.10   Toluene (FLUKA - 89677) by molecular sieving.
6.2.11   Sodium acetate (Merck ZA-6268)
6.2.12   Potassium dihydrogen phosphate (Merck ZA-4873)
6.2.13   Nitrogen (dried over silica gel)
6.2.14   Helium (very high purity, NSS, Carboxyque)
6.2.15   70% Perchloric acid ((Prolabo-20589293)
6.2.16   Sodium chloride (Merck-6404)
6.2.17   Isopropanol (Carlo-Erba-412421)
6.2.19   Nitrogen

6.3   Solutions
6.3.1   ß-agonists. Prepare stock solutions of the standards (6.1.1) in
            methanol (1 g per L and 100 mg per L) and store at -18°C.
6.3.2   ß-agonists. Prepare working solutions by dilution of stock
            solutions (6.3.1) with methanol to final concentrations of 10 µg
            and 1µg per mL. Store at -18°C in the dark.
6.3.3   0.2*M* Acetate buffer, pH 5.2, for hydrolysis of conjugates.
            Dissolve 16.4 g sodium acetate (6.2.11) in 900 mL water (6.2.3)
            and adjust the pH to 5.2 ± 0.1 with glacial acetic acid (6.2.2).
            Make up to 1 L with water and store at +4°C. Use for up to 1
            month.
6.3.4   0.1*M* Phosphate buffer, pH 6.0. Dissolve 13.6 ± 0.1 g potassium
            dihydrogen phosphate (6.2.12) in 900 mL water (6.2.3) and adjust
            the pH to 6.0 ± 0.1 with 1*M* potassium hydroxide (6.2.7). Make up

6.3.5   to 1 L with water and store at +4°C. Use for up to 1 month.
Mix ethyl acetate and 32% ammonium hydroxide 97:3 (v/v). 100 mL
does 16 samples. Stir/agitate the mixture prior to use and then
place into an ultra-sonic bath during step 9.13.3.

6.3.6   0.1*M* Perchloric acid (PCA) precipitating agent. Dilute 8.6 mL
70% perchloric acid to 1 L with water.

6.3.7   1*M* acetic acid; Dilute 5.6 mL glacial acetic acid (6.2.2) to 100
mL with water.

6.3.8   Isopropanol/ethyl acetate 40:60 v/v. Mix 400 mL of isopropanol
and 600 mL ethyl acetate.

7.0   EQUIPMENT
7.1.   Centrifuge
7.2   Rotary evaporator
7.3   Horizontal shaker
7.4   Stomacher (Cofralab-07555526) and plastic bags (Cofralab-
07556952)
7.5   Ultrasonic bath
7.6   Blender or mincer.
7.7   Vacuum filtration system (Vac-Elut from Analytichem
International)
7.8   Ultra-sonic probe (Cofralab-07580740)
7.9   Magnetic stirrer/agitator
7.10   Conical reaction vials for derivatisation
7.11   Heating block for reaction vials 7.10
7.12   Heating block with evaporation system using nitrogen
7.13   SPE-Columns; CLEAN SCREEN DAU 1M6 (Worldwide monitoring -
Horsham, PA, USA and sold by Technicol, Stockport, Cheshire, UK).
These columns contain 1000 mg of a mixed phase support which has
hydrophobic and ion-exchange properties.

7.14   GC-MS
7.14.1   GC; GC Hewlett Packard 5890.
Capillary column, 30 m X 0.25 mm i.d. with SE-30 stationary phase
of 0.25 μm thickness.
Injection mode; splitless over 1 minute
Injection volume; 2 μL
Injector temp. 250°C; Transfer temp. 280°C
Temp. programme;

              18° C/min   *5° C/min*
70°C (2 min) -----------> 200°C (0 min) ---------> 245°C (0 min)

      25° C/min
-----------> 300°C (12 min)

Gas; Helium at 1 mL per min and 5 psi.

7.14.2   MS; Hewlett Packard 5971 with UNIX station.
Electron Impact ionisation mode (70 eV)
Source temp. 190°C ± 5°C
Pressure, 30-40 mm Torr

Table 1.

ß-agonist	N	RT (min)	Selected ions	Mol. Ion
Tulobuterol	1	9.34	86, 194, 284	299
Mabuterol	1	10.36	86, 277, 296	382
Mapenterol	1	11.04	100, 277, 296	396
Terbutaline	3	11.67	86, 356	441
Clenbuterol	1	12.02	86, 243, 262 (264)	348
Cimaterol	1	12.14	72, 219	291
Salbutamol	3	12.27	86, 369	455
Cimbuterol	1	12.36	86, 219	305
Cimaterol	2	12.62	72, 291	363
Metoprolol (I.S)	1	12.7	72, 223	339
Cimbuterol	2	12.8	86, 291	377
Clenpenterol	1	12.86	100, 243, 262 (264)	362
Hydroxymethyl-clenbuterol (NA 1141)	2	14.05	174, 243, 262	436
Fenoterol	4	18.39	322, 356, 412	591
Ractopamine	3	18.63	250, 267	517

N is the number of TMS groups. RT are the retention times recorded in an analysis at LDH, Nantes.

8.   SAMPLES AND SAMPLING PROCEDURE.

N.B. Attention is drawn to section 6.3.1 and to ISO document 78/2-1982 and also the following notes derived from Annex II of 2052/VI/84-EN.

8.1.   Nature of the Sample; Samples shall be such as to enable the detection of residues in liver, kidney and meat as defined in Directive 64/433/EEC.

8.2.   Size of Sample; The size of the sample must be large enough to allow the method to be carried out and to allow repeat analysis where required. Each analysis needs a 10 g sample.

8.3.   The samples must be taken and packed in such a way as to allow proper identification in the laboratory.

8.4.   The method of packing, preservation and transport must maintain the integrity of the sample and not prejudice the result of the examination.
Samples for analysis within 48 h should be stored in the refrigerator otherwise they must be stored at temperatures below -18°C.

9.0.   PROCEDURE
9.1   Partially thaw the primary samples and transfer >15 g to a
          blender or mincer. Disrupt the tissues. This step is not
          necessary for liver samples.
9.2   Weigh 10 ± 1 g into a Stomacher bag. Add 15 mL acetate buffer,
          pH 5.2 (6.3.3) and disrupt for 5 min.
9.3   Transfer the contents to a 25 mL flask.
9.4   Sonicate the contents using the probe (7.8) for 0.5 sec. Wait 5
          sec and then sonicate again for 0.5 sec. Repeat this procedure
          for 10 times for liver and kidney samples (total time 50 sec) and
          20 times for meat (total time 100 sec).
9.6   Add 120 ng metoprolol as internal standard to all liver, kidney
          and meat samples including blank liver, kidney and meat samples.
          Concentration equivalent to 12 µg per kg.
9.7   To one blank liver, kidney and meat sample add 120 ng (equiv. 12
          ppb) of metoprolol and add 80 ng (equiv. 8 ppb) tulobuterol,
          fenoterol and ractopamine and 40 ng (equiv. 4 ppb) of the other
          ß-agonist standards (6.3.2).
9.8   Add 50 µL *Helix pomatia* juice (6.2.1) and incubate overnight at
          50°C (42-52°C) in a water bath or oven.
9.9   Transfer the hydrolysed liver, kidney and meats to a
          polypropylene centrifuge tube.
9.10   Add 10 mL 0.1*M* perchloric acid (6.3.6). Mix and and adjust the
          pH to 1 ± 0.3 with 70% PCA (6.2.15).
9.11   Centrifuge for 25 min at ≥7000 rpm and transfer the supernatant
          to a glass centrifuge tube.
9.12   Adjust the pH to 9.5 ± 0.3 with ammonium hydroxide (6.2.6).
9.13   Saturate the aqueous phase with sodium chloride.
9.14   Add 25 mL of a mixture of isopropanol/ethyl acetate (6.3.8) and
          shake for 15 min on a horizontal shaker.
9.15   Centrifuge at 3000 - 4000 rpm for 15 min to separate the phases.
9.16   Transfer the organic phase to a 250 mL rotary evaporation flask.
9.17   Repeat the extraction of the aqueous phase with the addition of
          15 mL of isopropanol/ethyl acetate (6.3.8). Combine the organic
          phases.
9.18   Evaporate the organic phase to dryness on a rotary evaporator at
          45 ± 5°C.
9.19   Resuspend the residue in 8 mL phosphate buffer (6.3.4) and
          transfer to a haemolysis tube. Rinse the flask with a further 4
          mL of phosphate buffer and pour into the haemolysis tube.
9.20   Centrifuge at 2000 - 3000 rpm for 15 min.
[Note This step is important when any solid material is present after the
evaporation step.]
9.21   Decant the liquid phase into a tube and add 3 mL phosphate buffer
          (6.3.4).
9.22   SPE Column extraction;
9.22.1   Place the columns on the Vac-Elut system and successively rinse
          with; 4 mL methanol; 4 mL water (6.2.3); 4 mL phosphate buffer
          (6.3.4).
9.22.2   Transfer the clear extracts with a pasteur pipette to the top of
          the column and allow to drain slowly using slight negative (ca.5
          cm Hg) pressure - it should take at least 10 min.
9.22.3   Rinse the columns using negative pressure of about 40 cm Hg with
          2 mL 1*M* acetic acid (6.2.8) and let the column dry for at least
          15 min then rinse with 12 mL methanol and dry the column under a
          strong vacuum for at least 10 min.
9.22.4   Place the ethyl acetate / ammonium hydroxide solution (6.3.5) in

	an ultra-sonic bath to agitate the mixture during step 9.22.3.
9.22.5	Elute the analytes with 12 mL the ethyl acetate / ammonium hydroxide solution (6.3.5)
9.23	Evaporate the eluate with nitrogen using an evaporation system and a heating block at 40 ± 5°C.
9.24	Dissolve the residue in 200 µL methanol with vigorous vortexing.
9.25	Transfer the solution to a reaction vial.
9.26	Dissolve and transfer to the reaction vial any remaining residue with a further 100 µL methanol and vortexing.
9.27	Evaporate the methanol to dryness using a heating block at 40° ± 5°C.
9.28	Derivatisation
9.28.1	Add 50 µL BSTFA (6.2.9) and vortex.
9.28.2	Place vials in heating block at 75°C ± 5°C for 90 ± 15 min.
9.28.3	Transfer the vials to a heating block at 40° ± 5°C. When the vials have cooled to room temperature (25°C) evaporate to dryness with nitrogen.
9.28.4	Add 25 µL toluene (6.2.10) and vortex vigorously.
9.28.5	The vials may be stored in a refrigerator at +4°C.
9.29	Inject 2 µL of 9.28.5 into the GC-MS.
9.30	GC-MS. The GC-MS is run in the selected ion monitoring mode. The ions and the retention times of the derivatives of the ß-agonists are shown in table 1.

10.0	INTERPRETATION OF RESULTS
10.1	Validity of Analysis; The criteria set out in EC Decision 256 must be fulfilled especially the following;-
10.1.1	The relative retention times for the TMS derivatives of the standard analytes in the appropriate matrix and the suspected ß-agonist must be the same.
10.1.2	The relative intensities of the selected ions to the base peak must be same as in the assay of spiked blank liver, kidney and meats and of standards.
10.1.3	The ions for the internal standard (metoprolol-monoTMS) **must** be present at the correct retention time.
10.1.4	The analysis of the blank liver, kidney and meat containing the internal standard **must** show NO evidence of carry-over of ß-agonists from the GC-MS system. This is a check for contamination of the system.

11.	SPECIAL CASES
12.	NOTES ON PROCEDURE.
13.	QUALITY CONTROLS

See section 8 of manual detailing the RMs for the ß-agonists.

14.	TEST REPORT
15.	LIST OF ABBREVIATIONS

A full list of abbreviations is given in Annex I, Section 12

16.	FLOW DIAGRAM

```
                              Homogenise
    Liver, kidney and meat ------------> PCA PRECIPITATION--------> EXTRACT
                                                                      |
                                      1. Solvent/solvent partition    |
                                      2. SPE column Chrom.            |
                                                                      |
                                                                      v
          INTERPRET RESULTS <----- GC-MS <------------ TMS DERIVATIVES
                                  (EI-mode)
```

Sg. 3.1.   ANTIBACTERIAL SUBSTANCES.   A SCREENING METHOD FOR THE DETECTION OF ANTIBACTERIAL SUBSTANCES IN FRESH MEAT USING A MODIFIED FOUR PLATE TEST.

WARNING AND SAFETY PRECAUTIONS

0.   INTRODUCTION

<u>Purpose</u>

The detection of the presence of antibacterial substances in samples of meat in compliance with the Residues Directive 86/469/EEC.

<u>Background</u>

The primary control of antibacterial substances has been carried out in the European Community using the four plate test method developed by Bogaerts and Wolf in 1980. There are several modifications to this test, this one is the official test to be used in France and developed by the Community Reference Laboratory at Fougeres in France.

1.   SCOPE

This method of analysis describes the detection but not the identification of antibacterial substances in fresh meat.

2.   FIELD OF APPLICATION.

The method is used for meat. The detection limit varies with the antibacterial substance under investigation. The sensitivity in µg per kg of the test for different antibiotics measured as the optimum sensity for detecting a 30 µL solution of standard on a 9 mm paper filter disc and giving a zone of inhibition of 12 mm is as follows;

<u>Penicillins;</u> Benzylpenicillin, 15; ampicillin, 50; cloxacillin, 400; amoxicillin, 80; oxacillin, 250; dicloxacillin, 200;
<u>Tetracyclins;</u> Oxytetracycline, 250; tetracyclin, 200; chlortetracycline, 30.
<u>Macrolides;</u> Spiramycin, 130; erythromycin, 30; tylosin, 250.
<u>Aminosides;</u> Dihydrostreptomycin, 400; gentamicin, 100.
<u>Sulphonamides;</u> All too insensitive in test.
<u>Quinolones;</u> Flumequin, 350.
<u>Chloramphenicol;</u> 8000

From Document UCM 90/01Rev.1

3.   REFERENCES.

Commission Decision, 93/256/EEC, laying down the methods for detecting residues of substances having a hormonal or thyreostatic action. [OJ. Nº L.118, 14.4.93. pp 64-74]

ISO Standard 78/2-1982 Layout for standards - Part 2: Standard for Chemical Analysis

Bogaerts, R. and Wolf, F., (1980), A standardised method for the detection of residues of anti-bacterial substances in fresh meat. Fleischwirtschaft, <u>60</u>, 672-673

Method of detecting residues of antibacterial substances in fresh meat.
Four plate test. (1993), Document UCM 90/01/Review 1. CNEVA, Lab. Med.
Vet., Fougeres, France.

4.   DEFINITIONS.

The detection of an antibacterial substance in meat is determined positive
when at least one of the four agar diffusion plates are considered to
contain residues of antibacterial substances determined according to the
described method.

5.   PRINCIPLE

An agar diffusion test is used in which:
-      an organism sensitive to antibacterial substances is inoculated
       in an agar medium in a Petri dish.
-      a disc of frozen meat is placed on the surface of the inoculated
       medium, which is incubated at the optimal temperature for growth
       of the test-organism.

Diffusion of any antibacterial substances present results in the formation
of a zone around the sample in which growth of the test-organism is
inhibited.

The following are the test-organisms;

       Bacillus subtilis at pH 6.0, pH 7.2 and pH 8.0 and *Micrococcus
       luteus* at pH 8.0.

In the agar diffusion method using *Bacillus subtilis* at pH 7.2, addition of
trimethoprim allows the detection of sulphonamides in meat due to
trimethoprim-sulphonamide synergy.

6.   MATERIALS

Note: The reagents (and equipment) for which examples of their source are
quoted are known to be satisfactory, nevertheless reagents and equipment
from other sources may be equally suitable. All the reagents must be of
analytical grade or better. Distilled water or water of comparable quality
should be used.

6.1.   CHEMICALS

6.1.1   Agar   (Difco 0140.01)
6.1.2   Sodium chloride (Merck 6404)
6.1.3   Pancreatic digest of casein (Difco 0123.01.1)
6.1.4   Tryptic digest of casein (Biomerieux 5.346.1)
6.1.5   Papaic digest of soya bean (Difco 0.436.01.3)
6.1.6   Beef extract (Pasteur 64355)
6.1.7   Nutrient agar (Pasteur 64487)
6.1.8   Glucose (Prolabo 24.370)
6.1.9   Manganese sulphate monohydrate (Prolabo 25.301)
6.1.10   Trimethoprim (Sigma, T7883)
6.1.11   Acetic acid Prolabo (20.104)
6.1.12   Penicillin G sodium (Sigma PEN-NA)
6.1.13   Sulphadimidine (Sigma S 6256)

6.1.14   0.1*M* Sodium hydroxide solution (Merck 6498)
6.1.15   Dihydrostreptomycin sulphate (Sigma S 6501)
6.1.16   Erythromycin   (Sigma E 6376)
6.1.17   Methanol (Prolabo 20.847)
6.1.18   Test agar pH 6.0.   (Merck dehydrated medium ref. 10663)
6.1.19   Test agar pH 7.2.   (Merck dehydrated medium ref. 15787)
6.1.20   Test agar pH 8.0.   (Merck dehydrated medium ref. 10664)

6.2   Solutions.
All solutions unless stated otherwise can be stored in the dark at +4° to
+6°C for up to six months.

6.2.1   Peptone-salt solution
          1 g Pancreatic digest of casein and 8.5 g sodium chloride are
          dissolved in water and made up to 1 L with a pH of 7.2 ± 0.1 at
          25°C.   The solution is autoclaved at 121°C for 15 min.
6.2.2   Tryptic soy agar (T.S.A.) (Difco - 0369)
          Dissolve 15 g pancreatic digest of casein (6.1.3), 5 g papaic
          digest of soya bean (6.1.5), 5 g sodium chloride and 15 g agar in
          water and make up to 1 L at pH 7.3 ± 0.2 at 25°C.
          The solution is autoclaved at 121°C for 15 min.
6.2.3   Culture broth for freezing of strains.
          Dissolve 5 g tryptic digest of casein (6.1.4) and 3 g beef
          extract (6.1.6) in water and make up to 1 L at pH 6.8 ± 0.2 at
          20°C.
          The solution is autoclaved at 121°C for 20 min.
6.2.4   Finley and Fields Medium.
          Dissolve 15 g nutrient agar (6.1.7), 5 g glucose (6.1.8) and 30
          mg manganese sulphate monohydrate (6.1.9) in water and make up to
          1 L at pH 7.0 ± 0.2 at 25°C.
          The solution is autoclaved at 121°C for 15 min.
6.2.5   Trimethoprim solution
          In a 500 mL volumetric flask dissolve 50 mg trimethoprim (6.1.10)
          in 5 mL 5% acetic acid (6.1.11) and dilute to 500 mL with water.
          Immediately before use, dilute this stock solution to 1/20 to
          give a final concentration of 0.005 mg per mL.   The stock
          solution can be stored for up to 2 weeks at +4°C to +6°C.
6.3   Standard Solutions.
6.3.1   Penicillin Solution
          Use a 100 mL volumetric flask. Dissolve a quantity of penicillin
          G sodium (6.1.12) equivalent to 100,000 I.U. (about 61 mg) in
          water and dilute to 100 mL with water. Immediately before use,
          dilute this stock solution to 1/100 and then again to 1/50 to
          give a final concentration of 0.02 I.U. per mL.   The stock
          solution can be stored for up to 4 days at +4°C to +6°C.
6.3.2   Sulphadimidine solution.
          Use a 50 mL volumetric flask. Dissolve a quantity of
          sulphadimidine (6.1.13) equivalent to 50 mg active substance in 5
          mL 0.1*M* sodium hydroxide (6.1.14) and dilute to 50 mL with water.
          Immediately before use, dilute this stock solution to 1/50 to
          give a final concentration of 0.02 mg per mL.   The stock solution
          can be stored for up to 2 weeks at +4°C to +6°C.
6.3.3   Dihydrostreptomycin solution.
          Use a 50 mL volumetric flask. Dissolve a quantity of
          dihydrostreptomycin sulphate (6.1.15) equivalent to 50 mg active
          substance (about 64 mg) in water and dilute to 50 mL with water.
          Immediately before use, dilute this stock solution to 1/200 to

give a final concentration of 5 μg per mL. The stock solution can be stored for up to one month at +4°C to +6°C.

6.3.4   Erythromycin solution.
Use a 50 mL volumetric flask. Dissolve a quantity of erythromycin (6.1.16) equivalent to 50 mg active substance (about 54 mg) in 3 mL methanol (6.1.17) and dilute to 50 mL with water. Immediately before use, dilute this stock solution to 1/200 and then again to 1/20 to give a final concentration of 0.25 μg per mL. The stock solution can be stored for up to 2 weeks at +4°C to +6°C.

6.4   Sensitive organisms
6.4.1   *Bacillus subtilis* test organism obtained as *Bacillus subtilis* B.G.A from Merck as ampoules containing a suspension of 8×10^6 to 5×10^7 spores per mL. (Ref № 10649)
6.4.2   *Micrococcus luteus* as test organism *Micrococcus luteus*, ATCC 9341 strain, available from the Institut Pasteur in freeze-dried form.

7.0   EQUIPMENT

7.1   Incubators capable of maintaining temperatures of 30° ± 1°C and 37° ± 1°C.
7.2   Freezer -18°C
7.3   Refrigerator at +4 to +6°C
7.4   Centrifuge (JOUAN JR4.11 or equivalent)
7.5   Water bath capable of operating from room temperature to 100°C
7.6   Vortex mixer
7.7   Balance sensitive to 0.1 mg
7.8   pH meter of calibration accuracy 0.1 pH unit at 20°C
7.9   Automatic micropipette, 10 to 100 μL
7.10   Disposable tips for pipette 7.9
7.11   Cork borer, 8 mm diameter
7.12   Sharpener for cork borer (7.11)
7.13   Scalpel and blades
7.14   Wire loop of nickel-chrome or Pasteur pipettes
7.15   Fine pointed forceps
7.16   Stainless steel trays
7.17   Discs of absorbent paper, diameter 6 mm (Durieux)
7.18   Flat-bottomed plastic Petri dishes, diameter 90 mm
7.19   Borosilicate glass bottles with screw tops, 125 mL, 250 mL and 500 mL
7.20   Roux flask, 1 L
7.21   Graduated borosilicate glass beakers, 1 L
7.22   Volumetric borosilicate glass flasks, 20 mL, 25 mL, 50 mL, 100 mL and 500 mL
7.23   Graduated borosilicate glass cylinders, 10 mL, 25 mL, 50 mL
7.24   Borosilicate glass culture tubes of 16 x 160 mm with and without screw tops
7.25   Sterile centrifuge tubes of at least 60 mL capacity, with caps
7.26   Sterile 10 mL pipettes graduated in 0.1 mL
7.27   Sterile and non-sterile 5 mL pipettes graduated in 0.1 mL
7.28   Sterile and non-sterile 2 mL pipettes graduated in 0.02 mL or 0.05 mL
7.29   Sterile and non-sterile 1 mL pipettes graduated in 0.01 mL
7.30   Glass beads diameter 3 mm
7.31   Plastic 1.5 mL tubes with caps (Eppendorf)

7.32   Phase-contrast microscope.

8.   SAMPLES AND SAMPLING PROCEDURE.

N.B. Attention is drawn to section 6.3.1 and to ISO document 78/2-1982 and
also the following notes derived from Annex II of 2052/VI/84-EN.

8.1.   Nature of the Sample; Samples shall be such as to enable the
           detection of residues in meat as defined in Directive 64/433/EEC.

8.2.   Size of Sample; The size of the sample must be large enough to
           allow the method to be carried out and to allow repeat analysis
           where required.

8.3.   The samples must be taken and packed in such a way as to allow
           proper identification in the laboratory.

8.4.   The method of packing, preservation and transport must maintain
           the integrity of the sample and not prejudice the result of the
           examination. When practicable the meat should be collected under
           sterile conditions.
           Samples for the analysis of antibacterial substances should be
           stored and transported at temperatures below -18°C.

9.   PROCEDURE
(Note; This four plate test is applicable to meat.)
9.1   Preparation of Sensitive Organisms.
9.1.1   *Bacillus subtilis*
9.1.1.1   *Bacillus subtilis* stock inoculum. Prepare enough to last for 2
           years.
           Use the suspension from the commercial source (6.4.1) to
           inoculate in streaks two T.S.A. (6.2.2) plates for isolation and
           confirmation of identification.
           Incubate for 16 to 18 h at 30°C
           From a few colonies removed from one of the plates, inoculate one
           or more tubes of culture broth for freezing of strains. Incubate
           at 30°C for 3 to 6 h.
           Divide the culture (which is in the exponential growth phase)
           into fractions of 0.5 to 1 ml in capped microtubes (7.31). Store
           at -18°C for up to two years.
9.1.1.2   Preparation of spore suspension. From the stock inoculum
           (9.1.1.1) perform three successive subcultures in slant T.S.A to
           reactivate the strain. In parallel inoculate in streaks two
           T.S.A. (6.2.2) plates for isolation and confirmation of
           identification.
           Incubate for 16 to 18 h at 30°C
           Harvest a culture of less than 24 h in the form of a suspension
           using about 10 glass beads and 2 mL of peptone salt solution
           (6.2.1).
           Transfer the suspension to the surface of 200 mL of Finley and
           Fields sporulation medium (6.2.4) prepoured into a Roux flask.
           Incubate at 30°C for at least five days, monitoring the advance
           of sporulation by observation of samples of the culture under a
           phase-contrast microscope (7.32). If necessary extend the
           incubation.
           After incubation, harvest the spores with glass beads and 50 mL

peptone-salt solution (6.2.1).
Centrifuge the spore suspension for 15 min at 4,400 g.
Discard the supernatant and resuspend the pellet in 50 mL
peptone-salt solution.
Centrifuge, discard the supernatant and resuspend the pellet in
50 mL peptone-salt solution.
Centrifuge and discard the supernatant and resuspend the pellet
in 30 mL peptone-salt solution and heat to 70°C for exactly 35
min.
Store the spore suspension at +4°C.

9.1.1.3 Enumeration of spore suspension. This is required in order to
determine the spore concentration. After suitable dilution to
10^{-10} in diluent (6.2.1) incubate at 30°C for 24 h before
enumeration.

9.1.1.4 Preparation of test plates.

9.1.1.4.1 pH 6.0 Agar
Inoculate the molten agar medium (6.1.18) cooled to 45°C with
pre-diluted spore suspension (9.1.1.2) to give a spore
concentration of 5×10^4 per mL. Transfer 5 mL of inoculated
medium to a Petri dish and allow the agar to cool on a cold
horizontal surface.
If not used on the day of preparation, these test plates may be
stored in a refrigerator (7.3) for up to one week.

9.1.1.4.2 pH 7.2 Agar
Inoculate the molten agar medium (6.1.19) cooled to 45°C with
pre-diluted spore suspension (9.1.1.2) to give a spore
concentration of 5×10^4 per mL. Add trimethoprim solution
(6.2.5) to the agar to a concentration of 1% (v/v). Transfer 5
mL of inoculated medium to a Petri dish and allow the agar to
cool on a cold horizontal surface.
If not used on the day of preparation, these test plates may be
stored in a refrigerator (7.3) for up to two days.

9.1.1.4.3 pH 8.0 Agar
Inoculate the molten agar medium (6.1.20) cooled to 45°C with
pre-diluted spore suspension (9.1.1.2) to give a spore
concentration of 5×10^4 per mL. Transfer 5 mL of inoculated
medium to a Petri dish and allow the agar to cool on a cold
horizontal surface.
If not used on the day of preparation, these test plates may be
stored in a refrigerator (7.3) for up to one week.

9.1.2   *Micrococcus luteus*

9.1.2.1 *Micrococcus luteus* stock inoculum. Prepare enough to last for 2
years.
Rehydrate the freeze dried strain (6.4.2) in 2 mL of peptone-salt
solution(6.2.1). Use the suspension to inoculate in streaks two
T.S.A. (6.2.2) plates for isolation and confirmation of
identification.
Incubate for at least 24 h at 37°C
From a few colonies removed from one of the plates, inoculate one
or more tubes of culture broth for freezing of strains. Incubate
at 37°C for 3 to 6 h.
Divide the culture (which is in the exponential growth phase)
into fractions of 0.5 to 1 ml in capped microtubes (7.31).

9.1.2.2 Preparation of test inoculum. From the stock inoculum (9.1.2.1)
perform three successive subcultures in slant T.S.A to reactivate
the strain. In parallel inoculate in streaks two T.S.A.

(6.2.2) plates for isolation and confirmation of identification. Incubate at 37°C for at least 24 h.
Harvest a culture of less than 24 h in the form of a suspension using about 10 glass beads and 2 mL of peptone salt solution (6.2.1).
Transfer the suspension to the surface of 200 mL of T.S.A. (6.2.2) prepoured into a Roux flask.
Incubate at 37°C for at least 24 h.
After incubation, harvest the culture with about 20 glass beads and 10 mL peptone-salt solution (6.2.1). Dilute to 50 mL in the bottle.
Store the suspension at +4° to 6°C for up to one month.

9.1.2.3   Enumeration of bacterial suspension. This is required in order to determine the germ concentration. After suitable dilution to 10^{-10} in diluent (6.2.1) incubate at 37°C for 24 to 48 h before enumeration.

9.1.2.4   Preparation of test plates.
Inoculate the molten agar medium (6.1.20) cooled to 45°C with pre-diluted bacterial suspension (9.1.2.2) to give a bacteria concentration of 5×10^{4} per mL. Transfer 5 mL of inoculated medium to a Petri dish and allow the agar to cool on a cold horizontal surface.
If not used on the day of preparation, these test plates may be stored in a refrigerator (7.3) for up to one week.

9.2   Preparation of samples.
Remove the samples from the deep-freeze a few minutes before use and place them on a stainless steel tray.
Remove from each sample a cylindrical plug 8 mm in diameter and two cm long using a cork borer.
Push the meat from the borer and cut into eight discs of 2 mm thickness using a scalpel.
Use forceps to place two discs opposite each other in each of the four test plates (9.1.1.4.1, 9.1.1.4.2, 9.1.1.4.3 and 9.1.2.4).
In this way it is possible to place in each plate up to six discs, corresponding to three test samples. The discs should form a circle about 1 cm from the rim of the plate.

9.3   Diffusion technique.
9.3.1   *Bacillus subtilis* at pH 6.0.
Use forceps to place a disc of filter paper (7.17) in the centre of the dish. Transfer 10 µL penicillin solution (6.3.1) to the disc.
Incubate the plates for at least 18 h. at 30°C.
After incubation, the disc impregnated with standard solution should present a zone of inhibition of minimum width 6 mm (the width is the distance between the edge of the disc and the outer limit of the zone of inhibition).

9.3.2   *Bacillus subtilis* at pH 7.2.
Use forceps to place a disc of filter paper (7.17) in the centre of the dish. Transfer 10 µL sulphadimidine solution (6.3.2) to the disc.
Incubate the plates for at least 18 h. at 30°C.
After incubation, the disc impregnated with standard solution should present a zone of inhibition of minimum width 6 mm.

9.3.3   *Bacillus subtilis* at pH 8.0.
Use forceps to place a disc of filter paper (7.17) in the centre of the dish. Transfer 10 µL dihydrostreptomycin solution (6.3.3)

9.3.4   *Micrococcus luteus* at pH 8.0.
to the disc.
Incubate the plates for at least 18 h. at 30°C.
After incubation, the disc impregnated with standard solution
should present a zone of inhibition of minimum width 6 mm.

9.3.4   *Micrococcus luteus* at pH 8.0.
Use forceps to place a disc of filter paper (7.17) in the centre
of the dish. Transfer 10 µL erythromycin solution (6.3.4) to the
disc.
Incubate the plates for at least 24 h. at 37°C.
After incubation, the disc impregnated with standard solution
should present a zone of inhibition of minimum width 6 mm.

10.0   CALCULATION OF RESULTS

The detection of an antibacterial substance in meat is determined positive
when at least one of the four agar diffusion plates is considered to
contain residues of antibacterial substances as shown by suitable duplicate
zones of inhibition of at least 2 mm in width.

11.   SPECIAL CASES

12.   NOTES ON PROCEDURE

12.1. The action level at which reanalysis of a suspected positive must be
decided (e.g only one positive zone of inhibition on a single plate). Also
similar decisions need to be taken when to proceed to a confirming method.

13.   QUALITY CONTROLS

14.   TEST REPORT

15.   LIST OF ABBREVIATIONS

A full list of abbreviations is given in Annex I, Section 12

16.   FLOW DIAGRAM

```
FROZEN MEAT ----> CORE ----> 8 DISCS -----> 2 DISCS/PLATE (4 PLATES)
                                                         |
                                                         |
                                                         |
                                                         ↓
         +ve or -ve RESULT <----- VIEW <---------- INCUBATE
```

Sg. 3.2.   SULPHONAMIDES - SCREENING METHOD USING HPTLC FOR THE DETECTION OF SULPHONAMIDES IN THE MEAT OF FARM ANIMALS.

WARNING AND SAFETY PRECAUTIONS

SAFETY

Organic solvents - all organic solvents must be treated as potentially   hazardous and all procedures using them must be performed in a fume cupboard.

FIRST AID
1. Solvents, acids and alkalis in contact with skin - wash with copious amounts of cold water. Splashes in the eye - irrigate with water and seek medical attention immediately.
2. Cuts - seek assistance of first aider immediately.
3. Burns and frostbite - run affected part under cold water (burns) or tepid water (frostbite) for 10 minutes and seek medical attention.

0.   INTRODUCTION

Sulphonamides are antibiotics widely used prophylactically and as growth enhancers.
To minimise risks from residues in the human diet, withdrawal periods are set. High residue levels exceeding the MRLs may occur if these periods are not adhered to. The MRL for sulphonamides is 100 μg per kg and for dapsone 25 μg per kg.

1.   SCOPE

This method of analysis describes the detection of sulphonamides and dapsone in meat.

2.   FIELD OF APPLICATION.

The method is described to be used for meat from adult cattle, calves, pigs and poultry. This method is used in The Netherlands to monitor residue levels in tissues taken at slaughter and is carried out in compliance with the Residues Directive (86/469/EEC). The minimum limit of determination for sulphonamides is 2 μg per kg of meat.

3.   REFERENCES.

Commission Decision, 93/256/EEC, laying down the methods for detecting residues of substances having a hormonal or thyrostatic action. [OJ. № L.118, 14.4.93. pp 64-74]

ISO Standard 78/2-1982 Layout for standards - Part 2: Standard for Chemical Analysis

Beek, W.M.J., Binnendijk, G.M., Smidt, R.A., Keukens, H.J. and de Vries, P.H.U. (1992), Vlees - Screening von sulfonamiden en dapson - HPTLC. RIKILT-DLO. SOP № A0644, DAM code; 0800302, Edition 2. Sept. 1992.

The USDA, USA, has developed a pig-side TLC test called the "Swine urine screen Sulfa-on-site" (SOS-test).

4.   DEFINITIONS.

Sulphonamides or dapsone content is taken to mean the amount of
sulphonamides or dapsone in meat determined according to the described
method and expressed as µg analyte per kg test sample.

5.   PRINCIPLE.

The method consists of four stages;-
    - Homogenisation and extraction with dichloromethane
    - Clean up with Sep-Pak silica cartridge using phosphate buffer
    - Back extraction to ethyl acetate
    - HPTLC chromatography on silica gel plates with flourescence detection.

6   MATERIALS

Note: The reagents (and equipment) for which examples of their source are
quoted are known to be satisfactory, nevertheless reagents and equipment
from other sources may be equally suitable. All the reagents must be of
analytical grade or better.

6.1   Chemicals
6.1.1   Acetone (Merck - 14)
6.1.2   n-butanol (Merck - 1990)
6.1.3   Chloroform (Merck - 2445)
6.1.4   Dichloromethane (Merck - 6050)
6.1.5   Di-potassium hydrogen phosphate (Merck - 5104)
6.1.6   Ethyl acetate, Uvasol grade, (Merck 863)
6.1.7   Fluorescamine (Sigma - F-9878)
6.1.8   Methanol (Merck - 6009)
6.1.9   Sodium hydroxide (Merck - 6495)
6.1.10   Sodium sulphate (Merck - 6649)
6.1.11   Light Petroleum (Merck - 909)
6.1.12   Distilled water
6.1.13   Orthophosphoric acid (Merck - 573)

6.2   Solutions
6.2.1   Sodium hydroxide 0.1M, Dissolve 4 g sodium hydroxide in 1 L
            water.
6.2.2   Phosphate buffer, 0.05M; pH = 10: Dissolve 4.36 g di-potassium
            hydrogen phosphate (6.1.5) in ca. 400 mL water. Adjust the pH to
            10 using sodium hydroxide solution (6.2.1) and make up to 1 L
            with water.
6.2.3   HPTLC solvent. Mix 4 volumes of chloroform with 1 volume of n-
            butanol. Prepare on day of analysis.
6.2.4   Fluorescamine solution; Dissolve 5 mg fluorescamine (6.1.7) in
            50 mL acetone. Solution is stable in the dark for up to two
            weeks.
6.2.5   Orthophophoric acid, 0.5M; Add about 50 mL water to a measuring
            cylinder and add carefully 3.4 mL orthophosphoric acid (6.1.13).
            Make up to 100 mL with water.

6.3   Standards.
6.3.1   Standards for Sulphonamides from Serva.
6.3.2   Stock solutions, ca. 100 µg per mL. Weigh accurately ca. 10 mg
            standard into a 100 mL graduated flask and make up to 100 mL with
            methanol (6.1.8). Store in the dark at 4 - 8°C . Stable not

6.3.3   Working standards, 1 μg per mL. Pipette 1 mL stock standard
        (6.3.2) into a 100 mL graduated flask and make up to 100 mL with
        methanol (6.1.8). Store in the dark at 4 - 8°C . Stable not
        longer than one month.
6.3.4   Spiking solution, 1 μg per mL.   Pipette 1 mL stock standard
        (6.3.2) into a 100 mL graduated flask and make up to 100 mL with
        water. Make fresh on day of analysis.

7   EQUIPMENT
7.1   Analytical balance
7.2   Balance
7.3   Vibromixer
7.4   Stomacher 400 (Labblender)
7.5   Ultrasonic bath (Bransonic 32)
7.6   Centrifuge
7.7   Glasswool or paper filters (S&S 595½ Φ 15 cm)
7.8   Sep-Pak^R silica cartridges (Waters - 51900)
7.9   Evacuator system for Sep-Pak cartridges
7.10   Heating block with nitrogen evaporation system.
7.11   HPTLC plates 10 x 10 cm, Kieselgel 60 without fluorescence
        indicator (Merck - 5631)
7.12   Micropipette, 5 μL
7.13   TLC tank system for 10 x 10 cm plates.
7.14   Kitchen blender (Moulinette or Waring)
7.15   Syringes, 50mL, 2 mL
7.16   Other standard laboratory glassware
7.17   Transilluminator (UV) at 366 nm
7.18   pH papers pH 5-9.
7.19   pH meter
7.20   Stomacher bags 1 L
7.21   Camag Unispray kit (Camag)
7.22   System for photographing the yellow-green fluorescent spots.
        Recommended filters for photography are Wratten № 2E, Kodak CC10M
        and Wratten 1A. Exposure 22.5 sec at f 8 on Polaroid 600 plus)

8.   SAMPLES AND SAMPLING PROCEDURE.

N.B. Attention is drawn to section 6.3.1 and to ISO document 78/2-1982 and
also the following notes derived from Annex II of 2052/VI/84-EN.

8.1. Nature of the Sample; Samples shall be such as to enable the
detection of residues in meat as defined in Directive 64/433/EEC.

8.2. Size of Sample; The size of the sample must be large enough to allow
the method to be carried out and to allow repeat analysis where required.

8.3. The samples must be taken and packed in such a way as to allow proper
identification in the laboratory.

8.4. The method of packing, preservation and transport must maintain the
integrity of the sample and not prejudice the result of the examination.
Samples for the analysis of Sulphonamides must be stored at temperatures
below -18°C.

9.   PROCEDURE
9.1   Quality controls; Meat from animals known not to have been
        treated or contaminated with sulphonamides or dapsone is blended
        to prepare a blank sample and a positive control sample and
        stored at -20°C until day of analysis. For the positive control
        add the equivalent of 10 µg per kg of sulphonamides and/or
        dapsone to the blank meat and wait 15 min before blending.
9.2   Meat samples for testing are blended and stored at -20°C until
        day of analysis.
9.3   Primary extraction
9.3.1   Poultry meat (chicken);
        Weigh 10 g blended meat for samples 9.1 and 9.2 and mix with 25
        mL dichloromethane in a Stomacher. Extract for 2 min with the
        Stomacher. Filter through glass wool into a 100 mL flask.
        Repeat this extraction step twice more. Proceed to 9.4.
9.3.2   Cattle and Pig meat;
        Weigh 10 g blended meat for samples 9.1 and 9.2 and mix with 25
        mL dichloromethane in a beaker. Place in an ultrasonic bath for
        10 min. Do not allow the temperature to exceed 40°C. Filter
        through glass wool into a 100 mL flask. Repeat this extraction
        step twice more.
9.4   Add 25 mL light petroleum to the combined dichloromethane
        extracts.
9.5   Sep-Pak clean up;
9.5.1   Connect a 50 mL reservoir to a Sep-Pak cartridge (7.8).
9.5.2   Put the whole contents of the primary extract (9.4) onto the
        column. Rinse the flask with 5 mL dichloromethane and transfer
        the solution to the column. [Note - the 50 mL volumne should
        pass through the column in about 15 min with slight suction.
9.5.3   Elute the sulphonamides with 5 mL phophate buffer, pH 10 (6.2.2).
        Collect the first three mL in a calibrated tube.
9.5.4   Control the pH with the aid of pH papers (7.18). Bring the pH of
        the collected eluate to 6.5 to 7 with phosphoric acid (6.2.5) or
        with sodium hydroxide (6.2.1).
9.6   Extract the eluate (9.5.4) with 1 mL ethyl acetate by mixing on a
        Vibromixer for 30 sec and then separating the phases using a
        bench centrifuge. Transfer 0.5 mL of the ethyl acetate phase to
        a 4 mL vial. Evaporate to dryness under a stream of nitrogen and
        take up the residue by vortexing in 50 µL ethyl acetate.
9.7   HPTLC
9.7.1   Using the plan in 9.7.1.1, pipette 10 µL of sample extract onto
        the plate, 1.5 cm from the bottom of the plate and with a
        distance of about 0.75 - 1 cm between the spotting places. Use a
        stream of nitrogen to control the evaporation on the plate.
        Place the extracts for quality controls, standards and a
        reference sample as in 9.7.1.1.
9.7.1.1 Order of spots on plate from left to right, 1.5 cm from bottom
        edge.
        1. Standard; 2. Blank; 3. Spiked blank; 4. test sample 1;
        5. test 2; 6. test 3; 7. standard; 8. test 4; 9. test 5;
        10. test 6; 11. reference standard; 12. standard

9.7.2   Place the solvent (6.2.3) in the tank to a depth of 0.5 cm and
        allow 30 min for equilibration.
9.7.3   Place the plate in the solvent and allow the system to run until
        the solvent front has moved 4 cm.

9.7.4 Remove the plate and mark the position of the solvent front with a pencil.

9.7.5 Dry the plate for 20 min in a fume cupboard. Spray the plate with the fluorescamine solution (6.2.4). After 5 min view the plates under UV light at 366 nm.

9.7.6 The sulphonamide spots can be seen to have a characteristic yellow-green colour.

9.7.7 Record the spots if positives are identified either by marking with a pencil or photographically (see 7.22).

10 INTERPRETATION OF RESULTS

10.1 The R_f values for the sulphonamides of interest and Dapsone are;- (data from RIKILT-DLO, NL)

Component	R_f
Sulphanilamide	0.33
Sulphathiazole	0.39
Mono-acetyl dapsone	0.43
Sulphadiazine	0.57
Dapsone	0.60
Sulphadimidine	0.64
Sulphachlorpyrazine	0.69
Sulphaquinoxaline	0.70
Sulphadimethoxine	0.78
Sulphadoxine	0.80

10.2 The sulphonamide spots can be seen to have a characteristic yellow-green colour.

10.3 The analytes in the spiked blanks must be detected.

10.4 Stability; The spots disappear very quickly if exposed to daylight and within 2 hours if kept in the dark. The plates should be viewed within 30 min of spraying with fluorescamine.

10.5 Identification of dapsone. The presence of dapsone is valid if its metabolite mono-acetyl dapsone is also detected on the plate.

11. SPECIAL CASES.

12. NOTES ON PROCEDURE.

The fluorescent spots are unstable in light.

13. SAMPLE CONTROLS

14. TEST REPORT

15. LIST OF ABBREVIATIONS.

See abbreviations in Annex I, Section 12 of Manual.

16. FLOW DIAGRAM

Homogenise meat -----> extract with dichloromethane -----> C18 Sep-Pak

Identify under UV light <-- Spray with fluorescamine <------- HPTLC

Sg 3.3.   CHLORAMPHENICOL - RIA SCREENING METHOD FOR THE DETECTION OF CHLORAMPHENICOL IN MEAT, MILK AND EGGS.

WARNING AND SAFETY PRECAUTIONS

SAFETY
Organic solvents - all organic solvents must be treated as potentially hazardous and all procedures using them must be performed in a fume cupboard.

0.   INTRODUCTION

Chloramphenicol (CAP) is a bacteriostatic with a broad spectrum of activity, frequently used for therapeutic and prophylolactic purposes in veterinary medicine. The EEC, through the CVMP, specifically does not recommend the use of CAP in laying hens and lactating cattle.

1.   SCOPE

The use of CAP is restricted throughout the EEC. To ensure that farmers are not continuing to use chloramphenicol in laying hens or lactating cattle, and to control the use in meat producing animals samples are collected on farms and at slaughterhouses and screened for the presence of this compound. Whenever there is a positive screening result, this must be confirmed.

2.   FIELD OF APPLICATION.

This method is used for confirmation of the presence of chloramphenicol in meat, milk and eggs. The detection limit for milk and eggs is 1 µg per L or kg of matrix and for meat 10 µg per kg, for Chloramphenicol.

3.   REFERENCES.

Commission Decision, 93/256/EEC, laying down the methods for detecting residues of substances having a hormonal or thyrostatic action. [OJ. № L.118, 14.4.93. pp 64-74]

ISO Standard 78/2-1982 Layout for standards - Part 2: Standard for Chemical Analysis

ISO Standard 5725 (1986)

Radioimmunoassay for the measurement of chloramphenicol residues in eggs, milk and meat. (1993) Bundesgesundheitsampt, Berlin.

Arnold, D., 1st Draft of the summary report of EEC Collaborative study "Chloramphenicol Methods", July 1987 - February 1988.

Arnold, D., vom Berg, D., Boertz, A.k., Mallik, U. and Somogyi, A. (1984), Radioimmunologische Bestimmung von Chloramphenicol-Rückständen in Musculatur, Milch und Eiern, Archiv. für Lebensmittel Hygiene, 35, 121-148

Preiß, A., Balizs, G., Bensch-Girke, Th., Gude, A., Boenke, A. and Kroker, R., (1993) Preparation of reference materials for chloramphenicol in muscle and milk - data on quality criteria. In Proc. Euroresidues II conference, Veldhoven, NL, Vol. 2. 558-562

4.	DEFINITIONS.

Chloramphenicol content is taken to mean the amount of chloramphenicol in
meat, eggs and milk determined according to the described method and
expressed as μg chloramphenicol per L or kg test sample.

5.	PRINCIPLE.

The method comprises three stages
 - Samples are extracted using ethyl acetate.
 - purification of extract with solvent-solvent partition (SPE for milk)
 - detection and quantification by RIA

6.	MATERIALS

6.1.	Chemicals

Note: The chemicals were all of analytical grade. Reagents of similar
quality may be used from other sources.

6.1.1	Ethyl acetate, (Merck 9623).
6.1.2	Methanol, (Merck 6009)
6.1.3	Chloroform, (Merck 2445)
6.1.4	n-Hexane, (Merck 4371)
6.1.5	Acetonitrile, (Merck 17)
6.1.6	Isooctane (Merck 4727)
6.1.7	Sodium Chloride (Merck 6404)
6.1.8	Ethanol (absolute) (Merck 983.25)
6.1.9	Sheep albumin (Sigma, A-3264)
6.1.10	Potassium dihydrogen phosphate (Merck 4871)
6.1.11	Disodium hydrogen phosphate (Merck 6586)
6.1.12	Sodium azide (Merck 6688)
6.1.13	Charcoal, Norit A pract. (Serva 30890)
6.1.14	Dextran, M.Wt ca 70,000 Daltons (Pharmacia 1702800)
6.1.15	Scintillation fluid compatible with aqueous phases (Beckmann
	270453721A)
6.1.16	Chloramphenicol (Sigma C-0378)

[Note;   The radiolabelled CAP (6.1.17) and the specific antiserum (6.1.18)
are not available commercially but may be purchased by negotiation with the
BGA, Berlin]
6.1.17	Radiolabelled Propionyl-CAP. 3-hydroxy-3-(4'-nitrophenyl)-2-
	($\underline{N}$/^{3}H/propionyl)-aminopropane-1-ol; specific activity, 61 Ci per
	mmol (2.26 TBq per mmol), TRQ 5394. (Custom synthesised for BGA).
	Supplied in ethanol at 14.47 μCi per mL. Store at -20°C.
6.1.18	Sheep antiserum against CAP (BGA)
6.1.19	Distilled water
6.1.20	Supply of ice.

6.2	CAP Standards.

6.2.1	Standard solution; 10 μg per mL chloramphenicol in ethanol.
	Store at 4°C. Stable for at least six months.

6.2.2	Working Standards	Within one week of use, dilute intermediate
	solutions with phosphate buffer (6.3.1) to give a set of 9

standards with concentrations in ng per mL equal to 10, 25, 50, 100, 125, 250, 500, 1250, 2500.
[Note; The performance characteristics of the assay were determined using 20 calibration points.]

6.3	Solutions.
6.3.1	Phosphate buffer, pH 7.45. Dissolve 3.4 g KH_2PO_4, 3.55 g Na_2HPO_4 and 0.5 g sodium azide in 950 mL water. Adjust the pH to 7.45 and make up to 1 L with water.
6.3.2	Antiserum predilution 1/200 (w/w); Contains 2.5 mg sheep antiserum (6.1.18) per mL phosphate buffer. Store at -20°C. If the material is in a lyophilised form supplied by BGA then; - centrifuge tube to prevent losses - add 1 mL water - shake overnight at 4°C to reconstitute the antiserum
6.3.3	Antiserum working solution, 1/75,000 (w/w); Dilute an aliquot of the antiserum predilution solution (6.3.2) 375 fold. Store at +4°C.
6.3.4	Radioligand working solution. An aliquot of the radiolabelled analogue (6.1.17) is diluted in phosphate buffer to give a 1.08 nanomolar solution. Prepare weekly and store at 4°C.
6.3.5	Charcoal suspension; Mix 3 g charcoal, 0.5 g dextran and 0.25 g sheep albumin in 1 L phosphate buffer, pH 7.45 (6.3.1).
6.3.6	Acetonitrile / 4% sodium chloride (1/1, v/v); Add an equal volume of acetonitrile to a 4% solution of sodium chloride in water.

7.   EQUIPMENT

7.1	Dispensing pipettes; 0-20 µL, 0-1000 µL, 0-5000 µL
7.2	Centrifuge tubes with stoppers, 10-12 mL, 15-20 mL (Schmidt, Germany)
7.3	Micro test tubes (Eppendorf 3812)
7.4	Universal vials, 10-20 mL with screw tops. (Beckmann)
7.5	Volumetric stoppered flasks, 10 mL and 100 mL
7.6	Automatic dispenser ("Dispensette", Brand, Germany)
7.7	Scintillation vials (beckmann)
7.8	Speed Vac (Savant, USA)
7.9	Stirrer for tubes, type HEIDOLPH "Top-mix"
7.10	Rotary stirrer with rotating plates, type HEIDOLPH "Reax 2"
7.11	Vortex mixer
7.12	Fume cupboards
7.13	Vacuum centrifuge (UniEquip, Germany)
7.14	Liquid scintillation counter (Beckmann)
7.15	Cold storage space, ca -18° to -20°C
7.16	Working cold room/refrigerator space
7.17	Pasteur pipettes
7.18	Tubes 75 mm x 12 mm
7.19	Analytical balance
7.20	Refrigerated centrifuge, (Sorvall, USA)
7.21	Bench centrifuge
7.22	C-18 cartridges (Sep-Pak, C-18, Waters-Millipore Cat.№ 519)

8.   SAMPLES AND SAMPLING PROCEDURE.

N.B. Attention is drawn to section 6.3.1 and ISO document 78/2-1982 and the following notes derived from Annex II of 2052/VI/84-EN.

8.1. Nature of the Sample; Samples of milk, meat and eggs shall be such
as to enable the detection of residues.

8.2. Size of Sample; The size of the sample must be large enough to allow
the reference method to be carried out and to allow repeat analysis where
required.

8.3. The sample must be cooled after collection and stored at $\leq$ -20°C
pending analysis.

9.   PROCEDURE

9.1.   Preparation of test sample;
9.1.1   Meat; Take a coherent part of muscle tissue and mince at 0-4°C.
           In the case of frozen meat add the excess liquid, produced when
           the meat is thawed, quantitatively to the minced meat and mix
           well. The sample can now be stored at 0-4°C fro analysis within
           the next 48 h. For prolonged storage, freeze aliquots at -20°C
           or preferably at -80°C to ensure stability.
9.1.2   Eggs. Should be homogenised.
9.1.3   Milk; Samples taken from raw milk or any type of homogeneous
           undenatured heated milk.
9.2   Primary extraction of Meat and Eggs;
9.2.1   Place 3 g of comminuted meat or homogenised eggs into a
           centrifuge tube.
9.2.2   To the egg samples add dropwise 5 mL acetonitrile while mixing.
           To the meat samples add 8 mL acetonitrile/4% sodium chloride
           solution (6.3.6).
9.2.3   Mix well or homogenise.
9.2.4   Centrifuge 10 min at 4000 g.
9.2.5   Weigh the supernatant into a universal vial.
9.2.6   Pipette ca. 1/6th (w/w) of the supernatant into a glass stoppered
           centrifuge tube.
9.2.7   Add 5 mL n-hexane and 2 mL water and mix well.
9.2.8   Centrifuge for 5 min at 1700 g
9.2.9   Discard the upper layer
9.2.10   Repeat steps 9.2.7 to 9.2.9.
9.2.11   Add 3.5 mL of water saturated ethyl acetate to the aqueous phase
           and mix well.
9.2.12   Centrifuge for 5 min at 1700 g
9.2.13   Separate the organic phase and evaporate it to dryness.

9.3   Extraction of Milk.
9.3.1   Mix 1 mL milk with 0.75 mL chloroform-isooctane (3/2, v/v) in a
           glass tube.
9.3.2   Centrifuge 15 min at 4000 g
9.3.3   Load 0.7 mL of the supernatant onto a C-18 cartridge conditioned
           as follows;
           Wash the cartridge in the following order with;-
           - 5 mL methanol; 5 ml chloroform; 5 mL methanol; 10 mL distilled
           water.
9.3.4   Wash test sample with 10 mL distilled water (6.1.19)
9.3.5   Elute the CAP with 5 mL acetonitrile/water (1/1, v/v).
9.3.6   Extract CAP from the column eluent with 5 mL of water saturated
           ethyl acetate. Centrifuge at 1700 g.

9.3.7   Transfer the upper layer and evaporate it to dryness using a
          Speed Vac.
9.3.8   Dissolve the residue in 0.7 mL phosphate buffer (6.3.1) and
          proceed directly to 9.5.2.

9.5   Radioimmunoassay.
[Note; All steps must be performed at 0°C using an ice bath.]
9.5.1   Dissolve the meat/eggs extract (9.2.13) with 450 µL phosphate
          buffer (6.3.1). For the meat extract it may be necessary to
          adjust the concentration of CAP to ca. 150 pg per 200 µL buffer
          by diluting up to 10 fold with buffer.
9.5.2   Combine in a glass tube;
          - 200 µL extract (9.5.1 or 9.3.8) or standard solutions (6.2.2)
          - 200 µL radioligand solution (6.3.4)
          - 400 µL antiserum working solution (6.3.3)
          Start the incubation by adding the antiserum last.
[Note; Two replicates are used for each test sample.]
9.5.3   Incubate overnight at +4°C
9.5.4   Pipette 1 mL of well stirred charcoal suspension into each tube.
          The additions must be completed within 5 min.
9.5.5   Incubate 30 min at 0°C
9.5.6   Centrifuge 10 min at 1700 g
9.5.7   Decant the supernatant to a sufficient amount of scintillation
          fluid.
9.5.8   Count the "radioactivity" for 10 min. or to a 2% statistical
          error.

10.0   CALCULATION OF RESULTS
10.1   It is strongly recommended to use non-linear curve fitting
          procedures for the calculation of the calibration curves.
[Note; For this RIA the CAP concentrations of the calibration standards and
"Bound"/"Total", (B/T), the fraction bound of the radioligand are the best
suited independent and dependant variables for the non-linear "least-
squares" curve fitting. Frequently only the central part of the
calibration curve can be linearized using the logit-log-transformation.]

For the calculation of the CAP contents of the test samples the following
data are required;
     A   The amount of CAP found per tube (mean of replicates). These
              values are determined from the calibration curve.
     F   The correction factor due to the fraction of the total residue
              transferred to the RIA tube.
     EA   The weight of the aliquot of the crude extract taken for extract
              clean up.
     EW   The weight of the crude extract.
     SW   The sample weight

For eggs
     F = 2.25 for analyses at 1 ppb
     EA = ca. 1/6th of EW, use exact value
     EW = typically 5 to 6.5 g, use exact value
     SW = ca. 3 g, use exact value
For meat
     F = 22.5 for analyses at 10 ppb
     EA = ca. 1/6th of EW, use exact value
     EW = typically 7.5 to 9 g, use exact value
     SW = ca. 3 g, use exact value

For milk
     F = 5 for analyses at 1 ppb
     EA = ca. 1 for analyses at 1 ppb
     EW = ca. 1 for analyses at 1 ppb
     SW = ca. 1 for analyses at 1 ppb

The results are calculated as; $F = \dfrac{A \times F \times EW}{1000 \times EA \times SW}$

10.2   Precision.
This was determined in an EEC collaborative trial using meat and milk. The results were;-

	Meat	Milk
True Content (µg per kg)	11.6	1.0
Mean level found[1] (µg per kg)	6.9	1.1
Repeatability (ng per g)	3.2	0.72
Repeatability CV%	16	23
Reproducibility (ng per g)	7.0	1.1
Reproducibility CV%	36	36
Between laboratory CV%	32	28

Superscript 1 is the value calculated without account of recovery.
The results were analyzed according to ISO standard 5725/1986.

10.3   Quality controls
Each assay must include duplicate assays for; reagent blanks, blank tissues, fortified (spiked) tissues and Reference Materials where available.

The total radioactivity pipetted into each assay tube should be determined.

The non-specific binding of the radioligand should be determined and should not exceed 8%

11.   SPECIAL CASES.

12.   NOTES ON PROCEDURE.

13.   SAMPLE CONTROLS.
Reference Materials for muscle, milk and eggs were prepared by the BGA and are undergoing the final intercomparison and certification procedures under the Measurement and Testing Programme of DG12.

14.   TEST REPORT

15.   LIST OF ABBREVIATIONS.
See abbreviations in Annex I, Section 12 of Manual.

16.   FLOW DIAGRAM
  MEAT/EGGS ---> SOLVENT EXTRACT ------------------------
                                                         ↓
  MILK ----->   SOLVENT EXTRACT ------> C-18 SPE -----> RIA --> RESULTS

Sg. 3.4.   NITROIMIDAZOLES AND NITROFURANS - ANALYSIS WITH DIALYSIS AND ON-LINE HPLC FOR DETERMINING RESIDUES OF NITROIMIDAZOLES AND NITROFURANS IN POULTRY (CHICKENS, DUCKS AND TURKEYS) MEAT.

WARNING AND SAFETY PRECAUTIONS

SAFETY
Organic solvents - all organic solvents must be treated as potentially hazardous and all procedures using them must be performed in a fume cupboard.

0.   INTRODUCTION

Nitroimidazoles (here dimetridazole and ronidazole) are coccidiostats used in poultry. The MRL for dimetridazole is 10 µg per kg and for ronidazole is 2 µg per kg. Both nitroimidazoles have a common metabolite, 1-methyl-2-hydroxymethyl-5-nitroimidazole. Nitrofurans (here furazolidone, and furaltadone) are antibacterial agents used in pigs and poultry.

1.   SCOPE

This work is carried out in compliance with the Residues Directive (86/469/EEC).

2.   FIELD OF APPLICATION.

This method is used for determining the presence of ronidazole and dimetridazole and their common metabolite 1-methyl-2-hydroxymethyl-5-nitroimidazole in poultry meat. The method also includes the monitoring of furazolidone and furadaltone in poultry meat. The method is operated at RIKILT-DLO in the Netherlands, as a routine monitoring method. The limit of detection is 2 µg per kg of matrix for nitroimidazoles and 1-methyl-2-hydroxymethyl-5-nitroimidazole and furazolidone. For furadaltone the limit of detection is 4 ug per kg.

3.   REFERENCES.

Commission Decision, 93/256/EEC, laying down the methods for detecting residues of substances having a hormonal or thyrostatic action. [OJ. Nº L.118, 14.4.93. pp 64-74]

ISO Standard 78/2-1982 Layout for standards - Part 2: Standard for Chemical Analysis

ISO Standard 5725 (1986)

Aerts, M.M.L., Beek,W.M.J. and Brinkman, U.A.Th., (1990), On-line combination of dialysis and column-switching liquid chromatography as a fully automated sample preparation technique for biological samples. Determination of nitrofuran residues in edible products. J.Chromatogr. <u>500</u>, 453-468

Elema, M.C., Beek, W.M.J. and Keukens, H.J. (1992), Kip-, kalkoen- en eendevlees - Bepaling van ronidazol, dimetridazol, furazolidon en furaltadon - CF-LC. RIKILT-DLO, SOP Nº A0656, RIKILT, Wageningen, NL.

Keukens, H.J., Elema, M.C., Beek, W.M.J. and Boekestein, A. (1993), Sample pretreatment based on dialysis; Determination of residues of nitroimidazoles in poultry meat. Proc. Euroresidues II, May 1993, pp 410-414.

4.   DEFINITIONS.

Nitroimidazoles/nitrofurans content is taken to mean the amount of nitroimidazoles in meat determined according to the described method and expressed as ug nitroimidazoles/nitrofurans per kg test sample.

5.   PRINCIPLE.

The method comprises four stages all carried out in the absence of daylight or white light.

- Meat is homogenised in water.
- Centrifugation
- purification of the supernatant extract by dialysis
- quantification by HPLC with UV detection at 320 nm.

6.   MATERIALS

6.1.   Chemicals

6.1.1   Methanol, Analytical grade (Merck - 6009)
6.1.2   Acetonitrile, HPLC grade (Merck - 3)
6.1.3   Anhydrous sodium acetate (Merck - 6268)
6.1.4   Glacial acetic acid (Merck - 63)
6.1.5   Demineralised water, filtered on Milli-Q purification system (Millipore, Milford, USA)

6.2.   Solutions
6.2.1   0.01M sodium acetate - acetic acid buffer; pH 4.3. Dissolve 0.82 g anhydrous sodium acetate (6.1.3) in about 800 mL water. Adjust the pH to 4.3 with glacial acetic acid (6.1.4). Make up the volume to 1 L with water.
6.2.2   HPLC eluent; Mix 850 mL of acetate buffer (6.2.1) with 150 mL acetonitrile (6.1.2). Filter the solution through a 0.22 μm Millipore filter and degas in an ultrasonic bath. The solution is stable for one month.

6.3   Standards
6.3.1   Ronidazole and dimetridazole (Sigma), 1-methyl-2-hydroxymethyl-5-nitroimidazole was a gift from Merck, Sharpe and Dohme. Furazolidone and furaltadone were obtained from Sigma, USA.
6.3.2   Stock standards; Make up stock solutions of nitroimidazoles, nitrofurans and 1-methyl-2-hydroxymethyl-5-nitroimidazole in methanol to give concentrations of ca. 100 μg per mL. The solution is stable for one month at 4° to 8°C in the dark.
6.3.3   Dilute Standards; Make up in a volumetric flask 1 mL of stock standard (6.3.2) to 100 mL with water.
6.3.4   Working Standards; A (5 ng per mL); Dilute 0.5 mL 6.3.3 to 100 mL with water. B (20 ng per mL); Dilute 2 mL 6.3.3 to 100 mL with water.

7   EQUIPMENT
7.1.   Glassware
7.1.1   Graduated pipettes,
7.1.2   Glass centrifuge tubes
7.1.3   Glass test tubes to take 6 mL samples.
7.1.4   Graduated volumetric flasks, 100 mL capacity
7.1.5   Normal laboratory glassware

7.2.   Apparatus
7.2.1   Automatic pipettes,
7.2.2   Analytical balance
7.2.3   Refrigerated centrifuge
7.2.4   Refrigerator at <-18°C
7.2.5   Vibromixer
7.2.6   Homogeniser, Model 400 Stomacher laboratory blender, (Lameris, NL)
7.2.7   Filter paper (Schleicher & Schuell 595½; ϕ 15 cm)
7.2.8   pH meter
7.2.9   Filter system for eluents; 0.22 µm (Millipore 83813)

7.3   Dialysis Equipment (see schematic representation)
An autosampler-dialysis module system consisted of a Model 232-401 Gilson autosampling injector, two automatic six-port valves (Rheodyne model 7010), a second Model 401 diluter , a Kel-F flat-plate dialyser block fitted with a Cuprophan membrane (10,000-15,000 Daltons cut-off) having a donor volume of 370 uL and an acceptor volume of 650 µL, a liquid chromatographic pump capable of maintaining a constant pulseless flow of 0.1-2 mL per min (model 305, Gilson). The diluters were equipped with two 5 mL syringes.
The sample tray of the injector device must be cooled to 4°C to keep the test samples at 4°C.

Schematic representation of dialysis and HPLC system.

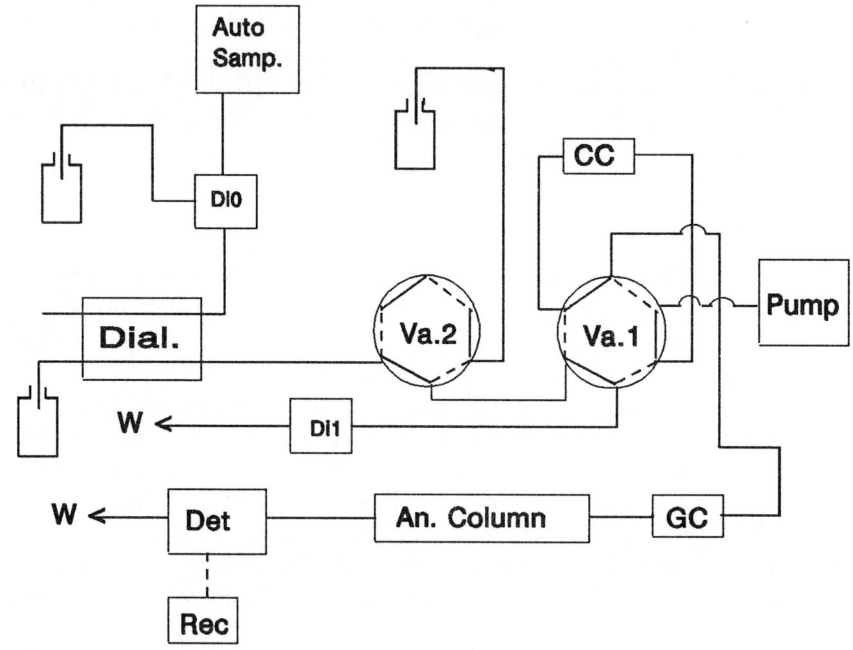

Sg 3.4 /3

7.4   HPLC equipment
Basic System : Gilson 305 and 805
Guard Column : Bondapack/Corasil 37-50μm, 10 mm x 2.1 mm i.d. (Millipore
                27248)
Analytical Column : Lichrosorb C-18 5 μm, 200 mm x 3.0 mm i.d. Chrompack)
Recorder : 10 mV, 0.5 cm per min   (Kipp BD-41)
Detector : UV at 320 nm. 0.002 Aufs, Rise time 2 sec. (ABI Type 785A)
Flow rate : 0.4 mL per min

8.   SAMPLES AND SAMPLING PROCEDURE.

N.B. Attention is drawn to section 6.3.1 and ISO document 78/2-1982 and
the following notes derived from Annex II of 2052/VI/84-EN.

8.1. Nature of the Sample; Samples of meat, milk and eggs shall be such
as to enable the detection of residues. Only samples which are not spoiled
by bacteria may be examined.

8.2. Size of Sample; The size of the sample must be large enough to allow
the reference method to be carried out and to allow repeat analysis where
required.

8.3. The samples must be cooled after collection and stored at $\leq$ -20°C
pending analysis.

9.   PROCEDURE
Note; All steps must be carried out in the absence of daylight or white
light.
9.1   Samples of meat are blended in a Waring blender or Moulinette.
9.2   Control and blank samples; Pipette into 10 g portions of blended
           meat 0, 100, 200 and 500 μL of each of the diluted standards
           6.3.3.
9.2   The control and blank samples and separate samples of 10 g of
           blended meat (test samples) are further blended for 3 min in a
           Stomacher (7.2.6) with 20 mL water.
9.3   Transfer the material to a centrifuge tube. Centrifuge at 4000 g
           for 5 min at 10 °C.
9.4   Filter through filter paper (7.2.7). The filtrate is ready for
           introduction into the dialysis system.
9.5   Dialysis-HPLC
9.5.1   The working standards are injected into the dialysis according to
           the following procedure until a stable base line and consistent
           peak height response(s) are observed.
           The samples are placed in the automatic sample injector and
           maintained at 4°C. Two sample doses (2 x 370 μL) are introduced
           into the dialysis block. Two mL of acceptor solvent (water) are
           sucked through the concentration column (CC) by the second
           diluter (Di1). After completion of the dialysis, the
           concentration column is flushed with water by switching the
           second six-port valve (Va.2). The enriched sample is backflushed
           with HPLC eluent (6.2.2) to the guard column and analytical
           column with the pump by switching the six-port valve (Va.1). The
           analytes are detected at 320 nm by UV detection.
[Note; This procedure (9.5) may be automated with home-made software
installed on the 232 mainframe.]

Sg 3.4 /4

10.   CALCULATION OF RESULTS

10.1   The content of the meat sample is given by the formula;-

$$\text{Conc. in meat (mg per kg)} = \frac{Hm}{Hst} \times Cst \times f$$

    Hm = peak height of analyte in sample
    Hst = peak height of standard added to blank sample
    Cst = concentration of standard in blank sample in mg per kg
    f   = Dilution factor

10.2   Recoveries;
Recoveries for meat were measured on the basis of the standards dissolved
in water. The values were;-

Conc.	recovery %				
μg per kg	2-OH-Metab	Ronidazole	Dimetridazole	Furazolidone	Furaltadone
5	82	91	90	109	84
10	89	90	92	99	85
20	94	93	93	96	76

10.3   The suspect peaks must have the same retention time as the
         standards as defined in the EC decision 93/256 (see section 5).

11.   SPECIAL CASES.

12.   NOTES ON PROCEDURE.

**NITROFURANS DECOMPOSE IN WHITE/DAY LIGHT. IT IS ESSENTIAL THAT ALL
PROCEDURES ARE CARRIED OUT IN THE ABSENCE OF DAYLIGHT AND WHITE LIGHT.**

13.   SAMPLE CONTROLS

14.   TEST REPORT

15.   LIST OF ABBREVIATIONS.

See abbreviations in Annex I, Section 12 of Manual.

16.   FLOW DIAGRAM

    MEAT ---------->   WATER EXTRACT ------> DIALYSIS
                                                   |
                                                   |
                                                   ↓
            CALCULATE RESULTS <--------- HPLC

Sg 3.5. CIPROFLOXACIN AND ENROFLOXACIN - ROUTINE SCREENING METHOD FOR THE DETERMINATION BY HPLC AFTER CATION-EXCHANGE COLUMN CHROMATOGRAPHY IN PIG MUSCLE, BACON AND BOVINE MUSCLE.

WARNING AND SAFETY PRECAUTIONS

SAFETY

Organic solvents - all organic solvents must be treated as potentially hazardous and all procedures using them must be performed in a fume cupboard.

FIRST AID

1. Solvents, acids and alkalis in contact with skin - wash with copious amounts of cold water. Splashes in the eye - irrigate with water and seek medical attention immediately.
2. Cuts - seek assistance of first aider immediately.
3. Burns and frostbite - run affected part under cold water (burns) or tepid water (frostbite) for 10 minutes and seek medical attention.

1.   INTRODUCTION

Purpose

The detection of the presence of Ciprofloxacin and Enrofloxacin in samples taken from cattle and pigs in compliance with the Residues Directive 86/469/EEC.

Background

Ciprofloxacin and Enrofloxacin are animal drugs with broad spectrum antibacterial activity.

1.   SCOPE

This method of analysis in use at MAFF, FSD, Norwich, UK, describes the determination of the total content of Ciprofloxacin and Enrofloxacin in pig muscle, bacon and bovine muscle.

2.   FIELD OF APPLICATION.

The method is described to be used for samples from pigs and cattle. It may be suitable for other species but would require validation. The limit of determination is not accurately defined but is taken to be 0.01 mg Ciprofloxacin or Enrofloxacin per kg although this may vary between samples because of variable background noise. Validation data are provided for 0.001 - 0.002 mg per kg.

3.   REFERENCES.

Commission Decision, 93/256/EEC, laying down the methods for detecting residues of substances having a hormonal or thyrostatic action. [OJ. № L.118, 14.4.93. pp 64-74]

ISO Standard 78/2-1982 Layout for standards - Part 2: Standard for Chemical Analysis

Determination of Ciprofloxacin and Enrofloxacin at residue levels in cattle muscle, pig muscle and bacon. (1993), MAFF, Food Safety Directorate, Food Science Lab. Norwich UK. SOP10(1)

4.   DEFINITIONS.

Ciprofloxacin or Enrofloxacin content is taken to mean the amount of Ciprofloxacin or Enrofloxacin in muscle or bacon determined according to the described method and expressed as µg Ciprofloxacin or Enrofloxacin per kg test sample.

5.0   PRINCIPLE

Ciprofloxacin and Enrofloxacin are extracted with solvents from homogenised samples into 1% acetic acid in ethanol. The extract is cleaned up using ion-exchange resin column chromatography and eluting with 25% methanolic - ammonia. End-point analysis is performed with reversed-phase HPLC and fluorescence detection.

6.   MATERIALS

Note: The reagents (and equipment) for which examples of their source are quoted are known to be satisfactory, nevertheless reagents and equipment from other sources may be equally suitable. All the reagents must be of analytical grade or better.

6.1.   <u>Chemicals</u>

6.1.1.   Acetonitrile (Rathburn Chem Ltd)
6.1.2.   Ammonia solution sp.gr. 0.88 (BDH Ltd.)
6.1.3.   Absolute alcohol (ethanol) (Hayman Ltd)
6.1.4.   Glacial acetic acid (FSA)
6.1.5.   Orthophosphoric acid   (BDH Ltd)
6.1.6.   Methanol (FSA)
6.1.7.   Triethylamine   (BDH)
6.1.8   Ciprofloxacin hydrochloride   (Sigma)
6.1.9.   Enrofloxacin   (Bayer)
6.1.10   Deionised water further processed by Elgastat UHP unit is used
           throughout.

6.2.   <u>Standards</u>
Store all solutions of standards in the refridgerator.
6.2.1   Stock standards.
6.2.1.1   Dissolve 5 mg Ciprofloxacin in 10 mL water. Prepare monthly.
6.2.1.2   Dissolve 5 mg Enrofloxacin in 10 mL water. Prepare monthly.
6.2.2   First intermediate standard (10 µg per mL). Take 200 µL of each
           stock (6.2.1.1 & 6.2.1.2), combine and dilute to 10 mL with
           methanol. Prepare daily.
6.2.3   Second intermediate standard (0.2 µg per mL). Take 200 µL of
           intermediate standard (6.2.2) and dilute to 10 mL with mobile
           phase (6.3.4). Prepare daily.
6.2.4   Working standards of concentrations 4 µg per mL and 20 µg per mL.
           Take 0.2 mL or 1.0 mL of the second intermediate standard
           solution and dilute to 10 mL with the HPLC mobile phase (6.3.4).
6.2.5   Tissue working standard (4 or 20 µg per mL). Redissolve the
           residue from the blank extract (blank extraction through to 9.13)
           in 1 mL working standard (6.2.4).

| 6.2.6 | Intermediate spiking solution. Take 200 µL of 10 µg per mL solution (6.2.2) and dilute to 10 mL with 1% acetic acid in ethanol (6.3.1). |
| 6.2.7 | Spiking solution. Take 0.2 mL or 1 mL of 0.2 µg per mL solution (6.2.3) and dilute to 10 mL with 1% acetic acid in ethanol (6.3.1). |

6.3	Solutions
6.3.1	1% acetic acid in ethanol; 10 mL acetic acid (6.1.4) made up to 1 L with ethanol (6.1.3)
6.3.2	25% ammonia in methanol; 125 mL ammonia solution (6.1.2) made up to 500 mL with methanol (6.1.6).
6.3.3	0.01M phosphate/TEA buffer, pH 3; 0.68 mL phosphoric acid (6.1.5) diluted to 1 L with water. Adjust the pH to 3.0 with triethylamine (6.1.7).
6.3.4	HPLC mobile phase. Mix 0.01M phosphate/TEA buffer and acetonitrile, 80:20 (v/v). Filter (7.14) and degas by ultrasonication (7.3) under reduced pressure.

7. EQUIPMENT

7.1	Centrifuge, Jouan CR422
7.2	Plastic centrifuge tubes, 50 mL and 100 mL capacity
7.3	Ultrasonic bath, L&R 140S
7.4	Glass vials and caps, 2 mL capacity
7.5	HPLC vials and caps, 0.3 mL capacity
7.6	All glass filter holder 47 mm. (Millipore UK Ltd)
7.7	Homogeniser (Ultra-Turrax or equivalent)
7.8	Test tubes 125 mm x 16 mm (to fit Speed mate 30 vacuum manifold)
7.9	Disposable syringes 1 mL capacity
7.10	Heater block assembly for evaporation using nitrogen
7.11	Vortex mixer(s)
7.12	Magnetic stirrer
7.13	Disposable syringe filters, Cameo 3N, 0.45 micron, 3 mm - (Jones Chromatography)
7.14	Membrane filter 0.45 µm "Durapore", 47 mm. (Millipore UK Ltd)
7.15	Refridgerator +4°C
7.16	Safety pipettes, 0.2 mL, 1.0 mL and 5.0 mL. (e.g. Gilson Pipetman)
7.17	Solid Phase extraction
7.17.1	Bond-Elut adapters
7.17.2	Bond-Elut SCX cartridges 500 mg in 2.8 mL (Jones Chromatography)
7.17.3	Bond-Elut reservoirs, 75 mL capacity
7.17.4	Speed Mate 30 vacuum manifold (Applied Separations)
7.17.5	Preparation SCX column; Wash the Bond-Elut SCX columns (7.17.2) with 5 mL 1% acetic acid in ethanol (6.3.1) prior to use.
7.25	HPLC Pump : Gilson 307 Injector: Gilson model 231, 20 µL injection Detector: Philips Scientific PU4027 fluorescence detector, excitation 278 nm, emission 445 nm. Column: 250 mm x 4.6 mm i.d. Zorbax RX-C8 column maintained at a constant 35°C in an oven. Mobile phase pumped at 0.5 mL per min.

8. SAMPLES AND SAMPLING PROCEDURE.

N.B. Attention is drawn to section 6.3.1 and to ISO document 78/2-1982 and also the following notes derived from Annex II of 2052/VI/84-EN.

8.1.   Nature of the Sample; Samples shall be such as to enable the detection of residues in meat as defined in Directive 64/433/EEC.

8.2.   Size of Sample; The size of the sample must be large enough to allow the method to be carried out and to allow repeat analysis where required.

8.3.   The samples must be taken and packed in such a way as to allow proper identification in the laboratory.

8.4.   The method of packing, preservation and transport must maintain the integrity of the sample and not prejudice the result of the examination.
          Samples for the analysis of Ciprofloxacin and Enrofloxacin must be stored and transported at temperatures below -18^{0}C.

9.0.   PROCEDURE

9.1.   Sample preparation
Samples may be processed in batches of up to eight. A control sample and/or one of the eight samples should be spiked at the limit of determination.

9.1.1   2 g thawed sample is sliced and placed into a 50 mL centrifuge tube.
9.1.2   20 mL of 1% acetic acid in ethanol (6.2.1) is added and the mixture homogenised for about 1 min and then placed in an ultrasonic bath for 3 min.
9.1.3   The tubes are centrifuged at 4500 rpm for about 5 min.
9.1.4   The supernatant is poured carefully into a 100 mL plastic centrifuge tube.
9.1.5   The residue is re-extracted with a further 20 mL of 1% acetic acid in ethanol (6.2.1)
9.1.6   The combined supernatants are centrifuged for 5 min at 4500 rpm.
9.2   Column Clean up;
9.2.1   The clear supernatant is passed through a prepared (7.17.5) Bond-Elut SCX column at a flow rate not exceeding 5 mL per min.
NOTE; The column should not be allowed to run dry at any stage during the washing loading and elution steps.
9.2.2   The column is washed with 5 mL methanol (6.1.6) follwed by 10 mL water and a further 5 mL methanol.
9.2.3   The Ciprofloxacin and Enrofloxacin are eluted with 5 mL 25% ammonia in methanol (6.3.2) into a test tube (7.8).
9.2.4   The test tube is stood a heated block for 5 min to equilibrate and the liquid phase evaporated to dryness under a stream of nitrogen. Acetonitrile may be added to assist evaporation of the last 1 to 2 mL extract.
9.2.5   The residue is redissolved in 1 mL HPLC mobile phase (6.3.4) by vortex mixing and ultrasonication for 3 min.
9.2.6   The extract is transferred to glass vial (7.4) and centrifuged for for 5 min at 4500 rpm.

9.2.7   The supernatant is transferred to a 1 mL disposable syringe and filtered through a Cameo 3N 0.45 μm syringe filter (7.13) into a HPLC vial (7.5).

9.3   HPLC

9.3.1   Using the conditions set out in 7.25 20 μL are injected onto the column using the automated injector.

9.3.2   Standards corresponding to 4 ng per mL (equiv. 2 μg per kg tissue conc.) or 20 ng per mL (equiv. 10 μg per kg tissue conc.) are injected in triplicate to determine the average peak height for both Ciprofloxacin and Enrofloxacin.

9.3.3   The peaks corresponding to Ciprofloxacin and Enrofloxacin and should be devoid of interfering peaks from the matrix.

9.3.4   The linearity of the detector response to Ciprofloxacin and Enrofloxacin can be checked by running a full calibration curve.

10.0   CALCULATION OF RESULTS

10.1   The concentration of Ciprofloxacin or Enrofloxacin in a sample is determined by interpolation from the spiked samples using the area of the peak corresponding to Ciprofloxacin or Enrofloxacin. If in doubt, suspect positive samples may be overspiked with standard Ciprofloxacin or Enrofloxacin solution. A resultant single peak indicates a positive (in screening) sample.

10.2   Screening procedure. A minimum of three injections of 20 μL of standard Ciprofloxacin or Enrofloxacin solution are carried out to determine the average peak height (see 9.3.2).

Uncorrected conc. of sample in μg per kg is given by

$$\frac{\text{peak height for sample}}{\text{peak height of standard}} \times 2.0 \times \text{standard conc. (as μg per kg tissue conc.)}$$

10.3   [Editors note. Positive samples will be rare and therefore a vigorous procedure to confirm the positive finding is recommended]. Quantitation of positive samples is carried out by performing a repeat duplicate analysis and interpolation from a full standard curve constructed over the suspect range. The curve should have at least 5 points (each point done in triplicate) and cover the range from 0 to 10% greater than the estimated concentration in the sample. Two blank samples fortified with Ciprofloxacin or Enrofloxacin to the same level as the suspected positive should also be analysed in the same batch.

10.4   Validation of method prior to use. Before adopting this method for use it it should be validated for in-house repeatability and reproducibility. Batches of up to 8 samples are spiked at the 0.002 and 0.01 mg per kg level using 1 mL of spiking solutions 6.2.7 (batches should include one blank sample and one blank sample for tissue working standard). Batches should be analysed on each of three separate days at each level. Recovery of analyte should fall within the range 45-110%. CV values should be less than 15% for inter and intra batch precision.

Typical results reported by FSD, Norwich were;
CPX is Ciprofloxacin; EFX is Enrofloxacin

<u>Bovine muscle</u> for intra-assay,
Bovine muscle fortified at 0.001 mg per kg; 80.9% ± 12.4% (CPX), 82.4 ±
7.5% (EFX); at 0.01 mg per kg; 73.1% ± 2.1% (CPX), 88.0 ± 4.0% (EFX), and
at 0.05 mg per kg 77.7 ± 2.5% (CPX), 90.2 ± 6.6% (EFX).
For inter-assay with 3 assays on separate days,
Bovine muscle fortified at 0.01 mg per kg; 74.9% ± 6.9% (CPX), 90.4 ±
5.6% (EFX)

<u>Pig muscle</u> for intra-assay,
Pig muscle fortified at 0.002 mg per kg; 52.8% ± 1.3% (CPX), 67.3 ± 4.9%
(EFX); at 0.01 mg per kg; 51.3% ± 3.5% (CPX), 75.6 ± 5.5% (EFX)
For inter-assay with 3 assays on separate days,
Pig muscle fortified at 0.01 mg per kg; 53.9% ± 4.4% (CPX), 74.8 ±
4.4% (EFX)

<u>Pig bacon</u> for intra-assay,
Pig bacon fortified at 0.002 mg per kg; 65.0% ± 3.9% (CPX), 85.0 ± 4.1%
(EFX); at 0.01 mg per kg; 63.2% ± 1.6% (CPX), 79.0 ± 1.1% (EFX)
For inter-assay with 3 assays on separate days,
Pig bacon fortified at 0.01 mg per kg; 63.2% ± 44.7 (CPX), 81.2 ±
5.9% (EFX)

11.   SPECIAL CASES

12.   NOTES ON PROCEDURE

12.1. The <u>action level</u> at which reanalysis of a suspected positive must be
decided. Also similar decisions need to taken when to proceed to a
confirming method.

13.   QUALITY CONTROLS
Batches must include at least two blank samples, one sample for use as
tissue standard, the other as the corresponding blank tissue. These will
act as the quality control reference samples for that batch and determine
whether the data obtained is acceptable. They will also be used to
estimate the overall recovery of analyte in any positive sample found in
the batch.

14.   TEST REPORT

15.   LIST OF ABBREVIATIONS

A full list of abbreviations is given in Annex I, Section 12

16.   FLOW DIAGRAM

    Tissue --> Extract into 1% acetic acid in ethanol ----> Ion exchange
                                                             chromatography
                                                                  |
                                                                  ↓
                        Calculate results <--------------- HPLC

Sg 3.6. GENTAMICIN AND NEOMYCIN - ROUTINE SCREENING METHOD FOR THE DETERMINATION BY HPLC IN MUSCLE OF CATTLE, SHEEP AND PIGS AND IN MUSCLE, LIVER, KIDNEY AND FAT OF VEAL CALVES.

WARNING AND SAFETY PRECAUTIONS

SAFETY   Organic solvents - all organic solvents must be treated as potentially hazardous and all procedures using them must be performed in a fume cupboard.

FIRST AID
1.   Solvents, acids and alkalis in contact with skin - wash with copious amounts of cold water. Splashes in the eye - irrigate with water and seek medical attention immediately.
2.   Cuts - seek assistance of first aider immediately.
3.   Burns and frostbite - run affected part under cold water (burns) or tepid water (frostbite) for 10 minutes and seek medical attention.

1.   INTRODUCTION

Purpose
The detection of the presence of Gentamicin and Neomycin in samples taken from cattle, sheep and pigs in compliance with the Residues Directive 86/469/EEC.
Background
Gentamicin and Neomycin are animal drugs with broad spectrum antibacterial activity. Gentamicin is composed of three major components, C_1, C_2 and C_{1a} which have similar antibacterial properties.

1.   SCOPE

This method of analysis in use at the Analytical Chemistry Laboratory, Faculty of Pharmacy, B.P.403, 54001 Nancy, Cedex-France, describes the determination of the total content of Gentamicin (all three components) and Neomycin in edible tissues.

2.   FIELD OF APPLICATION.

The method is described to be used for samples from pigs, sheep and cattle. It may be suitable for other species but would require validation. The limit of quantitation for gentamicin is 50 ng per g for muscle and fat and 100 ng per g for liver and kidney. The limit of quantitation for neomycin is 50 ng per g for muscle.

3.   REFERENCES.

Commission Decision, 93/256/EEC, laying down the methods for detecting residues of substances having a hormonal or thyrostatic action. [OJ. № L.118, 14.4.93. pp 64-74]

ISO Standard 78/2-1982 Layout for standards - Part 2: Standard for Chemical Analysis

Sar, F., Nicolas, A. and Archimbault, P., (1993), Development and Optimization of a liquid chromatographic method for the determination of gentamicin in calf tissues. Anal. Chim. Acta. 275, 285-293.

4.   DEFINITIONS.

Gentamicin or Neomycin content is taken to mean the amount of Gentamicin or
Neomycin in tissue determined according to the described method and
expressed as µg Gentamicin or Neomycin per kg test sample.

5.0   PRINCIPLE

The method consists of 5 stages;-
   -      Homogenisation
   -      Precipitation of protein with 5% trichloroacetic acid
   -      Clean up on Ion exchange column using CM-Sephadex.
   -      HPLC with post-column derivatisation.
   -      Interpolation of results

6.   MATERIALS

Note: The reagents (and equipment) for which examples of their source are
quoted are known to be satisfactory, nevertheless reagents and equipment
from other sources may be equally suitable. All the reagents must be of
analytical grade or better.

6.1.   Chemicals

6.1.1.   Disodium EDTA dihydrate   (Merck)
6.1.2.   Acetonitrile
6.1.3.   Sodium-*dl*-camphor-10-sulphonate (Aldrich)
6.1.4.   *o*-phthalaldehyde (Fluka)
6.1.5.   Boric acid (Merck)
6.1.6.   Sodium hydroxide
6.1.7.   Ethanol
6.1.8   Gentamicin sulphate, potency equiv. 620 µg per mg,   (Virbac SA,
          Carros, France)
6.1.9.   Neomycin   (Bayer)
6.1.10   Double distilled water further processed for HPLC by degassing
          with ultrasonication for 5 min before use and discarded if not
          used within 24 h.
6.1.11   2-mercaptoethanol (Aldrich)
6.1.12   Brij-35 (Sigma)
6.1.13   Trichloroacetic acid [TCA]
6.1.14   CM-Sephadex C-25 (Pharmacia)
6.1.15   Sodium azide
6.1.16   Sodium sulphate
6.1.17   Hydrophillic cotton (Pharmacopoeia grade)
6.1.18   1*M* hydrochloric acid
6.1.19   Dipotassium hydrogen phosphate
6.1.20   Methanol

6.2.   Standards
Store all solutions of standards in the refrigerator.
6.2.1   Stock standards.
6.2.1.1   Dissolve 162.1 mg Gentamicin in 100 mL water. Store in a
          polypropylene container. Prepare monthly.
6.2.1.2   Dissolve ca.320 mg Neomycin in 100 mL water. Prepare monthly.
6.2.3   Working standards and spiking solutions for muscle, liver and
          kidney; Prepare concentrations of free base of 0.5, 1.0, 1.5,
          2.0, 4.0, 8.0, 16.0 and 32.0 µg per mL by dilution with 1*mM* EDTA.

6.2.4   Spiking solution for fat. Prepare in acetonitrile : 1 *mM* EDTA
         (6.3.20) at the same concentrations as in 6.2.3.

6.3   Solutions
6.3.1   1*mM* EDTA. Dissolve 372 mg disodium EDTA (6.1.1) in 700 mL water
         and make up to 1 L with water.
6.3.2   1*mM* EDTA-Acetonitrile (1:1, v/v). Mix equal volumes of 1*mM* EDTA
         and acetonitrile (6.1.2).
6.3.3   5% trichloroacetic acid. Dissolve 50 g TCA (6.1.13) in 600 mL
         water and make up to 1 L with water.
6.3.4   EDTA/TCA. Dissolve 372 mg disodium EDTA in 1 L 5% TCA (6.3.3).
6.3.5   EDTA/0.2*M* Sodium sulphate/sodium azide. Dissolve 28.4 g sodium
         sulphate (6.1.16) and 200 mg sodium azide in 1 L EDTA solution
         (6.3.1)
6.3.6   0.1*M* buffer, pH 7.0. Dissolve 14.2 g sodium sulphate and 17.4 g
         dipotassium hydrogen phosphate in ca. 700 mL water. Adjust the pH
         to 7.0 if necessary and make up to 1 L with water.
6.3.7   0.5*M* camphor sulphonate. Dissolve 12.7 g camphor sulphonate
         (6.1.3) in water and make up to 100 mL with water.
6.3.8   Mobile phase for HPLC; Dissolve 12.7 g camphor sulphonate
         (6.1.3) in 100 mL 1*mM* EDTA ((6.3.1) and add ca. 500 mL degassed
         water. Adjust the pH to 2.2 with hydrochloric acid and make up
         to 1 L with degassed water. Mix with methanol in the ratio 55:45
         (v/v). Filter through a 0.2 μm filter before use.
6.3.9   OPA solution. Place 5.3 g boric acid (6.1.5) and 7.5 mL 30%
         sodium hydroxide in a 250 mL volumetric flask. Add ca. 200 mL
         water (6.1.10). Dissolve 0.2 g of *o*-phthalaldehyde in 10 mL of
         95% ethanol and add to flask. Add 0.5 mL mercaptoethanol and 1
         mL 30% Brij-35 solution (6.1.12). Adjust the volume to 250 mL
         with the degassed water. Use within 24 h.
6.3.10   HPLC flushing solution. Mix 300 mL methanol with 200 mL degassed
         water (6.1.10).

7.   EQUIPMENT

7.1   Refrigerated centrifuge, Jouan CR422
7.2   Teflon centrifuge tubes, 40 mL capacity
7.3   Ultrasonic bath, L&R 140S
7.4   Glass vials and caps, 2 mL capacity
7.5   HPLC vials and caps, 0.3 mL capacity
7.6   All glass filter holder 47 mm.   (Millipore UK Ltd)
7.7   Virtis blender (Virtis Model 45)
7.8   Virtis glass tubes, 50 mL capacity
7.9   Analytical balance.
7.10   Balance accurate to 0.1 g
7.11   Vortex mixer(s)
7.12   Magnetic stirrer
7.13   Mincer
7.14   Volumetric flasks, 50 mL, 250 mL, 100 mL and 1 L capacity.
7.15   Refrigerator +4°C
7.16   Safety pipettes, 0.2 mL, 0.5 mL, 1.0 mL. (e.g. Gilson Pipetman)
7.18   pH meter
7.19   Pasteur pipettes
7.20   Rubber bulbs for Pasteur pipettes
7.21   0.2 μm nylon filter

7.22   HPLC
-    Pump : Spectroflow 400 fitted with membrane pulse damper (Applied
     Biosystems, Foster City, USA)
-    Injector: Autosampler (Model 507 Beckmann) with 100 μL column
     loop.
-    Detector: Shimadzu Model RF-551 fluorescence detector equipped
     with a150-W xenon short arc lamp, excitation 340 nm, emission 440
     nm. Set sensitivity to "high" and gain to 1 (these values may be
     adjusted according to the concentration range tested for
     linearity).
-    Column: 125 mm x 4 mm i.d. LiChrospher 100 RP-18 (5 μm) end-
     capped column maintained at a constant 45°C in an oven. The
     column is regenerated on a weekly basis by initial flushing with
     methanol-water (6.3.10) and then running a gradient up to 100%
     methanol in 15 min and flushing with 100% methanol for 15 min at
     1.2 mL per min. Replace the column after 300 injections.
-    Post column derivatisation was done using a second similar pump
     and a low-dead-volume tee (Model 5-8283; Supelco, St. Germain-en-
     Laye, France) for the addition of the OPA solution (6.3.9).
-    Derivatisation took place in a Teflon knitted open tubular (KNOT)
     reactor (3 m x 0.5 mm i.d.) (Model 5-9206, Supelco) maintained
     at 45°C. The OPA is pumped at 0.5 mL per min.
-    Mobile phase is pumped at 1.2 mL per min.
-    Guard column, 4 mm x 4 mm i.d. (replace every 100 injections)

8. SAMPLES AND SAMPLING PROCEDURE.

N.B. Attention is drawn to section 6.3.1 and to ISO document 78/2-1982 and
also the following notes derived from Annex II of 2052/VI/84-EN.

8.1.   Nature of the Sample; Samples shall be such as to enable the
          detection of residues in meat as defined in Directive 64/433/EEC.
8.2.   Size of Sample; The size of the sample must be large enough to
          allow the method to be carried out and to allow repeat analysis
          where required.
8.3.   The samples must be taken and packed in such a way as to allow
          proper identification in the laboratory.
8.4.   The method of packing, preservation and transport must maintain
          the integrity of the sample and not prejudice the result of the
          examination.
          Samples for the analysis of Gentamicin and Neomycin must be
          stored and transported at temperatures below -18°C.

9.0.   PROCEDURE

9.1.   Sample preparation
Samples may be processed in batches. A control sample should be spiked at
the limit of determination.
9.1.1   Allow the sample to thaw and then mince the tissue.
9.1.2.1   Weigh 5 ± 0.1 g minced test sample into a 50 mL Virtis tube.
9.1.2.2   Weigh 5 ± 0.1 g minced blank sample into eight 50 mL Virtis tube.
9.1.3   Add 500 μL of spiking solutions (6.2.3 or 6.2.4 (fat)) to the
          blank samples (9.1.2.2). Allow the mixture to equilibrate for 30
          min.
9.1.4   Add 20 mL TCA/EDTA solution (6.3.4) and homogenise for 10 min in
          a Virtis blender with U-shaped blades.

9.1.5	Transfer the homogenate to a teflon centrifuge tube (7.2) and centrifuge at 8000 rpm (7000 g) for 15 min at 5°C.

9.1.6	The supernatant is poured carefully into a 50 mL volumetric flask.

9.1.7	Adjust the pH to 7.0 ± 0.1 with 30% sodium hydroxide and make up the volume to 50 mL with pH 7.0 buffer (6.3.6).

9.2	Column Clean up;

9.2.1	Preparation of columns.
Allow 5 g CM-Sephadex C-25 (6.1.14) to swell overnight in the sodium sulphate/EDTA/azide solution (6.3.5). Plug a Pasteur pipette with cotton (6.1.17) and fill the pipette with 1 mL of the swollen gel. Wash the gel with 2 x 1 mL of sodium sulphate/EDTA/azide solution (6.3.5).

9.2.2	Pipette 10 mL of extract 9.1.7 in 1 mL fractions onto the column. Wash with 2 x 1 mL of sodium sulphate/EDTA/azide solution (6.3.5), 1 mL water (6.1.10) and 250 µL 0.05M sodium hydroxide.

9.2.3	Elute the gentamicin and neomycin with 1 mL 0.05M sodium hydroxide applying pressure until the bed runs dry.

9.2.4	Add 100 µL 1M HCl and 100 µL camphor sulphonate solution (6.3.7).

9.3	Standards containing no biological material are processed in the same way but omitting the blending and centrifugation steps.

9.4	HPLC

9.4.1	Using the conditions set out in 7.22 100 µL are injected onto the column using the automated injector.

9.4.2	The peaks corresponding to Gentamicin and Neomycin and should be devoid of interfering peaks from the matrix.

9.4.3	The linearity of the detector response to Gentamicin and Neomycin is checked by running the full calibration curve.

9.4.4	The retention time for the combined peak of three components of gentamicin was 4.0 - 4.1 min and that for the peak for neomycin was 5.3 - 5.4 min.

10.0	CALCULATION OF RESULTS

10.1	The concentration of Gentamicin or Neomycin in a sample is determined by interpolation from the spiked samples using the area of the peak corresponding to Gentamicin or Neomycin. If in doubt, suspect positive samples may be overspiked with standard Gentamicin or Neomycin solution. A resultant single peak indicates a positive (in screening) sample.

10.2	[Editors note. Positive samples will be rare and therefore a vigorous procedure to confirm the positive finding is recommended]. Quantitation of positive samples is carried out by performing a repeat duplicate analysis and interpolation from a full standard curve constructed over the suspect range. The curve should have at least 5 points (each point done in triplicate) and cover the range from 0 to 10% greater than the estimated concentration in the sample. Two blank samples fortified with Gentamicin or Neomycin to the same level as the suspected positive should also be analyzed in the same batch.

10.3	Validation of method prior to use. Before adopting this method for use it should be validated for in-house repeatability and reproducibility. Batches of spiked samples should be analyzed

on each of three separate days at each level. Recovery of
analyte should fall within the range 45-110%. CV values should
be less than 15% for inter and intra batch precision.

Typical results reported by the Analytical Lab. Nancy for CALF tissues
fortified with gentamicin were;

Tissue	Corr. Coef (r) of curve n=7	Recovery at 0.1 µg/g (%)	Recovery at 0.8 µg/g (%)	SD at 0.1 µg/g (%)	SD at 0.8 µg/g (%)
Standard	0.9999	100	100	3.2	2.2
Liver	0.9986	98	70	11.8	5.6
Kidney	0.9974	68	83	12.7	8.2
Fat	0.9991	79	77	6.1	4.3
Muscle	0.9989	88	74	9.9	8.2

10.4   The HPLC parameters for the gentamicin and neomycin peaks were
calculated for standards at aconcentration of 0.5 µg per mL.

	Gentamicin	Neomycin
Retention time (min)	4.0 - 4.1	5.3 - 5.4
Capacity factor (k')	2.2	3.3
№ theoretical plates/m	16225	9784
Tailing factor	1.2	1.4
Selectivity factor (α)	1.5	1.5
Resolution (R_s)	2.1	2.1

11.   SPECIAL CASES

12.   NOTES ON PROCEDURE

12.1. The action level at which reanalysis of a suspected positive must be
decided. Also similar decisions need to taken when to proceed to a
confirming method.

13.   QUALITY CONTROLS

14.   TEST REPORT

15.   LIST OF ABBREVIATIONS

A full list of abbreviations is given in Annex I, Section 12

16.   FLOW DIAGRAM

Tissue --> Extract into trichloroacetic acid ----> Ion exchange
                                                    chromatography
                                                        |
                                                        ↓
                    Calculate results <--------------- HPLC

Sg. 4.1. TRANQUILLIZERS - AN HPLC METHOD WITH ON-LINE UV SPECTRUM IDENTIFICATION BY DIODE-ARRAY FOR RESIDUES IN PIG KIDNEYS.

WARNING AND SAFETY PRECAUTIONS

SAFETY
Organic solvents - all organic solvents must be treated as potentially
hazardous and all procedures using them must be performed in a fume
cupboard.
Dilute the concentrated sulphuric with care.

0.   INTRODUCTION

Tranquillizers and the ß-blocker carazolol are used to aid the management
of stress in many veterinary practices. Of particular interest for
residues is the treatment of pigs to prevent mortality and loss of meat
quality during transport to the slaughterhouse. The time between drug
administration and slaughter is usually not more than a few hours and this
can result in high residues in the edible tissues.

1.   SCOPE

The use of many of the tranquillizers and carazolol varies throughout the
EEC. To ensure that farmers are not using these drugs in non-approved
situations and to control the use in meat producing animals samples of
kidneys are taken at slaughterhouses and screened for the presence of these
compounds. Whenever there is a positive screening result, this must be
confirmed (see methods Cy 4.5 and Cy 4.6.   This work is carried out in
compliance with the Residues Directive (86/469/EEC) and is operated at
RIKILT-DLO in The Netherlands.

2.   FIELD OF APPLICATION.

This method is used for quantification and confirmation of the presence of
six tranquillizers and carazolol in pig kidney. The limits of
identification are 50 ug per kg kidney for the tranquillizers. Azaperone
forms a major metabolite, azaperol, and the two compounds appear together
as residues.

3.   REFERENCES.

Commission Decision, 93/256/EEC, laying down the methods for detecting
residues of substances having a hormonal or thyrostatic action. [OJ. №
L.118, 14.4.93. pp 64-74]

2052/VI/84 File 6.11 II-4, Scientific Veterinary Committee, Working
Group - "Reference Methods for Residues", General Criteria for the
establishment of Reference Methods for the Detection of Residues.

ISO Standard 78/2-1982 Layout for standards - Part 2: Standard for Chemical
Analysis

ISO Standard 5725 (1986)

Arneth, W. (1990), Multiresidue method for the residue-analysis of some
rtanquillizers and carazolol in animal tissue and urine. Proc.
Euroresidues I, Noorijkerhout, NL. May 1990, pp 101-104

Hoogland, H., Beek, W.M.J., Keukens, H.J. and Aerts, M.M.L. (1991),
Confirmation of tranquillizers in porcine kidney by GC-MS. Archiv. für
Lebensm. 42, 79-83

Keukens, H.J. and Aerts, M.M.L., (1989), Determination of residues of
carazolol and a number of tranquillizers in swine kidney by high-
performance liquid chromatography with ultraviolet and fluorescence
detection. J.Chromatog. 464, 149-161

Van Ginkel, L.A.. Schwillens, P.L.W.J. and Olling, M., (1989), Liquid
chromatographic method with on-line UV spectrum identification and off-line
thin-layer chromatographic confirmation for the detection of tranquillizers
and carazolol in pig kidneys. Anal. Chim. Acta. 225, 137-146

4.	DEFINITIONS.

Tranquillizers or carazolol content is taken to mean the amount of
tranquillizers or carazolol in kidney determined according to the described
method and expressed as ug tranquillizers or carazolol per kg test sample.

5.	PRINCIPLE.

The method comprises four stages

- Samples of kidney are extracted with acetonitrile
- clean-up with Sep-Pak C18 cartridges
- analysis and fractionation of eluate with HPLC using a UV or
  fluorescence detector
- identification of tranquillizers by diode-array of selected HPLC
  fractions.

6.	MATERIALS

6.1.	Chemicals

Note: The chemicals were all of analytical grade and obtained from Merck
unless stated otherwise. Reagents of similar quality may be used from
other sources.

6.1.1	Acetone (Merck-14)
6.1.2	Methanol (Merck-6009)
6.1.3	25% ammonia solution (Merck-5432)
6.1.4	n-Hexane (Merck-714)
6.1.5	Acetonitrile, HPLC grade (Merck-3)
6.1.6	Sodium chloride (Merck-6404)
6.1.7	Acetic acid (Merck-63)
6.1.8	Anhydrous sodium acetate (Merck-6268)
6.1.9	Conc. sulphuric acid (Merck-714)

6.2	Solutions

6.2.1	Sodium chloride solution; Dissolve 100 g sodium chloride in
	water and make up to 1 L.
6.2.2	Sulphuric acid solution, 0.01 - 0.05M; Mix 28 mL of sulphuric
	acid (6.1.9) in a beaker with 500 mL water. Allow the solution
	to reach room temperature and add water with mixing to 1 L.
	Transfer 20 to 100 mL of this solution to 250 mL water in a 1 L

	beaker. Fill the beaker with more water.

6.2.3   Acidic Acetonitrile : Add 1 mL of 0.01*M* sulphuric acid solution (6.2.2) to 100 mL acetonitrile.

6.2.4   HPLC-eluent; Weigh 2.46 g sodium acetate (6.1.8) into a 2 L beaker and add 450 mL water and 550 mL acetonitrile solution (6.2.3). Use measuring cylinders for these additions. Bring the pH to 6.4 with acetic acid. Filter the solution with the aid of a suction pump through a 0.22μm filter and place the filtrate in an ultrasonic bath for 10 min. to degas the solution. This solution is stable for 1 month.

6.3.   Standards; Acepromazine, Azaperol and Haloperidol (RIVM) Chlorpromazine hydrochloride, Propionylpromazine and xylazine (Sigma). Azaperone; (Janssen Pharm - Beerse, Belgium), Carazolol (AUU Cugijk)

6.3.1. Stock Standards. Weigh accurately 10 ± 1 mg of an individual standard (6.3) into a 100 mL graduated flask. Make up to 100 mL with methanol. The solution is stored in the dark at 4-8°C and is stable for up to one year.

6.3.2. Working Standards. Pipette 1 mL of stock standard for acepromazine and haloperidol, chlorpromazine hydrochloride, propionylpromazine and azaperone and 2 mL of the xylazine and 0.5 mL for the carazolol into a 100 mL graduated flask and make up to 100 mL with sulphuric acid solution, 0.01*M*, (6.2.2).

6.3.3. Working Standard for azaperone and azaperol; Pipette 1 mL of stock standard for azaperol and azaperone into a 100 mL graduated flask and make up to 100 mL with sulphuric acid solution, 0.01*M*, (6.2.2). Transfer 20 mL of this solution into another 100 mL graduated flask and make up to 100 mL with sulphuric acid solution, 0.01 - 0.05*M*, (6.2.2). The concentration of each standard is 0.2 mg per L.

6.4   Control Samples; Certified blank samples of pig kidneys should be spiked with the standards at concentrations of 20 and 50 μg per kg. Do this by pipetting 100 or 250 μL of the working standard 6.3.2 and/or 6.3.3 into an 80 mL centrifuge tube containing 5 g homogenised sample and allow to stand for 10 min. before extraction.

7.   EQUIPMENT

7.1   Analytical balances
7.2   Normal laboratory glassware including graduated volumetric flasks, 100 mL capacity
7.3   Centrifuge (MSE-Coolspin)
7.3.1   Polypropylene centrifuge tubes, capacity 80 mL
7.4   Ultrasonic bath
7.5   Sep-Pak C18 cartridges (Waters art. 51910)
7.6   Heating block with thermostat and evaporation system with nitrogen (Pierce Reacti Therm Module № 18790 and Pierce Reacti Vap № 18780)
7.7   Vibromixer
7.8   Food Processor (Moulinette)
7.9   Syringe, 50 mL (Terumo)

7.10   pH meter
7.11   HPLC
7.11.1   Basic system with pump (Waters 6000 A)
7.11.2   Automatic injection system with 50 μL injection volume (Waters
          WISP 710 B).
7.11.3   UV detector (Kratos 783 or diode-array Hewlett Packard HP 1040 A)
7.11.4   Fluorescence detector (Hewlett Packard HP 1046 A)
7.11.5   Recorder (Kipp BD 41)
7.11.6   Precolumn; Bondapak C18, 37-50 μm, 10 mm x 2.1 mm i.d. (Waters)
7.11.7   Analytical column; μ Bondapak C18, 10 μm, 300 mm x 3.9 mm i.d.
          (Waters)
7.11.8   Filtering unit for the eluent (Waters № 85124)
7.11.9   Eluent filter, 0.22 μm (Millipore № 83813)

8.   SAMPLES AND SAMPLING PROCEDURE.

N.B. Attention is drawn to section 6.3.1 and to ISO document 78/2-1982 and
also the following notes derived from Annex II of 2052/VI/84-EN.

8.1.   Nature of the Sample; Samples shall be such as to enable the
          detection of residues in meat as defined in Directive 64/433/EEC.

8.2.   Size of Sample; The size of the sample must be large enough to
          allow the method to be carried out and to allow repeat analysis
          where required.

8.3.   The samples must be taken and packed in such a way as to allow
          proper identification in the laboratory.

8.4.   The method of packing, preservation and transport must maintain
          the integrity of the sample and not prejudice the result of the
          examination.
          Samples for the analysis of tranquillizers must be stored and
          transported at temperatures below -18°C.

9.0   PROCEDURE
9.1   Homogenise the kidney sample in a food processor (7.8)
9.2   Weigh 5 g of the homogenised sample into an 80 mL centrifuge tube
          (7.3.1).
9.3   Place the samples and controls (6.4) in a Vibromixer (7.7) and
          spin at 750 rpm. Pipette 20 mL acetonitrile solution (6.2.3)
          into the tube and increase the speed to 1500 rpm for 45 sec.
          Transfer the tubes to an ultrasonic bath for 2 min. Centrifuge
          for 5 min at 4000 g.
9.4   Clean up with Sep-Pak cartridges;
9.4.1   Activate the cartridges (7.5) with 5 mL methanol and 5 mL water.
9.4.2   Drain the cartridges using a syringe (7.9).
9.4.3   Add 50 mL 10% sodium chloride solution (6.2.1) and 7.5 mL
          supernatant from the sample extract (9.3) together, mix and flush
          through the column.
9.4.4   Pass through the column 1 mL 0.01M sulphuric acid (6.2.2) and
          then 2 mL of air.
9.4.5   Prepare calibrated 10 mL test tubes by washing with ammonia
          solution (6.1.3), water, methanol and acetone.
9.4.6   Elute the analytes with 2 mL acidic acetonitrile solution (6.2.3)
          into the prepared test tubes (9.4.5).

9.4.7 Reduce the volume of the eluate to 300 µL by evaporation with nitrogen on a heating block at 70°C. <u>Do not dry.</u>

9.4.8 Add 1 mL n-hexane. Mix for 30 sec on a Vibromixer at 700 rpm and centrifuge at 2000 g for 5 min.

9.4.9 Transfer the aqueous phase with a Pasteur pipette to an injection vial for the HPLC.

9.5 HPLC

9.5.1 Conditions; Equipment as in 7.11
Flow rate; 1.2 mL per min
Injection volume; 50 µL
UV detector at 240 nm, 0.002 Aufs, Recorder 10 mV; 10 mm per min
Fluorescence detector; Excitation, 246 nm; Emission 351 nm, PMT gain, 12; Recorder, 10 mV, 10 mm per min.

9.5.2 Allow the system to equilibrate for 1 hour.

9.5.3 Inject the working standards (6.3.2 and 6.3.3) to achieve reproducible peak heights.

9.5.4 Inject 50 µL of the samples (9.4.9).

9.5.5 Use of Diode-array for suspected positive peaks.

9.5.5.1 Conditions ;
Detector ; HP1040A
Wave length; 240 nm
Bandwidth ; 4 nm
Reference wave length ; 450 nm
Band width for reference ; 100 nm
Threshold ; 1mAu
Spectrum aquisition ; top, slope, base
Spectrum range ; 225 - 400 nm
Spectrum step ; 2 nm

9.5.5.2 Suspect peaks observed during the HPLC separation are analyzed by diode-array to establish the identity of the analyte. The spectrum is compared with that of the standard.

10.0 INTERPRETATION OF RESULTS

10.1 The identity of an analyte is confirmed when;-
- The retention time of the suspect compound is within 5% of that of the standard.
- The diode-array spectra of the suspect peak and that of the standard on the top corrected for background must be similar within 15%.
- The maximum absorbance of the suspect analyte and that of the standard must be within 2 nm of each other.

10.2 QUANTIFICATION
The concentration of the tranquillizer or carazolol can be determined by using the equation;-

$$\text{Conc. in mg per kg} = \frac{Hm \times Cst \times Ve \times 100 \times}{Hst \times m \times R}$$

Hm = peak height of analyte
Hst = peak height of standard
Cst = conc. standard in working solution expressed as mg per L.
Ve = total volume of extract + water volume (23.5 mL)
m = initial weight of sample
f = dilution factor for sample
R = Recovery correction calculated from spiked samples

The percentage recoveries must be in the following ranges;
Carazolol, 84-113; xylazine, 24-80; azaperone, 74-124; haloperidol, 75-115;
acepromazine, 78-124; propionylpromazine, 77-113; chlorpromazine, 58-128.

11.   SPECIAL CASES.

12.   NOTES ON PROCEDURE.

The analytes are unstable in light. Keep all samples in the dark and work
only under an amber light.

13.   SAMPLE CONTROLS

14.   TEST REPORT

15.   LIST OF ABBREVIATIONS.
See abbreviations in Annex I, Section 12 of Manual.

16.   FLOW DIAGRAM

Homogenise kidney -----> extract with acetonitrile -----> C18 Sep-Pak
                                                                  |
                                                                  |
                                                                  |
                                                                  ↓
Identify <---- Diode-array <------ Suspect peaks <----------- HPLC

Sg 4.2.   CARBADOX AS QCA - ROUTINE SCREENING METHOD FOR THE DETERMINATION BY HPLC OF QUINOXALINE CARBOXYLIC ACID (QCA) IN PIG KIDNEY TISSUE.

WARNING AND SAFETY PRECAUTIONS

SAFETY

Organic solvents - all organic solvents must be treated as potentially hazardous and all procedures using them must be performed in a fume cupboard.

FIRST AID

1.   Solvents, acids and alkalis in contact with skin - wash with copious amounts of cold water. Splashes in the eye - irrigate with water and seek medical attention immediately.
2.   Cuts - seek assistance of first aider immediately.
3.   Burns and frostbite - run affected part under cold water (burns) or tepid water (frostbite) for 10 minutes and seek medical attention.

1.   INTRODUCTION

Purpose

The detection of the presence of QCA in samples taken from farm animals in compliance with the Residues Directive 86/469/EEC.

Background

Carbadox is an animal drug used to increase the rate of weight gain, improve feed efficiency and control swine dysentery and bacterial enteritis. Carbadox is a suspected carcinogen but is itself not normally found as a residue in edible tissues. The major metabolite quinoxaline-2-carboxylic acid (QCA) is found as a residue and may also be produced as an artefact during the assay for QCA. QCA is not a carcinogen.

1.   SCOPE

This method of analysis in use at MAFF, FSD, Norwich, UK, describes the determination of the total content of QCA in pig kidney.

2.   FIELD OF APPLICATION.

The method is described to be used for porcine kidney. The limit of determination is not accurately defined but is taken to be 0.01 mg QCA per kg although this may vary between samples because of variable background noise.

3.   REFERENCES.

Commission Decision, 93/256/EEC, laying down the methods for detecting residues of substances having a hormonal or thyrostatic action. [OJ. № L.118, 14.4.93. pp 64-74]

ISO Standard 78/2-1982 Layout for standards - Part 2: Standard for Chemical Analysis

Bygrave, J., Tarbin, J.A. and Rose, M.D. (1993), A method for the

development of quinoxaline carboxylic aacid (metabolite of carbadox) in pig
kidney by HPLC. MAFF, Food Safety Directorate, Food Science Lab, Norwich,
UK. Report. 93/6.

Farrington, W.H.H. The determination of QCA at residue levels in pig
kidney. (1993), MAFF, Food Safety Directorate, Food Science Lab, Norwich,
UK. SOP (1).

Standard operating procedure - CVL. Confirmation of a metabolite of
Carbadox in tissues by GC-MS. (1988)

Farrington, W.H.H., Bygrave, J., Croucher, J and Shearer, G. (1988),
Analysis of UK and imported porcine kidney for quinoxaline carboxylic acid,
a metabolic product of the drug carbadox. Food Science Lab. Report, 26th
April, 1988

4.   DEFINITIONS.

QCA content is taken to mean the amount of QCA in kidney determined
according to the described method and expressed as μg QCA per kg test
sample.

5.0   PRINCIPLE

QCA is extracted with solvents from homogenised kidney samples following
alkaline hydrolysis. The extract is cleaned up using ion-exchange resin
column chromatography and end-point analysis performed with reversed-phase
HPLC and UV detection.

6.   MATERIALS

Note: The reagents (and equipment) for which examples of their source are
quoted are known to be satisfactory, nevertheless reagents and equipment
from other sources may be equally suitable. All the reagents must be of
analytical grade or better.

6.1.   Chemicals
6.1.1.   2-Quinoxaline carboxylic acid (QCA) (Aldrich Chem. Co.)
6.1.2.   Conc. hydrochloric acid (BDH Ltd.)
6.1.3.   1M hydrochloric acid (see 6.3.5)
6.1.4.   Tetrabutylammonium phosphate (Sigma)
6.1.5.   Sodium hydroxide (BDH Ltd.)
6.1.6.   Methanol (Rathburn Chem. Ltd)
6.1.7.   Nitrogen
6.1.8   Ethyl acetate (Rathburn Chem. Ltd)
6.1.9.   Chloroform (Rathburn Chem. Ltd)
6.1.10   Deionised water further processed by Elgastat UHP unit is used
         throughout.
6.1.11   Potassium dihydrogen phosphate (BDH Ltd)
6.1.12   Dowex 50X8-200 cation exchange resin (Sigma)
6.1.13   Disodium hydrogen phosphate (BDH Ltd)

6.2.   Standards
Solid QCA may be obtained from Pfizer or Aldrich Chemical Co.(>97% pure).
6.2.1   A standard of concentration = 0.1 mg/L of QCA in methanol should
         be prepared using available QCA.

6.2.2   Working standards of concentrations = 0.025 µg/mL, 0.05 µg/mL,
         0.1 µg/mL, 0.2 µg/mL, 0.5 µg/mL should be prepared by dilution
         from the stock using the HPLC mobile phase (7.13.).

6.2.3   Spiking Solution; Dilute 0.25 mL of stock standard (6.2.1) to 50
         mL with water.

6.3   Solutions
6.3.1   1*M* Sodium hydroxide. 40 g sodium hydroxide (6.1.5) made up to 1
         L with water.
6.3.2   0.1*M* sodium hydroxide. 100 mL 1*M* Sodium hydroxide (6.3.1) made
         up to 1 L with water.
6.3.3   0.01*M* sodium hydroxide. 100 mL 0.1*M* Sodium hydroxide (6.3.2)
         made up to 1 L with water.
6.3.4   0.1*M* disodium hydrogen phophate buffer, pH 11.0.
         14.2 g disodium hydrogen phophate (6.1.13) is dissolved in 900 mL
         water, adjusted to pH 11.0 with 1*M* sodium hydroxide and made up
         to 1 L with water.
6.3.5   1*M* hyrdochloric acid. Add 86 mL of concentrated HCl to 900 mL
         water and make up to 1 L with water.

7.   EQUIPMENT

7.1   Centrifuge (low speed)
7.2   Separating funnels with teflon stopcock 100 mL, 250 mL
7.3   Screw topped plastic centrifuge tubes, 50 mL
7.4   Vortex mixer(s)
7.5   Magnetic stirrer
7.6   Glass chromatography column, 200 mm x 20 mm i.d. with sintered
         glass frit and stopcock.
7.7   Water bath
7.8   Round bottomed flask, 250 mL
7.9   Heater block assembly for evaporation using nitrogen
7.10   Refridgerator +4°C
7.11   Beakers 100 mL and 1 L capacity.
7.12   Pear-shaped flasks 50 mL
7.13   Bulb pipettes 10 mL fixed and graduated
7.14   All glass filter holder 47 mm.   (Millipore UK Ltd)
7.15   Measuring cylinders 50 mL and 100 mL capacity
7.16   Glass syringe with disposable needles
7.17   Volumetric flasks 50 mL and 100 mL capacity
7.18   Homogeniser (Ultra-Turrax or equivalent)
7.19   Ultrasonic bath
7.20   Rotary evaporator plus water bath
7.21   Disposable syringe filters 0.2 µm (Whatman)
7.22   Safety pipettes (e.g. Gilson Pipetman)
7.23   Membrane filter 0.45 µm "Durapore", 47 mm. (Millipore UK Ltd)
7.24   Preparation of Resin and Ion-exchange column;
         Prepare a slurry of 50 g resin (6.1.12) and 200 mL methanol in a
         1 L beaker. Stir using a glass rod or magnetic stirrer (7.5)
         Pour off the methanol and repeast the wash, then wash the resin
         twice with 200 mL water and twice with 200 mL 1*M* HCl.
         Transfer the resin to the chromatography columns. Pack the resin
         to a height of 50 mm and maintain the level of HCl just above the
         resin bed.

Sg 4.2/3

7.25   HPLC
          Pump : LKB 2150
          Injector: Waters WISP 710B, 50 μL injected
          Detector: Severn Analytical 6510 UV monitor, 320nm at 0.005 AUFS
          Integrator: Spectraphysics 4290
          Column: 200 mm x 3 mm i.d. cartridge columns (Chromsep,
          Chrompack) packed with Chromsher C18 with integral guard
          column packed with pellicular (30-40 μm) reverse phase.
          Mobile Phase: Dissolve 10.2 g tetrabutylammonium phosphate
          (6.1.4)
          and 1.4 g potassium dihydrogen phosphate (6.1.11) in 900 mL
          water. Adjust the pH to 7.5 with 1.0M sodium hydroxide solution
          (6.3.1). Make up to 1 L with water. Mix 650 mL of this buffer
          with 350 mL methanol and pass through a 0.45 μm filter (7.23)
          assisted by pressure.
          The mobile phase is pumped at 0.45 mL per min.

8.   SAMPLES AND SAMPLING PROCEDURE.

N.B. Attention is drawn to section 6.3.1 and to ISO document 78/2-1982 and
also the following notes derived from Annex II of 2052/VI/84-EN.

8.1.   Nature of the Sample; Samples shall be such as to enable the
          detection of residues in meat as defined in Directive 64/433/EEC.

8.2.   Size of Sample; The size of the sample must be large enough to
          allow the method to be carried out and to allow repeat analysis
          where required.

8.3.   The samples must be taken and packed in such a way as to allow
          proper identification in the laboratory.

8.4.   The method of packing, preservation and transport must maintain
          the integrity of the sample and not prejudice the result of the
          examination.
          Samples for the analysis of QCA must be stored and transported at
          temperatures below -18°C.

9.0.   PROCEDURE

9.1.   Sample preparation
Samples may be processed in batches of up to eight. A control sample
and/or one of the eight samples should be spiked with QCA at the 0.02 mg
per kg level.

9.1.1.   5 g thawed sample is minced and placed into a 50 mL centrifuge
          tube.
9.1.2.   10 mL of 0.1M sodium hydroxide is added and homogenised for about
          1 min. Add 4 mL conc. HCl.
9.1.3.   After capping the tubes 15 mL ethyl acetate is added and the
          mixture shaken for 1 min. before centrifuging at 3000 rpm for
          about 5 min to clarify the organic phase.
9.1.4   The ethyl acetate phase is transferred with a Pasteur pipette to
          a second 50 mL plastic centrifuge tube.
9.1.5   The aqueous phase is re-extracted with 2 additional 15 mL of
          ethyl acetate as in 9.1.3 and the ethyl acetate phases combined.

9.1.6   7 mL water is added and the mixture shaken for 1 minute. Centrifuge for 3 min at 3000 r.c.f. The upper ethyl acetate layer is transferred using a pasteur pipette to a 100 mL separating funnel.

9.1.7   Extract three times with 10 mL dihydrogen sodium phosphate, pH 11.0, buffer (6.3.4) by shaking vigorously for approx. 1 min. , running the lower aqueous phase off each time into a 50 mL plastic tube. Centrifuge for 3 min. at 3000 r.c.f. Remove any residual ethyl acetate by pasteur pipette, then bubble nitrogen through the extract for 30 min.. The extract may be refrigerated and stored overnight at this stage.

9.1.8   The aqueous phase is acidified with 6 mL conc. HCl.

9.2   Ion exchange Chromatography

9.2.1   The acidified extract is transferred to the ion-exchange column (7.24) and the column drained to the top of the bed. The resin is washed with 30 mL 1M HCl followed by 40 mL water and the eluent discarded. A 100 mL beaker is placed beneath the column and the column eluted with 75 mL 0.01M sodium hydroxide until the eluent reaches the top of the column bed.

9.2.2   1 mL conc HCl is added to the eluate and transferred to a 250 mL separating funnel. The eluate is extracted with 3 x 50 mL chloroform into a 250 mL round bottomed flask. The chloroform extract is evaporated to dryness using a rotary evaporator at 35-45°C. The residue is transferred to a 50 mL pear-shaped flask with 3 x 2 mL methanol. The volume is reduced to dryness under rotary evaporation at 35-45°C and taken up in 0.5 mL HPLC mobile phase (7.13.v). Use vortexing and ultrasonication to take up all the residue.

9.3   HPLC

9.3.1   Using the conditions set out in 7.25 50 µL are injected onto the column using the automated injector.

9.3.2   Standard QCA corresponding to 0.02 mg per kg is injected in duplicate.

9.3.3   The peak at ca. 7.1 min corresponds to QCA and should be devoid of interfering peaks from the matrix. A near full scale height peak should be found with 20 ng QCA and in the spiked samples.

9.3.4   The linearity of the detector response to QCA ca be checked by running 50 µL of each of the working standards.

10.0   CALCUALATION OF RESULTS

10.1   The concentration of QCA in a sample is determined by interpolation from the spiked samples using the area of the peak corresponding to QCA. If in doubt, suspect positive samples may be overspiked with standard QCA solution,. A resultant single peak indicates a positive (in screening) sample.

10.2   Screening procedure. A minimum of three injections of 50 µL of standard QCA solution (0.5 µg per mL) are carried out to determine the average peak height.

[Note; A 50 µL injection contains 25 ng and is equivalent to 50 µg per kg or 50 ppb tissue concentration.]

Uncorrected conc. of sample in µg per kg is given by

$$\frac{\text{peak height for sample}}{\text{peak height of standard}} \times 50$$

10.3   [Editors note. Positive samples will be rare and therefore a
        vigorous procedure to confirm the positive finding is
        recommended]. Quantitation of positive samples is carried out by
        performing a repeat duplicate analysis and interpolation from a
        full standard curve constructed over the suspect range. The
        curve should have at least 5 points (each point done in
        triplicate) and cover the range from 0 to 10% greater than the
        estimated concentration in the sample. Two blank samples
        fortified with QCA to the same level as the suspected positive
        should also be analysed in the same batch.

10.4   Recovery and intra-assay variation. Recovery is measured for
        each batch of analyses by calculating the recovery from spiked
        samples. For example this was measured four times using 6 single
        replicate spikes in kidney samples.

The results were; Fortified at 0.05 mg per kg; 79% ± 5.6%, 74 ± 5.6%, 72%
± 7.8% and at 0.01 mg per kg; 100% ± 9.8%. (MAFF, Food Safety Directorate,
Norwich, UK).

11.   SPECIAL CASES

11.1   Where the method is to be used for analysing tissues other than
        kidney, e.g. the method may be used for liver, then the method
        should be fully validated for this tissue.

12.   NOTES ON PROCEDURE

12.1.   The _action level_ at which reanalysis of a suspected positive must
        be decided. Also similar decisions need to taken when to proceed
        to a confirming method.

13.   QUALITY CONTROLS

14.   TEST REPORT

15.   LIST OF ABBREVIATIONS

A full list of abbreviations is given in Annex I, Section 12

16.   FLOW DIAGRAM

    Tissue --> add sodium hydroxide and homogenise ---> Extract EtAc
                                                              |
                                                              |
                                                              ↓
        Ion exclusion chrom. <-------- Extract to Na_2HPO_4, pH 11 buffer
            |
            |
            ↓
            HPLC -------> Calculate results

Sg 4.3. CARBADOX AS DESOXYCARBADOX - ROUTINE SCREENING METHOD FOR THE DETERMINATION BY HPLC OF CARBADOX AND DESOXYCARBADOX IN PIG MEAT, LIVER AND KIDNEY TISSUE.

WARNING AND SAFETY PRECAUTIONS
SAFETY
> Organic solvents - all organic solvents must be treated as potentially hazardous and all procedures using them must be performed in a fume cupboard.

FIRST AID
1. Solvents, acids and alkalis in contact with skin - wash with copious amounts of cold water. Splashes in the eye - irrigate with water and seek medical attention immediately.
2. Cuts - seek assistance of first aider immediately.
3. Burns and frostbite - run affected part under cold water (burns) or tepid water (frostbite) for 10 minutes and seek medical attention.

1.   INTRODUCTION

Purpose
The detection of the presence of Carbadox and Desoxycarbadox in samples taken from pigs in compliance with the Residues Directive 86/469/EEC.

Background
Carbadox is an animal drug used to increase the rate of weight gain, improve feed efficiency and control swine dysentery and bacterial enteritis. Carbadox is a suspected carcinogen but is itself not normally found as a residue in edible tissues. Desoxycarbadox is a metabolite of carbadox which persists for up to 15 days in treated animals. The toxicology of this metabolite is not fully evaluated but there is a possibility that it may be mutagenic/carcinogenic. The major metabolite quinoxaline-2-carboxylic acid (QCA) is found as a residue and may also be produced as an artefact during the assay for QCA. QCA is not a carcinogen. The assays for QCA are detailed in Sg 4.2 and Cy 4.3.

1.   SCOPE

This method of analysis in use at RIKILT-OLO, Wageningen, NL describes the determination of the total content of carbadox and desoxycarbadox in pig meat, liver and kidney. The suspect positives can be identified by rerunning the HPLC and using Diode-array detection.

2.   FIELD OF APPLICATION.

The method is described to be used for porcine meat, liver and kidney. The limit of determination is 1 µg per kg for carbadox and 2 µg per kg for desoxycarbadox.

3.   REFERENCES.

Commission Decision, 93/256/EEC, laying down the methods for detecting residues of substances having a hormonal or thyrostatic action. [OJ. № L.118, 14.4.93. pp 64-74]

ISO Standard 78/2-1982 Layout for standards - Part 2: Standard for Chemical Analysis

Aerts, M.M.L., Beek, W.M.J., Keukens, H.J. and Brinkman, U.A.Th., (1988),
Determination of residues of carbadox and some of its metabolites in swine
tissues by high performance liquid chromatography using on-line pre-column
enrichment and post-column derivatization with UV-Vis detection. J.
Chromatog. 456, 105-119

Binnendijk, G.M., Aerts, M.M.L., Keukens, H.J. and Brinkman, U.A.Th.,
(1991), Determination of residues of carbadox and metabolites in products
of animal origin; Stability studies in animal tissues. J. Chromatog. 541,
401-410

4.   DEFINITIONS.

Carbadox or desoxycarbadox content is taken to mean the amount of carbadox
or desoxycarbadox in meat, liver or kidney determined according to the
described method and expressed as μg carbadox or desoxycarbadox per kg test
sample.

5.0   PRINCIPLE

Carbadox and desoxycarbadox are extracted with solvents from homogenised
tissue samples. The extract is cleaned up using aluminium oxide - Florisil
column chromatography and end-point analysis performed with reversed-phase
HPLC and UV/Vis detection after post-column derivatization. The suspect
positives can be identified by rerunning the HPLC and using Diode-array
detection.

6.   MATERIALS

Note: The reagents (and equipment) for which examples of their source are
quoted are known to be satisfactory, nevertheless reagents and equipment
from other sources may be equally suitable. All the reagents must be of
analytical grade or better.

6.1.   Chemicals
6.1.1   Acetonitrile (Merck-3)
6.1.2   Aluminium oxide - Neutral activity 1 (Woelm-21190)
6.1.3   Acetic acid (Merck-63)
6.1.4   Florisil 0.150-0.250 mm (Merck-12518)
6.1.5   Sodium hydroxide (Merck-6498)
6.1.6   Methanol (Merck-6009)
6.1.7   Sodium acetate (Merck-6268)
6.1.8   Iso-octane (Merck-4727)
6.1.9   Helium
6.1.10   Nitrogen

6.2.   Standards
Solid Carbadox may be obtained from Pfizer.
Desoxycarbadox was a gift from Centr. Diergeneeskundig Instituut.
[Note; Use brown glassware for the standard solutions.]
6.2.1   Stock standard solutions (100 μg per mL). A concentration = 0.1
          mg/mL in acetonitrile/methanol (6.3.1) should be prepared
          separately 100 mL volumetric flasks using available carbadox and
          desoxycarbadox. Store the solution in the dark at 6-8°C.
6.2.2   Diluted standard (1 μg per mL). Dilute 1 mL of the stock
          solution 6.2.1 with water to 100 mL. The solution stored in the
          dark at 6-8°C is stable for 1 month.

| 6.2.3 | Working standards (0.1 μg per mL). Dilute 2 mL of the stock solution 6.2.1 with water to 20 mL. |
| 6.2.4 | Standar curves. Concentrations = 1 ng per mL, 2.5 ng per mL and 5 ng per mL should be prepared by dilution of 6.2.3 using water. |

6.3	Solutions
6.3.1	Acetonitrile/methanol. Mix 500 mL acetonitrile with 500 mL water.
6.3.2	0.5M Sodium hydroxide. 20 g sodium hydroxide (6.1.5) made up to 1 L with water. Degas the solution by passing helium through it for 15 min.
6.3.3	Sodium acetate buffer, 0.01M, pH = 6.0. Dissolve 0.82 g sodium acetate in ca 700 mL water. Adjust the pH to 6.0 with acetic acid and make up to 1 L with water.
6.3.4	HPLC Eluent 1. Mix 860 mL of acetate buffer (6.3.3) with 140 mL acetonitrile. Filter the solution through a 0.22 μm filter and degas the filtrate with helium. Use for not more than 2 weeks.
6.3.5	HPLC eluent 2 for diode-array detection. Mix 825 mL of acetate buffer (6.3.3) with 175 mL acetonitrile. Filter the solution through a 0.22 μm filter and degas the filtrate with helium. Use for not more than 2 weeks.

7.	EQUIPMENT
7.1.	Glassware
7.1.1	Graduated pipettes,
7.1.2	Glass centrifuge tubes
7.1.3	Glass test tubes to take 6 mL samples.
7.1.4	Brown graduated volumetric flasks, 100 mL capacity
7.1.5	Pear-shaped flasks 50 mL
7.1.6	Glass chromatography column, 300 mm x 10 mm i.d.
7.1.7	Normal laboratory glassware

7.2.	Apparatus
7.2.1	Automatic pipettes,
7.2.2	Analytical balance
7.2.3	Centrifuge (MSE 2000)
7.2.4	Refrigerator
7.2.5	Vibromixer
7.2.6	Homogeniser, Model 400 Stomacher laboratory blender, (Lameris, NL)
7.2.7	Blender (Moulinette)
7.2.8	pH meter
7.2.9	Filter system for eluents; 0.22 μm (Millipore 83813)
7.2.10	Acrodisc filters 0.45 μm (Gelman 4184)
7.2.11	Deep freeze.
7.2.12	Screw topped plastic centrifuge tubes, 80 mL
7.2.13	Vortex mixer(s)
7.2.14	Magnetic stirrer
7.2.15	Water bath
7.2.16	Rotary evaporator plus water bath at 40-50°C
7.2.17	Cotton wool
7.2.18	Stomacher bags, 1 L volume.

| 7.3 | Preparation of Aluminium oxide-Florisil column; Plug a glass column (7.1.6) with cotton wool. Add to the column 8 g aluminium oxide (6.1.2) and afterwards 2 g Florisil (6.1.4). |

7.4   HPLC
           Pumps: (Waters M-6000)
           Peristaltic pump (Skalar-2002)
           Injector: For 1 mL (Gilson 231/401)
           Detector: 390 nm at 0.001 AUFS (ABI 783)
           Recorder: (Kipp BD-41)
           Diode Array Detector: (HP-1040A)
           Teflon reaction spiral 2 m x 0.5 mm i.d., spiral diam. 1.5 cm
           RVS T-piece 1/16 x 0.75 mm (Valco)
           Guard Column : Bondapack/Corasil 37-50μm, 10 mm x 2.1 mm i.d.
           (Millipore 27248)
           Analytical Column : Chromspher C-18 5 μm, 100 mm x 3.0 mm i.d.
           Chrompack-028268)
           Concentration column : Sep-Pak C-18 (Waters-51910) 10 mm x 2.1
           mm, screens 20 μm (Chrompack-28240)
           The mobile phase, eluent 1 (6.3.4) is pumped at 0.5 mL per min.
           Water is pumped at 0.3 mL per min
           Peristaltic pump at 0.23 mL per min.

8.   SAMPLES AND SAMPLING PROCEDURE.

N.B. Attention is drawn to section 6.3.1 and to ISO document 78/2-1982 and
also the following notes derived from Annex II of 2052/VI/84-EN.

8.1.   Nature of the Sample; Samples shall be such as to enable the
           detection of residues in meat as defined in Directive 64/433/EEC.
8.2.   Size of Sample; The size of the sample must be large enough to
           allow the method to be carried out and to allow repeat analysis
           where required.
8.3.   The samples must be taken and packed in such a way as to allow
           proper identification in the laboratory.
8.4.   The method of packing, preservation and transport must maintain
           the integrity of the sample and not prejudice the result of the
           examination.
           Samples for the analysis of carbadox and desoxycarbadox must be
           stored and transported at temperatures below -18°C.

9.0.   PROCEDURE

9.1.   Sample preparation
Samples are processed in duplicate. Also assay a control sample in
duplicate and two control (blank) samples should be spiked with carbadox
and desoxycarbadox at the 10 μg per kg level.

9.1.1   Control (blank) sample is thawed and blended.
9.1.2   Weigh 10 g of 9.1.1 into a Stomacher bag, (7.2.18) and add 100 μL
           of the diluted carbadox standard (6.2.2). Proceed to step 9.1.5.
9.1.3   Weigh 10 g of 9.1.1 into a Stomacher bag, (7.2.18) and add 100 μL
           of the diluted desoxycarbadox standard (6.2.2). Mix the contents
           and allow to stand for 15 min.   Proceed to step 9.1.5.
9.1.4   The test samples are thawed and blended and 10 g are weighed into
           a Stomacher bag.
9.1.5   Add 40 mL extraction solution (6.3.1) and extract in the
           Stomacher for 3 min.
9.1.6   Transfer the contents of the bag into a 80 mL plastic centrifuge
           tube and centrifuge for 5 min at 2000 g.

9.2   Column Chromatography.
          Transfer the clear supernatant onto the prepared column (7.3) and
          collect the eluate into a 50 mL flask.
9.3   Pipette 10 mL into a calibrated test tube. Evaporate under a
          stream of nitrogen at 40-50°C down to a volume of 0.9-1.1 mL.
9.4   Make the volume up to 4 mL with water. Extract with 2 mL iso-
          octane using shaking for 30 sec on a Vibro-mixer and centrifuging
          at 2000 g for 5 min. Separate the aqueous phase and pass it
          through an Acrodisc filter (7.2.10).
9.5   Inject 1 mL of the aqueous filtrate into the HPLC system.
9.6   HPLC
9.6.1   The HPLC is equilibrated by injecting 1 mL of the 5 ng per mL
          standard solution (6.2.4) until both components give reproducible
          peaks and a stable base line.
9.6.2   The linearity of the detector response to carbadox and
          desoxycarbadox can be checked by running the standards 6.2.4.
          This should be done routinely after every 10 test samples.
9.6.3   Using the conditions set out in 7.4, 1.0 mL of the blank sample
          is injected onto the concentration column using the injector.
9.6.4   Inject 1 mL of the spiked blank samples. After flushing for 20
          min with water the concentration column is switched to the HPLC
          system.
[Note; The peaks for the spikes must be symmetrical (fAs<2) before
proceeding to step 9.6.5]
9.6.4   Inject 1 mL of the samples (9.5).

9.7   HPLC of suspect positive peaks using diode-array detection.
9.7.1   If the suspect peak is indicative of a concentration of either
          carbadox or desoxycarbadox >5 μg per kg then a spectrum using
          diode-array is determined.
9.7.2   Conditions for Detection.
          Eluent 2 (6.3.5) at 0.6 mL per min.
          Measuring wavelength : 350 nm, Bandwidth 4 nm.
          Reference wavelength : 450 nm, bandwidth 100 nm
          Stoptime 15 min after switching the concentration column in the
          HPLC system.
          Threshold : 0.5 mAu
          Spectrum : top, slope and base
          Spectrum range : 225 - 400 nm, step 2nm
9.7.3   Repeat steps 9.3 and 9.4 on 10 mL of eluate from the column.
          Inject as much as possible aqueous phase onto the concentration
          column in accordance with 9.6.3.
9.7.4   Examine the diode-array spectrum at the suspect peak.

10.0   CALCULATION OF RESULTS

10.1   The concentration of carbadox and desoxycarbadox in a sample is
          determined by interpolation from the spiked samples using the
          area of the peaks corresponding to carbadox and desoxycarbadox.
          If in doubt, suspect positive samples may be overspiked with
          standard Desoxycarbadox solution,. A resultant single peak
          indicates a positive (in screening) sample. Suspects are
          examined also by diode-array detection.

[Editors note. Positive samples will be rare and therefore a vigorous
procedure to confirm the positive finding is recommended].

The concentration of carbadox and desoxycarbadox in a sample is calculated using the formula;-

$$C_{an} = \frac{Om}{Ost} \times C_{st} \times \frac{Ve}{a} \times \frac{Va}{Vk} \times \frac{100}{R}$$

C_{an} = concentration of carbadox or desoxycarbadox in µg per kg
Om = peak area for test sample
Ost = peak area for standard
C_{st} = conc. of standard in µg per L
Ve = volume of extract + water content of sample in mL (normally 47 mL). The water content of the samples is usually 70 -75%).
Vm = volume of analysis solution (normally 4 mL)
Vk = Volume of aliquot from alumina column (normally 10 mL)
a   = weight in g of tissue
R   = recovery in %

Calculate the mean for the duplicate determinations.

10.2   Recovery is measured for each batch of analyses by calculating the recovery from spiked samples. Data reported by RIKILT-OLO for recovery for spikes of 10 µg per kg in 20 samples are >90% for carbadox and 95% for desoxycarbadox with a CV = 10.7%.

10.3   The limit of detection in meat, liver and kidney was 0.5 µg per kg for carbadox and 1.0 µg per kg for desoxycarbadox.

10.4   The sample was positive when according to the EEC criteria in EEC 93/256 (see section 5).
1. The concentration of carbadox or desoxycarbadox ≥ 5 µg per kg
2. The spectrum of carbadox or desoxycarbadox was confirmed by diode-array.

11.   SPECIAL CASES

12.   NOTES ON PROCEDURE

12.1.   The action level at which reanalysis of a suspected positive must be decided. In this method ≥ 5 µg per kg is the action level used in The Netherlands.

13.   QUALITY CONTROLS

14.   TEST REPORT

15.   LIST OF ABBREVIATIONS
A full list of abbreviations is given in Annex I, Section 12

16.   FLOW DIAGRAM

Tissue ---> Extract in acetonitrile/methanol ------> Alumina-Florisil
                                                        column
                                                          |
                                                          |
                                                          ↓
Calculate conc. <----- UV det.<------- Post column <------- HPLC
      | derivatization
      |
      ↓
If ≥ 5 µg/kg rerun HPLC with Diode Array to identify analyte.

Sg. 4.4 IONOPHORES - A ROUTINE METHOD FOR THE DETERMINATION OF RESIDUES OF IONOPHORES IN CHICKEN MEAT, LIVER AND KIDNEY, USING HPTLC.

WARNING AND SAFETY PRECAUTIONS

0.   INTRODUCTION
Ionophores are administered as in-feed additives to poultry and cattle.
They are used to prevent coccidiosis in poultry.
Ionophores are weak antibiotic substances which have growth enhancing
properties when used in poultry and ruminating cattle.

1.   SCOPE

This method of analysis describes the determination of the presence of
individual analytes for THREE ionophores, monensin, narasin and salinomycin
in samples of tissues of chickens. This work is carried out in compliance
with the Residues Directive (86/469/EEC) and the method is used routinely
in The Netherlands at RIKILT-DLO.

2.   FIELD OF APPLICATION.

The method is used to perform routine screening and confirmatory analyses
in chicken samples.

The limit of detection using UV detection is 0.02 mg per kg for meat, liver
and kidney. The limit of detection using autobiographical detection is
0.005 mg per kg for all samples.

3.   REFERENCES.

Commission Decision, 93/256/EEC, laying down the methods for detecting
residues of substances having a hormonal or thyrostatic action. [OJ. №
L.118, 14.4.93. pp 64-74]

ISO Standard 78/2-1982 Layout for standards - Part 2: Standard for Chemical
Analysis

RIKILT (1988), Diervoeders, kipmatrices- Bepaling van monensin, narasin and
salinomycin. Intern Analyseschrift A493 2e oplage 1988-03-07.

4.   DEFINITIONS.

Ionophore substance content is taken to mean the amount of ionophore
substance in the sample determined according to the described method and
expressed as mg ionophore substance per kg of test sample.

5.   PRINCIPLE

The methods comprises 7 stages;-

-        Homogenisation
-        Extraction using methanol.
-        Clean up of ionophore substance by aluminium oxide column
         chromatography
-        End point determination with TLC by derivatisation and UV light
or -   End point determination with TLC and Autobiography

-        The detection of ionophore substance is made by comparison with
         standards run on TLC.

6.   MATERIALS

Note: The reagents for which examples of their source are quoted are
known to be satisfactory, nevertheless reagents from other sources may be
equally suitable.

6.1.   Standards
6.1.1   Sodium monensin (Elanco)
6.1.2   Sodium narasin (Elanco)
6.1.3   Salinomycin   (Hoechst)

6.2   Chemicals
6.2.1   Methanol (Merck 6009)
6.2.2   Water (HPLC grade)
6.2.3   Ethyl acetate (Merck 9623)
6.2.4   Aluminium oxide (Alumina Woelm N, Art. I)
6.2.5   Sodium Chloride (Merck 6404)
6.2.6   p-anisaldehyde (Merck 822134)
6.2.7   Dextrose (Difco 0155-17-4)
6.2.8   Potassium dihydrogen phosphate (Merck 4873)
6.2.9   Disodium hydrogen phosphate. 2H$_2$0. (Merck 6580)
6.2.10   Sulphuric acid (Merck 732)
6.2.11   Acetic acid (Merck 63)
6.2.12   Triphenyltetrazoliumchloride (Merck 8380)
6.2.13   Stand II Nutrient agar (Merck 7883)
6.2.14   Micro-organism *Bacillus Subtilis* (BGA Berlin)

6.3   Solutions
6.3.1   90% Methanol; Mix 900 mL methanol with 100 mL water.
6.3.2   Ethyl acetate/1% water; Add 1 mL water to 100 mL ethyl acetate
          (6.2.3)
6.3.3   10% sodium chloride; Dissolve 100 g of sodium chloride in about
          700 mL water and make up the solution to 1 L.
6.3.4   Reaction mixture for dipping HPTLC plates. Mix 4 mL p-
          anisaldehyde (6.2.6) in 68 mL methanol (6.2.1). Add carefully 4
          mL sulphuric acid (6.2.10) and 2 mL acetic acid (6.2.11).
6.3.5   Triphenyltetrazoliumchloride.
          Mix 0.2 g triphenyltetrazoliumchloride (6.2.12) and 5 g dextrose
          (6.2.7) in 100 mL water.
6.3.6   Standards.
6.3.6.1   Stock solutions. Weigh accurately about 25 mg ionophore (6.1)
          and transfer with methanol to 100 mL volumetric flask. Make up
          to 100 mL with methanol.
6.3.6.2   Working solutions. Pipette into three 100 mL volumetric flasks,
          1 mL, 5 mL and 10 mL of stock solution (6.3.6.1) respectively.
          Make up to 100 mL with methanol. The concentrations in the
          flasks are;- 2.5; 12.5 and 25 µg per mL.

6.3.7   Solution for the Autobiography detection for 2 HPTLC plates.
          Into a round bottomed flask weigh 2.5 g nutrient agar (6.2.13),
          0.5 g sodium chloride (6.2.5), 1 g dextrose (6.2.7), 0.42 g
          potassium dihydrogen phosphate (6.2.8), 0.045 g disodium hydrogen
          phosphate (6.2.9). Add 100 mL water and dissolve the reagents in

a Magnetron for 15 sec. Sterilise the mixture for 15 min at 121
± 1°C. Stand the mixture in a water bath at 60°C and adjust the
pH to 6.0 ± 0.1 if necessary. Add 1 mL bacterial suspension
(6.2.14) and 1 mL diphenyltetrazoliumchloride solution (6.3.5).

7   EQUIPMENT

7.1   Ultra Turrax homogeniser or a Stomacher
7.2   Rotary evaporator
7.3   Vortex mixer(s)
7.4   HPTLC equipment for running HPTLC plates.
7.4.1   HPTLC silica gel plates, (Merck № 5631). The plates must be
        dried for 2 h at 110°C immediately before use.
7.5   UV lamp at 366 nm
7.6   Drying cabinet
7.7   Cabinet at 110°C for HPTLC plates
7.8   Centrifuge tubes, 300 mL capacity
7.9   Water bath at 60°C
7.10   Centrifuge
7.11   Erlenmeyer flasks, 100 mL capacity
7.12   Glass chromatography columns, 40 cm long x 10 mm i.d. with 2 mm
        outlet.
7.13   Petri dishes, ca 14 cm diam.
7.14   Shaking apparatus
7.15   pH meter
7.16   Incubator at 37 ± 1°C
7.17   Volumetric flasks, 100 mL
7.18   Evaporating system using nitrogen and heating. (Pierce)
7.19   Vacuum system for cartridges
7.20   Sterilisation apparatus
7.21   Paper filters.
7.22   Cotton wool
7.23   Baker C-18 SPE cartridges. Activate the columns by washing with
        5 mL methanol and 2 x 5 mL water.

8.   SAMPLES AND SAMPLING PROCEDURE.

N.B. Attention is drawn to section 6.3.1 and to ISO document 78/2-1982 and
also the following notes derived from Annex II of 2052/VI/84-EN. and EEC
93/256.

8.1.   Nature of the Sample; Samples shall be such as to enable the
        detection of residues in tissues as defined in Directive
        64/433/EEC.
8.2.   Size of Sample; The size of the sample must be large enough to
        allow the method to be carried out and to allow repeat analysis
        where required. Each analysis needs a 10 g sample.
8.3.   The samples must be taken and packed in such a way as to allow
        proper identification in the laboratory.
8.4.   The method of packing, preservation and transport must maintain
        the integrity of the sample and not prejudice the result of the
        examination.
        Samples for the analysis of ionophores must be stored at
        temperatures below -18°C.

9   PROCEDURE
9.1   Cut the sample into small pieces and weigh 10 g into a 100 mL
            Erlenmeyer flask.
9.2   Add 50 mL 90% methanol solution (6.3.1).
9.3   Primary extraction - For meat, liver and kidney homogenise with
            an Ultra Turrax for 3 min.
9.4   Centrifuge at 4000 rpm for 5 min.
9.5   Filter the supernatant through a cotton wool plug into a 100 mL
            Erlenmeyer flask .
9.6   Mix the sediment with 10 mL 90% methanol (6.3.1) using a
            vibromixer, centrifuge at 1000 rpm and decant the supernatant
            through a cotton wool filter into the Erlenmeyer flask.
9.7   Clean-up with Chromatography
9.7.1   Aluminium oxide columns. Use a cotton wool plug to act as filter
            for the columns. Add 7 g aluminium oxide (6.2.4) into a column
            (7.12). Pour the extract (9.5 & 9.6) onto the column. Use a 200
            mL flask to collect the eluate.
9.7.2   Rinse the flask containing any residual extract with 10 mL 90%
            methanol and transfer the solution onto the column.
9.7.3   Add to the collected eluate 60 mL 10% sodium chloride solution
            (6.3.3). Filter the mixture through a filter paper. Rinse.
9.7.4   Attach an activated Baker C-18 column (7.23) to a solvent
            reservoir. Pass the eluate (9.7.3) through the column with the
            aid of suction. Do not allow the column to run dry. Rinse the
            contents of the Erlenmeyer flask onto the column with 10 mL water
            and then 5 mL water. Allow the column to run dry and if
            necessary remove any residual water by centrifuging the
            cartridges.
9.7.5   Elute the columns with 6 mL methanol into a 10 mL tube.
9.8   Evaporate the methanol to dryness and redissolve the residue in
            400 μL methanol.
9.9   HPTLC
9.9.1   Transfer 20 μL of extract (9.8) onto a plate at 1.5 cm above the
            base of the plate using a stream of nitrogen to minimise the size
            of the spots. Use 10 mm distances between the spots for UV
            detection and 20 mm for Autobiography.
9.9.2   Add 20 μL of the working standards (6.3.6.2) onto the plate.
9.9.3   Pour the mobile phase, ethyl acetate/1% water (6.3.2), into the
            tank and allow 30 min for equilibration at room temperature.
9.9.4   Run the plates for 5 cm above the spotting places. After the run
            allow the plates to dry for 30 min at room temperature.
9.9.5   UV Detection.
9.9.5.1   Dip the dried HPTLC plate in the p-anisaldehyde solution (6.3.4)
            and stand to dry at room temperature for 1½ h. in a stream of
            air.
9.9.5.2   Detect the spots for the ionophores under UV light at 366 nm.
            Either mark the spots on the plate or photograph them.
9.9.6   Autobiography detection
9.9.6.1   Lie the plate in the bottom of a level petri dish. Pour 46 mL of
            the agar solution (6.3.7) over the plate. Allow the agar to
            solidify and cover the plate.
9.9.6.2   Incubate the plate at 37°C overnight and examine the plate for
            zones of inhibition.

10   INTERPRETATION OF RESULTS
10.1   Identification of the analytes on the HPTLC is obtained when the
           spots or zones of inhibition have the same R_f (and colours under
           UV) as the standards. The diameter of the measured zones are
           correlated with the logarithm of the concentration of the
           analyte.

11.   SPECIAL CASES

12.   NOTES ON PROCEDURE.

13.   QUALITY CONTROLS
Blank samples should be spiked with ionophore standards.

14.   TEST REPORT

15.   LIST OF ABBREVIATIONS

A full list of abbreviations is given in Annex I, Section 12

16.   FLOW DIAGRAM

```
             homogenise
   SAMPLE -------------> METHANOL  --------> ALUMINA COLUMN
             extract                                       |
                                              collect      |
                                              fraction     |
                                                           ↓
   IDENTIFY with UV <--------- HPTLC <------------ C-18 SPE
   or AUTOBIOGRAPHY
```

Sg 4.5. LEVAMISOLE - A ROUTINE METHOD FOR THE DETERMINATION OF RESIDUES OF LEVAMISOLE IN ANIMAL LIVERS BY GC-MS.
[Note; Method can be extended to a confirming method]

WARNING AND SAFETY PRECAUTIONS

Wear disposable gloves when handling tissues. All operations involving solvents must be conducted in a fume cupboard.

0.   INTRODUCTION

Levamisole is a broad spectrum anthelmintic drug used for the control of gastrointestinal and lungworm nematodes in ruminants, horses and pigs. The MRL set in the EEC is 10 µg per kg for edible tissues.

1.   SCOPE

This method of analysis describes the determination of the content of Levamisole in liver samples. The method is set out as a routine screening method but can easily be extended for use as a confirming method.

2.   FIELD OF APPLICATION.

The method was developed for monitoring liver tissue. The limit of determination following validation of the method is 5 µg per kg of liver.

3.   REFERENCES.

Commission Decision, 93/256/EEC, laying down the methods for detecting residues of substances having a hormonal or thyrostatic action. [OJ. № L.118, 14.4.93. pp 64-74]

ISO Standard 78/2-1982 Layout for standards - Part 2: Standard for Chemical Analysis

Neate, S. (1993), The determination of levamisole in liver by gas chromatography - mass spectrometry. Standard Operating Proc. ACU 0267A, CVL., UK.

Porter, S., Patel, R., Neate, S. and Osso, P. (1993). Determination of levamisole in liver by gas chromatography - mass spectrometry. Euroresidues II, Proc. Residues of veterinary drugs in food. Ed. Haagsma, N., Ruiter, A. & Czediik-Eysenberg, P.B., Veldhoven, NL. pp 548-552.

4.   DEFINITIONS.

Levamisole content is taken to mean the amount of Levamisole in the substance in question, regardless of the chemical form, determined according to the described method and expressed as µg Levamisole per kg of test sample.

5.   PRINCIPLE

The methods comprises 4 stages;-

-       Homogenisation of tissue samples in alkali and ethyl acetate.
-       Clean up with liquid/liquid partition.
-       GC-MS in EI-PI mode.
-       The amount of Levamisole is calculated by interpolation from a
        standard curve and taking into account the recovery of
        Levamisole.

6.   CHEMICALS

6.1.1   Chloroform (BDH)
6.1.2   Ethyl acetate (BDH)
6.1.3   Potassium hydroxide (BDH)
6.1.4   Methanol, HPLC grade (BDH)
6.1.5   Concentrated Hydrochloric acid (BDH)
6.1.6   Sodium sulphate anhydrous granular (BDH)
6.1.7   Ethyl acetate (BDH)
6.1.8   Water Deionised and filtered 0.2 μm.

6.2.   Solutions
6.2.1   50% Potassium hydroxide. Carefully dissolve 250 g of KOH in 400
         mL water. Make up to 500 mL when cool.
6.2.2   0.5M Hydrochloric acid. Carefully add 22 mL conc. HCl to 400 mL
         water and make up to 500 Ml when cool.

6.3.   Standards

6.3.1.   Levamisole hydrochloride (Sigma - L9756)
6.3.2.   Stock standards; Dissolve 50 mg Levamisole in methanol and
         dilute to 50 mL. Make fresh monthly.
6.3.3   Working standards;
6.3.3.1 Dilute 1 mL stock to 100 mL with chloroform. Final concentration
         is 10 μg per mL. Make fresh daily.
6.3.3.2 Dilute 1,2 and 5 mL 6.3.3.1 to 10 mL with chloroform. Final
         concentrations are 1, 2 and 5 μg per mL respectively. Make fresh
         daily. These are equivalent to 1, 2 and 5 times the MRL.

6.5.   Spiking Procedure

         Using separately the working standards (6.3.6.1 & 6.3.6.2) spike
         5 g sample with 1 mL of solution. Allow to stand for 15 minutes.

7.   EQUIPMENT

7.1   Centrifuge tubes 50 mL capacity, Sarsted polypropylene with screw
         cap.
7.2   Conical centrifuge tubes, Polypropylene, 12 mL, with push cap.
7.3   Conical centrifuge tubes, glass, 10 mL, with plastic stopper
7.4   Measuring cylinders, 25 mL, 500 mL and 1 L
7.5   Volumetric flasks, 10 mL, 25 mL, 50 mL 100 mL and 500 mL.
7.6   Glass pipettes, 1 mL, 2 mL and 5 mL.
7.7   Glass beakers, 100 mL, 250 mL, 500 mL and 1 L.
7.8   Sartorius cellulose acetate, 0.2 μm
7.9   Short tipped Pasteur pipettes.

Sg 4.5/2

7.10   Glass microsyringes, 100 µL (SGE UK)
7.11   Mixer (Vortex)
7.12.   Centrifuge - MSE Mistral 2L or equivalent
7.13   Homogeniser (Silverson heavy duty sealed unit)
7.14   Shaker, mechanical flat bed (Denley)
7.15   Glass microvials, 1.5 mL with crimp-on metal caps and inserts.
7.16   Falcon 710S bottle top (Becton Dickinson)
7.17   200 µL microvial (Chromacol, Type 02-CVTG)
7.18   Balances
7.19   Heating blocks and accompanying nitrogen evaporation system.
7.20   Adjustable pipettes 200 µL, 1000 µL and 5000 µL

7.21   GC-MS
        Mass selective detector (Hewlett Packard - HP5970) coupled to HP-
        5890 gas chromatograph and linked to HP Vectra 486/33U PC or
        equivalent. The GC-MS was equipped with an autosampler (Hewlett
        Packard 7673A).
        GC column; 15 m x 0.25 mm i.d. with a phase of DB5 film, 0.25 µm
        thickness (J&W Scientific)

8.   SAMPLES AND SAMPLING PROCEDURE.

        Note; Attention is drawn to section 6.3.1 and ISO document 78/2-
        1982 and the following notes derived from Annex II of 2052/VI/84-
        EN.

8.1.   Nature of the Sample; Samples shall be such as to enable the
        detection of residues in meat, as defined in Directive
        64/433/EEC.

8.2.   Size of Sample; The size of the sample must be large enough to
        allow the reference method to be carried out and to allow repeat
        analysis where required.

8.3.   The samples must be taken and packed in such a way as to allow
        proper identification in the laboratory.

8.4.   The method of packing, preservation and transport must maintain
        the integrity of the sample and not prejudice the result of the
        examination.

        Samples for the analysis of Levamisole must be stored and
        transported at temperatures below -18°C.

9.   PROCEDURE

9.1   Samples are prepared in batches of up to 13 test samples, plus 2
        control spikes at the MRL and 1 control blank.
9.2   Weigh out 10 ± 0.09 g of liver tissue into a Sarsted tube (7.1)
9.3   To each of two control livers add 100 µL of 1 µg per mL standard
        (6.3.3.2) using a 100 µL syringe.
9.4   To each tube add 5 g of anhydrous sodium sulphate, spreading it
        evenly over the tissue surface.
9.5   Add 1 mL of 50% KOH to each tube and 15 mL ethyl acetate.
9.6   Homogenise at maximum speed for 2 min.
9.7   Attach samples to the horizontal shaker (7.14) and shake for 15
        min.
9.8   Centrifuge for 15 min at 2500-3500 rpm.

9.9   Remove the ethyl acetate into clean Sarsted tubes.
9.10   Add 15 mL ethyl acetate to the precipitate and break up the tissue residue with a metal spatula and repeat stages 9.8 and 9.9.
9.11   Pool and mix the second ethyl acetate fraction with the first.
9.12   Transfer a 20 mL aliquot to a clean labelled Sarsted tube (7.1)
9.13   Add 5 mL 0.5M HCl shake by hand vigorously for 2 min and then centrifuge at 3000 rpm for 5 min.
9.14   Draw off the upper ethyl acetate layer with a Pasteur pipette connected via a vacuum line. Discard the ethyl acetate fraction.
9.15   Transfer the acid layer to a clean glass centrifuge tube. Add 1 mL 50% KOH to each of the tubes and vortex mix.
[Note; If necessary these extracts can be stored overnight at 4°C]
9.16   Add 100 μL chloroform, shake vigorously by hand for one min. Allow to stand for 10 min.
9.17   Centrifuge at 3000 rpm for 5 min.
9.18   Remove and discard most of the upper aqueous phase with a Pasteur pipette.
9.19   Using a 100 μL syringe transfer all of the organic phase to 200 μL microvial. Rinse the syringe with 100 μL chloroform and transfer the rinsing to the microvial.
9.20   Evaporate to dryness using a stream of nitrogen.
[Note; The sample can be stored for up to five days at -18°C]
9.21   Add 100 μL chloroform and redissolve with vortexing.
9.22   Inject 1 μL into the GC.

9.23   <u>GC-MS Analysis</u>

9.23.1.   The GC parameters are set up as follows;

COLUMN: see 7.21
INJECTIONS: 1 μl manual injections.
TEMPERATURES: Interface: 240°C
                Injector: 240°C
OVEN TEMPERATURES:

from temp (°C)	to temp (°C)	rate (°C/min)	time (min)	total time (min)
60	60	-	2.0	2.0
60	240	25.5	7.06	9.06
240	240	-	7.0	16.06

CARRIER GAS: Helium
         flow rate   = 1 cm^3/min   column head pressure = 70 Kpa.

The retention time for Levamisole in this system is 8.47 min

9.23.2 The mass spectrometry parameters are

IONISER: Electron-Impact

Calibration of the mass axis plus tuning of the ion source is carried out using the "autotune programme", using the calibration compound perfluorotributylamine (PFTBA).

10.   CALCULATION OF RESULTS

10.1   The presence of Levamisole is suspected if
-           The retention of the analyte in the GC is within 5 sec of the
            retention time of the Levamisole standard.
-           The presence of the ion at m/z 204 is observed.

10.2   Confirmation procedure.
        Examine the spectra for the ions at m/z 121, 148, 203 and 204.
        Calculate their ratios in relationship to the base peak, m/z 148.
        The ratios must be within 10% of those of the reference standard
        Levamisole. This was shown to hold true for ions two ions, 203
        and 204 (Porter et al., 1993) and acceptable for ion 121;-

ION m/z	Relative Abundance %		CV%	
	Standard	Spike	Standard	Spike
121	29.9	30.0	9.1	13
203	40.6	44.8	6.1	4.1
204	90.2	100.7	13.2	7.3

10.3.   Quantitation.
        A calibration curve is constructed of peak height against
        concentration for a range of standards. A linear curve was
        obtained over the range 5 - 100 µg per kg liver (Porter et al.,
        1993). The quantity of Levamisole in each sample injection is
        then calculated from the measured peak height

$$\% \text{ recovery} = \frac{\text{amount of Levamisole found}}{\text{amount of Spike added}} \times 100$$

Concentration of Levamisole in sample (µg/kg) =

$$\text{µg Levamisole (from calibration curve)} \times \frac{10}{\text{mass of sample}}$$

        For samples containing Levamisole at concentrations beyond the
        range of the standard curve, a dilution of the extract is
        prepared and chromatographed, and the appropriate volumetric
        correction is applied.

10.4.   SENSITIVITY
        The minimum limit of determination of Levamisole by this method
        is 5 µg/kg.

10.5.   QUALITY ASSURANCE PROCEDURES.

        Recovery of the analyte should fall within 50-80%.

11.   SPECIAL CASES.

12.   NOTES ON PROCEDURE.

        The method should be validated in-house especially if its use is
        extended to confirming procedures.

13.   SAMPLE CONTROLS

The blank samples were obtained from a sample previously analyzed
and found to contain no Levamisole.

14.   TEST REPORT

15.   LIST OF ABBREVIATIONS.

See abbreviations in Annex I, section 12 of Manual.

16.   FLOW DIAGRAM

Tissue ---→ add ethyl acetate ------→ Homogenise ------> Solvent/solvent
                                                            |
                                                            ↓
            Calculate results <---- Confirm <------- GC-MS

Cy 1.1. ANABOLIC AGENTS - A MODULAR METHOD FOR THE ANALYSIS OF BIOLOGICAL MATERIALS FOR RESIDUES OF ANABOLIC AGENTS (STEROID-LIKE GROWTH PROMOTERS).

WARNING AND SAFETY PRECAUTIONS

Pentafluorobenzyl bromide is a strong lachrymator agent.

0.   INTRODUCTION

Throughout the EEC the use of xenobiotic anabolic agents is prohibited in food-producing animals. Also the MRL for residues of these anabolics in animal products imported into or produced within the Community is zero. Preparations of natural steroids or their esters may be used in farm animals under strictly controlled conditions (see EEC Directive 86/469/EEC) and the maximum concentrations of natural steroids allowed in plasma are set (see section 2) but the levels permitted in edible tissues have not yet been defined (August 1991).

1.   SCOPE

This modular method of analysis describes the detection and confirmation of the presence of individual analytes for a large number of Anabolic Agent(s) (AnAg) in samples of animal origin - the method has been mainly tested for residues in urine and muscle including minced meat for the gestagens. This work is carried out in compliance with the Residues Directive (86/469/EEC).

2.   FIELD OF APPLICATION.

The method is used to perform routine screening and confirmatory analyses in bovine urine and muscle samples.
The method can be adapted for fish and also for biological material such as animal organs, biological fluids and faeces. This modular method is suitable for testosterone*, trenbolone*, oestradiol, zeranol, taleranol, diethylstilboestrol, hexoestrol, dienoestrol, 19-nortestosterone*, methyltestosterone, boldenone, ethinyloestradiol*, medroxyprogesterone acetate, chlormadinone acetate and megestrol acetate,

*   either the 17α- or the 17ß- hydroxy compounds.

The limit of detection is below 1 ug per L or ug per kg for all compounds. The limit of detection is based on the detection of the most abundant ion with a response at the correct retention time exceeding the average noise ± 3 SD. The limit of identification ranges from 0.5 - 2.0 ug per kg or L depending on the analyte and the matrix. The limit of identification equals the limit of detection as based on the fourth diagnostic ion.

3.   REFERENCES.

Commission Decision, 93/256/EEC, laying down the methods for detecting residues of substances having a hormonal or thyrostatic action. [OJ. № L.118, 14.4.93. pp 64-74]

2052/VI/84 File 6.11 II-4, Scientific Veterinary Committee, Working Group - "Reference Methods for Residues", General Criteria for the establishment of Reference Methods for the Detection of Residues.

ISO Standard 78/2-1982 Layout for standards - Part 2: Standard for Chemical
Analysis

Bagnati, R., Castelli, M.G., Airoldi, L., Oriundi, M.P., Ubaldi, A. and
Fanelli, R. (1990), Analysis of diethylstilboestrol, dienoestrol and
hexoestrol in biological samples by immunoaffinity extraction and gas-
chromatography - negative ion chemical ionization mass spectrometry
detection. J. Chromatogr. <u>527</u>, 267-278

Bagnati, R. and Fanelli R. (1991). Determination of trace levels of 19-
nortestosterone, testosterone and trenbolone by Gas-chromatography -
Negative ion mass spectrometry after a new derivatization procedure.
J.Chromatogr. (submit)

Bagnati, R., Oriundi, M.P., Russo, V., Danese, M., Berti, F. and Fanelli,
R. (1991). Determination of Zeranol and ß-Zearalanol in calf urine by
immunoaffinity extraction and gas chromatography - mass spectrometry after
repeated administrations of zeranol. J.Chromatogr. <u>564</u>, 493-502

Cunningham, N., Communication to EEC, DGVI, of GC-MS methods for detection
of Stilbenes, Zeranol, and 17α-Trenbolone in bile, CVL, Weybridge, UK, 17th
August, 1988.

Daeseleire, E., De Guesquiere, A. and Van Peteghem, C., (1991),
Derivatization and gas chromatographic-mass spectrometric detection of
anabolic steroid residues isolated from edible muscle tissues. J.
Chromatogr. <u>562</u>, 673-679

Van Ginkel, L.A., Stephany, R.W., Van Rosum, H.J., Steinbuch, H.M., Zomer,
G., Van De Heeft, E. and De Jong, P.J.M. (1989), Multi-immunoaffinity
Chromatography: A simple and highly selective clean-up method for multi-
anabolic residues of meat. J. Chromatogr. <u>489</u>, 111-120.

4.   DEFINITIONS.

AnAg content is taken to mean the amount of AnAg in the substance in
question, regardless of the chemical form, determined according to the
described method and expressed as ug AnAg per kg or litre of test sample.

5.   PRINCIPLE

5.1. The methods comprises 4 stages;-
    1. preparation of a primary extract
    2. extract purification and concentration using IAC and/or HPLC.
[Note; GC-MS methods from CVL, UK, for measuring residues of stilbenes,
trenbolone and zeranol in bile are described elsewhere in this section (Cy
1.3, Cy 1.4, Cy 1.5).
    3. detection and identification by GC-MS
    4. calculation of results.

The method allows choice of biological material, equipment, reagents and
the procedures.

TABLE. 5.I.

AnAg	Sample	IAC		HPLC	Derivative for GCMS			
		RIVM	GENEGO		TMS	HFB	PFB	PFB/TMS
DES	U,M	+	+	+	++	+c	+	
HEX	U,M	+	+	+	++	+c	+	
DE	U,M	+	+	+	++	+c	+	
β-E$_2$	M	+	+	+	+	++		+
EE	U,M			+	+	++		
Z	U,M	+	+	+	++	+c		+
Taleranol	U		+					+
17β-TB	U,M	+	+	+	+c			
17α-TB	U	+		+	+c			
β-NT	U,M	+	+	+	+	++		
α-NT	U	+		+	+	++		
MT	U,M	+	+	+	+			
17α-T	U	+		+	+	++		
17β-T	U	+	+	+	+	++		
Boldenone	U			+	+	++		
MPA	Fat			+		+		
MGA	Fat			+		+		
CMA	Fat			+		+		

++ indicates that it is the most suitable derivative when RIVM compared the
TMS and HFB derivatives. c refers to the derivatives made for extracts of
bile used in the CVL method (M 1.2).

5.2.   THE MODULAR STEPS AND THE OPTIONS.

5.2.1.   Choice of modules for different analytes for clean-up and GCMS.

5.2.2.   THE OPTIONS FOR PROCEDURES.

STEP	OPTIONS		NOTES.
1. Select tissue	a. U,Bi,		2,3,4a
	b. Fc	Required steps	2,3,4a,5a
	c. M	between 2 and 5	2,3,(4b),5a/b
	d. L, K		2,3,4a,5a
	e. F		3,5c
	f. Mi,		2,3
	g, Eg		2,3,

  Use incurred and blank RMs if available.   as per matrix

2. Dilute   Select buffer

3. Internal Standard. Select and add internal standard (IS).

4. Hydrolyse   a. enzyme for conjugates,   Glucuronides, SO_4
                   b. alkali for esters   Especially injection sites
                   Select time, temp, pH.

5. Homogenise   a. Mechanical (e.g. Ultra-Turrax)
                   b. Enzymatic; Select time, temp, pH
                   c. Dissolve in lipophilic solvent   Fat only

6. Solvent Extract. Select solvents and quantities. Omit if possible.
Note; In the method for muscle (Daeseleire et al. 1991) further clean-up is
achieved by passing an ether extract through disposable C-18 cartridges.
   Recoveries were >97% for T, EE, MPA, MT and NT and 85% for $E_2\beta$.

7. Go to step 8 or 9

8. IAC.   Select column (see Table 1)
                   Follow instructions of suppliers.
                   Collect analyte fractions.
                   Omit step 9

9. HPLC   Select column, solvent and conditions
 (omit 8)   Determine R_T with Ref. Compounds.
                   Collect analyte fractions.

10. Derivatives   Select derivatives (TMS/HFB/PFB)
                   Make derivatives of analyte in fraction
                   Make derivatives of Ref. Compounds
                   Use off-line derivatisation.

11. GC-MS   Select instruments and operating conditions
                   Run Reference compounds as derivatives.
                   Run derivatised analyte fraction.
                   Check analytes for correct R_T on GC as derivatives
                   Check at least four ions for correct abundance in MS

12. Results   Determine recovery from IS data.
                   Determine accuracy and precision using RM.
                   Decide if analyte present.
                   Determine amount of analyte in sample.
                   Present results as required.

14. Decisions.   a. Did method meet criteria   section 5
                   b. Was the analyte present
                   c. How much analyte in sample.   mass per kg or L
                   d. Should the analysis be repeated?

6.   MATERIALS

[Note: The reagents for which examples of their source are quoted are
known to be satisfactory, nevertheless reagents from other sources may be
equally suitable.]

6.1.   Reference Compounds and Standard Solutions.

6.1.1   <u>As used at IRFMN</u>

Stock solution containing; 0.4 mg cis-$DESD_8$, 0.75 mg @-$DESD_8$ and 1 mg trans-$DESD_8$.

Stock solution containing 1.16 mg zeranol-D_2 and 0.78 mg ß-zearalanol-D_2 per mL ethyl acetate.

Stock solution containing 1 mg zeranol-D_2 per mL ethyl acetate.

Stock solution containing 1 mg ß-oestradiol-D_2 per mL ethyl acetate

6.1.2.   <u>As used at RIVM.</u>

Pure standards of steroids and anabolics are those listed in Section 8. d-medroxyprogesterone and d-17ß-testosterone are recommended as the internal standards for the HPLC module.

6.2.   <u>Chemicals</u>

6.2.1.   As used at RIVM.
All listed chemicals are of Pro Analyze quality or better, unless otherwise stated.

6.2.1.1   Acetone (Merck, art. no. 14)
6.2.1.2   Ethanol (Merck, art. no. 983)
6.2.1.3   Hexane (Baker, art. no. 8044)
6.2.1.4   Methanol (Merck, art. no. 6007)
6.2.1.5   Toluene (Merck, art. no. 8325)
6.2.1.6   Acetonitrile (Merck, art. no. 30)
6.2.1.7   tert-Butylmethylether (Merck, art. no. 1845)
6.2.1.8   Sodium hydroxide (Merck, art. no. 6498)
6.2.1.9   Hydrochloric acid, 37% solution (Merck, art. no. 317)
6.2.1.10   Ethyl acetate (Merck, art. no. 9623)
6.2.1.11   Acetic acid (Merck, art. no. 63)
6.2.1.12   Sodium acetate (merck, art. no. 6268)
6.2.1.13   Sodium chloride (Analar BDH art. no. 10241)
6.2.1.14   Potassium hydroxide (Merck, art. no 9033)
6.2.1.15   Disodium hydrogenphosphate (Merck, art. no. 6568)
6.2.1.16   Potassium dihydrogenphosphate (Merck, art. no. 4873)
6.2.1.17   Beta-glucuronidase/sulphatase (suc'Helix Pomatia containing
           100,000 units beta-glucuronidase and 1 million units sulphatase
           per mL, Industrie Biologique, France, code IBF 213473)
6.2.1.18   Subtilisin A (Sigma, P-5380)
6.2.1.19   Derivatization reagents: - N,0-
           bis(trimethylsilyl)trifluoracetamide (BSTFA) with 10% TMCS
           (Pierce art. no.8253).
           Heptafluorobutyric acid anhydride (HFBA), (Pierce art. no.
           63163).

6.2.1.20   Buffer-solutions
6.2.1.20.1 Phosphate buffered saline (PBS), 0.02 mol/L, pH 7.4
           Dissolve in 800 mL water 2.278 g disodium hydrogenphosphate,
           0.416 g potassium dihydrogenphosphate and 9.0 g sodium chloride.

Cy 1.1/5

Adjust the pH at 7.0 ± 0.1 and add water to a final volume of
1000 mL.

6.2.1.20.2   Acetate buffer, 2 mol/L , pH 5.2
Dissolve 25.2 g acetic acid and 129.5 g anhydrous sodium acetate
in 1000 mL water.

6.2.1.20.3 Tris buffer, 0.1 mol per L, pH 9.5, Dissolve 12.1 g
Tris(hydroxymethyl)aminomethane in 800 mL water. Adjust the pH
to 9.5 ± 0.1 and add water to final volume of 1 L.

6.2.1.21 Other solutions

6.2.1.21.1 IAC-eluting solution; Add to 50 mL of ethanol water to a final
volume of 100 mL.

6.2.1.21.2 IAC-washing solution; Add to 80 mL of ethanol water to a final
volume of 100 mL.

6.2.1.21.3 Alkaline hydrolysis solution; Dissolve 5.6 g KOH in 50 mL
ethanol.

6.2.1.21.4 Acidic buffer; Mix 1.70 mL hydrochloric acid with 5 mL 2 mol/L
acetate buffer (pH = 5.2) and add water to a final volume of 100
mL.

6.2.1.22 Solutions of Standards.

6.2.1.22.1 Stock solutions of standards containing 0.01 g/L in ethanol,
stored at -20°C in the dark.

6.2.1.22.2 Working solutions of standards containing 0.01 g/L in ethanol,
stored at +4°C for a maximum period of 2 weeks. N.b. smallest
volume pipetted out of the stock solution is 0.1 mL.

6.2.2. As used at IRFMN, Milan.

6.2.2.0   Chemicals

6.2.2.1   Acetone (Merck, art. no. 14)

6.2.2.2   Acetonitrile (Merck, art. no. 30)

6.2.2.3   ß-glucuronidase/arylsulphatase (Boehringer, art no. 127060)

6.2.2.4   Ethanol absolute (Merck, art. no. 983)

6.2.2.5   KOH (Farmitalia Carlo Erbna, art no. 472057)

6.2.2.6   N,O-bis(trimethylsilyl)trifluoroacetamide (BSTFA), Pierce, art
no. 38830)

6.2.2.7   Pentafluorobenzyl bromide (PFBBr) (Aldrich art no. 10,105-2)

6.2.2.8   Disodium hydrogen phosphate dihydrate (Na_2HPO_4) (Farmitalia Carlo
Erbna, art. no. 480226)

6.2.2.9   Potassium dihydrogen phosphate (KH_2PO_4) (Farmitalia Carlo Erbna,
art no. 471686)

6.2.2.10 Sodium acetate trihydrate (Farmitalia Carlo Erbna, art no.
478137)

6.2.2.11 Thiomersal (Sigma, art no. T 5125)

6.2.2.12   Buffer Solutions.

6.2.2.12.1 Phosphate buffer, 0.05M, pH 7.4
Dissolve in about 900 mL water 1.51 g KH_2PO_4 and 6.92 g
$Na_2HPO_4.2H_2O$. Adjust the pH to 7.4 and dilute to a final volume
of 1 L.

6.2.2.12.2 Acetate buffer, 0.05M, pH 4.5
Dissolve in about 900 mL water 3.5 g sodium acetate trihydrate
and 1.5 mL glacial acetic acid. Adjust the pH to 7.4 and dilute
to a final volume of 1 L.

6.2.2.12.3 Phosphate buffer, 0.05M, pH 7.4, 0.02% thiomersal
Dissolve 0.2 g thiomersal in 1 L phosphate buffer, 0.05M, pH 7.4,

6.2.2.13 Other Solutions.

6.2.2.13.1 IAC eluting and washing solution; add 5mL water to 95 mL
          acetone.
6.2.2.13.2 Derivatization solutions; PFBBr is diluted 1 to 40 with
          acetonitrile and stored at 4°C.
6.2.2.13.3 KOH/ethanol; 40 mg KOH is dissolved in 10 mL anhydrous ethanol
          and stored at 4°C. Make fresh every month.

6.2.2.14 Solutions of Standards.
6.2.2.14.1 Standard solutions; Stock solutions of standards containing
          1 mg per mL in acetonitrile or ethanol are stored in the dark at
          -18°C;
6.2.2.14.2 Working solutions of standards containing 100 ng per mL or 10
          ng per mL in ethanol are stored in the dark at4°C.

7.   EQUIPMENT

Reference to a company and/or product is for purposes of information and
identification only. Equivalent types or products also may be suitable.

7.1.1.   Glass round bottomed flasks, 150 mL (Corex, art. no. 8422-A).
7.1.2.   Glass Pasteur capillary pipettes.
7.1.3.   Automatic pipettes (Gilson P20, P200, P1000 and P5000) .
7.1.4.   Refrigerated centrifuge (RC-3, Sorvall).
7.1.5.   Bench-top centrifuge (GLC-4, Sorvall).
7.1.6.   Centrifuge tubes, glass (55 mm x 11,5 mm) (Renes, RB55)
7.1.7.   Electric water bath with thermostat adjustable to 50 ± 2°C (GFL,
          Salm & Kipp) with nitrogen facility.
7.1.8.   Vortex (Vortex-genic, Wilton & Co).
7.1.9.   Ultrasonic water bath (Bransonic 32).
7.1.10.   Glass derivatization vials (chromacol 250 (A)) with screw caps
          (chromacol 85c) and septa (chromacol 8-ST15).
7.1.11.   Incubator 60° C (Seelvis).
7.1.12.   Heating module for derivatization vials (Pierce no. 18790) with
          nitrogen facility.
7.1.13.   Glass injection vials (Chrompack, art. no. 10201) with glass
          inserts (Chrompack, art. no. 10381).
7.1.14.   Aluminium caps (Chrompack, art. no. 10210).
7.1.15.   GC-MS equipment.
7.1.15.1 Gas chromatograph (Hewlett Packard, type 5890).
7.1.15.2 Automatic injector (Hewlett Packard, type 7637A).
7.1.15.3 Mass selective detector (Hewlett Packard, type 5970).
7.1.15.4 Workstation (Hewlett Packard, type 59970).
7.1.15.5 Printer (Hewlett Packard, ink jet).
7.1.15.6 GC-column, fused silica permaband SE-52, 25 m x 0,25 mm ID, film
          thickness 0,25 μm (Machery-Nagel, art. no. 723054).
7.1.16   Rotavapor with water bath at 40 ± 2° C (Rotavapor).

7.1.17.   IRFMN, Milan

7.1.17.1 Conical tubes
7.1.17.2 Water bath
7.1.17.3 Drying apparatus using nitrogen or dry air
7.1.17.4 Hamilton syringes 10uL, 100uL
7.1.17.5 Heating module for derivatization in vials and conical tubes.
          (Pierce)

7.2.   IAC-COLUMNS

RIVM - The columns are glass (100 mm x 9 mm i.d.) and contain 1 mL gel. A
multi-analyte column was successfully tested and is moving towards
commercial development. The column has a capacity of at least 20 ng per
analyte. The analytes tested are DES, Z, 17α-TB, 17ß-TB, NT, MT, T, E_2.
The internal standards were the deuterated anabolic agents.(see Section 8
of manual for availability)

GENEGO, 34170 Gorizia, Italy - This company market three multi-analyte
columns claiming a capacity of at least 20 ng or 100 ng (high capacity
column) per analyte. The products are -
        Multi-Prep I for DES, HEX, DE, Z, Taleranol ß-E_2, NT, T, MT, and
        TB
        Multi-Prep II for DES, HEX, DE, Z, NT, MT,T, TB and Taleranol
        Multi-Prep III for Clenbuterol, salbutamol, terbutaline,
        carbuterol and marbuterol all ß-agonists.

These columns are marketed as a complete kit, comprising the enzyme and the
buffer for the digestion of samples, extraction and washing buffers and
detailed instructions.

IFRMN give a method for use with Genego columns (9.2.1.3)

LABORATORY OF HORMONOLOGY - MARLOIE, Rue de Point de Jour, 8, B-6900,
Marloie, Belgium.

Antibodies are available against; for testosterone[*], oestradiol[*],
oestrone, androstenedione, dehydroepiandrosterone, cortisol,
desoxycorticosterone, 17α-hydroxyprogesterone and progesterone,
trenbolone[*], zeranol, diethylstilboestrol, 19-nortestosterone[*],
methyltestosterone, ethinyloestradiol[*], medroxyprogesterone acetate,
dexamethasone

[*] either the 17α- or the 17ß- hydroxy compounds.

Gels for immunoaffinity chromatography are available (minimum quantity 1
mL) prepared from high affinity antisera and with a minimum capacity of 50
ng per mL for; Nortestosterone, methyltestosterone, trenbolone,
ethinyloestradiol, diethylstilboestrol

7.3 GCMS

There are several suitable GCMS machines available. The equipment used
must be capable of fulfilling the criteria for GCMS detailed in the
criteria document (see section 5 of this manual).   The machines used
are;-

RIVM
        GC   HP 5890
        column   Macherey-Nagel Permabond[r] SE 52
        injection   1-5 mL splitless 225°C
        programme   100°C - 280°C at 20°C/min.
        temperature transfer line   280°C
        MS   HP 5970

IRFMN, Milan
    GC-MS   HP 5890 coupled to a VG TS-250
  or GC-MS   DANI 6500 GC coupled to
                                      Finnigan 4000 MS
      Negative ion CI mode with ammonia or methane as reacting gas.
      Column   CP Sil 5 CB 25 m X 0.32 mm
                                      film thickness 0.12 μm
(Chrompack)
      Injection   1 - 2 μL splitless 240°C
      programme   160°C (1 min) - 20°C /min - 220°C - 12°C/min - 300°C
      temperature transfer line   280°C
      Acquisition   see 9.2.4.2

  Note:
  CVL
      The mass spectrometer is a Finnigan MAT, coupled to a gas
      chromatograph using a J&W fused Silica capillary column (SE-54, 15 m
      X 0.25 mm) and linked to an INCOS data system.
  University of Ghent,
      The mass spectrometer is a Hewlett Packard HP 5970 mass-selective
      detector coupled to a HP 5890 gas chromatograph using an HP Ultra-2
      (5% phenylmethyl silicone) fused silica capillary column (25 m X 0.20
      mm) and an all-glass moving needle injection system. Carrier gas was
      helium at a flow rate of 0.47 mL per min. The injection and
      interface temperatures were maintained at 290°C. The oven
      temperature was programmed from 200-280°C at 5°C per min, the final
      temperature was held for 10 min.   The ionization voltage was 70 eV.

  7.4. HPLC

  A variety of HPLC machines for the analysis of anabolic agents are suitable
  but the one chosen must fulfil the criteria for HPLC laid down in the
  criteria document, (see Section 5). The following reversed phase system
  used at RIVM has proven to be adequate for extract purification prior to
  GC-MS:

  pre-column   chromguard-reversed phase cartridge
  analytical column   ODS-hypersil C18 (150 x 7.5 (mm x mm))
  eluent   acetonitrile:water::45:55 V/V (see also 9.2.2.1)
  flow-rate   1.5 mL/min

  At the University of Ghent the HPLC conditions were

  pre-column - 75 mm chromguard-pellicular reversed phase cartridge,30-50 μm
  analytical column - Li-Chrospher RP-18 (Merck) (125 mm x 4 mm i.d., 5 μm)
  eluent - methanol:water, 65:35 V/V
  flow-rate - 1.0 mL/min

  8. SAMPLES AND SAMPLING PROCEDURE.

  N.B. Attention is drawn to section 6.3.1 and ISO document 78/2-1982 (E)
  and the following notes derived from Annex II of 2052/VI/84-EN.

  8.1. Nature of the Sample; Samples shall be such as to enable the
  detection of residues in meat as defined in Directive 64/433/EEC. Failing
  this biological fluids or faeces may constitute the samples for the
  detection of residues.

8.2. Size of Sample; The size of the sample must be large enough to allow
the reference method to be carried out and to allow repeat analysis where
required.

In this method for Anabolics the sizes shall not be less than

   5 g muscle, liver, kidney or fat
   0.5 - 2 mL urine (IRFMN), 5 mL urine (RIVM)

8.3. The samples must be taken and packed in such a way as to allow proper
identification in the laboratory.

8.4. The method of packing, preservation and transport must maintain the
integrity of the sample and not prejudice the result of the examination.

Samples for the analysis of AnAg must be stored and transported at
temperatures below -18°C.

9.   PROCEDURE.

9.1   Preparation of a primary extract

9.1.1   Liquid samples
For extraction of liquid samples liquid-liquid partition is most frequently
used. Alternatives like direct application to immunoaffinity (IAC)
materials and HPLC column switching, however, can be suitable or preferable
in particular cases.

9.1.1.1   Urine samples
From the laboratory sample a test portion of 5.0 mL is taken to which the
internal standards are added, preferably the isotopically substituted
analyte (e.g. in the case of nortestosterone (NT) 5 ng of trideutero-NT
(NT-d3)). The pH is adjusted to 5.2 with acetic acid (HAc) and 1.0 mL 2.0
mol/L HAc/NaAc is added. To deconjugate glucuronide- and sulphate
conjugates of the analytes 0.1 mL ß-glucuronidase/sulphatase (e.g.
suc'Helix Pomatia containing 100,000 units ß-glucuronidase and 1 million
units sulphatase per mL) is added and the sample is incubated for 2 hours
at 37°C.

After incubation the test portions are cooled to room temperature and
extracted twice with 5 mL t-butylmethylether (TBME). The combined extracts
are evaporated to dryness under a stream of nitrogen in a water bath at
50°C.

9.1.1.2 Bile samples
The procedure for bile is the same as for urine with the exception that the
test portion for analysis is a mixture of 1 mL of the laboratory sample and
4 mL of water.   Note; CVL method uses 5 mL bile.

9.1.2   Tissue samples
Two different procedures are considered, the first is an enzymatic
procedure which uses a protease, the second a mechanical procedure. The
advantage of the enzymatic procedure is the protein digestion frees
analytes from cells and from conjugates with proteins (non covalently
protein bound residues). However, some analytes are not stable under the
conditions used (pH 9.5, 60°C) and therefore sometimes a mechanical
procedure has to be used. As far as data are available (based on incurred

tissues) enzymatic digestion results in slightly higher values of analyte contents.
Remark: It should be noted that internal standards do <u>not</u> give adequate information about the extractability of incurred residues.

9.1.2.1 Enzymatic digestion

From the laboratory sample a test sample of 50-100 g is homogenized thoroughly and a test portion of 5.0 g is weighted into a 50 mL glass centrifuge tube. Internal standards are added and mixed with the test portions at least 30 minutes prior to the addition of 20 mL 0.1 mol/L Tris buffer, pH 9.5, containing 5 mg Subtilisin A (e.g. Sigma P-5380). The mixture is shaken a few times and incubated for 2 hours at 55°C, shaking at least every 30 minutes. After the samples are cooled to room temperature the mixture is washed with 20 mL hexane (shaking one minute and centrifuging for 5 minutes at 1600 g) and extracted twice with TBME. The combined extracts are evaporated to dryness under a stream of nitrogen in a water bath at 50°C. The dry residue is dissolved in 10 mL methanol/water (4:1, V/V) and washed twice with 10 mL petroleum ether. Subsequently the methanol/water phase is evaporated to dryness.

9.1.2.2 Mechanical extraction

From the laboratory sample a test sample of 50-100 g is homogenized thoroughly and a test portion of 5.0 g is weighted into a 20 mL glass vial. Internal standards are added and mixed with the test portions at least 30 minutes prior to the addition of 10 mL methanol. The samples are shaken thoroughly during 15 minutes and subsequently placed in an ultrasonic water bath for 15 minutes. The supernatant is removed (centrifuging 5 minutes at 1600 g) and the extraction procedure is repeated. The combined extracts are evaporated to dryness under a stream of nitrogen in a water bath at 50°C. The dry residue is dissolved in 10 mL methanol-water (4:1,V/V) and washed twice with 10 mL petroleum ether. Subsequently the methanol/water phase is evaporated to dryness.

9.1.3 Alkaline hydrolyses

In the case of analysis for compounds which might be present in the form of small esters (e.g. the gestagens and trenbolone acetate) an additional basic hydrolysis is applied. The residue obtained is dissolved in 0.2 mL methanol and 0.2 mL of a solution of 5.6 g potassium hydroxide in 50 mL ethanol is added. This mixture is incubated at 37°C for 30 minutes. The hydrolyses is ended by the addition of 1.0 mL acidic buffer (6.2.1.3). This mixture is extracted twice with t-butylmethylether. The combined extract is evaporated to dryness under a stream of nitrogen. In some cases it is necessary to repeat the above described procedure for defatting.

9.2. Extract clean-up

To allow detection and identification of low concentrations of analytes in extracts of biological samples adequate extract clean-up is necessary. One of the most powerful techniques is immunoaffinity chromatography (IAC), however, other alternatives like high performance liquid chromatography (HPLC) are also suitable.

9.2.1 Immunoaffinity chromatography. (DES, HEX, DE, Z, Taleranol, 17α-TB, 17ß-TB, NT, MT, T, E_2)

9.2.1.1. RIVM method.

The procedure for sample preparation by IAC depends on the characteristics

of the IAC-material used. The following procedure is used at RIVM and is
suitable for the polyclonal rabbit antibodies tested.
The IAC materials usually have a capacity of 20 ng or more per mL of gel.
For multi-residue analysis combinations of gels can be made.
The primary extract is dissolved in 0.05 mL ethanol. Subsequently 5 to 10
mL water is added and the total mixture is applied to the IAC column. After
sample application the column is washed with 5 mL water and eluted with 5
mL ethanol-water (1:1,V/V) mixture. The eluate is evaporated to dryness
under a cold stream of nitrogen in a water bath at 50°C or alternatively
extracted twice with 5 mL TBME.
The dry residue is suitable for analysis with gas chromatography-mass
spectrometry

9.2.1.2. GENEGO method.

Full details of the use of the Multi-Prep columns are supplied with the
columns by the company.

The columns are washed with a buffer solution and the fraction containing
the analytes is eluted with 1 mL acetone/water, 95:5, v/v.   The dry
residue is suitable for derivatization and analysis with gas
chromatography-mass spectrometry

9.2.1.3. IRFMN method.

The centrifuged samples (0.5 - 2 mL urine) are diluted with 2 mL acetate
buffer (0.05M, pH 4.5) into polystyrene tubes and digested by the addition
of 25 -100 µL glucuronidase/arylsulphatase and incubated for 2 hour at 37°C
or overnight at room temperature. The digested urines are diluted 8 mL
with phosphate buffer (0.05M, pH 7.4) and directly applied to the IAC
columns. After allowing 4 minutes for binding and with gentle mixing of
the gel, the urines are left to elute and the gel is washed with 2 X 10 mL
phosphate buffer and 2 mL distilled water. The analytes are eluted into
conical glass tubes with 2 X 1.5 mL acetone:water 95:5 v/v, and the eluate
is evaporated to dryness under a stream of air at 60°C. The dry residue is
suitable for derivatization.
The IAC columns are washed with 10 mL acetone water, 2 mL distilled water
and finally 5 mL phosphate buff containing 0.02% thiomersal. The columns
are stored in this buffer in the dark at 4°C.

9.2.2 High performance liquid chromatography

A variety of HPLC systems for the analysis of anabolic agents has been
described. The following reversed phase system used at RIVM has proven to
be adequate for extract purification prior to GC-MS:

pre-column	chromguard-reversed phase cartridge
analytical column	ODS-hypersil C18 (150 x 7.5 (mm x mm))
eluent	acetonitrile:water (45:55,V/V)
flow-rate	1.5 mL/min
detector	UV at 254 nm and 330 nm.

The residue is dissolved in 0.10 mL of the HPLC eluent of which
subsequently 0.09 mL is injected into the system. The fractions of interest
are collected, usually starting 0.5 minutes before the retention time of
the analyte and ending 1 minute later. Sometimes it is possible or
advantageous to combine different analytes in a single fraction. The eluent

is removed under a cold stream of nitrogen in a water bath at 50°C

Where the deuterated-compound of the analyte of interest is not available other deuterated anabolics may be used (RIVM recommend d-ß-T and d-medroxyprogesterone). The fraction containing these compounds is collected and is needed for the estimation of recoveries (see Calculation of Results. 10).

9.2.2.1 Retention times on HPLC systems.

Data provided by RIVM for R_T of anabolics in three separate solvent systems.
This data should only be used as a guideline for the development of one's own system using standards.

Anabolic Agent.	Retention Time. (min)	UV wavelength nm.	UV Max. nm
System A: Acetonitrile:water::45:55 V/V			
Ethinyloestradiol	4.99	280	197
Boldenone	3.22	254	
Medroxyprogesterone	8.99	254	245
Chlormadinone	8.28	280	
Megestrol	7.39	280	
System B: Methanol:water::65:35 V/V			
DES	5.27	254	195
HEX	6.16	280	195
DEN	5.66	254	195
ß-oestradiol	4.45	280	197
ß-NT	4.34	254	243
α-NT	7.0	254	243
ß-T	5.34	254	245
α-T	7.62	254	245
MT	6.69	254	254
System C: Methanol:acetonitrile:water:::4:38:58			
ß-trenbolone	3.49	350	350
α-trenbolone	4.13	350	350
zeranol	4.80	265	215

At University of Ghent the following retention windows were used to collect fractions containing anabolic agents.

AnAg	Retention window (min)	AnAg	Retention window (min)
TbOH,	3.5 - 3.5	MT	8.5 - 10.0
EE	5.17 - 6.17	MGA	10.0 - 12.0
E_2ß, NT	5.5 - 6.5	CMA	11.0 - 13.0
T	6.5 - 8.0	MPA	11.5 - 13.5

9.2.3 Gas chromatography-mass spectrometry

For GC-MS analysis on the system described below both the TMS- and HFB-derivatives are suitable.

9.2.3.1 Preparation of TMS-derivatives

The residue obtained after extract clean-up is transferred to a derivatization vial with 0.5 mL absolute ethanol. The ethanol is evaporated and 0.05 mL 10% TMS in BSTFA (e.g Pierce no 8253) is added. The vial is vortexed and the reaction mixture incubated during 1 hour at 80°C. After incubation the reaction mixture is evaporated to dryness under a stream of nitrogen at 50°C and the derivatized residue is dissolved in 0.025 mL isooctane.

9.2.3.2 Preparation of HFB-derivatives

The residue obtained after extract clean-up is transferred to a derivatization vial with 0.5 mL absolute ethanol. The ethanol is evaporated and 0.1 mL HFBA (e.g. Pierce no 63163) in acetone (1:4,V/V) is added. The vial is vortexed and incubated during 1 hour at 80°C. After incubation the reaction mixture is evaporated to dryness under a stream of nitrogen at 50°C and the derivatized residue is dissolved in 0.025 mL isooctane.

9.2.3.3 Preparation of PFB-TMS derivatives

The dried samples (equiv. to 0.5-2 mL urine) from the IAC-columns were reacted with 50 µL of a solution of PFBBr in acetonitrile(1:20, v/v) and 50 µL of a solution of KOH in anhydrous EtOH (8 mg/mL) in a conical tube at 60°C for 30 min. After evaporation of the solvents the samples were redissolved in 50 µL of BSTFA, heated for 30 min. and then injected into the gas chromatograph.

Under these conditions PFBBr reacts with phenolic groups and BSTFA with the remaining aliphatic hydroxyl groups. BSTFA also is also used as the solvent for the GC injection.

9.2.4 GC-MS analysis

The following conditions are used during GC-MS analysis at RIVM.

GC	HP 5890
column	Macherey-Nagel Permabond[r] SE 52
injection	1-5 mL splitless 225°C
programme	100°C - 280°C at 20°C/min.
temperature transfer line	280°C
MS	HP 5970
acquisition:	see table

IRFMN, Milan
GC-MS   HP 5890 coupled to a VG TS-250
or GC-MS   DANI 6500 GC coupled to Finnigan 4000 MS
Mode   Negative ion CI mode with ammonia or methane as reacting gas.
Column   CP Sil 5 CB 25 m X 0.32 mm film thickness 0.12 µm (Chrompack)
Injection 1 - 2 µL splitless 240°C

Programme   160°C (1 min) - 20°C /min - 220°C - 12°C/min - 300°C
Temperature transfer line; 280°C
Acquisition see 9.2.4.2

9.2.4.1. Retention times on GC systems.

The following times in minutes are observed at IRFMN, they will vary
slightly with day to day operation.

cis-DES, 7.67; @-DES, 7.97; trans-DES, 8.38; DE, 8.22; Hex, 8.25;
β-E$_2$, 7.93; E^3, 8.85; Z, 10.18; Taleranol, 10.29

9.2.4.2. Selected Ions.

Ions monitored during GC-MS analysis. Most suitable derivative is indicated
(++). The ion used during initial screening is underlined

	derivative		IONS of ++ derivative (RIVM)				derivative	IONS					
	TMS	HFB					IRFMN	NI-CI		EI			
17β-NT	+	++	<u>666</u>	453	306	133							
17α-NT	+	++	<u>666</u>	453	306	133							
17β-T	+	++	<u>680</u>	467	355	320							
17α-T	+	++	<u>680</u>	467	355	320							
MT	(+)	++	480	<u>465</u>	369	355							
Bol	+	++	<u>678</u>	464	369	169							
17β-TB	++		<u>342</u>	252	237	211							
17α-TB	++		<u>342</u>	252	237	211							
EE2	+	++	<u>474</u>	459	446	353							
MPA		++	<u>479</u>	331	317	147							
CMA		++	540	<u>497</u>	462	440							
MGA		++	520	<u>477</u>	421	381							
ZER	+	++	538	<u>433</u>	335	307	PFB$_2$/TMS	573	393	754	664	566	523
TAL	+	++	538	<u>433</u>	335	307	PFB$_2$/TMS	573	393	754	664	566	523
DES	++	+	<u>412</u>	397	383		PFB2	447	427	628	447	238	181
DE	++	+	<u>410</u>	395	381		PFB$_2$	445	425	626	445	249	181
HEX	++	+	<u>207</u>	191	179		PFB$_2$	449	429	315	287	181	
17β-E$_2$			<u>664</u>	451	409	356	PFB/TMS	343		524	393	253	181
17α-E$_2$	+	++	<u>664</u>	451	409	356							
E$_3$							PFB/TMS$_2$	431		612	494	453	419

10. CALCULATION OF RESULTS.

10.1. PRECISION. To take into account the Criteria document (89/610 EEC)
and will explain how the precision of the method is determined using the
standards available.

11. SPECIAL CASES. e.g. if a particular species presents unique problems.

12. NOTES ON PROCEDURE. The procedure chosen will depend on the
availability of reagents,reference compounds and equipment.

13. QUALITY CONTROL. STANDARDS, REFERENCE MATERIALS AND ANTIBODIES.
A description of the source and quality of the key reagents and standards
is given in Section 8.

13.1 IAC. Follow the instructions relating to the storage and procedures
as recommended by the supplier.

13.2. Source of IAC columns and gel packings.

GENEGO S.p.A., Via Ressel S. Andrea zona ind., 34170 Gorizia, Italy

LABORATORY OF HORMONOLOGY - MARLOIE, Rue de Point de Jour, 8, B-6900,
Marloie.
Gels for immunoaffinity chromatography are available (minimum quantity 1
mL) prepared from high affinity antisera and with a minimum capacity of 50
ng per mL for; nortestosterone, methyltestosterone, trenbolone,
ethinyloestradiol, diethylstilboestrol

13.3. Deuterated standards.

Deuterated standards are held at RIVM (see section 8). The supply is
limited and available to approved laboratories against payment.

14. TEST REPORT.
To give the indications necessary for the identification of the sample, the
reference to the method employed, the results and the form in which these
are expressed, any particular points observed in the course of the test and
any operations not specified in the method or regarded as optional which
might affect the results.

15. LIST OF ABBREVIATIONS
A list of the most important abbreviations is given in Annex I section 12.

16. FLOW DIAGRAM.

```
   Tissue --→ add buffer and recovery standard   --→ Homogenise
                                                         |
                                                         |
                                                         |
   Fluid (urine, bile, plasma, serum)                    |
      |                                                   |
      ↓                                                   ↓
   add buffer and recovery standard ------------→ Hydrolyse
                                                         |
                                                         |
                                                         |
                                                         ↓
      Calculate ←---- GCMS ←------ IAC or SPE ←----- organic solvent
        results                   and/or HPLC                extraction
```

Cy 1.2 ANABOLIC AGENTS - A MULTI-RESIDUE METHOD USING GC-MS FOR DETERMINING RESIDUES OF ANABOLIC AGENTS (ANDROGENS, OESTROGENS AND GESTAGENS) IN ANIMAL TISSUES .

WARNING AND SAFETY PRECAUTIONS

0.   INTRODUCTION

Throughout the EEC the use of xenobiotic anabolic agents is prohibited in food producing animals. Also the MRL for residues of these anabolics in animal products imported into or produced within the Community is zero. Preparations of natural steroids or their esters may be used in farm animals under strictly controlled conditions (see EEC Directive 86/469/EEC) and the maximum concentrations of natural steroids allowed in edible tissues is defined (see section 2, 2.3).

1.   SCOPE

This multiresidue method of analysis describes the detection and confirmation of the presence of individual analytes for a large number of Anabolic Agents in samples of animal origin - the method has been mainly tested for residues in edible tissues. This work is carried out officially in Germany in compliance with the Residues Directive (86/469/EEC).

2.   FIELD OF APPLICATION.

The method is used to perform routine screening and confirmatory analyses in edible tissue samples.
This method is suitable for testosterone[*], oestradiol[*], oestriol, oestrone, diethylstilboestrol, hexoestrol, dienoestrol, ethinyloestradiol[*], 19-nortestosterone[*], methyltestosterone, androsterone, boldenone, chlorotestosterone, medroxy-progesterone acetate, progesterone, hydroxyprogesterone.

[*] either the 17α- or the 17β- hydroxy compounds.

The data obtained in interlaboratory comparison in 7 German laboratories have shown that in veal, DES and DE may be determined in concentrations >0.5 μg per kg and EE and NT in concentrations > 1 μg per kg.

3.   REFERENCES.

Commission Decision, 93/256/EEC, laying down the methods for detecting residues of substances having a hormonal or thyrostatic action. [OJ. № L.118, 14.4.93. pp 64-74]

2052/VI/84 File 6.11 II-4, Scientific Veterinary Committee, Working Group - "Reference Methods for Residues", General Criteria for the establishment of Reference Methods for the Detection of Residues.

ISO Standard 78/2-1982 Layout for standards - Part 2: Standard for Chemical Analysis

Official Collection of Methods of Analysis according to § 35 of the Foods Act (LM8G) Examination of Foodstuffs. Germany. (1989) Bundesgesundhbl. _2,_ 76-80.

Bergner-Lang, B. and Kächele, M. (1981). Anabolica in Kalbfleisch -
Nachweis und Bestimmung, Befunde und Beobachtungen. Dtsch. Lebensm. -
Rundschau, 77, 305-313

Bergner-Lang, B. and Kächele, M. (1987). Anabolica in Kalbfleisch -
Nachweis und Bestimmung, Befunde und Beobachtungen. Dtsch. Lebensm. -
Rundschau, 83, 349-351

Bergner-Lang, B. and Kächele, M. (1989). Anabolica in Kalbfleisch -
Nachweis und Bestimmung, Befunde und Beobachtungen. Dtsch. Lebensm. -
Rundschau, 85, 78-79

4.   DEFINITIONS.

Anabolic agent content is taken to mean the amount of anabolic agent in the
substance in question, regardless of the chemical form, determined
according to the described method and expressed as µg anabolic agent per kg
of test sample.

5.   PRINCIPLE

5.1. The methods comprises 8 stages;-
    1. preparation of a primary extract
    2. hydrolysis of conjugates with enzyme.
    3. extraction with organic solvent partition.
    4. clean up using XAD-2 column
    5. separation into androgens, oestrogens and gestagens using Extrelut
        celite and Al_2O_3 columns
    6. derivatisation to TMSi ethers
    7. detection and identification by GCMS
    8. calculation of results.

6.   MATERIALS

Note: The reagents for which examples of their source are quoted are
known to be satisfactory, nevertheless reagents from other sources may be
equally suitable. Unless specified otherwise chemicals are of AR grade.

6.1.   Reference Compounds and Standard Solutions.
6.1.1   Solutions of 2 µg per mL methanol, stored in brown glass bottles
            in the dark at +4°C
6.1.2   Internal standard for oestrogen fraction is 1 µg Dichlorophene
            per mL methanol.
6.1.3   Internal standard for androgen-gestagen fraction is 2 µg 3,4-
            13-C_2-testosterone per mL methanol.
Pure standards of steroids and anabolics are those listed in Section 8.

6.2.   Chemicals
6.2.1.   Acetone (Merck, art. no. 14)
6.2.2.   Ethanol (Merck, art. no. 983)
6.2.3.   Hexane (Baker, art. no. 8024)
6.2.4.   Methanol (Merck, art. no. 9623)
6.2.5.   Toluene (Merck, art. no. 8325)
6.2.6.   Chloroform
6.2.7.   Dichloromethane
6.2.8.   Diethyl-ether (peroxide free)

6.2.9.   Isooctane; 2,2,4-trimethylpentane
6.2.10   Acetonitrile (Merck, art. no. 30)
6.2.11   Acetic acid (Merck, art. no. 63)
6.2.12   Sodium acetate (Merck, art. no. 6268)
6.2.13   Potassium hydroxide 0.25 mol per L (Merck, art. no 9033)
6.2.14   Beta-glucuronidase/sulphatase (suc'Helix Pomatia containing
          100.000 units beta-glucuronidase and 1000.000 units sulphatase
          per mL, Industrie Biologique, France, code IBF 213473) or
          Boehringer Mannheim, Germany, art No. 127060 or 127698

6.3   Derivatization reagents:
6.3.1   60 parts (v/v) of acetonitrile are mixed with 40 parts N-methyl-
          N-trimethylsilyl-trifluoracetamide (MSTFA) containing 5% by mass
          trimethylchlorosilane (TMCS) as a catalyst. The mixture must be
          freshly prepared.
6.3.2   200 mg dithioerythritole (Sigma - D8255) and 100 mg ammonium
          iodide (Merck - 1173) are dissolved in 5 mL N-methyl-N-trimethyl-
          silyltrifluor-(0)-acetamide (MSTFA) (Macherys Nagel - 70127) in a
          headspace vial in an oven at 60°C. 1 part (v/v) of this solution
          is mixed with 9 parts of MSTFA . (Stable for up to 1 month stored
          in the dark). Before use for silylation mix one part of this
          solution with 1 part acetonitrile (v/v).
6.3.3   Heptafluorobutyric acid anhydride (HFBA), (Pierce art. no.
          63163).

6.4   Buffer-solutions
6.4.1   Acetate buffer, 0.04 mol/L , pH 5.2
          Dissolve 25.2 g acetic acid and 43.0 g sodium acetate.3H$_2$0 in
          1000 mL water.

6.5.   Packings for Chromatography Columns
6.5.1   Amberlite XAD-2 (300-1000 um) (Serva Ltd)
          Pretreatment - low molecular weight and turbid substances are
          eliminated by allowing the resin to sediment in methanol. 50 g
          resin is added to 250 mL methanol and stirred for 3 minutes.
          After sedimentation for 2 minutes in a 500 mL measuring cylinder
          the supernatant is removed by suction. The resin is resuspended
          in 250 mL water and decanted after standing for 5 minutes. The
          resin is stored in a humid state.
6.5.2   Celite Granulate; (Extrelut Merck art No. 11738). Store in
          desiccator over drying agent (e.g. calcium chloride)
6.5.3   Aluminium oxide (neutral; Brockmann stage activity 1).
          Pretreatment; 20 g Al$_2$0$_3$ are treated with 1.2 mL distilled water
          in a wide-necked bottle provided with a glass stopper. After
          violent shaking the mixture is allowed to stand overnight at room
          temperature.

7.   EQUIPMENT

Reference to a company and/or product is for purposes of information and
identification only. Equivalent types or products also may be suitable.

7.1.1.   Beakers, 250 mL
7.1.2.   Glass Pasteur capillary pipettes.
7.1.3.   Automatic pipettes (e.g.Gilson P20, P200, P1000 and P5000)   .
7.1.4.   Centrifuge (e.g. RC-3, Sorvall).

7.1.5.   Centrifuge tubes, minimum volume 250 mL if stainless steel
7.1.6   pH meter with glass electrode.
7.1.7.   Electric water bath with adjustable thermostat.
7.1.8.   Vortex (Vortex-genic, Wilton & Co).
7.1.9   Small filter funnels
7.1.10   Separating funnels, 500 mL
7.1.11.   Glass derivatization vials (chromacol 250 (A)) with screw caps
            (chromacol 85c) and septa (chromacol 8-ST15) or alternatively
            pointed flasks or conical tubes with glass stoppers.
7.1.12.   Heating module for derivatization vials (Pierce no. 18790) with
            nitrogen facility.
7.1.13.   Glass injection vials (Chrompack, art. no. 10201) with glass
            inserts (Chrompack, art. no. 10381).
7.1.14.   Aluminium caps (Chrompack, art. no. 10210).
7.1.15   Pointed flasks, 100 mL
7.1.16   Rotavapor with water bath at 40 ± 2°C (Rotavapor).
7.1.17   Ultra-Turrax (or similar) homogeniser.
7.1.18   Desiccator or vacuum oven at 40°C.
7.1.19   Round bottomed flasks, 500 mL
7.1.20.   GC-MS equipment.
7.1.20.1   Capillary gas chromatograph with all glass injector at up to
            250°C and splitless operation.
7.1.20.2   Automatic injection for GC - not compulsory
7.1.20.3   A mass spectrometer with a low resolution and a mass range of at
            least 600 amu. It must be possible to apply the MID (multiple
            ion detection) mode, also a mass specific detector and an ion
            trap detector.
7.1.20.4   Workstation (e.g. Hewlett Packard, type 59970).
7.1.20.5   Printer
7.1.20.6   GC-column, fused silica OV-1, SE-30 or SE 54, 25 m x 0.32 mm ID,
            film thickness 0.30 - 0.50 um
7.1.20.7   The coupling of GC-MS may be by means of a fused silica capillary
            heated to 280°C using the direct or open principle.

7.2.   COLUMNS
7.2.1   The columns require glass frits, a stopcock and ground glass
            joints and stoppers.   The sizes are
            Extrelut and XAD-2 250 mm x 8-10 mm i.d., Al_2O_3 150 mm x 8-10
            mm. i.d.
7.2.2   Amberlite-XAD2 column; 8 g resin (6.5.3) was suspended in 30 mL
            water and the suspension used to form a column about 8 cm long.
            The resin was washed with 50 mL water.
7.2.3.   Extrelut celite granulate; Treat 1.5 g pretreated celite
            granulate (6.5.2) with 0.75 mL KOH (6.2.13.) in a stoppered flask
            and shake vigorously. After standing for 15 minutes fill one
            half of a column with a toluene:hexane::1:9 (v/v) and add through
            a funnel the prepared celite. The column is washed with a
            further 20 mL toluene:isooctane.   The column must not run dry.
7.2.4   Aluminium oxide column; 4 g prepared aluminium oxide (6.5.3) was
            mixed with 10 mL toluene and the suspension poured into a column.
            After draining the bed was washed with 15 mL
            toluene:isooctane::1:9 (v/v). The tap was closed when the level
            of liquid is 3 to 4 cm above the top of the bed.
7.2.5   The Extrelut column was fixed onto the top of the aluminium oxide
            column so that the eluate from the Extrelut dropped directly onto
            the oxide column.

8.   SAMPLES AND SAMPLING PROCEDURE.

N.B. Attention is drawn to section 6.3.1 and ISO document 78/2-1982 (E)
and the following notes derived from Annex II of 2052/VI/84-EN.

8.1.   Nature of the Sample; Samples shall be such as to enable the
            detection of residues in meat as defined in Directive 64/433/EEC.
            Failing this biological fluids or faeces may constitute the
            samples for the detection of residues.
8.2.   Size of Sample; The size of the sample must be large enough to
            allow the reference method to be carried out using 50 g and to
            allow repeat analysis where required.
8.3.   The samples must be taken and packed in such a way as to allow
            proper identification in the laboratory.
8.4.   The method of packing, preservation and transport must maintain
            the integrity of the sample and not prejudice the result of the
            examination. Samples for the analysis of anabolic agent must be
            stored and transported at temperatures below -18°C. If samples
            are analyzed within 48 hours of collection then they may be
            stored and transported at 0 to +4°C.

9.   PROCEDURE.
9.1.   Preparation of a primary extract
9.1.1   Homogenisation and Enzymatic digestion
            From the laboratory sample a test sample of 50 g is mixed with 50
            ml acetate buffer (6.4.1) in a 250 mL beaker. 100 µL internal
            standards are added and the mixture homogenised using an Ultra-
            Turrax machine. Fat tissues are melted at 80°C and then
            homogenised with 80 mL acetate buffer. The pH is readjusted to
            5.2 using a glass electrode and 0.25 mL enzyme solution (6.2.14)
            and a few drops of chloroform added. The mixture is incubated
            overnight at 37°C. The hydrolysis may be omitted for fat tissues

9.1.2.   Extract clean-up
9.1.2.1   The mixture is transferred to a centrifuge tube, mixed with 180
            mL methanol and rehomogenised. The homogenate is centrifuged for
            10 minutes at ca. 2000g.
            The supernatant is decanted into a separating funnel and
            extracted (defatted) with 2 x 50 mL hexane. The hexane fraction
            is discarded.
[Note; The methanol phase may remain turbid but this does not have a
detrimental effect.]
9.1.2.2   The methanol phase is extracted with, 150, 90 and 90 mL
            dichloromethane. The dichloromethane phases are combined in a
            round bottomed flask and evaporated to dryness using a rotary
            evaporator at 45°C. The residue is taken up in 20 mL water.
[Notes; Water (5-10 mL) may be added to assist the separation of the
phases. Foaming in the evaporator can be reduced by the addition of a few
drops of methanol.]

9.2   Column Chromatography.
9.2.1   The aqueous extract is added to the top of the Amberlite XAD-2
            column with a drop rate of ca. 2 mL per minute. The flask is
            rinsed twice with 20 mL water and the rinsings passed through the
            column at ca. 5 mL per minute. The water eluates are discarded.
            The anabolic agents are eluted from the column with 40 mL
            methanol. The methanol is evaporated to dryness at 45°C. The

9.2.2   5 ml toluene and 9 ml isooctane are added to the chloroform
         extract (9.2.1) and the solution transferred quantitatively to
         the assembled Extrelut and Al_2O_3 columns (7.2.4). The residues
         are rinsed twice with 5 mL toluene/isooctane and the rinsings
         passed through the column. The flow should be about 0.5 mL per
         minute. The columns are separated.
9.2.3   The Extrelut column is washed with 20 mL toluene/isooctane
         mixture and the oestrogens eluted at 1 mL per minute with 70 mL
         of water-washed ether into a flask containing 1 mL ethanol. The
         ether is evaporated to dryness in a rotary evaporator at 45°C.
9.2.4   The Al_2O_3 column is washed with 25 mL toluene and the androgens
         and gestagens eluted with 30 mL toluene:ethanol::99:1 (v/v)
         mixture. After addition of 1 mL ethanol the mixture is
         evaporated to dryness in a rotary evaporator at 45°C.
9.2.5   The dry extracts from the columns are transferred with 3 x 1 mL
         acetone to the derivatization vessels (7.1.11). The solvent is
         evaporated under nitrogen.

9.3.   Derivatisation.
9.3.1   The extracts (9.2.5) are dried carefully in a vacuum oven or a
         heated desiccator at 40°C. 100 μL silylation mixture (6.3) are
         added and heated in a metal block at 60°C for 10 minutes. The
         resulting mixture is used for injection onto the GC column.
9.3.2   The extracts 9.2.5 are dried carefully in a vacuum oven or a
         heated desiccator at 40°C. 100 μL silylation mixture (6.3.2) are
         added shaken very carefully. The sample is transferred in a
         conical derivatization vial and heated in an oven at 60°C for 15
         min.
[Note; The silylation should be tested for uniformity by means of standard
solutions. With hexoestrol and perhaps other compounds further
confirmation may be necessary and the hexafluorabutyrate (HFB) derivative
can be prepared and evaluated (see also M 1.1.)]
9.3.3   Preparation of HFB-derivatives
         The residue obtained after extract clean-up is transferred to a
         derivatization vial with 0.5 mL absolute ethanol. The ethanol is
         evaporated and 0.1 mL HFBA (e.g. Pierce no 63163) in acetone
         (1:4,V/V) is added. The vial is vortexed and incubated during 1
         hour at 80°C. After incubation the reaction mixture is evaporated
         to dryness under a stream of nitrogen at 50°C and the
         derivatized residue is dissolved in 0.025 mL isooctane. The
         resulting solution is used for injection onto the GC column.

9.4.   Gas chromatography-mass spectrometry
         For GC-MS analysis on the system described below both the TMS-
         and HFB-derivatives are suitable.
9.4.1.   The following conditions are used during GC-MS analysis.
         GC   Capillary GC (HP 5840)
         column   SE 54, 25 m x 0.32 mm, film 0.5 um
         injection   2 μL splitless 250°C
         carrier gas   Helium at 2.5 mL per minute
         Initial column pressure 0.68 bar
         programme   160°C for 1 min., 160°C - 300°C at 20°C/min.
         temperature transfer line   280°C
         Under these conditions retention times are; Dichlorophene 8.6 min
         and 3,4-^{13}C-testosterone ca. 13.3 min.

9.4.2.1 Selected Ions.
        Ions monitored during GC-MS analysis.
        TMS-derivatives after silylation with 6.3.1.
        Oestrogens;
        Dichlorophene (ISTD)   412, 414, 377, 413
        DES   412, 413, 397, 383
        HEX   207   as HFB 303, 331
        DE   410, 395, 381, 411
        Ethinyloestradiol   425, 440, 300, 285
        Oestradiol (α or β)   285, 416, 231, 232, 326
        Oestriol   504, 345, 324, 386
        Oestrone   342, 257, 218, 244
        Androgens;
        3,4-^{13}C-testosterone (I.S.)   362, 272, 228, 347

        Testosterone   360, 270, 226, 345
        Androsterone   362, 347, 272, 246
        Androstenedione   286, 201, 148, 124
        Boldenone   358, 268, 237, 194, 147, 122
        Methyltestosterone   143, 284, 240, 269, 304
        19-nortestosterone   346, 331, 256, 215
        Trenbolone (α or β)   342, 252, 237, 211

        Gestagens;
        Progesterone   314, 272
        Medroxyprogesterone   373, 283, 265, 145
        Hydroxyprogesterone   359, 269, 227, 145

9.4.2.2   Ions monitored during GC-MS analysis after silylation with 6.3.2.

        Oestrogens as TMS-derivatives
        Dichlorophene (I.S.)   412, 413, 414, 377
        cis-DES   412, 413, 397, 383
        trans-DES   412, 413
        Hexoestrol   207
        Dienoestrol   410, 395, 381, 411
        Oestradiol   416, 285, 231, 326
        Oestriol   504, 345, 324, 386
        Oestrone   414, 399, 309, 270

        Androgens and Gestagens as TMS-enol-TMS derivatives
        3,4-^{13}C-testosterone (I.S) 434, 419, 303, 211
        Testosterone   432, 417, 301, 209
        Androstenedione   430, 234, 209
        4-chlorotestosterone   466, 468
        Boldenone   430, 431, 206, 299
        Methyltestosterone   446, 301, 314, 356
        19-nortestosterone   418, 403, 287

        Progesterone   458, 353, 443
        Medroxyprogesterone   315, 330, 455

[Notes; 1) values for TMS and HFB derivatives are also given in method Cy
1.1. 2) Trenbolone TMSi-ethers are not stable and must be injected
immediately after silylation. 3) Trenbolone TMS-enol-TMS-derivative is not
produced, possibly trenbolone is destroyed during this silylation.]

10.   CALCULATION OF RESULTS.

10.1.   Expression of Results.

Correction factors have to be determined and applied to the TMS
derivatives, because the responses of the peak areas are not identical when
compared with the internal standards (ISTD). It is essential that the
determination of the correction factors is performed within the
concentration range expected for the anabolics. 1 to 10 ng of the
derivatives of the internal standards has to be injected. The correction
factors are based on the common peak area method.

The following formula is applied

$$g_x = f \times \frac{g_{st} \times F_x}{F_{st} \times E}$$

where g_x = anabolic content (ug per kg)
        g_{st} = quantity of ISTD (ng) added
        F_x = area of anabolic derivative
        F_{st} = area of ISTD
        f = correction factor
        E = quantity sample (g) used

10.2.   Quality Assurance Procedure

10.2.1   Validation; Batches of two blanks and five blank samples spiked
at the 2 µg per kg level for the analytes of interest are required.
Recovery of the analyte should be within 50-120% with a CV value <30%.

10.2.2   Examples of quality assurance data obtained by Bergner-Lang, B.
and Kächele, M. (Dt. Lebensm. Rundschau, 1989, 85, 78-79) for the recovery
of 10 anabolic agents added to homogenised kidney tissue are shown below;

Agent	n	spike (ug per kg)	mean	Recovery (%)	CV (%)
DES	5	2	1.3	65	12.2
DEN	5	2	1.34	67	18.0
HEX	5	2	1.34	67	14.5
EE	5	2	1.26	63	15.5
$E_2\alpha$	5	2	1.20	60	33.3
$E_2\beta$	5	2	1.16	58	16.8
E_1	5	2	1.38	69	15.7
E_3	5	2	1.16	56	20.8
NT	6	3	1.53	52	40.3
MT	6	3	2.12	70	7.0

10.3.   Reliability

The method has been verified with good success in seven laboratories in
Germany having experience with the analysis of anabolic agents. The
results met the criteria of the EEC set out in section 5.

The data obtained in the interlaboratory comparison have shown that in
veal, DES and DE may be determined in concentrations >0.5 µg per kg and EE
and NT in concentrations > 1 µg per kg. Similar results and statistical
data were obtained in one of the laboratories for the substances, HEX, α-
and ß- oestradiol, oestrone, oestriol and methyltestosterone.

11.   SPECIAL CASES. e.g. if a particular analyte presents problems
with the TMS derivatives then the HFB derivatives should also be prepared
and analyzed.
If a "Baby" food is analyzed the starting material will contain less meat
and 100 g should be used.
The silylation (9.3.2) produces TMS-enol-TMS-derivatives. This procedure
allows good results also in problematical samples with dirty extracts and
small traces of hormones, especially for oestrone, gestagens and androgens.
The TMSi-ethers of trenbolone are unstable. The method is only applicable
for trenbolone if the TMSi-ethers are injected onto the GC after their
preparation. The TMS-enol-TMS-derivatives of trenbolone are not produced.

The method is not suitable for zeranol because the Extrelut column is not
useful for separating zeranol.

12.   NOTES ON PROCEDURE. The procedure chosen will depend on the
availability of reagents,reference compounds and equipment.

13.   QUALITY CONTROL. STANDARDS, REFERENCE MATERIALS AND ANTIBODIES.
A description of the source and quality of key reagents and standards is
given in Section 8.

14.   TEST REPORT.
To give the indications necessary for the identification of the sample, the
reference to the method employed, the results and the form in which these
are expressed, any particular points observed in the course of the test and
any operations not specified in the method or regarded as optional which
might affect the results.

15.   LIST OF ABBREVIATIONS
A list of the most important abbreviations is given in Annex I section 12.

16.   FLOW DIAGRAM.
    Tissue ---→ add buffer and recovery standard ---→ Homogenise
                                                            |
                                                            |
                                                            ↓
    XAD-2 column <------- solvent extraction <---- Hydrolyse
        |
        |
        |
        ↓
    Extrelut column and Al$_2$O$_3$ columns
        | |
        | |
        | |
        ↓   ↓
    Oestrogens   Androgens and Gestagens
        | |
        | |
        |____________________|
                 ↓
          Derivatize --------> GC-MS --------> Calculate results

Cy 1.3. STILBENES - CONFIRMATION OF STILBENES IN BILE BY GAS CHROMATOGRAPHY-MASS SPECTROMETRY.

SAFETY - When using ammonia CI, ensure that there are no leaks in the system and that there is adequate ventilation. If you feel unwell leave the room and get some fresh air.

0.   INTRODUCTION

<u>Purpose</u>

To confirm the presence and identity of stilbene compounds in bile sampled from farm animals. This work is carried out in compliance with the Residues Directive (86/469/EEC).

<u>Background</u>

Stilbenes are administered to animals because of their growth promoting properties. Three stilbene compounds commonly in use are: diethylstilboestrol (DES), dienoestrol (DE) and hexoestrol (HEX).

In 1981 the administration of stilbene growth promoters to animals was prohibited throughout the EEC. The presence of these compounds in slaughtered animals is monitored under the National Surveillance Scheme which is now carried out in compliance with the Residues Directive (86/469/EEC).

1.   SCOPE

With effect from 1 January 1988, the use of hormonal growth promoters was prohibited throughout the EEC. To ensure that farmers are not continuing to use stilbenes, bile is sampled at slaughterhouses and screened for the presence of these compounds using a radioimmunoassay technique. Whenever there is a positive screening result, this must be confirmed. In the UK this is done using this gas chromatography-mass spectrometry (GC-MS) method.

2.   FIELD OF APPLICATION.

This method is used for confirmation of the presence of stilbenes in bile samples found positive in the UK. The detection limit in bile is 5 µg/L for DES and 1 µg/L for Hexoestrol.

3.   REFERENCES.

Commission Decision, 93/256/EEC, laying down the methods for detecting residues of substances having a hormonal or thyrostatic action. [OJ. № L.118, 14.4.93. pp 64-74]

ISO Standard 78/2-1982 Layout for standards - Part 2: Standard for Chemical Analysis

CVL (1990) Standard operating procedure for Confirmation of stilbenes in bile by GC-MS. 27th June 1990

Bates, M.L., Warwick, M.J. and Shearer, G. (1985), Determination of synthetic growth promoters in bile. Food Additives Contaminants. $\underline{2}$, 37-46

Covey,T.R., (1985), Quantitative secondary ion monitoring gas chromatography/mass spectrometry of diethylstilbestrol in bovine liver. Biomed. Mass Spectrometry, $\underline{12}$,

Day, E.W., Vanatta, L.E. and Sieck, R.F. (1975), The confirmation of diethylstilbestrol residues in beef liver by gas chromatography-mass spectrometry. J.A.O.A.C. $\underline{58}$, 520-527

Van Peteghem, C.H., Lefevere, M.F. Van Haver, G.M. and De Leenheer, A.P., (1987).Quantification of diethylstilbestrol residues in meat samples by gas chromatography-isotope dilution mass spectrometry. J. Agric. Food Chem. $\underline{35}$, 228-231.

4. DEFINITIONS.

Stilbenes content is taken to mean the amount of stilbenes in the substance in question, regardless of the chemical form, determined according to the described method and expressed as µg stilbenes per litre of test sample.

5. PRINCIPLE.

The method of analysis comprises six stages:

(1)	Overnight hydrolysis of the bile.
(2)	Extrelut column clean-up.
(3)	Double Bond-Elut column purification.
(4)	Derivatisation.
(5)	Post-derivatisation clean-up.
(6)	Analysis by gas chromatography-mass spectrometry (GC-MS).

6.0.   MATERIALS

6.1.	Glucuronidase	Boehringer BCL (Cat No. 127051)
6.2.	Dichloromethane	Fisons Distol grade (stabilised with aniline)
6.3.	Diethyl ether	Fisons Distol grade
6.4.	Petroleum ether	Fisons Distol grade (40-60°C fraction)
6.5.	Methanol	Fisons Distol grade
6.6.	Heptafluorobutyrate (HFBA)	Phase Sep Ltd (Cat No. 940851)
6.7.	Extrelut columns	Merck BDH
6.8.	Bond-Elut columns	500 mg CN, Jones Scientific (Cat No. 613303)
6.9.	Bond-Elut columns	500 mg NH_2, Jones Scientific (Cat No. 611303)
6.10	Phosphate buffer	pH 7 (0.06M) [3.3 g Na_2HPO_4 + 5.75 g NaH_2PO_4 made up to 1 litre]
6.11	Phosphate buffer	pH 6 (1.0M) [35 g NaH_2PO_4 + 3g NaH_2PO_4 made up to 1 litre]
6.12	Hexane	Distol grade
6.13	Heptane	Distol grade
6.14	Perfluorotributylamine	Finnigan MAT.

6.15.   <u>Standards</u>

    DES   Sigma
    Hexoestrol   Sigma
    Dienoestrol   Sigma

These should be made up in methanol to a concentration of 1 mg/mL and diluted to working standards of concentrations of 10 µg/mL, 1 µg/mL, 100 ng/mL, 10 ng/mL and 1 ng/mL.

7.   EQUIPMENT

7.1.	Universal bottles	20 mL
7.2.	Techni Dri-block	
7.3.	Quick-fit tubes	50 mL (MF-24)
7.4.	Quick-fit expansion adaptor	(34/35-24/29)
7.5.	Screw cap tubes	J Bibby (Cat No. 5142-10)
7.6.	Water bath	
7.7.	Manifold	Supplying oxygen-free nitrogen
7.8.	GC vials and caps	
7.9.	Mass spectrometer	Finnigan MAT, coupled to a gas chromatograph and linked to an INCOS data system.

8. SAMPLES AND SAMPLING PROCEDURE.

N.B. Attention is drawn to section 6.3.1 and ISO document 78/2-1982(E) and the following notes derived from Annex II of 2052/VI/84-EN.

8.1. Nature of the Sample; Samples shall be such as to enable the detection of residues in meat as defined in Directive 64/433/EEC. Failing this biological fluids (in this method bile) or faeces may constitute the samples for the detection of residues.

8.2. Size of Sample; The size of the sample must be large enough to allow the reference method to be carried out and to allow repeat analysis where required.

This method for Stilbenes uses 5 mL bile therefore the size shall not be less than 20 mL bile

8.3. The samples must be taken and packed in such a way as to allow proper identification in the laboratory.

8.4. The method of packing, preservation and transport must maintain the integrity of the sample and not prejudice the result of the examination.

Samples for the analysis of stilbenes must be stored and transported at temperatures below -18°C.

9.0.   PROCEDURE

9.1.   <u>Hydrolysis</u>

Place 5 mL bile, 15 mL of phosphate buffer pH 7 and 50 µL of glucuronidase in a 20 mL universal bottle and incubate overnight at 37°C.

9.2.   Extrelut Clean-up

Prepare an Extrelut column according to the maker's instructions. Onto a 50 mL (MF-24) Quick-fit tube place a 34/35-24/29 Quick-fit expansion adaptor and place the column in the adaptor.

Add the bile/buffer mix and leave for 30 minutes before eluting the column with 2 x 35 mL of diethyl ether.

Reduce the ether under nitrogen to approximately 5 mL before washing into a 10 mL conical centrifuge tube and drying under nitrogen. A small residue is normally left after drying. Resuspend the extract in 2 mL of 40% (v/v) dichloromethane/hexane.

9.3.   Bond-Elut Purification

The CN Bond-Elut columns should be prepared by washing twice with 2 mL of methanol and twice with 2 mL of petroleum ether. Before the columns are dry add the extract and wash with 2 mL of dichloromethane/hexane (70:30 v/v).

Prepare the NH_2 columns by washing twice with methanol then twice with 2 mL of petroleum ether. Fill the NH_2 column with diethyl ether and attach the CN column to the top of it. Elute the CN column into the NH_2 column using 3 mL of diethyl ether. Discard the CN column. Wash the NH_2 column with 2 mL of 2% (v/v) methanol in dichloromethane.

Elute the NH_2 column into a screw cap centrifuge tube with 3 mL of 33% (v/v) methanol in dichloromethane.

9.4.   Derivatisation

Dry the methanol/dichloromethane extract and resuspend in 1 mL heptane and 100 μL of HFBA (from a fresh ampoule). Cap the tube and incubate the extract at 80°C for 20 minutes in the Techni Dri-block. Shake after 3 minutes to ensure adequate mixing of the two layers. After 20 minutes remove the tubes and allow to cool.

Concurrently run stilbenes standards through the derivatisation steps. Standard concentrations = 1 ng, 10 ng, 50 ng, 100 ng, 500 ng, 1 μg, 10 μg/mL.

9.5   Post-Derivatisation Column Clean-up

To improve chromatography, clean up the derivatised extracts by adding 5 mL of phosphate buffer pH 6. Shake vigorously for exactly 30 seconds, then allow layers to settle. (If necessary, spin at 2000 rpm for 5 minutes). Carefully pipette off the upper heptane layer, using a Multipette set to 0.7 mL and vial up ready for GC-MS. The vials should be capped immediately.

9.6   <u>GC-MS Analysis</u>

9.6.1.   The GC parameters are set up as follows;

COLUMN: J&W fused silica capillary column, SE-54, 15 m x 0.25 mm.
INJECTIONS: 0.5 µl manual injections.
TEMPERATURES: Interface: 230°C
               Injector: 220°C
OVEN TEMPERATURES:

from temp (°C)	to temp (°C)	rate (°C/min)	time (min)	total time (min)
55	55	-	1.0	1.0
55	240	20	9.2	10.2
240	240	-	10.0	20.2

         Capillary   close = 0.00   open = 0.7
         Divert   close = 0.00   open = 20.7
CARRIER GAS: Helium
           flow rate   = 1 cm^3/min   injector pressure = 10 psi.

9.6.2 The mass spectrometry parameters are

IONISER:
       Mode: Chemical ionisation (CI)
       Temperature: 130°C
       Pressure;   50 Torr
MANIFOLD TEMPERATURE: 90 (± 5) °C
ELECTRON MULTIPLIER: 1.2 kV
ELECTRON ENERGY: 70 electron volts.
MAKE-UP GASES; DES use methane, DE and HEX use ammonia

Other parameters should be set up by adjusting the instrument controls to
give the optimum peak height and shape for a suitable calibration compound.
The CVL uses perfluorotributylamine (PFTBA).
9.6.3   In CI mode, using ammonia as the make-up gas, and scanning
between m/z = 50 and 700, run (a) a blank hexane (b) 10 µg in 100 µL
stilbenes standard. Collect 1000 scans.
9.6.4.   Focus in on the GC peak of the stilbene standard. Find the exact
masses in the spectrum for the three selected ions:

       DES   464, 465, 661 (using CH$_4$ CI)
       Dienoestrol   462, 480, 676 (using CH$_4$ CI)
       Hexoestrol   466, 484, 680 (using CH$_4$ CI)

9.6.5.   Use these masses to set up or modify a multiple ion detection
(MID) scan list. Create the scan list.
9.6.6.   Rerun hexane to ensure there is no carry over of the stilbene.
9.6.7.   Using the scan list just created, analyse the sample and the
standards on the GC-MS. It is advisable to:
(a)   Analyse the 100 µg standard first to ensure that the MID is set
          up correctly. Follow this with hexane.
(b)   Analyse standards in order of increasing concentration.
(c)   Switch the filament on 100 scans before the peak is due to elute
          from the column and enter the source and turn it off 100 scans
          afterwards.
(d)   Run hexane between each injection.

Cy 1.3/5

10.0.   RESULTS

The presence of the suspected stilbene in a sample is confirmed if the GC-
MS data agree with the following criteria:

1.   The peak has the same retention time on GC as the standards.
2.   All the selected ions are present in the mass spectrum of that
          peak after subtraction of the background.
3.   The selected ions are present in the same ratio to one another as
          seen in the standard.

If the stilbene is present in a sample, and satisfies the above criteria,
then an estimate of the quantity present may be calculated using one of two
methods:
1.   Use the data system to calculate peak areas and create a
          quantitation list. Use a relevant standard to set up a
          quantitation library, or use a range of standards. Refer the
          sample to this and obtain a quantitation report. This is the
          preferred method.
2.   Measure the peak area of the sample and a relevant standard. The
          concentration of stilbene in the TOTAL sample submitted is then
          found using the equation:

$$\frac{\text{peak height sample}}{\text{peak height standard}} \quad x \quad \text{concentration of standard}$$

              Limit of detection: DES 5 µg per L of bile
                         Hexoestrol 1 µg per L of bile.

11.   SPECIAL CASES
12.   NOTES ON PROCEDURE
13.   QUALITY CONTROL.   STANDARDS AND REFERERENCE MATERIALS.
14.   TEST REPORT.
To give the indications necessary for the identification of the sample, the
reference to the method employed, the results and the form in which these
are expressed, any particular points observed in the course of the test and
any operations not specified in the method or regarded as optional which
might affect the results.
15.   LIST OF ABBREVIATIONS
A list of the most important abbreviations is given in Annex I section 12.

16.   FLOW DIAGRAGM.

          enzyme hydrolysis   ether eluate
  BILE ----------------------> EXTRELUT COLUMN ---------------> DRY --->

                                      elute   elute
  ---->CH_2Cl_2/MeOH -----> CN-BOND-ELUT -----------> NH_2-BOND-ELUT ------>
                             COLUMN   COLUMN

  ----> CH_2Cl_2/MeOH -----> DERIVATISE WITH HFBA -------> CLEAN UP WITH
                                                       PHOSPHATE BUFFER -->

  ----> GC-MS OF HFB DERIVATIVES -----------------> CALCULATE RESULTS

Cy. 1.4.. TRENBOLONE - CONFIRMATION OF TRENBOLONE IN BILE BY GAS CHROMATOGRAPHY-MASS SPECTROMETRY

SAFETY

Take care when handling the BSTFA-TMCS. It is irritating to eyes, respiratory system and skin. After contact with skin wash immediately with water. There is also a danger of cumulative effects.

0.   INTRODUCTION

Purpose

The confirmation of the presence of trenbolone (TB) in bile samples taken from farm animals in compliance with the Residues Directive (86/469/EEC).

Background

Trenbolone is a synthetic steroid with androgenic activity used to promote growth in farm livestock. With effect from 1 January 1988, the use of hormonal substances for fattening purposes was prohibited throughout the EEC.

Metabolism

Trenbolone is administered to farm animals as the ester trenbolone acetate. The active ingredient is 17ß-hydroxy-TB (ßTB) which is the major residue in muscle and blood.   ßTB is metabolised in the liver to 17α-hydroxy-TB (αTB) and this is the most abundant residue in bile, urine and faeces.   This method is capable of measuring the total content of both isomers but the αTB accounts for most of the residue in bile.

1.   SCOPE

To ensure that farmers are not continuing to use trenbolone, bile is sampled at slaughterhouses and screened for the presence of this compound using an ELISA technique. Whenever there is a positive screening result, this must be confirmed (in the UK) by gas chromatography-mass spectrometry (GC-MS).   This work is carried out in compliance with the Residues Directive (86/469/EEC).

2.   FIELD OF APPLICATION.

This method is used for confirmation of the presence of trenbolone in bile samples found positive in the UK. The detection limit for trenbolone is 1 ng of TOTAL bile.

3.   REFERENCES.

Commission Decision, 93/256/EEC, laying down the methods for detecting residues of substances having a hormonal or thyrostatic action. [OJ. № L.118, 14.4.93. pp 64-74]

2052/VI/84 File 6.11 II-4, Scientific Veterinary Committee, Working Group - "Reference Methods for Residues", General Criteria for the establishment of Reference Methods for the Detection of Residues.

ISO Standard 78/2-1982 Layout for standards - Part 2: Standard for Chemical
Analysis

CVL (1990) Standard operating procedure for Confirmation of trenbolone in
bile by GC-MS. 27th June 1990

Other references;
Hsu, S.S., Eckerlin, R. and Henion J. (1988) Identification and
quantification of trenbolone in bovine tissue by gas chromatography-mass
spectrometry. J. Chromatog. <u>424</u>, 219-225

Daeseleire, E., De Guesquiere, A. and Van Peteghem, C., (1991),
Derivatisation and gas chromatographic-mass spectrometric detection of
anabolic steroid residues isolated from edible muscle tissues. J.
Chromatog. <u>562</u>, 673-679

4.   DEFINITIONS.

Trenbolone content is taken to mean the amount of trenbolone in the
substance in question, regardless of the chemical form, determined
according to the described method and expressed as µg trenbolone per kg or
litre of test sample.

5.   PRINCIPLE.

The method of analysis comprises six stages:
            (1)   Overnight hydrolysis of the bile.
            (2)   Extrelut column clean-up.
            (3)   Double Bond-Elut column purification.
            (4)   Derivatisation.
            (5)   Post-derivatisation clean-up.
            (6)   Analysis by gas chromatography-mass spectrometry (GC-MS).

6.0.   CHEMICALS
Note: The reagents (and equipment) for which examples of their source are
quoted are known to be satisfactory, nevertheless reagents and equipment
from other sources may be equally suitable. All the reagents should be of
analytical grade or better.

6.1.   Bis-(trimethylsilyl) trifluoroacetamide [BSTFA] with 1%
            trimethylchlorosilane [TMCS] (Pierce Chemical Company)
6.2.   Diethyl ether, Distol grade
6.3   Acetonitrile, HPLC grade
6.4   Iso-octane (trimethylpentane) Distol grade
6.5   Perfluorotributylamine   (Finnigan MAT)

6.6.   Standards
            17∝-trenbolone (Roussel Uclaf)
            17∝-trenbolone in methanol; 10 µg/mL, 1 µg/mL, 100 ng/mL, 10
            ng/mL.

7.0.   EQUIPMENT
7.1.   Centrifuge tubes, screw capped (J Bibby)
7.2.   Dri-block (Techni)
7.3   Water bath
7.4.   Manifold supplying oxygen-free nitrogen

7.5.   GC mini-vials, (Chromacol, Cat No. 03-CV)
7.6.   Vial caps, (Chromacol, Cat No. 8-AC3)
7.7.   GC column, SE54 (Jones Chromatography)
7.8   Sonic water bath (or Whirlimixer)
7.9   Mass spectrometer, Finnigan MAT Model 4600 coupled to GC and
         linked to an INCOS data system.

8. SAMPLES AND SAMPLING PROCEDURE.

N.B. Attention is drawn to section 6.3.1 and ISO document 78/2-1982 and
the following notes derived from Annex II of 2052/VI/84-EN.

8.1. Nature of the Sample; Samples shall be such as to enable the
detection of residues in meat as defined in Directive 64/433/EEC. Failing
this biological fluids (in this method bile) or faeces may constitute the
samples for the detection of residues.

8.2. Size of Sample; The size of the sample must be large enough to allow
the reference method to be carried out and to allow repeat analysis where
required.

This method for Trenbolone uses 5 mL bile therefore the size shall not be
less than 20 mL bile

8.3. The samples must be taken and packed in such a way as to allow proper
identification in the laboratory.

8.4. The method of packing, preservation and transport must maintain the
integrity of the sample and not prejudice the result of the examination.

Samples for the analysis of trenbolone must be stored and transported at
temperatures below -18°C.

9.0   PROCEDURE
9.1.   Hydrolysis
Place 5 mL bile, 15 mL of phosphate buffer pH 7 and 50 μL of glucuronidase
in a 20 mL universal bottle and incubate overnight at 37°C.

9.2.   Extrelut Clean-up
Prepare an Extrelut column according to the maker's instructions. Onto a 50
mL (MF-24) Quick-fit tube place a 34/35-24/29 Quick-fit expansion adaptor
and place the column in the adaptor.

Add the bile/buffer mix and leave for 30 minutes before eluting the column
with 2 x 35 mL of diethyl ether.

Reduce the ether under nitrogen to approximately 5 mL before washing into a
10 mL conical centrifuge tube and drying under nitrogen. A small residue
is normally left after drying. Resuspend the extract in 2 mL of 40% (v/v)
dichloromethane/hexane.

9.3.   Bond-Elut Purification
The CN Bond-Elut columns should be prepared by washing twice with 2 mL of
methanol and twice with 2 mL of petroleum ether. Before the columns are
dry add the extract and wash with 2 mL of dichloromethane/hexane (70:30
v/v).

Prepare the NH$_2$ columns by washing twice with methanol then twice with 2 mL of petroleum ether. Fill the NH$_2$ column with diethyl ether and attach the CN column to the top of it. Elute the CN column into the NH$_2$ column using 3 mL of diethyl ether. Discard the CN column. Wash the NH$_2$ column with 2 mL of 2% (v/v) methanol in dichloromethane.

Elute the NH$_2$ column into a screw cap centrifuge tube with 3 mL of 33% (v/v) methanol in dichloromethane.

9.4.   Derivatisation:

9.4.1.   Resuspend the dried sample in 5 mL ether. Sonicate for a few
           seconds then transfer to a screw capped centrifuge tube using a
           Pasteur pipette.
9.4.2.   Evaporate to dryness under nitrogen.
9.4.3.   Add 200 μL BSTFA-TMCS and cap IMMEDIATELY. Place in Techi Dri-
           block and incubate at 60°C for 1 hour.

[NOTE: The derivatising reagent absorbs water very easily. Do not open vial until you are ready to use it and seal it immediately if there is any left. The derivatisation will not work if there is any water present.

9.4.4.   Allow to cool, then add 200 μL acetonitrile. Evaporate as an
           azeotropic mixture. Gently take to dryness under nitrogen.
9.4.5.   Resuspend in 200 μL iso-octane. Sonicate briefly, then transfer
           to a GC mini-vial.
9.4.6.   Evaporate to dryness under a very gentle stream of nitrogen.
9.4.7.   Resuspend in 20 μL iso-octane and sonicate briefly.
9.5.   Concurrently run trenbolone standards. Concentrations of 1 ng, 5
           ng, 10 ng, 50 ng, 100 ng and 10 μg/mL should be taken to dryness
           and the same procedure followed.

9.6.   GC-MS Analysis
9.6.1.   The GC parameters are

COLUMN: J&W fused silica capillary column, SE-54, 15 m x 0.25 mm.
INJECTIONS: 0.5 μL manual injections.
TEMPERATURES: Interface: 230°C;   Injector: 220°C
OVEN TEMPERATURES:

from temp (°C)	to temp (°C)	rate (°C/min)	time (min)	total time (min)
55	55	-	1.0	1.0
55	240	20	9.2	10.2
240	240	-	10.0	20.2

GC Valves:

Capillary	close = 0.00	open = 0.7
Divert	close = 0.00	open = 20.2

Carrier Gas:
          Helium;   Flow rate   = 1 cm^3/min
                    Injector pressure = 10 psi

9.6.2   Set up the MS parameters as shown below. The MS should be tuned
           in using a suitable calibrant (e.g. PFTBA).

Ionizer: Mode   = EI positive ion
                            Temperature = 150°C.
Manifold: Temperature: 90 (±5°C).
Electron Multiplier: 1.2 kV
Electron Energy: 70 electron volts.
Various settings: These parameters should be optimised by calibrating the
instrument using PFTBA. The actual values will depend upon the instrument
and the condition of source etc but default values may be found in the
instrument manual.

9.6.3.   Operate the MS in EI mode and scan between m/z = 50 and 400.
          Analyze:
          (a) Hexane
          (b) 10 µg in 200 µL trenbolone standard.
          Collect 1000 scans. After 7 minutes turn on the filament.

9.6.4. The trenbolone peak elutes between 10-13 minutes after injection.
Focus on the GC peak and find the exact masses (to 3 decimal places) for at
least the ions:
          $m/z = 211, 237, 252, 342.$

9.6.5. Use these ions to set up or modify a multiple ion detection (MID)
scan list. Create the scan list.

9.6.6. Re-run hexane to ensure there is no carry over of trenbolone.

9.6.7. Using the scan list just created, analyze the standards and the
sample on GC-MS. It is advisable to:

(a)   analyze the 1 µg standard first to ensure that the MID is set up
        correctly. Follow this by hexane.
(b)   analyze the standards in order of increasing concentration.
(c)   switch the filament on 100 scans before the trenbolone is due to
        elute from the column and turn it off 100 scans afterwards.
(d)   run hexane between each injection.

10.   RESULTS
10.1.   Rationale
Dried bile extracts, prepared by column chromatography, are derivatised
with BSTFA-TMCS and the derivatised extract is analyzed by GC-MS.

Three criteria must be satisfied for the positive confirmation of
trenbolone:
1.   The GC retention time of trenbolone must be the same as that of
        the standard.
2.   All the characteristic ions must be detected after subtraction of
        the background.
3.   The characteristic ions must be present in the spectrum of the
        sample in the same ratios as in the spectrum of the standard.

If trenbolone is present in the sample, and satisfies the above criteria,
then an estimate of the quantity present may be calculated using one of two
methods:

1.   Use the data system to calculate peak areas and create a
        quantisation list. Use a relevant standard to set up a
        quantisation library, or use a range of standards. Refer the

sample to this and obtain a quantisation report. This is the
preferred method.

2.   Measure the peak area of the sample and a relevant standard. The
concentration of trenbolone in the TOTAL sample submitted is then
found using the equation:

$$\frac{\text{peak height sample}}{\text{peak height standard}} \times \text{concentration of standard}$$

Limit of detection: 1 ng trenbolone per L bile.

11.   SPECIAL CASES

12.   NOTES ON PROCEDURE

13.   QUALITY CONTROL.   STANDARDS AND REFERENCE MATERIALS.

14.   TEST REPORT.

To give the indications necessary for the identification of the sample, the
reference to the method employed, the results and the form in which these
are expressed, any particular points observed in the course of the test and
any operations not specified in the method or regarded as optional which
might affect the results.

15.   LIST OF ABBREVIATIONS

A list of the most important abbreviations is given in Annex I section 12.

16.   FLOW DIAGRAM.


```
             enzyme hydrolysis                            ether eluate
 BILE ----------------------> EXTRELUT COLUMN --------------> DRY --->


                                          elute                       elute
 ---->CH2Cl2/MeOH -----> CN-BOND-ELUT -----------> NH2-BOND-ELUT ------>
                             COLUMN                    COLUMN


 ----> CH2Cl2/MeOH -----> DERIVATISE WITH HFBA -------> CLEAN UP WITH
                                                        PHOSPHATE BUFFER -->


 ----> GCMS OF HFB DERIVATIVES ----------------> CALCULATE RESULTS
```

Cy 1.5. ZERANOL - CONFIRMATION OF ZERANOL IN BILE BY GAS CHROMATOGRAPHY-MASS SPECTROMETRY.

WARNING AND SAFETY PRECAUTIONS

When using ammonia CI, ensure that there are no leaks in the system and that there is adequate ventilation. If you feel unwell leave the room and get some fresh air.

0.   INTRODUCTION

Zeranol is a synthetic anabolic agent with weak oestrogenic activity. It is structurally related to the naturally occurring oestrogenic mycotoxin zearalenone which was originally isolated from mouldy maize. Like other anabolic compounds, zeranol is used to promote growth in farm livestock.

1.   SCOPE

With effect from 1 January 1988, the use of hormonal growth promoters was prohibited throughout the EEC. To ensure that farmers are not continuing to use zeranol, bile is sampled at slaughterhouses and screened for the presence of this compound using a radioimmunoassay technique. Whenever there is a positive screening result, this must be confirmed (in the UK) by gas chromatography-mass spectrometry (GC-MS). This work is carried out in compliance with the Residues Directive (86/469/EEC).

2.   FIELD OF APPLICATION.

This method is used for confirmation of the presence of zeranol in bile samples found positive in the UK. The detection limit is 2 µg/litre of bile for zeranol.

3.   REFERENCES.

Commission Decision, 93/256/EEC, laying down the methods for detecting residues of substances having a hormonal or thyrostatic action. [OJ. № L.118, 14.4.93. pp 64-74]

2052/VI/84 File 6.11 II-4, Scientific Veterinary Committee, Working Group - "Reference Methods for Residues", General Criteria for the establishment of Reference Methods for the Detection of Residues.

ISO Standard 78/2-1982 Layout for standards - Part 2: Standard for Chemical Analysis

CVL (1990) Standard operating procedure for Confirmation of zeranol in bile by GC-MS. 27th June 1990

4.   DEFINITIONS.

Zeranol content is taken to mean the amount of zeranol in the substance in question, regardless of the chemical form, determined according to the described method and expressed as µg zeranol per kg or litre of test sample.

5.   PRINCIPLE.

The method of analysis comprises six stages:
           (1)   Overnight hydrolysis of the bile.
           (2)   Extrelut column clean-up.
           (3)   Double Bond-Elut column purification.
           (4)   Derivatisation.
           (5)   Post-derivatisation clean-up.
           (6)   Analysis by gas chromatography-mass spectrometry (GC-MS).

6.0.	CHEMICALS	
6.1.	Glucuronidase	Boehringer BCL (Cat No. 127051)
6.2.	Dichloromethane	Fisons Distol grade (stabilised with aniline)
6.3.	Diethyl ether	Fisons Distol grade
6.4.	Petroleum ether	Fisons Distol grade (40-60°C fraction)
6.5.	Methanol	Fisons Distol grade
6.6.	Heptafluorobutyrate (HFBA)	Phase Sep Ltd (Cat No. 940851)
6.7.	Extrelut columns	Merck BDH
6.8.	Bond-Elut columns	500 mg CN, Jones Scientific (Cat No. 613303)
6.9.	Bond-Elut columns	500 mg NH_2, Jones Scientific (Cat No. 611303)
6.10	Phosphate buffer	pH 7 (0.06M) [3.3 g Na_2HPO_4 + 5.75 g NaH_2PO_4 made up to 1 litre]
6.11	Phosphate buffer	pH 6 (1.0M) [35 g NaH_2PO_4 + 3g NaH_2PO_4 made up to 1 litre]
6.12	Hexane	Distol grade
6.13	Heptane	Distol grade
6.14	Perfluorotributylamine	Finnigan MAT.

6.15.   Standards

Zeranol   International Minerals & Chemical Corp.

The standard should be made up in methanol to a concentration of 1 mg/mL and diluted to working standards of concentrations of 100 μg/mL, 10 μg/mL, 1 μg/mL, 100 ng/mL, 10 ng/mL and 1 ng/mL.

7.   EQUIPMENT

7.1.	Universal bottles	20 mL
7.2.	Techni Dri-block	
7.3.	Quick-fit tubes	50 mL (MF-24)
7.4.	Quick-fit expansion adaptor	(34/35-24/29)
7.5.	Screw cap tubes	J Bibby (Cat No. 5142-10)
7.6.	Water bath	
7.7.	Manifold	Supplying oxygen-free nitrogen
7.8.	GC vials and caps	
7.9.	Mass spectrometer	Finnigan MAT, coupled to a gas chromatograph and linked to an INCOS data system.

8.   SAMPLES AND SAMPLING PROCEDURE.

N.B. Attention is drawn to section 6.3.1 and ISO document 78/2-1982 and the following notes derived from Annex II of 2052/VI/84-EN.

8.1. Nature of the Sample; Samples shall be such as to enable the detection of residues in meat as defined in Directive 64/433/EEC. Failing this biological fluids (in this method bile) or faeces may constitute the samples for the detection of residues.

8.2. Size of Sample; The size of the sample must be large enough to allow the reference method to be carried out and to allow repeat analysis where required.

This method for Zeranol uses 5 mL bile therefore the size shall not be less than 20 mL bile

8.3. The samples must be taken and packed in such a way as to allow proper identification in the laboratory.

8.4. The method of packing, preservation and transport must maintain the integrity of the sample and not prejudice the result of the examination.

Samples for the analysis of zeranol must be stored and transported at temperatures below -18°C.

9.   PROCEDURE

9.1.   Hydrolysis
Place 5 mL bile, 15 mL of phosphate buffer pH 7 and 50 μL of glucuronidase in a 20 mL universal bottle and incubate overnight at 37°C.

9.2.   Extrelut Clean-up
Prepare an Extrelut column according to the maker's instructions. Onto a 50 mL (MF-24) Quick-fit tube place a 34/35-24/29 Quick-fit expansion adaptor and place the column in the adaptor.

Add the bile/buffer mix and leave for 30 minutes before eluting the column with 2 x 35 mL of diethyl ether.

Reduce the ether under nitrogen to approximately 5 mL before washing into a 10 mL conical centrifuge tube and drying under nitrogen. A small residue is normally left after drying. Resuspend the extract in 2 mL of 40% (v/v) dichloromethane/hexane.

9.3.   Bond-Elut Purification
The CN Bond-Elut columns should be prepared by washing twice with 2 mL of methanol and twice with 2 mL of petroleum ether. Before the columns are dry add the extract and wash with 2 mL of dichloromethane/hexane (70:30 v/v).

Prepare the NH_2 columns by washing twice with methanol then twice with 2 mL of petroleum ether. Fill the NH2 column with diethyl ether and attach the CN column to the top of it. Elute the CN column into the NH_2 column using 3 mL of diethyl ether. Discard the CN column. Wash the NH_2 column with 2 mL of 2% (v/v) methanol in dichloromethane.

Elute the NH_2 column into a screw cap centrifuge tube with 3 mL of 33% (v/v) methanol in dichloromethane.

9.4.   Derivatisation

Dry the methanol/dichloromethane extract and resuspend in 1 mL heptane and 100 μL of HFBA (from a fresh ampoule). Cap the tube and incubate the extract at 80°C for 20 minutes in the Techni Dri-block. Shake after 3 minutes to ensure adequate mixing of the two layers. After 20 minutes remove the tubes and allow to cool.

Concurrently run zeranol standards through the derivatisation steps. Standard concentrations = 1 ng, 10 ng, 50 ng, 100 ng, 500 ng, 1 μg, 10 μg/mL.

9.5   Post-Derivatisation Column Clean-up

To improve chromatography, clean-up the derivatised extracts by adding 5 mL of phosphate buffer pH 6. Shake vigorously for exactly 30 seconds, then allow layers to settle. (If necessary, spin at 2000 rpm for 5 minutes). Carefully pipette off the upper heptane layer, using a Multipette set to 0.7 mL and vial up ready for GC-MS. The vials should be capped immediately.

9.6   GC-MS Analysis

9.6.1.   The GC parameters are

COLUMN: J&W fused silica capillary column, SE-54, 15 m x 0.25 mm.
INJECTIONS: 0.5 μl manual injections.
TEMPERATURES: Interface: 230°C
               Injector: 220°C
OVEN TEMPERATURES:

from temp (°C)	to temp (°C)	rate (°C/min)	time (min)	total time (min)
55	55	-	1.0	1.0
55	240	20	9.2	10.2
240	240	-	10.0	20.2

CARRIER GAS: Helium
          flow rate   = 1 cm^3/min
          injector pressure = 10 psi.
GC Valves: Capillary   close: 0.00   open: 0.7
              Divert   close: 0.00   open: 20.2

9.6.2   Set up the MS parameters as shown below. The MS should be tuned in using a suitable calibrant (e.g. PFTBA).

Ionizer:
          Mode: chemical ionisation (CI)
          Temperature: 130°C.
          Pressure: 50 Torr
Manifold: Temperature: 90 (± 5)°C.
Electron Multiplier: 1.2 kV
Electron Energy: 70 electron volts.
Make-up Gas: Ammonia

Other parameters should be optimised by calibrating the instrument. Further details on setting up the instrument may be found in the instrument manual.

9.6.3   In CI mode, using ammonia as the make-up gas, and scanning

between m/z = 50 and 700, run
(a)   a blank hexane
(b)   10 µg in 100 µL zeranol standard.
Collect 1000 scans.

9.6.4   Focus in on the GC peak from the zeranol standard. Find the
exact masses in the spectrum for the selected ions: 279, 296, 519, 536.

9.6.5   Use these masses to set up or modify a multiple ion detection
(MID) scan list. Create the scan list.

9.6.6   Re-run hexane to ensure there is no carry over of the zeranol.

9.6.7   Using the scan list just created, analyze the sample and the
standards on the GC-MS. It is advisable to:

(a)   analyze the 100 µg standard first to ensure that the MID is set up
correctly. Follow this with hexane.
(b)   analyze standards in order of increasing concentration.
(c)   switch the filament on 100 scans before the peak is due to elute from
the column and enter the source and turn it off 100 scans afterwards.
(d)   run hexane between each injection.

10.   CALCULATION OF RESULTS

The presence of zeranol in a sample is confirmed if the GC-MS data agree
with the following criteria:

1.   The peak has the same retention time on GC as the standards.

2.   All the selected ions are present in the mass spectrum of that
          peak after subtraction of the background.

3.   The selected ions are present in the same ratio to one another as
          seen in the standard.

If zeranol is present in a sample and satisfies the above criteria, then an
estimate of the quantity present may be calculated using one of two
methods:
1.   Use the data system to calculate peak areas and create a
          quantisation list. Use a relevant standard to set up a
          quantisation library, or use a range of standards. Refer the
          sample to this and obtain a quantisation report. This is the
          preferred method.
2.   Measure the peak area of the sample and that of the relevant
          standard. The concentration of zeranol in the TOTAL sample
          analyzed is given by the equation:

$$\frac{\text{peak height sample}}{\text{peak height standard}} \quad \times \quad \text{concentration of standard}$$

Limit of detection: 2 µg per L of bile.

TMS derivatisation used for trenbolone (refer to trenbolone Standard
Operating Procedure) can also be used for zeranol. In this case the MS is
operated in the EI mode and the ions focused on are: 307, 335, 433, 538.

11.   SPECIAL CASES

12.   NOTES ON PROCEDURE

13.   QUALITY CONTROL.   STANDARDS AND REFERENCE MATERIALS.
Reference materials for zeranol are being prepared under the Measurement
and Testing Programme of DG12.

14.   TEST REPORT.
To give the indications necessary for the identification of the sample, the
reference to the method employed, the results and the form in which these
are expressed, any particular points observed in the course of the test and
any operations not specified in the method or regarded as optional which
might affect the results.

15.   LIST OF ABBREVIATIONS
A list of the most important abbreviations is given in Annex I section 12.

16.   FLOW DIAGRAM.


```
          enzyme hydrolysis                    ether eluate
  BILE ----------------------> EXTRELUT COLUMN --------------> DRY --->



                                     elute                  elute
  ---->CH2Cl2/MeOH -----> CN-BOND-ELUT -----------> NH2-BOND-ELUT ------>
                              COLUMN                    COLUMN


  ----> CH2Cl2/MeOH -----> DERIVATISE WITH HFBA -------> CLEAN UP WITH
                                                         PHOSPHATE BUFFER -->


  ----> GCMS OF HFB DERIVATIVES ----------------> CALCULATE RESULTS
```

Cy 1.6.   ZERANOL - METHOD FOR MEASUREMENT OF RESIDUES OF ZERANOL IN ANIMALS AND ANIMAL TISSUES USING RADIOIMMUNOASSAY (RIA)

WARNING AND SAFETY PRECAUTIONS

1.   INTRODUCTION.

Throughout the EEC the use of zeranol is prohibited in food producing animals. Also the MRL for residues of zeranol in animal products imported into or produced within the Community is zero.

2.   SCOPE AND FIELD OF APPLICATION

This method of analysis describes the determination of the total content of zeranol in foodstuffs and samples of animal origin. The method can be used for meat and fish and also for biological material such as animal organs, biological fluids and faeces. The detection limit, defined as three times the standard deviation of the blank determination, is 0.1 - 1 µg per kg or litre of sample for zeranol.

3.   REFERENCES.

Commission Decision, 93/256/EEC, laying down the methods for detecting residues of substances having a hormonal or thyrostatic action. [OJ. № L.118, 14.4.93. pp 64-74]

2052/VI/84-EN File 6.21 II-4, Scientific Veterinary Committee, Working Group - "Reference Methods for Residues", General Criteria for the establishment of Reference Methods for the Detection of Residues.

ISO Standard 78/2-1982 Layout for standards - Part 2: Standard for Chemical Analysis

Method based on modifications of methods described by;-

Dixon, S.N. and Russel, K.L. (1983), Radioimmunoassay of the anabolic agent zeranol. II. Zeranol concentrations in the urine of sheep and cattle implanted with zeranol (Ralgro). J.Vet. Pharmacol. Therap. $\underline{6}$, 173-179.

Dixon, S.N. and Mallinson, C,B. (1986), Radioimmunoassay of the anabolic agent Zeranol. III. Zeranol concentrations in the faeces of steers implanted with zeranol Ralgro). J.Vet. Pharmacol. Therap. $\underline{9}$, 88-93.

Dixon, S.N. and Russel, K.L. (1986), Radioimmunoassay of the anabolic agent zeranol.IV. Zeranol concentrations in the tissues of sheep and cattle implanted with zeranol (Ralgro). J.Vet. Pharmacol. Therap. $\underline{9}$, 94-100.

Determination of zeranol in bile by HPLC/RIA. (1989). Central Veterinary Laboratory, Surrey, KT15 3NB.

Other references;
Bates, M.L., Warwick,M.J. and Shearer, G., (1985) Determination of synthetic growth promoters in bile. Food Add. Contaminants, $\underline{2}$, 37-46

Duchatel, J.P., (1985), Free and conjugated zeranol residues determined by radioimmunoassay in urine and plasma of calves treated with Forplix. ANN. rech. Vet. $\underline{16}$, 93-97

4.   DEFINITIONS.

Zeranol content is taken to mean the amount of zeranol in the substance in question, regardless of the chemical form, determined according to the described method and expressed as µg zeranol per kg or litre of test sample.

5.   PRINCIPLE

The methods comprises 6/7 stages;-

- Homogenisation of tissue samples in buffer or diluting biological fluid in buffer
- Hydrolysis of conjugates in buffer/homogenate with enzyme
- Extraction of zeranol with organic solvents
- Purification on Sep-Pak 18 minicolumn (optional)
- Purification of zeranol by HPLC
- End point determination with RIA
- The amount of zeranol is calculated by interpolation from a standard curve and taking into account the recovery of zeranol, especially from tissue samples.

6.   REAGENTS FOR EXTRACTION OF TISSUES

N.B.:   The reagents for which examples of their source are quoted are known to be satisfactory, nevertheless reagents from other sources may be equally suitable.

6.1.   FOR ALL TISSUES
6.1.1.   Acetone
6.1.2.   Dry ice
6.1.3.   Diethyl-ether (peroxide free and very high purity) Methyl tert-butyl ether can be substituted for diethyl ether.
6.1.4.   Double distilled water

6.2.   REAGENTS SPECIFIC FOR LIVER, KIDNEY, BILE AND URINE.
6.2.1.   Phosphate buffer pH 7.0 (as 6.5.4.).
6.2.2.   B-glucuronidase (e.g. Sigma G-0876) diluted with ten volumes double distilled water. This enzyme works at pH 7.
6.2.3.1. Quality control urine or bile from cattle treated with zeranol.
6.2.3.2. Quality control urine or bile from cattle not treated with zeranol.

6.3.   REAGENTS SPECIFIC FOR MUSCLE AND FAECES
6.3.1.   Chloroform
6.3.2.   1*M* sodium hydroxide
6.3.3.   90% acetic acid
6.3.4.   Methanol 3.4.1. Methanol:water 60:40 (v/v)
6.3.4.2   Methanol:water 30:70 (v/v)
6.3.5.   Quality control faeces from untreated cattle

6.4.   REAGENTS SPECIFIC FOR MUSCLE, LIVER, KIDNEY AND FAT.
6.4.1.   Tritiated zeranol recovery solution prepared from stock solution (6.5.6.1.) by evaporation and redissolving in buffer (6.5.4.) to 1000 cpm/0.1 mL, prepared immediately before use.
6.4.2.   Quality Controls
6.4.2.1   Quality control 1. Muscle, liver, kidney and fat from cattle not

treated with zeranol.
Quality control 2. Muscle, liver , kidney and fat from cattle
treated with zeranol.

6.5.   REAGENTS FOR RIA PROCEDURE.
6.5.1.   Zeranol standard solutions in methanol (6.3.4.) stored at +4°C.

Number   1   2   3   4   5   6   7   8   9   10   11   12
pg/0.1mL 0   25   50   75   100   150   200   300   400 600   800 1000

6.5.2.   Scintillation solution suitable for mixing with 1.5 mL aqueous
          solution. e.g. 4.5 g 2,5,diphenyl oxazone (PPO) (e.g.
          Hopkin/Williams scintillation grade). 500 mL triton X-114 (e.g.
          Koch Light Scintillation grade). 1.5 litres toluene (6.5.9.).
6.5.3.   Charcoal suspension - 5 g charcoal (e.g. Sigma Norit-A). 0.5 g
          dextran (e.g. Pharmacia T70). Made up in 1 litre double
          distilled water.
6.5.4.   Phosphate-gelatin buffer - 4.68 g sodium dihydrogen
          orthophosphate anhyd. (e.g. Analar BDH). 8.66 g disodium
          hydrogen orthophosphate anhyd. (e.g. Analar BDH). 9.0 g sodium
          chloride (e.g. Analar BDH). 0.1 g thiomersal (e.g. BDH) or 1.0 g
          sodium azide. 1.0 g gelatin (e.g. BDH). Made up to 1 litre (pH
          7.0) with double dist. water, stored at +4°C
6.5.5.   Pure zeranol for making standard solutions.
6.5.6.   Tritiated zeranol stored at -20°C. from which stock solutions
          (6.5.6.1.) are prepared. e.g. 3H-Zeranol from Amersham
          International (custom synthesis).
6.5.6.1   Dilute solutions (6.5.6) with methanol to yield stock solution of
          3H-zeranol with approximate activity of 1 uCi/mL methanol. Store
          at -20°C.
6.5.6.2   Tritiated zeranol assay solution, prepared from stock solution
          6.5.6.1. by evaporation and redissolving in buffer (6.5.4.) to
          give approximately 10,000 cpm/0.1 mL. Prepared on day of use.
6.5.6.3   The non-specific binding (NSB) of the 3H-zeranol must be
          determined and if it exceeds 10% of the total count (T) of
          3H-zeranol should be repurified or replaced.
6.5.7.   Antiserum against zeranol stored at -20°C. (see section 13)
6.5.7.1   Prepare solution of antibody in buffer (6.5.4.). It will be
          necessary to follow the instructions pertaining to the individual
          antibody preparations.   The concentration of antibody in buffer
          should be 7x greater than the concentration needed in the final
          RIA incubation mixture (see 9.5.2.1.- 9.5.2.3.).
6.5.8   Siliconising fluid (e.g. Serva 35130).
6.5.9   Toluene.

7.   EQUIPMENT.
7.1.   Liquid scintillation Counter, with automatic sample changer.
7.2.   Homogeniser (Silverson type).
7.3.   Cold storage space.
7.3.1.   Cold room/refrigerator space.
7.3.2.   Deep freeze -20°C.
7.4.   Fume cupboards.
7.5.   Centrifuges.
7.5.1.   Refrigerated centrifuge with large capacity for small tubes.
7.5.2.   Bench centrifuge.
7.6.   Heating units.
7.6.1.   37°C water bath/incubator.

7.6.2.   40/45°C water bath.
7.6.3.   110°C oven.
7.7.   Glassware.
7.7.1.   Glass tubes 75 mm x 16 mm.
7.7.2.   Glass conical centrifuge tubes.
7.7.3.   Glass universal bottles, approx 25 mL with plastic screw tops.
7.7.4.   Glass tubes 7.7.1. were siliconised by rinsing with siliconising
          fluid and baking for 1 hour at 100°C.
7.8.   Scintillation vials.
7.9.   Vortex mixer.
7.10.   Pipettes and dispensers.
7.10.1.   Semi-automatic pipettes with disposable tips.
7.10.2.   Pasteur pipettes.
7.10.3.   Tilt measures (10 mL and 5 mL for diethyl ether).
7.10.4.   Dispenser for scintillator.
7.11.   Apparatus suitable for evaporation of solvents. e.g.
          Compressed nitrogen supply and evaporation manifold.
7.11.1.   Facilities for evaporating at temperatures not exceeding 50°C.
7.12.   Magnetic stirrer.
7.13.   Measuring cylinder, 25 mL.
7.14.   HPLC apparatus. Reference to a company and/or product is for
          purposes of information and identification only. Equivalent
          types or products also may be suitable.
7.14.1.   Injector (Reodyne, model 7125) equipped with a 0.25 mL sample
          loop.
7.14.2.   HPLC-pump (Waters Ass., model 510 or LKB, model 2150). 7.14.3.
          UV-detector, variable or fixed wave-length at 254 or 240 nm
          (Waters Ass., model 440)
7.14.4.   Fraction collector (LKB, model Redirac), see note 2. 7.14.5.
          HPLC-column (150mm x 4.6mm I.D.) with Valco fittings (Chrompack)
          packed with Hypersil ODS, 5 μm or a column (100mm x 4.6mm) packed
          with CP microsphere C18, 3 μm (Chrompack). 7.14.6.
          Recorder-printer.

8.   SAMPLES AND SAMPLING PROCEDURE.

N.B. Attention is drawn to section 6.3.1 and ISO document 78/2-1982 and
the following notes derived from Annex II of 2052/VI/84-EN.

8.1. Nature of the Sample; Samples shall be such as to enable the
detection of residues in meat as defined in Directive 64/433/EEC. Failing
this biological fluids or faeces may constitute the samples for the
detection of residues.

8.2. Size of Sample; The size of the sample must be large enough to allow
the reference method to be carried out and to allow repeat analysis where
required.

In this method for zeranol the sizes shall not be less than

    20 g muscle, liver, kidney or fat; 10 g faeces; 20 mL blood
      5 mL urine; 1 mL bile

8.3. The samples must be taken and packed in such a way as to allow proper
identification in the laboratory.

8.4. The method of packing, preservation and transport must maintain the integrity of the sample and not prejudice the result of the examination.

Samples for the analysis of zeranol must be stored and transported at temperatures below -18°C.

9.0.   PROCEDURE

9.1.   EXTRACTION PROCEDURE
[Note; For all samples recovery of zeranol is measured by addition of tritiated zeranol before the extraction procedure and determining the recovery of tritiated zeranol in an aliquot of extract before the RIA stage.]

9.1.1. URINE AND BILE
The method measures the total concentration of zeranol. The conjugated form of the zeranol in the samples is hydrolysed to the free form and the total residue of zeranol is extracted into ether. The extract can be further purified by HPLC step before proceeding to the RIA step.

9.1.2.   Into universal bottles (7.7.3.) place 2.0 mL double distilled water (6.1.4.) and 0.1 mL tritiated recovery solution (6.4.1.)
9.1.2.1   Add 0.1 mL recovery solution (6.4.1.) to 2 scintillation vials (7.8.).
9.1.3.   Into universal bottles from 9.1.2. add 0.05 mL bile or urine (if the concentration of zeranol is extremely high a smaller aliquot of bile or urine may be used). All samples are assayed in duplicate.
9.1.4.   Into 2 other universal bottles from 9.1.2. add 0.05 mL quality control urine or bile (6.2.3.1. or 6.2.3.2.).
9.1.5.   Two universal bottles from 9.1.2. are used as solvent blanks.
9.1.6.   Add to universals 9.1.3.-9.1.5. 100 µL enzyme (6.2.2.) and incubate for 2 h at 37°C.
9.1.7   Allow to cool and add 5 mL diethyl-ether (6.1.3.), vortex mix for 15 seconds.
9.1.8.   Freeze samples in dry ice/acetone bath (6.1.1., 6.1.2.) and decant ether phase into glass tubes.
9.1.9.   Evaporate to dryness.(7.11.1).
9.1.10.   HPLC step.
9.1.10.1 Dissolve the dry residue in 0.25 mL methanol/water (30:70 v/v)
9.1.10.2 Apply the redissolved extract (9.1.10.1) to the HPLC-system.
9.1.10.3 Operate the HPLC-system isocratically using methanol/water (60:40 v/v) as mobile phase with a flow of 1-2 mL per min.
9.1.10.4 Collect one fraction of 5 min around the retention time of zeranol as determined for standards of zeranol and related compounds shortly before the run with the extract (9.1.10.1). Separation of zeranol from related compounds should be complete.

Notes on HPLC.   1. For tissue extracts an additional Sep-Pak C18 clean-up is recommended prior to HPLC purification to save the HPLC column. 2. Fraction collector can be operated manually or by an electric pulse from the injection to the fraction collector.

9.1.10.5 Evaporate the solvent from the single fraction.
9.1.11. Add 1.0 mL buffer (6.5.4.) and vortex mixed.
9.1.12. Proceed as 9.3.17 - 9.3.21.

9.2.   FAECES
The principal of the method is to extract free zeranol from faeces using
ether. The ether extract is further purified by   solvent/solvent
partition systems before RIA.

9.2.1.   Into universal bottles (7.7.3.) are weighed 1 g faeces in
          duplicate.
9.2.2.   Into 2 universal bottles are weighed 1 g of quality control
          faeces (6.3.5.).
9.2.3.   Into 2 universal bottles and universal bottles 9.2.1. and 9.2.2.
          are added 5 mL water.
9.2.4.   Add 0.1 mL zeranol recovery solution (4.1.) to universals
          9.2.1.,9.2.2.,9.2.3. and vortex mix for 15 seconds. 9.2.4.1. Add
          0.1 mL of zeranol recovery solution to 2 scintillation vials
          (7.8.).
9.2.5.   Add 10 mL diethyl-ether, vortex mix for 15 seconds, centrifuge at
          2000-3000 rpm for 10 minutes.
9.2.6.   Freeze the universal bottles in dry ice/acetone (6.1.1., 6.1.2.)
          and decant the ether phase into glass conical centrifuge tubes
          (7.7.2.).
9.2.7.   Thaw the aqueous phase and repeat procedures 9.2.5. and 9.2.6.
9.2.8.   Evaporate the combined ether phases to dryness.(7.11.1).
9.2.9.   Dissolve the residue in 1 mL chloroform (6.3.1.).
9.2.10.   Extract zeranol from the chloroform using 1 x 3 mL (1M) sodium
          hydroxide (6.3.2.). Vortex mix for 15 seconds and centrifuge at
          1000g for 10 minutes. Pipette the upper sodium hydroxide phase
          into universal bottles (7.7.3.).
9.2.11   Repeat 9.2.10.
9.2.12.   The combined alkaline extracts are acidified with 0.6 mL of 90%
          acetic acid (6.3.3).
9.2.13.   Extract zeranol from the aqueous phase with 1 x 10 mL
          diethyl-ether separate the ether phase by freezing in dry
          ice/acetone (9.2.6). Each step was facilitated by vortex mixing
          and gentle centrifugation prior to freezing if required.
9.2.14.   Evaporate the combined ether extracts to dryness.
9.2.15.   HPLC step (see 9.1.10. to 9.1.10.5.)
9.2.16.   Dissolve the residue in 1 mL MeOH (6.3.4.).
9.2.16.1 Transfer 0.2 mL to a scintillation vial (7.8.) and proceed
          9.3.16. - 9.3.18. to measure recovery.
9.2.17.   Prepare aliquots of 1/50 to 1/10 sample for RIA as in 9.2.16.1.
9.2.17.1 Transfer 0.1 mL MeOH extract (9.2.15.) to siliconised glass tubes
          (7.7.4.) and evaporate to dryness under nitrogen. Add 0.5 mL
          buffer (6.5.4.) for RIA stage (9.5.1.to 9.5.10.)

9.3.   MUSCLE, LIVER, KIDNEY.
The method is based on further purification by ether extraction of muscle
followed by solvent/solvent partition and HPLC. Liver and kidney require an
additional hydrolysis step prior to the extraction.

9.3.1.   1 g tissue is cut into small pieces and weighed in universal
          bottles (7.7.3.).
9.3.2.   Add 2 mL water and homogenise (7.2).
9.3.3.   Repeat 9.3.1.-9.3.4. using quality control tissue (6.4.2.1-2).
9.3.4.   Add 2 mL water to two universal bottles which serve as solvent
          blanks.
9.3.5.   Add 0.1 mL radiolabelled zeranol recovery solution (6.4.1.) to
          universals 9.3.2., 9.3.3., and into 2 scintillation vials (7.8.)

and homogenise the contents of the universals.
9.3.6.   For liver and kidney add 0.1 mL of enzyme (6.2.2.) to each universal and incubate for 2 hours at 37°C.
9.3.7.   Add 10 mL diethyl ether, vortex mix for 30 seconds, centrifuge at 2000-3000 rpm at 18°C.
9.3.7.1   Freeze the universal bottles in dry ice/acetone (6.1.1., 6.1.2.) and decant the ether phase to glass conical centrifuge tubes (7.7.2.).
9.3.8.   Thaw the aqueous phase and add 5 mL diethyl ether to aqueous phase and repeat extraction as in 9.3.7.
9.3.9.   Pool ether extracts and evaporate to dryness (7.11.1).
9.3.10.   Dissolve residue in 1 mL chloroform (6.3.1.).
9.3.11.   Extract zeranol with 1 x 3 mL of 1M sodium hydroxide (6.3.2.) (30 seconds vortex mixing and centrifugation, 1000g for 10 min at 18°C).
9.3.12.   The sodium hydroxide extract is pipetted into a universal bottle (7.7.2.) containing 90% acetic acid (250 µL) (6.3.3.).
9.3.13.   Extract zeranol with 5 mL diethyl-ether (vortex mix and gentle centrifugation). Freeze the universals in dry ice/acetone and decant the ether phase into glass conical centrifuge tubes (7.7.2.).
9.3.14.   Evaporate to dryness (7.11.1).
9.3.15.   HPLC step.(9.1.10. to 9.1.10.5.).
9.3.16.   Add 1 mL gelatin-phosphate buffer (6.5.4.) and vortex mix for 30 seconds.
9.3.17.   Transfer 0.25 mL of 9.3.16. into scintillation vial (7.8.).
9.3.18.   Add 10 mL scintillation fluid to 9.3.17 and 2 scintillation vials containing recovery solution (see 9.3.5., 9.2.4.1. and 9.1.2.1.).
9.3.19.   Add 10 mL scintillator to 2 scintillation vials (7.8) containing 0.2 mL gelatin-phosphate buffer (6.5.4.). This is for the background count.
9.3.20.   Count vials 9.3.18. and 9.3.19. for 20 minutes on B-counter (7.1.)
9.3.21.   Transfer 0.5 mL of 9.3.16 into siliconised tube (7.7.4.) for RIA step (see 9.5.1. to 9.5.10.).

9.4.   FAT
9.4.1.   1 g fat is cut into small pieces and weighed into universal bottles (7.7.3).
9.4.2.   Add 2 mL double distilled water (6.1.4)
9.4.3.   Repeat 9.4.1 and 9.4.2 using quality control fat (6.4.2.1-2)
9.4.4.   Add 0.1 mL radiolabelled recovery solution (6.4.1) to universals 9.4.2, 9.4.3.
9.4.5.   Add to all universals (9.4.2, 9.4.3) 10 mL of diethyl ether and vortex for 1 minute.
9.4.6.   Centrifuge all universals at 1000g for 10 minutes and separate the two phases by freezing at -20°C in a deep freeze (7.3.2).
9.4.7.   Decant the ether phase into glass tubes (7.7.2).
9.4.8.   Add 5 mL diethyl ether to all universals and repeat the extraction (9.4.5, 9.4.6).
9.4.9.   Pool ether extracts and evaporate to dryness (7.11.1). 9.4.10. Dissolve residue in 2 mL chloroform (6.3.1).
9.4.11.   Proceed as from 9.3.10.

9.5.   RADIOIMMUNOASSAY PROCEDURE.
The method chosen for separation of antibody-bound and free ligand uses charcoal. The RIA procedure is the same for all extracts obtained from bile, urine, faeces, muscle, liver, kidney or fat.

Cy 1.6/7

9.5.1.   Into 4 siliconised tubes (7.7.4.) pipette 0.1 mL methanol (zero
          standard tubes). Into siliconised tubes (7.7.4.) pipette in
          duplicate 0.1 mL of zeranol standard solutions (6.5.1.) to give
          range 0-1000 pg per tube. Evaporate methanol to dryness
          e.g.under nitrogen (7.11.1.).
9.5.2.1   Add 0.5 mL gelatin-phosphate buffer (6.5.4.).
9.5.2.2   Add to 9.5.2.1. and to test samples (see 9.1.11, 9.2.16.
          9.2.16.2.,9.3.20.) 0.1 mL tritiated zeranol solution (6.5.6.2.).
9.5.2.3   Add 0.1 mL antibody (6.5.7.1.) to all tubes except 2 of the zero
          standard tubes to which is added 0.1 mL buffer (6.5.4.) (NSB
          tubes).
9.5.3.   Vortex mix for a few seconds. Incubate overnight at 41°C.
9.5.4.   Add 0.5 mL charcoal suspension (6.5.3) at 4°C.
9.5.5.   Shake all tubes gently by hand for 1 minute and stand at 4°C for
          10 minutes.
9.5.6.   Centrifuge at 2000-3000 rpm at 4°C for 10 minutes. 9.5.7.
          Decant supernatant into scintillation vial (7.8.), at 4°C.
9.5.8.   Add 10 mL scintillator (6.5.2.) to all vials including 2 vials
          containing 0.1 mL tritiated zeranol solution (6.5.6.2.) and 0.1
          mL gelatin-phosphate buffer (6.5.4.).
9.5.9.   Stand vials in dark for at least 20 minutes before counting.
9.5.10.   Place samples in liquid scintillation counter (7.1) and count
          (preset time or counts) e.g. 10000 counts or 4 minutes.

10.   CALCULATION OF RESULTS.

10.1.   METHOD OF CALCULATION.
Prepare calibration curve by plotting cpm 3H-zeranol bound (cpm bound to
antibody for vials containing standards 0-1000 pg (see 6.5.1) against pg
standard.

[Note.: Two corrections are needed, one for the radioactivity carried into
the RIA from the recovery solution and another for the recovery of
zeranol.]

10.2.   Correction equation for cpm

$$\text{corrected cpm} = \frac{\text{cpm bound} \times \text{cpm 3H-zeranol (T)}}{\text{cpm 3H-zeranol (T)} + N(\text{cpm recovery} - \text{cpm Bg})}$$

$$N = \frac{\text{Volume of sample to RIA}}{\text{Volume of sample to recovery determination}}$$

cpm bound = cpm bound for test sample
cpm 3H-zeranol (T) = cpm for 0.1 mL 3H-Zeranol solution (6.5.6.2) used in
RIA incubations (see 9.5.10).
cpm recovery = cpm for 0.25 mL extract of test sample (9.3.17).
cpm Bg is cpm for background (see 9.3.19).

10.3.   Read off calibration curve pg zeranol against corrected cpm for
          test samples and solvent blanks.

10.4.   Calculation for concentration of zeranol in sample

Cy 1.6/8

pg zeranol in sample i.e. 1 g muscle, 50 μL bile and 50 μL urine.

$$pg = \frac{(\text{curve pg} - \text{blank pg})(\text{recovery stnd.} - \text{cpm Bg})}{N(\text{cpm recovery} - \text{cpm Bg})}$$

curve pg = pg obtained in step 10.3.
blank pg = pg for solvent blanks obtained in step 10.3.
recovery standard = cpm for 0.1 mL 3H-zeranol recovery solution (6.4.1.).

cpm recovery = cpm for volume of extract of test sample used for recovery estimation (9.2.16.1., 9.3.17)
cpm Bg = cpm for background (9.3.19).

10.5.   Alternative calculations.

B = cpm bound to antibody - cpm for NSB (NSB tubes 9.5.2.3.).
Bo = cpm bound to antibody in zero standard tubes - cpm for NSB. Bo should be between 40-60% of total cpm (cpm 3H-zeranol(T)) (see 10.2.).

10.5.1. Prepare calibration curve by plotting B/Bo against pg standard.

10.5.1.1 If a microcomputer programme is possible then a best line plot of log pg standard against Ln Z/(1-Z) where

Z = B/Bo (LOGIT plot) can be used to interpolate results.

10.5.2. Calculate B/Bo for test sample and for the solvent blank using corrected cpm - NSB (see 10.2.) and estimate pg zeranol from calibration curve.
10.5.3. Proceed as 10.4.
10.5.4. The original counting data should be included with the final results.

10.6.   PRECISION. To take into account the Criteria document (89/610 EEC) and will explain how the precision of the method is determined using the standards available.

11.   SPECIAL CASES

This method is an alternative method to spectroscopic methods. However it is strongly emphasised that the spectroscopic methods (e.g. GC-MS) are preferred (see EEC 93/256 1.2.3.1 {section 5}).

12.   NOTES ON PROCEDURE
In order to have even greater certainty when positives are found it is recommended to repeat the HPLC separation using an alternative column with different properties (e.g. different polarity).

11.   SPECIAL CASES. e.g. if a particular species presents unique problems.

12.   NOTES ON PROCEDURE.

13.   QUALITY CONTROL. STANDARDS, REFERENCE MATERIALS AND ANTIBODIES.
A description of the source and quality of the key reagents and standards.

13.1   ANTIBODIES. Follow the instructions relating to the storage and
dilution of the antibody as recommended by the supplier.

13.2.   Source of antibodies.
Commercial suppliers;-

Laboratoire d'Hormonologie, C.E.R, Rue de Carmel 1, B-5406, Marloie,
Belgium

Genego, Via Ressel S Andrea zona ind., 34170, Gorizia, Italy

14.   TEST REPORT.   To give the indications necessary for the
identification of the sample, the reference to the method employed, the
results and the form in which these are expressed, any particular points
observed in the course of the test and any operations not specified in the
method or regarded as optional which might affect the results.

15.   LIST OF ABBREVIATIONS

A list of the most important abbreviations is given in Annex I section 12
and also in section 5 (criteria).   NSB is non-specific binding.

16.   FLOW DIAGRAM.

    Tissue ---→ add buffer and recovery standard   ---→ Homogenise
                                                             |
                                                             |
                                                             |
    Fluid (urine, bile, plasma, serum) |
        | |
        | |
        ↓   ↓
    add buffer and recovery standard ------------→ Hydrolyse
                                                        |
                                                        |
                                                        |
                                                        ↓
       Calculate ←------ RIA ←------ HPLC ←------ organic solvent
         results   extraction

Cy 1.7. STILBENES - METHOD FOR THE MEASUREMENT OF RESIDUES OF DIETHYLSTILBOESTROL, HEXOESTROL AND DIENOESTROL IN ANIMALS AND ANIMAL TISSUES ON THE BASIS OF HPLC/RIA.

WARNING AND SAFETY PRECAUTIONS.

1.   INTRODUCTION.

Throughout the EEC the use of stilbenes is prohibited in food producing animals. Also the MRL for residues of stilbenes in animal products imported into or produced within the Community is zero.

2.   SCOPE AND FIELD OF APPLICATION

This method of analysis describes the determination of the total content of diethylstilboestrol (DES), hexoestrol (HEX) or dienoestrol (DEN) in foodstuffs and samples of animal origin. The method can be used for meat and fish and also for biological material such as animal organs, biological fluids and faeces. The detection limit, defined as three times the standard deviation of the blank determination, is 0.1-1 µg/kg or litre of sample for the stilbene.

3.   REFERENCES.

ISO Standard 78/2-1982 Layout for standards - Part 2: Standard for Chemical Analysis

EEC Interim Report of Scientific Veterinary Committee, Working Group on Reference Methods for Residues. Draft reference method for the measurement of stilbenes in animals and animal tissues 2526/VI/84-EN File 6.21 II-4

Bates, M.L., Warwick, M.J. and Shearer, G. (1985), Determination of synthetic growth promoters in bile. Food Additives & Contaminants. 2, 37-46

Gaspar, P. and Maghuin-Rogister, G., (1985), Rapid extraction and purification of diethylstilboestrol in bovine urine hydrolysates using reversed phase C 18 columns before determination by radioimmunoassay. J. Chromat. 328, 413-416

Harwood, D.J., Heitzman, R.J. and Jouquey, A., (1980), A radioimmunoassay method for the measurement of residues of the anabolic agent hexoestrol in tissues of cattle and sheep. J.Vet. Pharmacol. & Therapeutics, 3, 245-254

Heitzman, R.J. and Harwood, D.J. (1983), Radioimmunoassay of hexoestrol residues in faeces, tissues and body fluids of bulls and steers. Vet. Rec. 112, 120-123

Jansen, E.H.J.M., (1985), A highly specific detection method for diethylstilboestrol in bovine urine by radioimmunoassay following high performance liquid chromatography. Food Additives & Contaminants. 2, 271-281

Richou-Bac, L., (1977), Recherche et dosage par radioimmunologie d'estradiol-17α, d'estrone et de DES sur les jeunes bovines traites uax anabolisants. Bull Acad. Vet. de France. 50, 359-363

Vogt, von K., (1985), Vereinfachte Absicherung des radioimmunologischen Nachweises von Diethylstilbestrol in Fleischhaltigen Konserven und tierischen Ausscheidungen. Arch. fur Lebensm.hygiene. _36_, 1-24

4.   DEFINITIONS.

DES, HEX or DEN content is taken to mean the amount of DES, HEX or DEN in the substance in question, regardless of the chemical form, determined according to the described method and expressed as µg DES, HEX or DEN per kg or litre of test sample.

5.   PRINCIPLE

The method comprises 6 stages;-

-        Homogenisation of tissue samples in buffer or diluting biological fluid in buffer
-        Hydrolysis of conjugates in buffer/homogenate with enzyme
-        Extraction of DES, HEX or DEN with organic solvents
-        Purification of DES, HEX or DEN by HPLC
-        End point determination with RIA
-        The amount of DES, HEX or DEN is calculated by interpolation from a standard curve and taking into account the recovery of DES, HEX or DEN, especially from tissue samples.

6.   REAGENTS FOR EXTRACTION OF TISSUES.

Note: The reagents for which examples of their source are quoted are known to be satisfactory, nevertheless reagents from other sources may be equally suitable.

6.1.   FOR ALL TISSUES

6.1.1.   Acetone
6.1.2.   Dry ice
6.1.3.   Diethyl-ether (peroxide free and very high purity)

6.2.   Reagents specific for bile and urine
6.2.1.   Phosphate buffer pH 7.0 (as 6.5.4. but omit gelatin).
6.2.2.   B-glucuronidase (e.g. Sigma G-0876) diluted with two volumes double distilled water. This enzyme works at pH 7. If an Arylsulphatase - glucuronidase preparation from Helix Pomatia is used then the hydrolysis stage (9.1.6.) is performed in buffer adjusted to pH 4.7.
6.2.3.1   Quality control urines or biles from cattle treated with stilbenes.
6.3.   Reagents specific for muscle and faeces
6.3.1.   Chloroform
6.3.2.   1_M_ sodium hydroxide
6.3.3.   6_M_ hydrochloric acid
6.3.4.   Methanol
6.3.4.1   Methanol:water 75:25 (v/v)
6.3.5.1   Quality control faeces from untreated calf
6.3.5.2   Quality control faeces from untreated steer

6.4.   Reagents specific for muscle
6.4.1.   Tritiated stilbene recovery solution prepared from stock solution

6.4.1. (6.5.6.1.) by evaporation and redissolving in buffer (5.4.) to 1000 cpm/0.1 mL stored at 4°C.
6.4.2. Petroleum ether bp 40°-60°C (or 50-70°C) for method 1.
6.4.3. Diethyl-ether:n-butanol 9:1 (v/v) method 2.
6.4.4. 1M hydrochloric acid for method 2.
6.4.5. Quality control muscle tissue.
6.4.5.1 Quality control 1. Muscle from untreated cattle.
6.4.5.2 Quality control 2. Muscle from cattle treated with stilbene.
6.5. Reagents for RIA procedure
6.5.1. Stilbene standard solutions in methanol (6.3.4.) stored at +4°C.

Number	1	2	3	4	5	6	7	8	9
pg/0.1 mL	0	20	50	100	200	400	600	800	1000

6.5.2. Scintillation solution suitable for mixing with 1.5 mL aqueous solution. e.g. 4.5 g 2,5,diphenyl oxazone (PPO) (e.g. Hopkin/Williams scintillation grade). 500 mL triton X-114 (e.g. Koch Light Scintillation grade). 1.5 litres toluene (6.5.9.).
6.5.3. Charcoal suspension - 5 g charcoal (e.g. Sigma Norit-A). 0.5 g dextran (e.g. Pharmacia T70). Made up in 1 litre double distilled water.
6.5.4. Phosphate-gelatin buffer - 4.68 g sodium dihydrogen phosphate anhyd. (e.g. Analar BDH). 8.66 g disodium hydrogen phosphate anhyd. (e.g. Analar BDH). 9.0 g sodium chloride (e.g. Analar BDH). 0.1 g thiomersal (e.g. BDH) or 1.0 sodium azide. 1.0 g gelatin (e.g. BDH). Made up to 1 litre (pH 7.0) with double distilled water, stored at +4°C.
6.5.5. Pure DES, HEX and DEN (e.g. Sigma) for making standard solutions.
6.5.6. Tritiated stilbenes stored at -20°C from which stock solutions (6.5.6.1.) are prepared. e.g. 3H-DES from Amersham International.
6.5.6.1 Dilute solutions (6.5.6) with methanol to yield stock solution of 3H-stilbene with approximate activity of 1 uCi/mL methanol. Store at +4°C.
6.5.6.2 Tritiated stilbene assay solution, prepared from stock solution 6.5.6.1. by evaporation and redissolving in buffer (6.5.4.) to give 10,000 cpm/0.1 mL. Prepared on day of use.
6.5.6.3 The non-specific binding (NSB) of the 3H-stilbene must be determined and if it exceeds 10% of the total count (SA) of 3H-stilbene should be repurified or replaced.
6.5.7. Antiserum against stilbenes stored at -20°C.
6.5.7.1 Prepare solution of antibody in buffer (6.5.4.). It will be necessary to follow the instructions pertaining to the individual antibody preparations. The concentration of antibody in buffer should be 8x greater than the concentration needed in the final RIA incubation mixture (see 9.5.2.1.-9.5.2.3.)
6.5.8. Siliconising fluid (e.g. Serva 35130).

7. EQUIPMENT.

7.1. Liquid scintillation Counter, with automatic sample changer.
7.2. Homogeniser (Silverson type).
7.3. Cold storage space.
7.3.1. Cold room/refrigerator space.
7.3.2. Deep freeze -20°C.
7.4. Fume cupboards.
7.5. Centrifuges.
7.5.1. Refrigerated centrifuge with large capacity for small tubes.

7.5.2.   Bench centrifuge.
7.6.   Heating units.
7.6.1.   37°C water bath/incubator.
7.6.2.   40/45°C water bath.
7.6.3.   110°C oven.
7.7.   Glassware.
7.7.1.   Glass tubes 75 mm x 12.5 mm.
7.7.2.   Glass stoppered tubes 100 mm x 16 mm.
7.7.3.   Glass universal bottles, approx 25 mL with plastic screw tops.
7.7.4.   Glass tubes 7.7.1. were siliconised by rinsing with siliconising
          fluid and baking for 1 hour at 105°C.
7.8.   Scintillation vials.
7.9.   Vortex mixer.
7.10.   Pipettes and dispensers.
7.10.1.   Semi-automatic pipettes with disposable tips.
7.10.2.   Pasteur pipettes.
7.10.3.   Tilt measures (10 mL for diethyl ether).
7.10.4.   Dispenser for scintillator.
7.11.   Apparatus suitable for evaporation of solvents. e.g. Compressed
          nitrogen supply and evaporation manifold or rotary film
          evaporator.
7.11.1.   Solvent should be evaporated at temperatures not exceeding 50°C
          using e.g. either a stream of nitrogen or a rotary film
          evaporator.
7.12.   Magnetic stirrer.
7.13.   Measuring cylinder, 25 mL.
7.14.   HPLC apparatus.

Reference to a company and/or product is for purposes of information and
identification only. Equivalent types or products also may be suitable.

7.14.1.   Injector (Reodyne, model 7125) equipped with a 0.25 mL sample
          loop.
7.14.2.   HPLC-pump (Waters Ass., model 510 or LKB, model 2150).
7.14.3.   UV-detector, variable or fixed wave-length at 254 or 240 nm
          (Waters Ass., model 440)
7.14.4.   Fraction collector (LKB, model Redirac), see note 2.
7.14.5.   HPLC-column (150mm x 4.6mm I.D.) with Valco fittings (Chrompack)
          packed with Hypersil ODS, 5um or a column (100mm x 4.6mm) packed
          with CP microsphere C18, 3um (Chrompack).
7.14.6.   Recorder-printer.

8.   SAMPLES AND SAMPLING PROCEDURE.

N.B. Attention is drawn to section 6.3.1 and ISO document 78/2-1982 and
the following notes derived from Annex II of 2052/VI/84-EN.

8.1. Nature of the Sample; Samples shall be such as to enable the
detection of residues in meat as defined in Directive 64/433/EEC. Failing
this biological fluids or faeces may constitute the samples for the
detection of residues.

8.2. Size of Sample; The size of the sample must be large enough to allow
the reference method to be carried out and to allow repeat analysis where
required.

In this method for stilbenes the sizes shall not be less than

        20 g muscle, liver, kidney or fat
        10 g faeces
        20 mL blood
         5 mL urine
         1 mL bile

8.3. The samples must be taken and packed in such a way as to allow proper
identification in the laboratory.

8.4. The method of packing, preservation and transport must maintain the
integrity of the sample and not prejudice the result of the examination.

Samples for the analysis of stilbenes must be stored and transported at
temperatures below -18°C.

9.   PROCEDURE.

9.1.- 9.4. EXTRACTION PROCEDURE.
Note: For all samples recovery of stilbene is measured by addition of
tritiated stilbene before the extraction procedure and determining the
recovery of tritiated stilbene in an aliquot of extract before the RIA
stage.
9.1.   URINE AND BILE.
9.1.1.   The method measures the total concentration of stilbenes. The
           conjugated form of the stilbenes in the samples is hydrolysed to
           the free form and the total residue of stilbene is extracted into
           ether. The extract is further purified by a chromatography step
           before proceeding to the RIA step.
9.1.2.   Into universal bottles (7.7.3.) place 1.0 mL buffer (6.5.4.) and
           0.1 mL tritiated recovery solution (6.4.1.).
9.1.2.1   Add 0.1 mL recovery solution (6.4.1.) to 2 scintillation vials
           (7.8.).
9.1.3.   Into universal bottles from 9.1.2. add 0.05 mL bile or urine (if
           the concentration of stilbene is extremely high a smaller aliquot
           of bile or urine may be used). All samples are assayed in
           duplicate.
9.1.4.   Into 2 other universal bottles from 9.1.2. add 0.05 mL quality
           control urine (6.2.3.1. or 6.2.3.2.).
9.1.5.   Two universal bottles from 9.1.2. are used as solvent blanks.
9.1.6.   Add to universals 9.1.3.- 9.1.5. 10 µL enzyme (2.2.) and incubate
           for 2 h at 37°C.
9.1.7.   Allow to cool and add 5 mL diethyl-ether (6.1.3.), vortex mix for
           15 seconds.
9.1.8.   Freeze samples in dry ice/acetone bath (6.1.1., 6.1.2.) and
           decant ether phase into glass tubes.
9.1.9.   Evaporate to dryness.(7.11.1).
9.1.10.   HPLC step.(see also 9.2.14; 9.3.21; 9.4.12)
9.1.10.1   Dissolve the dry residue in 0.25 mL methanol/water (60:40 v/v)
9.1.10.2   Apply the redissolved extract (9.1.10.1) to the HPLC-system
9.1.10.3   Operate the HPLC-system isocratically using methanol/water (60:40
           v/v) as mobile phase with a flow of 1-2 mL per min.
9.1.10.4   Collect three fractions of 1 min around the retention times as
           determined for standards of DES,DEN and HEX shortly before the
           run with the extract (9.1.10.1). Separation of DES, DEN and HEX
           should be complete (see note 3).
9.1.10.5   Evaporate the solvent of the three fractions under nitrogen.
9.1.10.6   For each fraction continue with 9.1.11.

Notes on HPLC.
1. For tissue extracts an additional LH-20 column clean-up is recommended prior to HPLC purification to save the HPLC column.
2. Fraction collector can be operated manually or by an electric pulse from the injection to the fraction collector.
3. For typical examples see: E.H.J.M.Jansen, R Both-Miedema, H. van Blitterswijk and R.W.Stephany; J Chromatography, 1984, _299_, 450-455

9.1.11.   1.0 mL buffer (6.5.4.) are added and vortex mixed.
9.1.12.   Proceed as 9.3.23 - 9.3.27.

9.2.   FAECES.

The principal of the method is to extract free stilbene from faeces using ether. The ether extract is further purified by solvent/solvent partition systems before RIA.

9.2.1.   Into universal bottles (7.7.3.) are weighed 1 g faeces in duplicate.
9.2.2.   Into 2 universal bottles are weighed 1 g of quality control faeces (6.3.5.1. or 6.3.5.2.).
9.2.3.   Into 2 universal bottles and universal bottles 9.2.1. and 9.3.2.2. are added 5 mL water.
9.2.4.   Add 0.1 mL stilbene recovery solution (6.4.1.) and vortex mix for 1 minute.
9.2.4.1   Add 0.1 mL recovery solution to 2 scintillation vials (7.8.).
9.2.5.   Add 10 mL diethyl-ether, vortex mix for 30 seconds, centrifuge at 2000-3000 rpm for 5 minutes.
9.2.6.   Separate ether phase into glass tubes (7.7.2.).
9.2.7.   Repeat procedures 9.2.5. and 9.2.6. using 5 mL diethyl-ether.
9.2.8.   Evaporate the combined ether phases to dryness (7.11.1).
9.2.9.   Dissolve the residue in 1 mL chloroform (6.3.1.).
9.2.10.   Extract stilbene from the chloroform using 1 x 2 mL M sodium hydroxide and 1 x 1 mL M sodium hydroxide. In each case the samples are vortex mixed and then separated by gentle centrifugation.
9.2.11.   Adjust pH of the combined alkaline extracts to about pH 8 with 6M HCl and to pH 7-8 with 1M HCl.
9.2.12.   Extract stilbene from the aqueous phase with 3 x 2 mL diethyl-ether. Each step was facilitated by vortex mixing and gentle centrifugation.
9.2.13.   Evaporate the combined ether extracts to dryness.
9.2.14.   HPLC step (see 9.1.10.)
9.2.15.   Dissolve the residue in 1 mL MeOH (6.3.4.).
9.2.15.1. Transfer 0.2 mL to a scintillation vial (7.8.) and proceed
9.3.23. - 9.3.26. to measure recovery.
9.2.16.   Prepare aliquots of 1/50 to 1/10 sample for RIA as in 9.2.16.1. or 9.2.16.2.
9.2.16.1   Method for veal calves: dissolve 0.1 mL MeOH extract (9.2.15.) in 6 mL buffer (6.5.4.) and transfer 0.6 mL to siliconised tubes (7.7.4.) for RIA stage.
9.2.16.2   Method for other farm animals: transfer 0.1 mL MeOH extract (9.2.15.) to siliconised glass tubes (7.7.4.) and evaporate to dryness under nitrogen (9.1.9.). Add 0.6 mL buffer (6.5.4.) for RIA stage.

9.3.   MUSCLE - method 1

Two methods are described and appear equally reliable. The method is based
on further purification by ether extraction of muscle followed by
solvent/solvent partition and HPLC.

9.3.1.   5 g muscle is cut into small pieces and weighed in universal
          bottles (7.7.3.).
9.3.2.   Add 15 mL water and homogenise.
9.3.3.   Transfer to measuring cylinder and adjust volume to 20 mL with
          water.
9.3.4.   Transfer in duplicate (or more if capacity allows) 4 mL of
          homogenate 9.3.3. to universal bottles (7.7.3.).
9.3.5.   Repeat 9.3.1.- 9.3.4. using quality control muscle (6.4.5.1, 2, 3
          or 4).
9.3.6.   Add 4 mL water to two universal bottles which serve as solvent
          blanks.
9.3.7.   Add 0.1 mL radiolabelled stilbene recovery solution (6.4.1.) to
          universals 9.3.4. to 9.3.6. and into 2 scintillation vials
          (7.8.).
9.3.8.   Add 10 mL diethyl ether, vortex mix for 30 seconds, centrifuge at
          2000-3000 rpm at 4°C and transfer ether phase to glass tube
          (7.7.2.).
9.3.9.   Add 5 mL diethyl ether to aqueous phase and repeat extraction as
          in 9.3.8.
9.3.10.   Pool ether extracts and evaporate to dryness (7.11.1).
9.3.11.   Dissolve residue in 1 mL chloroform (6.3.1.).
9.3.12.   Extract stilbene with 1 x 2 mL and 2 x 1 mL volumes of 1M sodium
          hydroxide (30 seconds vortex mixing and gentle centrifugation).
9.3.13.   Pool sodium hydroxide extracts and reduce pH to about pH 8 with
          6M hydrochloric acid and to pH 7-8 with 1M HCl.
9.3.14.   Extract stilbene with 3 x 2 mL diethyl-ether (vortex mix and
          gentle centrifugation).
9.3.15.   Pool ether extracts and evaporate to dryness (7.11.1).
9.3.16.   Add 1 mL methanol:water: 3:1 (v/v, 6.3.4.1.).
9.3.17.   Wash aqueous methanol with 2 x 2 mL petroleum ether
          (6.4.2.)(vortex mix and gentle centrifugation).
9.3.18.   Evaporate aqueous methanol phase to dryness.
9.3.19.   Add 1 mL water and extract stilbene with 3 x 2 mL diethyl-ether.
9.3.20.   Pool ether extracts and evaporate to dryness (7.11.1.).
9.3.21.   HPLC step.(see 9.1.10.).
9.3.22.   Add 1 mL gelatin-phosphate buffer (6.5.4.) and vortex mix for 30
          seconds.
9.3.23.   Transfer 0.2 mL of 9.3.22. into scintillation vial.
9.3.24.   Add 10 mL scintillation fluid to 9.3.23 and 2 scintillation vials
          containing recovery solution (see 9.3.7., 9.2.4.1. and 9.1.2.1.).
9.3.25.   Add 10 mL scintillator to 2 scintillation vials containing 0.2 mL
          gelatin-phosphate buffer (6.5.4.). This is for the background
          count.
9.3.26.   Count vials 9.24. and 9.25. for 20 minutes on B-counter (7.1.).
9.3.27.   Transfer 0.6 mL of 9.3.22 into siliconised tube (7.7.4.) for RIA
          step.

9.4.   MUSCLE - method 2

9.4.1.   Proceed as from 9.3.1. to 9.3.10.
9.4.2.   Add 1 mL 1M NaOH and dissolve residue by vortex mixing. 9.4.3.

Add to all tubes 4.0 mL diethyl-ether:n-butanol: 9:1 (v/v) and vortex for 5 seconds.

9.4.4.   Centrifuge for 5 minutes at 3000 rpm.

9.4.5.   Freeze the aqueous phase in dry ice-acetone bath and discard the organic phase.

9.4.6.   Add 4.0 mL diethyl-ether and vortex for 2 seconds. Repeat 9.4.5. once.

9.4.7.   Repeat 9.4.6. once.

9.4.8.   Acidify all tubes with 1.2 mL 1M hydrochloric acid.

9.4.9.   Add 8.0 mL diethyl-ether and extract on a shaking machine, 15 min.

9.4.10.   Freeze the aqueous phase in dry ice-acetone bath.

9.4.11.   Decant ether phase and evaporate to dryness.

9.4.12.   HPLC step.(see 9.1.10.).

9.4.13.   Proceed as 9.3.23. to 9.3.27.

9.5.   RADIOIMMUNOASSAY.

The method chosen for separation of antibody-bound and free ligand uses charcoal. The RIA procedure is the same for all extracts obtained from bile, urine, faeces or muscle.

9.5.1.   Into 4 siliconised tubes (7.7.4.) pipette 0.1 mL methanol (zero standard tubes). Into siliconised tubes (7.7.4.) pipette in duplicate 0.1 mL of stilbene standard solutions (6.5.1.) to give range 20-1000 pg per tube. Evaporate methanol to dryness e.g.under nitrogen (9.1.9.).

9.5.2.1   Add 0.6 mL gelatin-phosphate buffer (6.5.4.).

9.5.2.2   Add to 9.5.2.1. and to test samples (see 9.1.11, 9.2.16., 9.3.27. and 9.4.13) and 0.1 mL tritiated stilbene solution (6.5.6.2.).

9.5.2.3   Add 0.1 mL antibody (6.5.7.1.) to all tubes except 2 of the zero standard tubes to which is added 0.1 mL buffer (6.5.4.) (NSB tubes).

9.5.3.   Vortex mix for a few seconds.

9.5.4.   Either - place in water bath at 37°C for 15 minutes and then incubate overnight at +4°C. Or place in water bath at 37°C for 1 hour and then cool in ice bath to 0-4°C.

9.5.5.   Add 0.5 mL charcoal suspension (5.3) at 4°C.

9.5.6.   Shake all tubes gently by hand for 1 minute and stand at 4°C for 5 minutes.

9.5.7.   Centrifuge at 2000-3000 rpm at 4°C for 10 minutes.

9.5.8.   Decant supernatant into scintillation vial (7.8.).

9.5.9.   Add 10 mL scintillator (6.5.2.) to all vials including 2 vials containing 0.1 mL tritiated stilbene solution (6.5.6.2.) and 0.1 mL gelatin-phosphate buffer (6.5.4.).

9.5.10.   Place samples in liquid scintillation counter (7.1) and count (preset time or counts) e.g. 10000 counts or 4 minutes.

10.   CALCULATION OF RESULTS.

Note: The example given is for the calculation using DES. The calculation for hexoestrol is the same.

10.1.   Prepare calibration curve by plotting cpm H3-DES bound (cpm bound to antibody for vials containing standards 0-1000 pg (see 6.5.1) against pg standard.

Note: Two corrections are needed, one for the radioactivity carried into
the RIA from the recovery solution and another for the recovery of
stilbene.
10.2. Correction equation for cpm -

corrected cpm = $\dfrac{\text{cpm bound x cpm 3H-DES}}{\text{cpm 3H-DES (SA)} + 3(\text{cpm recovery} - \text{cpm Bg})}$

 cpm bound = cpm bound for test sample
 cpm 3H-DES (SA) = cpm for 0.1 mL 3H-DES solution (6.5.6.2) used in RIA
incubations (see 9.5.10).
 cpm recovery = cpm for 0.2 mL extract of test sample (see 9.3.23).
 cpm Bg is cpm for background (see 9.3.25).

10.3.   Read off calibration curve pg DES against corrected cpm for test
           samples and solvent blanks.

10.4.   Calculation for concentration of stilbene (as DES) in sample -
            pg stilbene in sample i.e. 1g muscle, 50uL bile, 50uL urine and
            either 20mg (from 9.2.16.1.) or 100mg (from 9.2.16.2.) faeces.

           $= \dfrac{(\text{curve pg} - \text{blank pg})(\text{recovery stnd.} - \text{cpm Bg})}{3(\text{cpm recovery} - \text{cpm Bg})}$

       curve pg = pg obtained in step 10.3.
       blank pg = pg for solvent blanks obtained in step 10.3.
       recovery standard = cpm for 0.1 mL 3H-DES recovery solution (6.4.1.).
          cpm recovery = cpm for extract of test sample (9.5.11).
             cpm Bg = cpm for background (9.3.25).

10.5.   Alternative calculations.

 B = cpm bound to antibody - cpm for NSB (NSB tubes 9.5.2.3.).
 Bo = cpm bound to antibody in zero standard tubes - cpm for NSB.

 Bo should be between 40-60% of total cpm (cpm 3H-DES(SA)) (see 10.2.).

10.5.1. Prepare calibration curve by plotting B/Bo against pg standard.

10.5.1.1 If a microcomputer programme is possible then a best line plot of
          log pg standard against Ln Z/(1-Z) where
          Z = B/Bo (LOGIT plot) can be used to interpolate results.

10.5.2. Calculate B/Bo for test sample and for the solvent blank using
          corrected cpm - NSB (see 10.2.) and estimate pg DES from
          calibration curve.
10.5.3. Proceed as 10.4.

10.5.4. The original counting data should be included with the final
          results.

11.   SPECIAL CASES

This method is an alternative method to spectroscopic methods. However it
is strongly emphasised that the spectroscopic methods (e.g. GC-MS) are
preferred (see EEC 93/256 1.2.3.1 {section 5}).

Cy 1.7/9

12.   NOTES ON PROCEDURE

This method in which the separation of the stilbenes by HPLC and the
measurement by RIA has been compared with a GC-MS procedure at RIVM,
Bilthoven. No discrepancies between positives and negatives for both
methods were observed. However for even greater certainty when positives
are found it is recommended to repeat the HPLC separation using an
alternative column with different properties (e.g. different polarity).

13.   ANTIBODIES

Some antibodies are commercially available but recommend up to date
information is obtained from the Community Reference Laboratories.

14.   QUALITY CONTROLS

See section 8 of manual detailing the RMs available for the stilbenes.

15.   LIST OF ABBREVIATIONS

NSB, non-specific binding; SA, standard addition; Bg, background
counts/min
A full list of abbreviations is given in Annex I, Section 12

16.   FLOW DIAGRAM

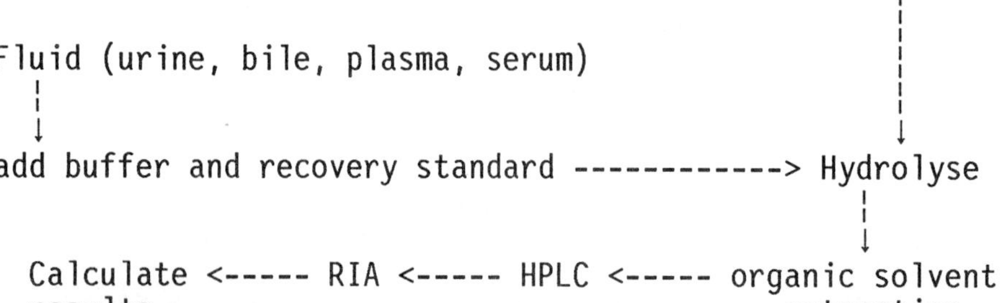

Cy 1.8. ETHINYLOESTRADIOL - METHOD FOR THE MEASUREMENT OF RESIDUES OF ETHINYLOESTRADIOL IN CATTLE URINE BY GC-MS.

WARNING AND SAFETY PRECAUTIONS

0.   INTRODUCTION

Throughout the EEC the use of xenobiotic anabolic agents is prohibited in food producing animals.

1.   SCOPE

This method of analysis describes the detection and confirmation of the presence of ethinyloestradiol in urine of cattle

2.   FIELD OF APPLICATION.

The method is used to perform routine screening and confirmatory analyses in bovine urine samples. The detection limit of ethinyloestradiol was 0.7 μg per L.

3.   REFERENCES.

Commission Decision, 93/256/EEC, laying down the methods for detecting residues of substances having a hormonal or thyrostatic action. [OJ. № L.118, 14.4.93. pp 64-74]

ISO Standard 78/2-1982 Layout for standards - Part 2: Standard for Chemical Analysis

Daeseleire, E., De Guesquiere, A. and Van Peteghem, C, (1991), Detection of the illegal use of ethinyloestradiol in cattle urine by gas chromatography-mass spectrometry. J. Chromatog. <u>564</u>, 469-475

4.   DEFINITIONS.

Ethinyloestradiol content is taken to mean the amount of ethinyloestradiol in bovine urine, regardless of the chemical form, determined according to the described method and expressed as μg ethinyloestradiol per L urine.

5.   PRINCIPLE

5.1. The methods comprises 7 stages;-

        1. Concentration using C18 column
        2. Hydrolysis of conjugates with enzyme.
        3. Clean up using linked C18 and amino SPE columns
        4. Purification on HPLC
        5. Derivatisation to diTMSi ethers
        6. Detection and identification by GCMS
        7. Calculation of results.

6.   MATERIALS

Note: The reagents for which examples of their source are quoted are
known to be satisfactory, nevertheless reagents from other sources may be
equally suitable. Unless specified otherwise chemicals are of AR grade.

6.1.   Reference Compounds and Standard Solutions.
              Ethinyloestradiol was from Sigma, USA
              Solutions of 1 mg per mL methanol, stored in brown glass bottles
              in the dark at +4°C
6.2.   Sodium acetate
6.3   Glacial acetic acid
6.4.   Methanol, HPLC grade (Alltech Assoc, USA)
6.5.   Water, HPLC grade (Alltech Assoc, USA)
6.6.   Helix Pomatia extract (ß-glucuronidase plus aryl sulphatase from
              Boehringer, Mannheim, Germany).
6.7.   Nitrogen
6.8.   Ethyl acetate (Janssen, Belgium)
6.9.   Pyridine (Pierce, USA)
6.10.   N-methyl-N-trimethylsilyltrifluoroacetamide (MSTFA) (Aldrich,
              USA)
6.11.   Trimethylchlorosilane (TMCS) (Fluka, Buchs, Switzerland)
6.12.   Helium (L'Aire Liqiude, Liege, Belgium)
6.13.   n-hexane
6.14.   Dimethyldichlorosilane (Merck)
6.15.   Toluene (Merck)
6.16.   Acetate buffer solution 3 mol/L , pH 4.6
              Dissolve 18.015 g acetic acid and 40.83 g sodium acetate.$3H_2O$ in
              100 mL water.
6.17.   Acetate buffer solution 0.2 mol/L , pH 4.6, The acetate buffer
              (6.16) is diluted 15 times with water.
6.18.   Derivatization reagents: 10 parts (v/v) of pyridine are mixed
              with 3 parts N-methyl-N-trimethylsilyl-trifluoracetamide (MSTFA)
              and 1 part trimethylchlorosilane (TMCS) as a catalyst. The
              mixture must be freshly prepared.

7.   EQUIPMENT.

Reference to a company and/or product is for purposes of information and
identification only. Equivalent types or products also may be suitable.

7.1.   Glass Pasteur capillary pipettes.
7.2.   Automatic pipettes
7.3   pH meter with glass electrode.
7.4.   Electric water bath with adjustable thermostat.
7.5.   Vortex Mixer
7.6   Small filter funnels
7.7   Glass derivatization vials (Chromacol 250 (A)) with screw caps
              (Chromacol 85c) and septa (Chromacol 8-ST15) or alternatively
              pointed flasks or conical tubes with glass stoppers. The vials
              were silanised with dimethyldichlorosilane (6.14) before use.
7.8.   Heating module set at 60°C for derivatization vials (Pierce no.
              18790) with nitrogen facility.
7.9.   SPE Columns.
7.9.1.   C18 column; (6 mL disposable, Baker, USA). The column was
              conditioned by washing with 2 x 5 mL methanol and 2 x 5 mL water.

7.9.2.   Amino column; (3 mL disposable, Baker, USA). The column was
           conditioned by washing with 2 x 3 mL ethyl acetate.

7.10.   HPLC equipment
7.10.1.   The system consisted of a pump (Waters 6000A), automatic injector
           (Waters Wisp 710B), a fraction collector (2212 Helirac,
           Pharmacia), and a UV detector (Pye Unicam, PU 4020) set at 280
           nm.
7.10.2.   The column was a LiChospher RP18, 125 mm x 4 mm i.d., (Merck)
           protected by a guard column of pellicular reversed phase 30-50
           um, 75 mm x 2.1 mm i.d., (Chrompack, Cat no.28603, Middelburg,
           NL).
7.10.3.   The mobile phase was methanol:water (65:35, v/v) pumped at a flow
           rate of 1 mL per min.
7.10.4.   The time-window for collecting ethinyloestradiol is established
           by first running 25 ng of ethinyloestradiol.

7.11.   GC-MS equipment.
7.11.1.   Capillary gas chromatograph with all glass injector maintained at
           290°C. (Hewlett Packard HP 5890)
7.11.2.   Automatic injection for GC - not compulsory
7.11.3.   A mass spectrometer with a low resolution and a mass range of at
           least 600 amu. It must be possible to apply the MID (multiple
           ion detection) mode, also a mass specific detector and an ion
           trap detector. (Hewlett Packard HP 5970)
7.11.4.   Workstation (e.g. Hewlett Packard, type 59970).
7.11.5.   Printer
7.11.6.   GC-column,
7.11.7.   The carrier gas was helium
7.11.8.   The coupling of GC-MS may be by means of a fused silica capillary
           heated to 290°C.

8.   SAMPLES AND SAMPLING PROCEDURE.

N.B. Attention is drawn to section 6.3.1 and ISO document 78/2-1982 and
the following notes derived from Annex II of 2052/VI/84-EN.

8.1. Nature of the Sample; Samples of urine shall be such as to enable
the detection of residues.

8.2. Size of Sample; The size of the sample must be large enough to allow
the reference method to be carried out and to allow repeat analysis where
required.

8.3. The urine must be cooled after collection and stored at $\leq$ -20°C
pending analysis.

9. PROCEDURE

9.1.   10 mL of urine sample is adjusted to pH 4.6 with acetate buffer
           (6.16).
9.2.   The urine is put on to the C18 column (7.9.1), washed with 2 x 5
           mL water and eluted with 2 mL methanol.
9.3.   The methanol is evaporated to dryness under a stream of nitrogen
           at 40°C
9.4.   The residue is taken up in 100 μL methanol and 5 mL 0.2M acetate
           buffer (6.17) added and 50 μL Helix Pomatia juice added.

Cy 1.8/3

9.5.   The sample is incubated for 16 hours at 37°C.
9.6   After cooling to room temperature, the sample is added to the
           previously used and reconditioned C18 column. The amino column
           (7.9.2) is connected beneath the C18 column.
9.7.   Ethinyloestradiol is eluted from both columns with 2 x 1 mL of
           ethyl acetate.
9.8.   The ethyl acetate is evaporated to dryness under a stream of
           nitrogen at 40°C
9.9.   The residue is taken up in 100 μL methanol and 50 μL injected
           into the HPLC system. The methanol-water fraction collected
           between 4 and 7 min (3 mL) was evaporated to dryness under a
           stream of nitrogen.
9.10.   The residue is dissolved in 100 μL of derivatizing agent (6.18)
           and heated at 60°C for 1 hour. After evaporation of the excess
           reagent, the final residue is dissolved in 50 μL of n-hexane, 2
           μL of which is injected into the GC-MS system.

9.11.   The following conditions are used during GC-MS analysis.

9.11.1. GC System

           GC   Capillary GC (HP 5890)
           column   fused silica HP Ultra-2 (5% phenylmethyl-
                                 silicone) 25 m x 0.2 mm ID, film thickness
                                 0.33 um
           injection   2 μL all-glass moving needle at 290°C
           carrier gas   Helium at 0.47 mL per minute
           programme   200°C - 280°C at 5°C/min. 280°C for 10 min.
           transfer line temp.   290°C
           initial column pressure 1.2 bar

           Under these conditions retention times for ethinyloestradiol-
           diTMS is 28.43 expressed as methylene-unit values.

9.4.2.   MS Conditions.

The MS was run in the SIM mode using dwell times of 100 msec.

The selected ions for ethinyloestradiol-diTMS were 440, 425, 300 and 285.

10.   CALCULATION OF RESULTS.

A sample is declared positive when all ions simultaneously appeared at the
right retention times, and checked with retention behaviour of an
ethinyloestradiol-diTMS standard.

The detection limit (Daeseliere et al, 1991) is 0.7 μg per L based on all
ions being present at a value greater than 3 times the signal to noise
ratio for ion m/z 440.

No false negative results were found in a collaborative trial (see
Daeseliere et al, 1991).

11.   SPECIAL CASES.

12.   NOTES ON PROCEDURE.

13.   SAMPLE CONTROLS.

14.   TEST REPORT

15.   LIST OF ABBREVIATIONS.

See abbreviations in Annex I, Section 12 of Manual.

16.   FLOW DIAGRAM

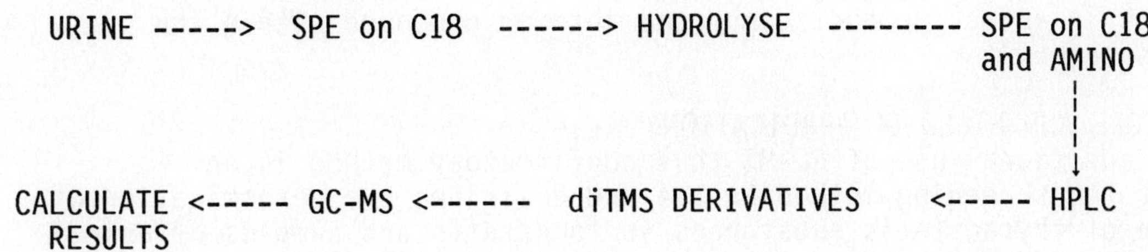

Cy 1.9. THYREOSTATS - METHOD FOR THE MEASUREMENT OF RESIDUES OF THYREOSTATIC SUBSTANCES IN ANIMALS AND ANIMAL TISSUES ON THE BASIS OF HIGH PERFORMANCE THIN LAYER CHROMATOGRAPHY (HPTLC) AND GAS CHROMATOGRAPHY - MASS SPECTROMETRY (GC-MS).

WARNING AND SAFETY PRECAUTIONS.

1.   INTRODUCTION.

Throughout the EEC the use of thyreostatic (anti-thyroid) substances is prohibited in food producing animals. Also the MRL for residues of thyreostatics in animal products imported into or produced within the Community is zero.

2.   SCOPE AND FIELD OF APPLICATION
Through the additional use of GC-MS this confirmatory method is an extension of the screening method Sg 1.4 and describes the determination of the presence of thyreostatic substances in foodstuffs and samples of animal origin. The method can be used for meat and also for biological material such as animal organs, biological fluids and excreta. The limit of detection for 2-thiouracil (TU); 4(6)-Methyl-2-thiouracil (MTU) and 4(6)-n-propyl-2-thiouracil (PTU) is about 25 μg per kg or L. Because the recovery of 4(6)-phenyl-2-thiouracil (PhTU) and 1-methyl-2-mercaptoimidazole (tapazole, TAP) from the mercurated column is less efficient the limit of detection for these two compounds is about 100 μg per kg or L.

3.   REFERENCES.

ISO Standard 78/2-1982 Layout for standards - Part 2: Standard for Chemical Analysis

Commission Decision, 93/256/EEC, laying down the methods for detecting residues of substances having a hormonal or thyrostatic action. OJ. № L.118, 14.4.93, pp 64-74.

EEC Working paper VI/3186/84-EN, File 6.21 II-4. Method of analysis for detecting anti-thyroid substances in fresh muscle tissue using a selective mercurated column.

De Brabander, H.F. and Verbeke, R. (1984), Determination of methylthiouracil and analogous thyreostatic drugs. Proc. 30th Eur. Meat Res. Workers, Bristol, 387-388.

De Brabander, H.F., Batjoens, P. and Van Hoof, J. (1992), Determination of thyreostatic drugs by HPTLC with confirmation by GC-MS. J. Planar Chrom. <u>5</u>, 124-130

4.   DEFINITIONS.

Thyreostatic substances detected in this assay are;

    2-thiouracil (TU);   4(6)-Methyl-2-thiouracil (MTU);
    4(6)-n-propyl-2-thiouracil (PTU);   4(6)-phenyl-2-thiouracil (PhTU);
    1-methyl-2-mercaptoimidazole (tapazole, TAP);

5.   PRINCIPLE

The method comprises 4 stages from the screening method;
 - Homogenisation of tissue samples or diluting fluids in methanol
 - Percolation of supernatant through mercurated ion-exchange resin
      chromatographic column
 - Derivatization
 - Separation and identification by two dimensional HPTLC

and then 3 stages for confirmation;
 - scrape spots from plate
 - derivatise with MSTFA
 - GC-MS

6.   CHEMICALS

Note: The reagents for which examples of their source are quoted are
known to be satisfactory, nevertheless reagents from other sources may be
equally suitable. All the reagents must be of analytical grade.

6.1. - 6.12. The chemicals for the screening part of the assay,
              i.e. to the point of identification of the thyreostats on an
              HPTLC plate are described in method Sg 1.4.
6.13.   Derivatising agent, N-methyl-N-trimethylsilyl-trifluoroacetamide,
              (MSTFA). (Pierce, art № 70127 or Machery-Nagel, Düren, Germany)
6.14.   A standard mixture of the thyreostatic drugs (20 ng per μL) was
              prepared and 10 μL of this solution was transferred to an
              autosampler vial (7.16) evaporated to dryness and heated with 50
              μL MSTFA at 60°C for 15 min.

7.   EQUIPMENT.

7.1. - 7.14. The chemicals for the screening part of the assay, i.e. to
              the point of identification of the thyreostats on an HPTLC plate
              are described in method Sg 1.4.

7.15.   GC-MS equipment was performed with an ITS40 ion trap mass
              spectrometer (Finnigan MAT, San Jose, CA, USA).
7.15.1.   Gas chromatograph column was a 30 m x 0.25 mm with 0.25 μm film
              of DB-5 (J&W). The oven temperature for splitless injection was
              100°C; this was maintained for 2 min, programmed at 5°C per min
              to 150°C and then 20° per min to 250°C, which was held for 3 min.
              (total programme 20 min).
7.15.2.   Positive CI spectra (reagent gas, butane) between m/z 90 and 400
              were aquired for 20 min at 1 scan per sec (filament, multiplier
              delay 600 sec).
7.15.3.   The retention times and the ions used for tracing the peaks after
              full-scale aquisition are shown in table 1.
7.15.4.   Workstation
7.15.5.   Printer
7.16.   Autosampler vials (100 μL)
Reference to a company and/or product is for purposes of information and
identification only. Equivalent types or products also may be suitable.

Drug	R_t (min)	ion 1	ion 2	ion 3 (MH^+)
TAP	13.2	171	186	259
TU	13.4	257	273	345
MTU	14.3	271	287	359
DMTU	15.2	285	301	373
PTU	15.6	299	315	387

8. SAMPLES AND SAMPLING PROCEDURE.

N.B. Attention is drawn to section 6.3.1 and to ISO document 78/2-1982 and also the following notes derived from Annex II of 2052/VI/84-EN.

8.1. Nature of the Sample; Samples shall be such as to enable the detection of residues in meat as defined in Directive 64/433/EEC. Failing this biological fluids or faeces may constitute the samples for the detection of residues.

8.2. Size of Sample; The size of the sample must be large enough to allow the method to be carried out and to allow repeat analysis where required.

8.3. The samples must be taken and packed in such a way as to allow proper identification in the laboratory.

8.4. The method of packing, preservation and transport must maintain the integrity of the sample and not prejudice the result of the examination. Samples for the analysis of thyreostatic substances must be stored and transported at temperatures below -18°C.

9.   PROCEDURE.

9.1 to 9.14.   2 g tissue, 2 mL urine, plasma or skim milk, are homogenised in 10 mL methanol and processed through to the formation and identification of the thyreostats on HPTLC plates as descibed in the screening method (see Sg 1.4)

9.15.   The spot suspected of containing the drug was removed from the plate by careful scraping and transferred to an autosampler vial (7.16). 25 µL MSTFA was added, the contents mixed, and the vial heated to 100°C for 15 min. After sedimentation of the silica gel, 1-2 µL of the clear supernatant was analysed by GC-MS.

9.16.   1 µL standard mixture (6.14) was analysed by GC-MS.

10.   CALCULATION OF RESULTS.

10.1.   IDENTIFICATION.

Identification of the unknown compounds was performed by matching the retention times on the GC and the specta on the MS with the standards.

10.1.   RECOVERIES.
The recoveries of the thyreostats from the mercurated column is >78% for
TU, MTU, PTU and DMTU but only about 17% for PhTU and 60% for TAP.

The recoveries of the internal standard, DMTU, from meat, plasma and milk
are shown in table 2;

Table 2; Recoveries of 100 µg per kg spike of DMTU.

Sample.	Concentration found ± SD (ug per kg)		
	PTU	MTU	TU
Meat	106 ± 5.5	102 ± 13.7	97 ± 21.8
Plasma	84 ± 6.2	98 ± 5.0	76 ± 5.7
Milk	88 ± 6.9	105 ± 3.6	85 ± 8.0

Recoveries from the GC-MS steps were not determined.

10.2.   PRECISION

10.2.1. Reproducibility; The reproducibility of the analysis of meat
spiked at the 100 µg per kg level was recorded for each step of the assay.
The results obtained by De Brabander and Verbeke (1984), Ghent, are shown
in table 3 in method Sg 1.4.

11.   SPECIAL CASES

12.   NOTES ON PROCEDURE

13.   QUALITY CONTROLS

See section 8 of manual detailing the RMs available for the thyreostatics.

14.   TEST REPORT

15.   LIST OF ABBREVIATIONS

A full list of abbreviations is given in Annex I, Section 12

16.   FLOW DIAGRAM

```
    Tissue --> add methanol and internal standard ---> Homogenise
                                                           |
                                                           |
                                                           ↓
      HPTLC <------- Derivatise <------- percolate through Hg column
        |
        |
        ↓
      Measure fluorescence at 366 nm -------> Elute spot from plate
                                                           |
                                                           |
                                                           ↓
      Calculate results <------ GC-MS <-------TMS derivatives
```

Cy 2.1.   ß-AGONISTS - A METHOD FOR THE DETECTION AND IDENTIFICATION OF ß-AGONISTS IN BIOLOGICAL SAMPLES AND ANIMAL FEED.

1.   SCOPE

This method of analysis describes the detection and confirmation of the presence of individual β-agonists in samples of animal origin and animal feed. The method has been mainly tested for residues of clenbuterol and salbutamol. This work is carried out in compliance with the Residues Directive (86/469/EEC).

2.   FIELD OF APPLICATION

The method is used to perform routine screening and confirmatory analyses in urine and liver from veal calves, cattle and pigs as well as in animal feed. Routinely the method is used to test for the presence of residues of clenbuterol, salbutamol, terbutaline, cimaterol and mabuterol but is in principle also suitable for the detection and confirmation of other t-butyl or isopropyl-β-agonists like carbuterol, pirbuterol and tulobuterol. The detection limit, defined as three times the standard deviation of the blank determination, measured in μg per kg or litre of sample is well below 1 for compounds during initial screening. The limit of detection for confirmation according to the EC criteria for reference methods is 0.5 to 1.5 μg per kg or L but depends on the ionisation technique and equipment used.

3.   REFERENCES

Courtheyn R, Verne R, Schilt R, Hooijerink H, Desaever C and Bakeroot V, 1988. Detectie en identificatie van clenbuterol en cinesterol op HPLC. Benelux Working Group "Hormones and anti-Hormones". Brussels, document SP/LAB/h (88) 43.

Foerster, H.J., Rominger, K.L., Ecker, E., Peil, H. and Wittrock, A. (1988), Quantification of clenbuterol in biological fluids using ammonia CI and automated capillary GC-MS. Biomed. Environ. Mass Spec. 17, 417-420

Ginkel L.A. van, Blitterswijk H. van, Zoontjes P.W., Bosch D. van den and Stephany R.W., 1988. Assay for trenbolone and its reduced metabolite 17 α-trenbolone in bovine urine based on immunoaffinity chromatographic clean-up and off-line high performance liquid chromatography/thin layer chromatography, Journal Chrom., 445:385-392.

Ginkel L.A. van, Stephany R.W., Rossum H.J., (1992). Development and validation of a multi-residue method for β-agonists in biological samples and animal feed. J. Ass. Off. Anal. Chem. Int, 75, 554-560

Ginkel C.A. van, Stephany R.W., Rossum H.J. van and Farla J., 1990 Multi residue test for beta-agonists in slaughter animals. IMAC Symposium on "New Trends in Veal Calf Production", Wageningen, the Netherlands, 1990. Proceedings of the Symposium.

Ginkel C.A. van, Stephany, R.W., Rossum, H.J. van, Steinbuch, H.M., Zomer, G., Heeft, E van der, and De Jong, A.P.J.M. 1989. Multiimmunoaffinity chromatography: a simple and highly selective clean-up method for multi-anabolic residues in meat. J. Chrom. 489, 111-120

Girault, J., Gobin, P. and Fourtillan, J.B. (1990), Quantitative
measurement of clenbuterol at the femtomole level in plasma and urine by
combined gas chromatography/negative ion chemical ionisation mass
spectrometry. Biomed. Environ. Mass Spectrometry. $\underline{19}$, 80-88

Yamamoto I and Iwalak, 1982 Enzyme immunoassay for clenbuterol, a β-2-
adrenergic stimulant. Journal of Immunoassay, $\underline{3}$, 15-?

4.   DEFINITIONS

ß-agonists content is taken to be the amount of β-agonists in the substance
in question determined according to the described method and expressed as
µg β-agonists per kg or litre of test sample.

5.   PRINCIPLE

The method comprises 4 stages;
1. preparation of a primary extract
2. extract purification and concentration using immunoaffinity
    chromatography
3. detection by GC-MS
4. calculation and evaluation of results

6. MATERIALS

6.1. Chemicals and reagents
6.1.1. Reference compounds.

The following standard compounds are used.

Compound	CAS-No	mol formula	Mol. Wt.
clenbuterol	37148-27-9	$C_{12}H_{18}C_{12}N_2O$	277.18
salbutamol	18559-94-9	$C_{13}H_{21}NO_3$	239.31
terbutaline	23031-25-6	$C_{12}H_{19}NO_3$	235.29
cimaterol	54239-37-1	$C_{12}H_{17}N_3O$	219.29
mabuterol	56341-08-3	$C_{13}H_{18}ClF_3N_2O$	310.75

and additional β-agonists if desired.

It is preferred to use isotope labelled internal standards, e.g.
clenbuterol-d6, salbutamol-d6 or clenbuterol-$^{37}Cl_2$. It is foreseen that
these reference compounds will be made available through BCR.

6.1.2.   IAC-materials
The immunogens used were prepared as described earlier by coupling
diazonium-clenbuterol and diazonium-cimaterol to bovine serum albumin (BSA,
Sigma) (Yamamoto et al., 1982). The respective antisera used to prepare
the IAC-matrices were obtained by immunizing rabbits four times over a
period of 5 months, with 2 mg of immunogen each time. The isolation of the
antiserum immunoglobulin-G (IgG) fraction and coupling of this fraction to
the activated matrix were performed as described previously (Ginkel et al.,
1989). The final columns have a capacity >100 ng for the compounds
mentioned (6.1.1).

6.1.3.   Ethanol (Merck, art. no. 983).
6.1.4.   Methanol (Merck, art. no. 9623).
6.1.5.   Toluene (Merck, art. no. 8325).
6.1.6.   Acetonitrile (Merck, art. no. 30).

6.1.7.   Dichloromethane (Merck, art. no. 6050).
6.1.8.   Hydrochloric acid (Merck, art. no. 317).
6.1.9.   Ethyl acetate (Merck, art. no. 9623).
6.1.10.   Acetic acid (Merck, art. no. 63).
6.1.11.   Sodium acetate (Merck, art. no. 6268).
6.1.12.   Sodium chloride (Analar BDH art. no. 10241).
6.1.13.   Extrelut^R (Merck, art. no. 11737; refills art. no. 11738)
6.1.14.   Acetate buffer 0.1 mol/L, pH 4.0.
           Mix 4.92 g acetic acid (6.1.10) with 800 mL water, add 2.45 g
           sodium acetate (6.1.11.) and 29.25 g sodium chloride (6.1.12.).
           Adjust the pH at 4.0 ± 0.1 and add water to a final volume of
           1000 mL.
6.1.15.   IAC-eluting buffer.
           Mix 400 mL of ethanol (6.1.3.) with 75 mL water and 25 mL acetate
           buffer (6.1.14).
6.1.16.   Disodium hydrogen phosphate (Merck, art. no. 6586).
6.1.17.   Potassium dihydrogen phosphate (Merck, art. no. 4873).
6.1.18.   Phosphate buffer, 0.02 mol/L, pH = 7.0.
           Dissolve in 800 mL water 2.278 g disodium hydrogen phosphate
           (6.1.16.), 0.416 g potassium dihydrogen phosphate (6.1.17.) and
           9.09 sodium chloride (6.1.12.). Adjust the pH at 7.0 ± 0,1 and
           add water to a final volume of 1000 mL.
6.1.19.   Stock solutions of standards containing 1 g/L in ethanol, stored
           at -20°C in the dark.
6.1.20.   Working solutions of standards containing 0.01 g/L in ethanol,
           stored at +4°C for a maximum period of 2 weeks.
           Smallest volume pipetted out of the stock solution is 0.1 mL.
6.1.21.   Derivatization reagent: N_2O-bis (trimethylsilyl)
           trifluoracetamine (BSTFA) with 1% TMS (Pierce, art. no. 38832).
6.1.22.   Beta-glucuronidase/sulphatase (suc'Helix Pomatia, containing
           100,000   units β-glucuronidase and 1 million units sulphatase per
           mL, Industrie Biologique, France, code IBR 213473)

7.   EQUIPMENT
7.1.   Glass round bottomed flasks, 150 mL (Corex, art. no. 8422-A).
7.2.   Glass Pasteur capillary pipettes.
7.3.   Automatic pipettes (Gilson P20, P200, P1000 and P5000).
7.4.   Refrigerated centrifuge (RC-3, Sorvall).
7.5.   Bench-top centrifuge (GLC-4, Sorvall).
7.6.   Centrifuge tubes, glass (55 mm x 11.5 mm) (Renes, RB55)
7.7.   Electric water bath with thermostat adjustable to 50 ± 2°C (GFL,
           Salm & Kipp) with nitrogen facility.
7.8.   Vortex (Vortex-genic, Wilton & Co).
7.9.   Ultrasonic water bath (Bransonic 32).
7.10.   Glass derivatization vials (chromacol 250 (A)) with screw caps
           (chromacol 85c) and septa (chromacol 8-ST15).
7.11.   Incubator 60°C (Seelvis).
7.12.   Heating module for derivatization vials (Pierce no. 18790) with
           nitrogen facility.
7.13.   Glass injection vials (Chrompack, art. no. 10201) with glass
           inserts (Chrompack, art. no. 10381).
7.14.   Aluminium caps (Chrompack, art. no. 10210).
7.15.   GC-MS equipment.
7.15.1.   Gas chromatograph (Hewlett Packard, type 5890).
7.15.2.   Automatic injector (Hewlett Packard, type 7637A).
7.15.3.   Mass selective detector (Hewlett Packard, type 5970).

Cy 2.1/3

7.15.4. Workstation (Hewlett Packard, type 59970).
7.15.5. Printer (Hewlett Packard, think yet).
7.15.6. GC-column, fused silica permabond SE-52, 25 m x 0.25 mm ID, film
         thickness 0.25 um (Machery-Nagel, art. no. 723054).
7.15.7. Rotavapor with water bath at 40 ± 0.2°C (Rotavapor).

8.   SAMPLES AND SAMPLING PROCEDURE.

N.B. Attention is drawn to section 6.3.1 and ISO document 78/2-1982(E) and
the following notes derived from Annex II of 2052/VI/84-EN.

8.1. Nature of the Sample; Samples shall be such as to enable the
detection of residues in meat as defined in Directive 64/433/EEC. Failing
this biological fluids or faeces may constitute the samples for the
detection of residues.

8.2. Size of Sample; The size of the sample must be large enough to allow
the reference method to be carried out and to allow repeat analysis where
required.
In this method for ß-agonists the amount required for a single
determination is
     3 g liver;   10 mL urine;   10 g animal feed

8.3. The samples must be taken and packed in such a way as to allow proper
identification in the laboratory.

8.4. The method of packing, preservation and transport must maintain the
integrity of the sample and not prejudice the result of the examination.

Samples for the analysis of ß-agonists must be stored and transported at
temperatures below -18°C. Feed samples should be stored at +4°C.

9.   ANALYTICAL PROCEDURE

Several procedures based on either c.q. sublitizin digestion or ultrasonic
extraction may be used for the extraction of liver samples.. Studies at
RIVM revealed no significant difference between the methods when samples
obtained from treated animals were analyzed. However, ultrasonic
extraction is simpler and results in less interfering compounds and is the
preferred technique.

9.1.   Extraction procedures.
9.1.1.   Animal feed.
          Accurately weigh 10.0 g of animal feed into a glass flask and add
          50.0 mL of water. Place the flask in an ultrasonic water bath and
          extract for 30 minutes. Subsequently shake or vortex the flask for
          10 seconds. Centrifuge the flask for 10 minutes (1800 g) and
          pipette 19 mL into a clean flask. Adjust to pH 9.8 ± 0.2 with 1
          mol/L NaOH and add water to adjust the volume to 20 mL.
9.1.2.   Liver
          Accurately weigh 3.0 g of liver into a 20 mL glass flask and add
          15 mL 0.01 mol/L HCl. Place the flask in an ultrasonic water bath
          and extract for 15 minutes. Subsequently shake or vortex the flask
          for 10 seconds. Centrifuge the flask for 10 minutes (1800 g) and
          decant the supernatant into a clean flask. Adjust the pH to 5.2 ±
          0.2 with 1 mol/L NaOH and add water to adjust the volume to 20 mL.

9.1.3. Urine.
Accurately pipette 10.0 mL of urine into a 20 mL glass flask.
Adjust the pH to a value of 5.2 ± 0.2 with 1 mol/L NaOH and add
water to adjust the volume to 20 mL.

9.2. Enzymatic Hydrolysis
Samples of urine and primary extracts of liver are enzymatically
hydrolysed. To the aqueous samples 0.1 ml Helix Pomatia (6.1.22)
is added. All samples are incubated overnight at 37°C. After
incubation the samples are cooled to room temperature and the pH
is adjusted to 9.2 ± 0.2. The volume of the urine samples is
adjusted to 20 ml with water.

9.3. Extrelut^R extraction
The aqueous extract (20 mL) is applied to an Extrelut^R extraction
centrifuge. After equilibration for 15 minutes the water is
extracted with 60 mL ethyl acetate and the extract is evaporated
on a rotation vaporizer at 50°C.

9.4. Sample clean-up; immunoaffinity chromatography.
The IAC-columns are washed with at least 10 mL of water. The dry
residue is dissolved in 0.1 mL ethanol. Subsequently 50 mL water
is added and the residue is further dissolved by placing the flask
in an ultrasonic water bath for at least 1 minute. The aqueous
extract is applied to the IAC column and flushed through with a
flow of 2 mL/minute. Subsequently the column is washed with 5 mL
of water after which the β-agonists are eluted with 5 mL IAC-
eluting buffer. The eluate is evaporated to dryness in a water
bath at 50°C under a cold stream of nitrogen. The IAC column is
regenerated by washing it with 5 mL IAC eluting buffer, 25 mL of
water and 25 mL PBS.

9.5. Desalting of the IAC eluate.
The dry residue is resuspended in 0.5 mL of cold ethanol and
centrifuged for 5 minutes (1800 g) at 4°C. The supernatant is
removed into a derivatization vial and the ethanol is evaporated
using a heating block at 50°C under a cold stream of nitrogen.

9.6. Derivatization.
The dry residue is dissolved in 0.1 mL derivatization reagent
(6.1.21). The mixture is incubated for 1 hour at 60°C (7.11). The
reagent is evaporated (7.12) and the dry derivatized residue is
dissolved in 0.025 mL toluene (6.15). The toluene solution is
transferred to a derivatization vial (7.10) and subjected to GC-
MSD analysis and confirmed as in 10.1.
GC-MSD settings:

injection volume	2 μL.
injection temperature	260°C
injection mode	splitless
starting temperature	70°C
gradient	25°C/min
first firal temperature	200°C/min (6 minutes)
gradient	25°C/min
second firal temperature	300°C/min (2 minutes)
ions monitored (screening)	m/Z = 86 (t-butyl-β-agonists)
	m/Z = 72 (isopropyl-β-agonists)

10.0.   CALCULATION OF RESULTS

The procedure used for calculation results (quantification) depends on the
internal or external standards used.
Where isotope labelled standards are available a linear calibration curve
can be fitted with the ID-ratio as dependent and the concentration of
standard (e.g. ng/injection vial) as dependent variable.
This procedure yields linear calibration curves which give an intercept
deviating not significantly from 0.

For other ß-agonists quantification is less straight forward. In practice
however recovery for most compounds is equal to the recovery of
clenbuterol, both for muscle and liver. The only compound with
significantly different analytical recovery is salbutamol. For this
compound however an internal standard is available (see validation).

For confirmation the simultaneous detection of at least four ions response
ratios have to be calculated for both standards and unknown compounds.

10.1.   CONFIRMATION

For purposes of confirmation additional (fragment)-ions have to be
monitored. Beta-agonists fragment according to the scheme shown below:
The ions are shown in order (A to F) of intensity.

	N	M.W	M.WD.	[A]	[B]	[C]	[D]	[E]	[F]
terbutaline	3	225	441	86	356	336	426	370	280
salbutamol	3	239	455	86	369	350	440	384	294
clenbuterol	1	276	348	86	262	243	333	277	187
cimaterol	1	219	291	72	219	186	276	234	
	2	219	363	72	291	258	348		
mabuterol	1	310	382	86	296	277	367	311	221

N = number of TMS-groups; M.W.= molecular weight of pure compound
M.WD = molecular weight after derivatization

For identification according to the EC-criteria it is mandatory that at
least 4 ions are monitored. Each response should fulfil the criterium that
the maximum exceeds the average noise ± 3 SD. If this criterium is
fulfilled for all ions monitored the 3 different ratios are calculated. The
same ratios are calculated for the standard analyte, preferably at the corresponding concentration. For positive identification the responses
obtained for the unknown samples should all be within ± 10% of the average
value for the standard.
Note: Frequently the variability of the MS-equipment does not allow this
criterium to be strictly applied. In this case the criterium is replaced by
a criterium based on the experimental variability. The response ratios for
the unknown sample should be within the corresponding standard ± 3 SD.

10.1.1.   Fragmentation pattern for ß-agonists (See figure 1).

10.2.   Validation.
A number of studies was undertaken to validate the analytical
procedure.Most of these experiments were within laboratory experiments
(repeatability and within laboratory reproducibility). In addition the
method was validated in a cooperative study on animal feed, organized by
the EC and demonstrated during an EC workshop, April 22-26, 1991, at RIVM.

Figure 1

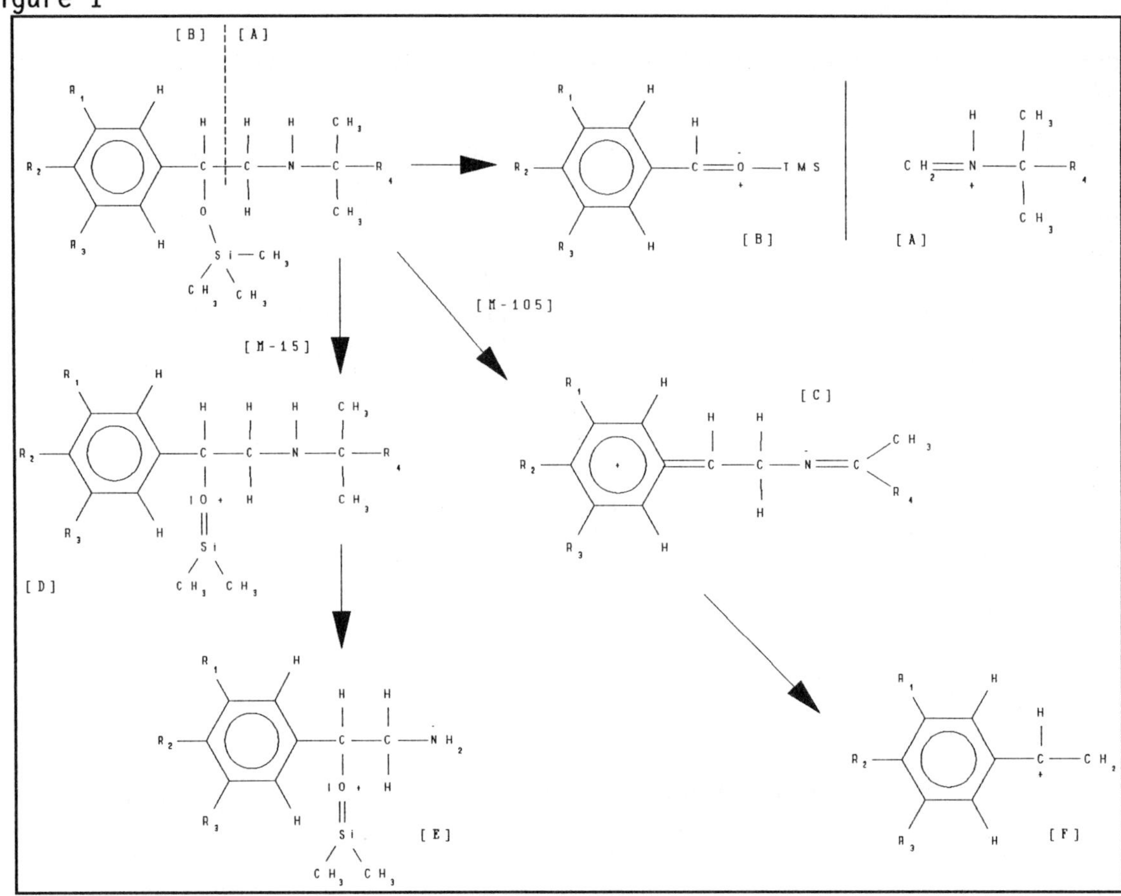

10.2.1.   Analytical recovery during IAC

Each newly prepared batch of IAC material has to be tested for its capacity
to retain relevant components. Typical results are given below (200 ng
applied):

Compound	recovery during IAC %
clenbuterol	95
mabuterol	111
salbutamol	103
cimaterol	96

10.2.3.   Analytical recovery of the procedure

When the IAC materials were demonstrated to be suitable the procedure was
validated by determining the analytical recovery of components spiked to
blank urine. The internal standard was added after the analysis for
corrections during derivatization and GC-MSD analysis.

Compound	analytical recovery % (average ± SD, N = 2)
clenbuterol	102 ± 8
salbutamol	56 ± 5
mabuterol	115 ± 4
cimaterol	100 ± 5

10.2.4. Repeatability and reproducibility

Repeatability and within laboratory reproducibility were determined for
clenbuterol and salbutamol by analyzing samples of urine and liver obtained
from treated animals (urine from veal calves and liver from a pig).The
samples were analyzed on three different occasions, each time in duplicate.

Salbutamol in liver

individual values $\mu g/kg$		within assay variability	between assay
3.6	3.3	$s_2 = 0.016$	$s_2 = 0.065$
3.4	3.3	$s = 0.13$	$s = 0.25$
3.7	3.7	%RSD = 3.7	%RSD = 7.1

Clenbuterol in liver

individual values $\mu g/kg$		within assay variability	between assay variability
13.8	11.2	$s_2 = 1.31$	$s_2 = 2.63$
12.9	12.6	$s = 1.14$	$s = 1.62$
15.1	14.1	%RSD = 8.5	%RSD =12.1

Clenbuterol in urine

individual values $\mu g/kg$		within assay variability	between assay variability
4.4	4.3	$s^2 = 0.035$	$s^2 = 0.122$
4.2	4.6	$s = 0.19$	$s = 0.35$
4.7	4.9	%RSD = 4.2	%RSD = 7.8

Salbutamol in urine

individual values $\mu g/kg$		within assay variability	between assay variability
2.0	2.0	$s = 0.007$	$s = 0.020$
1.8	2.0	$s = 0.08$	$s = 0.14$
2.1	2.1	%RSD = 4.0	%RSD = 7.0

10.2.5. Sensitivity.

The sensitivity depends on whether the method is used for screening where
only the most abundant ion (m/Z = 86 or 72) is monitored or for
confirmation when four ions must be monitored. In the latter case the
sensitivity is reduced to the limit of detection for the weakest of the
four ions.

11.   SPECIAL CASES.

This procedure includes a special step for deconjugation of ß-agonists
which might be present in the form of glucuronide- or sulphate-esters. For
clenbuterol all data available lead to the conclusion that no conjugates
are formed. For salbutamol the presence of sulphate-esters is described.
Studies at RIVM show that in cattle salbutamol is more than 95% conjugated.
The use of prolonged incubations and relative large amounts of enzymes is
needed. Based on these results it was concluded that in routine it is
necessary to perform a deconjugation step during multi residue sample
preparation. For the specific analysis of clenbuterol the hydrolysis step
can be omitted. For other β-agonists no data are available at the moment.

12.   NOTES ON PROCEDURE. The procedure chosen will depend on the
availability of reagents,reference compounds and equipment.

13.   QUALITY CONTROL. STANDARDS, REFERENCE MATERIALS AND ANTIBODIES.
A description of the source and quality of the key reagents and standards
is given in Section 8. In-house standards were prepared at RIVM by spiking
blank bovine liver with clenbuterol at 1 or 2 µg per kg and preparing a
hompgenious batch of lyophilized samples. Using these samples the inter-
assay variation for was 13% at 1 µg per kg and 8.6% at 2 µg per kg and the
average value was 85-100% of the target value.

13.1   IAC. Follow the instructions relating to the storage and
procedures as recommended by the supplier.

13.2.   Source of IAC columns and gel packings.
Commercial suppliers;-

Laboratory of Hormonology - Marloie, Rue de Point de Jour, 8, B-6900,
Marloie, Belgium.
Gels for immunoaffinity chromatography are available (minimum quantity 1
mL) prepared from high affinity antisera and with a minimum capacity of 50
ng per mL for;
        ß$_2$-agonists; Clenbuterol, Salbutamol (single or combined)

GENEGO S.p.A., Via Ressel S. Andrea zona ind., 34170 Gorizia, Italy
This company market three multi-analyte columns claiming a capacity of at
least 20 ng or 100 ng (high capacity column) per analyte. The products
are -
        Multi-Prep I for DES, HEX, DE, Z, Taleranol ß-E$_2$, NT, T, MT, and
        TB
        Multi-Prep II for DES, HEX, DE, Z, NT, MT,T, TB and Taleranol
        Multi-Prep III for Clenbuterol, salbutamol, terbutaline,
        carbuterol and marbuterol all ß-agonists.

These columns are marketed as a complete kit, comprising the enzyme and the
buffer for the digestion of samples, extraction and washing buffers and
detailed instructions.

13.3.   Deuterated standards.
Deuterated ß-agonists are held at RIKILT.

14.   TEST REPORT.
To give the indications necessary for the identification of the sample, the
reference to the method employed, the results and the form in which these
are expressed, any particular points observed in the course of the test and
any operations not specified in the method or regarded as optional which
might affect the results.

15.   LIST OF ABBREVIATIONS
A list of the most important abbreviations is given in Annex I section 12.

16.   FLOW DIAGRAM.

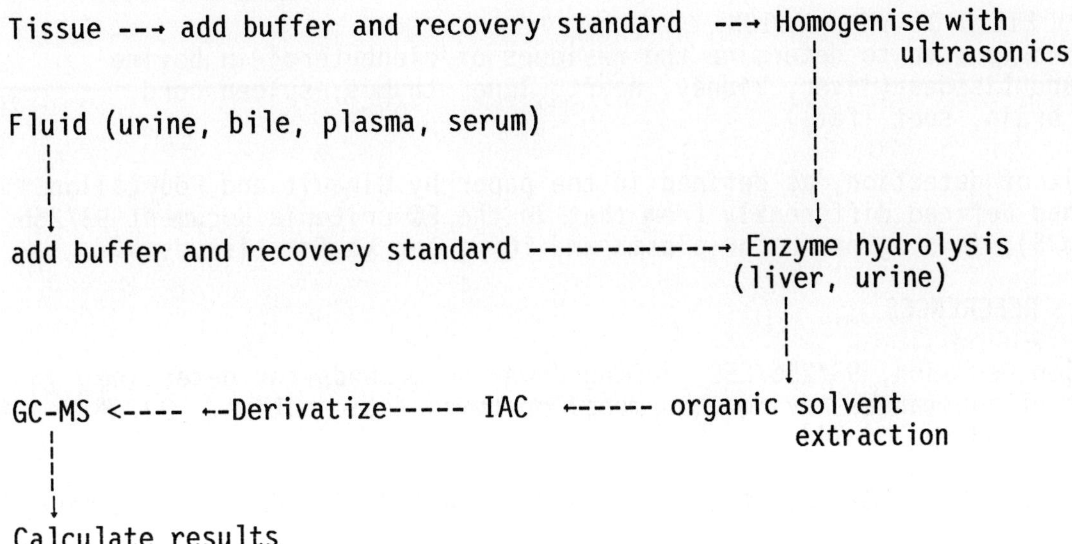

Cy 2.2.   CLENBUTEROL - DETERMINATION OF CLENBUTEROL AT RESIDUE LEVELS IN BOVINE PLASMA AND TISSUES BY GC-MS.

1.   SCOPE

Clenbuterol is a potent ß-agonist used as a bronchodilator in humans and also a repartitioning agent in farm animals. Clenbuterol may be administered orally or parentally. The oral dose is usually administered as a feed supplement equivalent to approximately 3 mg per kg feed.

This method of analysis describes the detection and confirmation of the presence of clenbuterol in bovine plasma and tissue samples.

2.   FIELD OF APPLICATION

The method is used to determine the residues of clenbuterol in bovine plasma and tissues (liver, kidney, heart, lung, thymus, spleen cord, muscle, brain, suet {fat}).

The limit of detection, as defined in the paper by Girault and Fourtillan (1990) and defined differently from that in the EC criteria document 93/256 (Section 5), is 5 ng per L for plasma and 10 ng per kg for tissues.

3.   REFERENCES

Commission Decision, 93/256/EEC, laying down the methods for detecting residues of substances having a hormonal or thyrostatic action. [OJ. № L.118, 14.4.93. pp 64-74]

ISO Standard 78/2-1982 Layout for standards - Part 2: Standard for Chemical Analysis

Foerster, H.J., Rominger, K.L., Ecker, E., Peil, H. and Wittrock, A. (1988), Quantification of clenbuterol in biological fluids using ammonia CI and automated capillary GC-MS. Biomed. Environ. Mass Spec. 17, 417-420

Ginkel L.A. van, Stephany R.W., Rossum H.J., (1992). Development and validation of a multi-residue method for β-agonists in biological samples and animal feed. J. Ass. Off. Anal. Chem. Int, 75, 554-560

Ginkel C.A. van, Stephany R.W., Rossum H.J. van and Farla J., 1990 Multi residue test for beta-agonists in slaughter animals. IMAC Symposium on "New Trends in Veal Calf Production", Wageningen, the Netherlands, 1990. Proceedings of the Symposium,

Girault, J., and Fourtillan, J.B. (1990), Determination of clenbuterol in bovine plasma and tissues by gas chromatography-negative-ion chemical ionization mass-spectrometry. J. Chromatogr. 518, 41-52

Girault, J., Gobin, P. and Fourtillan, J.B. (1990), Quantitative measurement of clenbuterol at the femtomole level in plasma and urine by combined gas chromatography/negative ion chemical ionisation mass spectrometry. Biomed. Environ. Mass Spectrometry. 19, 80-88

4.   DEFINITIONS

Clenbuterol content is taken to be the amount of clenbuterol in the substance in question determined according to the described method and expressed as µg clenbuterol per kg or litre of test sample.

5.   PRINCIPLE

The method comprises five stages;
1.   preparation of a primary extract
2.   extract purification and concentration using solvent partition
3.   derivatisation as perfluoroacyl derivatives
4.   detection by GC-MS
5.   calculation and evaluation of results

6.   MATERIALS

6.1.   Chemicals and reagents

6.1.1.   Ethyl acetate (Merck, art. no. 9623).
6.1.2.   Acetone (Merck).
6.1.3.   Double distilled water
6.1.4.   Methanol (Merck, art. no. 9623)
6.1.5.   2*M* sodium hydroxide
6.1.6.   Sodium hydrogen carbonate
6.1.7.   Hexane (Merck)
6.1.8.   0.2*M* Sulphuric acid (Merck,)
6.1.9.   Anhydrous sodium sulphate (Merck)
6.1.10. Nitrogen
6.1.11. Pentafluoropropionic anhydride (PFPA) (Pierce, Rockford, Ill,
         USA)
6.1.12. Human plasma free of clenbuterol

6.2.   Reference compounds.
6.2.1.   Clenbuterol is from Chiesi Farmaceutici Laboratories,
         Parma,Italy.
6.2.2.   The internal standard is the isotope labelled standard,$[^2H_9]$
         clenbuterol from Chiesi Farmaceutici Laboratories, Parma,Italy.
6.2.3.   Stock solution of clenbuterol standard containing 0.1 g/L in
         methanol, stored at -20°C in the dark.
6.2.4.   Stock solution of $[^2H_9]$ clenbuterol standard containing 0.1 g/L
         in methanol, stored at -20°C in the dark.
6.2.5.   Working solutions of standards (6.2.3., 6.2.4.) are made by
         diluting the stock solutions in distilled water. The solutions
         are protected from light by wrapping the flasks in aluminium foil
         and are stored at +4°C until used.

6.3.   Solutions.
6.2.1.   2*M* sodium hydroxide buffered at pH 12 with sodium hydrogen
         carbonate.
6.2.2.   Sorensen buffer, pH 7

7. EQUIPMENT

Note; All glassware is cleaned with a mechanical scaling brush, then left
overnight in a chromic acid bath (CrO_3-H_2SO_4) and finally rinsed with
double distilled water.

7.1.   Mechanical scaling brush
7.2.   Polytron tissue grinder powered by overhead stirrer.
7.3.   Automatic pipettes
7.4.   Refrigerated centrifuge

7.5.   Reciprocating shaker
7.6.   Centrifuge tubes, 10 mL with PTFE screw-caps
7.7.   Water bath with nitrogen evaporator facility.
7.8.   Vortex
7.9.   Rotavapor with water bath.
7.10.   Glass derivatization tubes, 10 mL, with seals/stoppers
7.11.   Glass Pasteur capillary pipettes.
7.12.   Quick-fit type glass tubes with stoppers. (10 mL and 20 mL)
7.13.   GC-MS equipment.
7.13.1.   Gas chromatograph (Hewlett Packard, type HP 5985 B).
7.13.2.   Moving/Falling needle injection system. One end of the capillary
            column is connected to the glass solid injector 1 mm from the
            bottom of the moving needle. The other end is introduced
            directly near the ion source of the mass spectrometer via a
            1/16th inch stainless-steel transfer line, the temperature of
            which is held at 280°C.
7.13.3.   Mass selective detection operating in NICI mode
7.13.4.   Workstation
7.13.5.   Printer
7.13.6.   GC-column, fused silica capillary column, 25 m x 0.35 mm o.d/0.22
            mm i.d., coated with OV-1701, film thickness 0.11 um.

8.   SAMPLES AND SAMPLING PROCEDURE.

N.B. Attention is drawn to section 6.3.1 and ISO document 78/2-1982(E) and
the following notes derived from Annex II of 2052/VI/84-EN.

8.1. Nature of the Sample; Samples shall be such as to enable the
detection of residues in meat as defined in Directive 64/433/EEC. Failing
this biological fluids may constitute the samples for the detection of
residues.

8.2. Size of Sample; The size of the sample must be large enough to allow
the method to be carried out and to allow repeat analysis where required.

In this method for clenbuterol the amount required for a single
determination is 1 mL plasma or 0.2 g tissue.

8.3. The samples must be taken and packed in such a way as to allow proper
identification in the laboratory.

8.4. The method of packing, preservation and transport must maintain the
integrity of the sample and not prejudice the result of the examination.

Samples for the analysis of clenbuterol must be stored at temperatures
below -18°C.

9.   ANALYTICAL PROCEDURE

9.1.   Extraction procedures.

9.1.1.   Plasma.
9.1.1.1   Plasma samples (1 mL) spiked as stated in 9.2. are placed in 20
            mL screw-capped tubes and mixed with 1 mL pH 12 buffer (6.2.1).
9.1.1.2   6 mL ethyl acetate are added and the mixture shaken for 10 min on
            a reciprocating shaker.
9.1.1.3   Centrifuge for 5 min at 1,600 g.

9.1.1.4   Transfer the organic layer into a 10 mL screw-capped tube containing 1 mL of 0.2M sulphuric acid.

9.1.1.5   The mixture is shaken for 10 min on a reciprocating shaker and centrifuged for 5 min at 1,600 g.

9.1.1.6   The organic phase is evaporated under vacuum and to the residual aqueous phase 4 mL of ethyl acetate-hexane (2:1, v/v) is added.

9.1.1.7   The mixture is shaken for a short period and then gently centrifuged. The upper organic layer is discarded.

9.1.1.8   The sulphuric acid phase is made alkaline with 1 mL 2M sodium hydroxide and extracted with 5 mL ethyl acetate.

9.1.1.9   The organic solvent is decanted into a 10 mL glass tube (7.10) and evaporated to dryness at 40°C under nitrogen.

9.1.2.   Tissue Samples.

9.1.2.1   Tissue samples are accurately weighed and placed in a 20 mL glass tube with 3 mL Sorensen buffer, pH 7, (6.2.2.) and 500 pg[^{2}H$_9$] clenbuterol. The sample is homogenised for 1 min with a Polytron homogeniser (7.2).

9.1.2.2   After centrifuging for 15 min at 1,800 g the supernatant is decanted into another 20 mL screw-capped tube. The aqueous phase is made alkaline by adding 1 mL 2M sodium hydroxide and then extracted with 6 mL ethyl acetate by shaking for 10 min on a reciprocating shaker.

9.1.2.3   The samples are then processed as for the extraction of plasma, steps 9.1.1.3. to 9.1.1.9.

9.2.   Spiking of Quality Controls.

9.2.1.   Plasma; Aliquots of drug-free human plasma are fortified with 50 μL of a 10 ng per mL [^{2}H$_9$] clenbuterol solution in water (6.2.5) and various amounts of clenbuterol ranging from 5 - 250 pg per mL. Blanks are prepared by adding only the [^{2}H$_9$] clenbuterol to 1 ml plasma.

9.2.2.   Tissues; 0.2 g tissue are fortified with 50 μL of a 10 ng per mL [^{2}H$_9$] clenbuterol solution in water (6.2.5) and various amounts of clenbuterol ranging from 10 - 500 pg per g. Blanks are prepared by adding only the [^{2}H$_9$] clenbuterol to 0.2 g tissue.

9.3.   Derivatization.
To eliminate moisture in the derivatization tubes, the insides of the tubes (7.10) are rinsed with acetone previously dried over anhydrous sodium sulphate. The acetone is evaporated and 40 μL PFPA added. The tubes are tightly capped and stood at room temperature until analysis.

9.4.   GC-MS.

9.4.1.   GC settings:

9.4.1.1

injection volume	1 μL of derivatized sample (9.2).
injection temperature	290°C
injection mode	moving/falling needle
starting temperature	180°C
gradient	8°C/min
first firal temperature	230°C/min
gradient	20°C/min
second firal temperature	290°C/min

9.4.1.2   The retention times of clenbuterol is 5.22 min and the $[^2H_9]$
          clenbuterol 5.16 min (Data from Girault and Fourtillan, 1990)

9.4.2.   MS settings

          Ioniser;
          Mode   negative ion - chemical ionization
          Temperature   180°C
          Emission current   300 μA
          Electron energy   100 eV

          ions monitored   m/2 = 368 (clenbuterol)
                               m/2 = 377 (internal standard)
          Reagent gas - methane at source pressure ca. 0.8 Torr

          Tuning; The instrument is tuned using the fragments m/Z 414, 595,
          and 633 from the perfluorotributylamine calibrant gas..

9.4.3.   Determination of clenbuterol content.
          The NICI spectra are recorded for Clenbuterol and $[^2H_9]$
          clenbuterol by scanning the quadrupole mass filter every 1.1 sec
          from m/Z 250 to 450. Determination of clenbuterol is performed
          by focusing the instrument in the single-ion monitoring mode in
          order to measure the fragments of m/Z 368 (clenbuterol) and 377
          ($[^2H_9]$ clenbuterol). The dwell time is 100 msec for each mass
          range.

9.4.4.   Confirmation of Clenbuterol (see 10.1).

10.0.   CALCULATION OF RESULTS

10.1.   Calibration Curves.
The procedure used for the calculation of results (quantification) uses a
linear calibration curve which can be fitted with the $[^2H_9]$ clenbuterol-
ratio as dependent and the concentration of standard (e.g. pg/injection
vial) as the dependent variable.
This procedure using 7 points yields linear calibration curves (r = 0.9998)
which give an intercept deviating not significantly from 0. The slopes of
the plasma calibration curves were reproducible from day to day, with a
relative standard deviation of 4%. (Data from Girault and Fourtillan,
1990)

10.2.   Recoveries.
The yield of the extraction was about 80% and all sources of variability
are reduced by including $[^2H_9]$ clenbuterol as internal standard.

10.3.   Accuracy and Precision.
The precision of the method was measured by Girault and Fourtillan, (1990),
in tissues and plasma and the results are shown in table 1.

Table 1.

Sample	Theoretical concentration (pg/mL or g)	n	Mean Observed concentration (pg/mL or g)	SD	CV (%)	Error (%)
Plasma						
	200	10	196.3	5.89	3.0	-1.9
	100	5	99.3	3.41	3.4	-0.7
	20	5	20.0	0.74	3.7	+0.2
	5	10	4.8	0.61	12.8	-4.3
Tissue (kidney)						
	200	10	212.7	15.6	7.3	+6.4
	20	10	18.9	1.7	9.0	-5.5

10.1. CONFIRMATION

For confirmation the simultaneous detection of at least four ions response
ratios have to be calculated for both standards and unknown compounds.

The ions are shown below for the monofluoroacyl derivatives.

	M.W	M.WD.	----------Ions----------				
clenbuterol-PFA	276	404	368	297	312	350	404
[^{2}H$_9$] clenbuterol-PFA	285	413	377	297	313	359	413

M.W.= molecular Wt. of pure compound
M.WD = molecular weight after derivatization

For identification according to the EC-criteria it is mandatory that at
least 4 ions are monitored. Each response should fulfil the criterium that
the maximum exceeds the average noise $\pm$ 3 SD. If this criterium is
fulfilled for all ions monitored the 3 different ratios are calculated. The
same ratios are calculated for the standard analyte, preferably at the corresponding concentration. For positive identification the responses
obtained for the unknown samples should all be within $\pm$ 10% of the average
value for the standard.
Note: Frequently the variability of the MS-equipment does not allow this
criterium to be strictly applied. In this case the criterium is replaced by
a criterium based on the experimental variability. The response ratios for
the unknown sample should be within the corresponding standard $\pm$ 3 SD.

11.   SPECIAL CASES.
12.   NOTES ON PROCEDURE.
13.   QUALITY CONTROL. STANDARDS, REFERENCE MATERIALS AND ANTIBODIES.
14.   TEST REPORT.
15.   LIST OF ABBREVIATIONS
A list of the most important abbreviations is given in Annex I section 12.
16.   FLOW DIAGRAM.

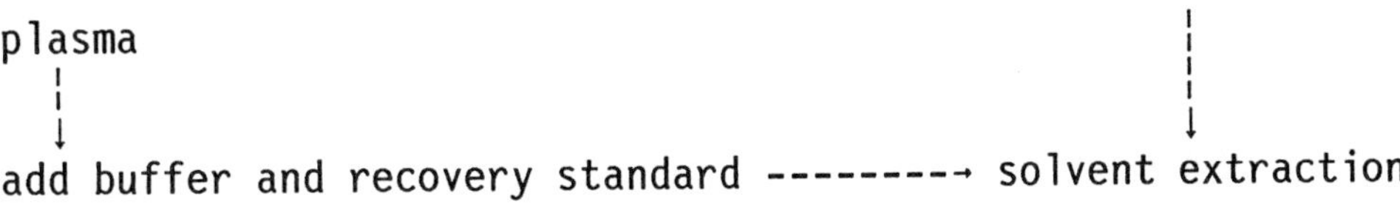

Cy 2.3.   ß-AGONISTS - A METHOD FOR CONFIRMING THE DETECTION OF ß-AGONISTS IN BOVINE URINE BY GC-MS IN THE POSITIVE CHEMICAL IONISATION MODE FOR THE TRIMETHYLSILYL DERIVATIVES.

1.   SCOPE

This method of analysis describes the confirmation of the presence of individual β-agonists in samples of urine of veal calves and adult cattle. The method is used officially in France and is carried out in compliance with the Residues Directive (86/469/EEC).

2.   FIELD OF APPLICATION

The method is used to confirm positives found during the routine screening of urine from veal calves and adult cattle. The method is used to confirm the presence of residues of clenbuterol, clenpenterol, hydroxymethyl-clenbuterol, salbutamol, terbutaline, cimaterol, cimbuterol, mabuterol, mapenterol, tulobuterol, fenoterol and ractopamine.

The detection limit, defined as a signal noise ratio >3 is below 1 μg per L

It is important to note that the method is applied specifically to the confirmation of an already suspected known ß-agonist. Thus the analysis is targeted at compounds with specific retention times on the GC and with known spectra.

3.   REFERENCES

Commission Decision, 93/256/EEC, laying down the methods for detecting residues of substances having a hormonal or thyrostatic action. [OJ. № L.118, 14.4.93. pp 64-74]

Montrade, M-P., Le Bizec, B., Monteau, F., Siliart, B. and André, F. (1993), Multi-residue analysis for ß-agonistic drugs in urine of meat-producing animals by gas chromatography - mass spectrometry. Anal. Chim. Acta. <u>275</u>, 253-268

Montrade, M-P., Le Bizec, B. and André, F. (1992), Methode de recherche urinaire (screening) d'agonistes ß-adrenergiques par chromatographie gazeuse couplee à la spectrometie de masse (GC-MS) en mode impact electronique. Document LDH/92/01 Lab. Dosage Hormonaux, Nantes, DGAL/SDHA/№.92-8066

Montrade, M-P., Le Bizec, B. and André, F. (1993), Research and identification of ß-agonistic drugs in biological samples by gas chromatography coupled with mass spectrometry. Confirmation method in positive ion chemical ionisation. Document LDH/93/05 Lab. Dosage Hormonaux, Nantes, DGAL/SDHA/№.93-8065.

4.   DEFINITIONS

ß-agonists content is taken to be the amount of β-agonists in the substance in question determined according to the described method and expressed as ug β-agonists per litre of test sample (urine).

5.   PRINCIPLE

The method comprises 6 stages;
 1. hydrolysis of conjugates
 2. methanol precipitation (optional), particulary for "dirty" urine of
     adult cattle
 3. extract purification and concentration using mixed solid-phase
     extraction (SPE) chromatography
 4. derivatisation
 5. detection by GC-MS in positive chemical ionisation mode using methane
     as the react gas
 6. calculation and evaluation of results

6.   MATERIALS

Note: The reagents (and equipment) for which examples of their source are
quoted are known to be satisfactory, nevertheless reagents and equipment
from other sources may be equally suitable. All the reagents should be of
analytical grade or better.

6.1   Reference compounds and Standards.

6.1.1   The following standard compounds are used.

Clenbuterol hydrochloride (Interchim, Montlucon, France)
Salbutamol hemisulphate, Terbutaline hemisulphate, metoprolol tartrate and
meterproterenol hemisulphate (Sigma)
Cimaterol, Clenpenterol (NAB 760), mabuterol, fenoterol hydrobromide and
hydroxymethyl clenbuterol (NA1141) (Boehringer Ingleheim)
Tulobuterol hydrochloride (Abbott)
Ractopamine hydrochloride (Eli Lilly)
Cimbuterol and marpenterol were synthesised by Chem Dept, University of
Rennes, France

Isotope labelled internal standards, clenbuterol-d6 and salbutamol-d6 were
obtained as a gift from RIKILT, Wageningen, The Netherlands. It is
foreseen that these reference compounds will be made available through the
Measurement and Testing Programme of DGXII.

6.2   Chemicals
6.2.1   *Helix pomatia* juice (ß-glucuronidase-arylsulfatase, Merck-4114)
6.2.2   Glacial acetic acid   (Panreac - 131008 or Merck-62)
6.2.3   Ultra-pure water (>14 M Ω.cm)
6.2.4   Methanol (Carlo-Erba RS CLHP-412002 or Merck-6009)
6.2.5   Ethyl acetate (Merck ZA-9623)
6.2.6   32% Ammonium hydroxide (Merck 5426)
6.2.7   1*M* Potassium hydroxide (Merck ZA-9018920)
6.2.8   1*M* Acetic acid
6.2.9   N-O-bis(trimethylsilyl)trifluoracetamide (BSTFA) (Regisil-270111
          or FLUKA - 15244)
6.2.10   Toluene (Fluka - 89677) on molecular sieve.
6.2.11   Sodium acetate (Merck ZA-6268)
6.2.12   Potassium dihydrogen phosphate (Merck ZA-4873)
6.2.13   Nitrogen (dried over silica gel)
6.2.14   Helium (very high purity) (N55, Carboxyque)
6.2.15   Methane (very high purity) (N45, Carboxyque)

6.3   Solutions
6.3.1   ß-agonists. Prepare stock solutions of the standards (6.1.1) in methanol (1 g per L and 100 µg per L) and store at -18°C.
6.3.2   ß-agonists. Prepare working solutions by dilution of stock solutions (6.3.1) with methanol to final concentrations of 10 µg and 1µg per L. Store at -18°C.
6.3.3   2M Acetate buffer, pH 5.2, for hydrolysis of conjugates. Dissolve 164 g sodium acetate (6.2.11) in 900 mL water (6.2.3) and adjust the pH to 5.2 ± 0.1 with glacial acetic acid (6.2.2). Make up to 1 L with water and store at +4°C. Use for up to 1 month.
6.3.4   0.1M Phosphate buffer, pH 6. Dissolve 13.6 ± 0.1 g potassium dihydrogen phosphate (6.2.12) in 900 mL water (6.2.3) and adjust the pH to 6.0 ± 0.1 with 1M potassium hydroxide (6.2.7). Make up to 1 L with water and store at +4°C. Use for up to 1 month.
6.3.5   Mix ethyl acetate and 32% ammonium hydroxide 97:3 (v/v). 100 mL does 16 samples. Stir/agitate the mixture prior to use and then place into an ultra-sonic bath during step 9.13.3.

7.0   EQUIPMENT
7.1.   Centrifuge
7.2   Rotary evaporator
7.3   Vortex mixer
7.4   pH meter
7.5   Pipettes
7.6   Balance
7.7   Vacuum filtration system (Vac-Elut from Analytichem International)
7.8   Ultra-sonic bath
7.9   Magnetic stirrer/agitator
7.10   Conical reaction vials for derivatisation
7.11   Heating block for reaction vials 7.10
7.12   Heating block with evaporation system
7.13   SPE-Columns; CLEAN SCREEN DAU (Worldwide monitoring - Horsham, PA, USA and sold by Technicol, Stockport, Cheshire, UK). These columns of 6 mL volume contain 500 mg of a mixed phase support which has hydrophobic and ion-exchange properties.
7.14   GC-MS
7.14.1 GC; GC Hewlett packard 5890.
        Capillary column, 30 m X 0.25 mm i.d. with SE-30 (or OV-1 or HP-1) stationary phase of 0.25 µm thickness.
        Injection mode; splitless over 1 minute
        Injection volume; 2 µL
        Injector temp. 250°C; Transfer temp. 280°C
        Temp. programme;

                        18° C/min   *5° C/min*
        70°C (2 min) -----------> 200°C (0 min) ---------> 245°C (0 min)

            25° C/min
        ---------------> 300°C (12 min)

        Gas; Helium at 1 mL per min and 5 psi.

7.14.2 MS; Hewlett Packard 5971 with UNIX station.
        Positive Chemical ionisation mode (70 eV)
        Source temp. 190° ± 5°C

Cy 2.3/3

The reactant gas is methane:- regulate the flow of reactant gas
in such a way as to obtain a pressure in the ion source of
6×10^{-5} to 1×10^{-4} Torr, according to the functioning
conditions of the apparatus.

8.   SAMPLES AND SAMPLING PROCEDURE.

N.B. Attention is drawn to section 6.3.1 and to ISO document 78/2-1982 and
also the following notes derived from Annex II of 2052/VI/84-EN and EEC
93/256.

8.1.   Nature of the Sample; Samples shall be such as to enable the
          detection of residues in urine as defined in Directive
          64/433/EEC.
8.2.   Size of Sample; The size of the sample must be large enough to
          allow the method to be carried out and to allow repeat analysis
          where required. Each analysis needs a 10 mL sample.

8.3.   The samples must be taken and packed in such a way as to allow
          proper identification in the laboratory.

8.4.   The method of packing, preservation and transport must maintain
          the integrity of the sample and not prejudice the result of the
          examination.
          Samples for the analysis of ß-agonists must be stored at
          temperatures below -18°C.

9.0.   PROCEDURE

Note; The steps 9.1 to 9.20 are identical to those reported in the
screening method, M.Sg. v.v.

9.1   Thaw the primary samples and transfer more than 10 mL to a
          centrifuge tube. Centrifuge at 3000 rpm for 15 min. Pipette 10
          mL to a screw-topped tube (e.g. scintillation counting vial).
9.2   Add 60 ng metoprolol as internal standard to all urines including
          two blank urines.
9.3   To one of the blank urines (9.2) add 40 ng (equiv. 4 ppb)
          tulobuterol, fenoterol and ractopamine and 20 ng (equiv. 2 ppb)
          of the other ß-agonist standards (6.3.2).
9.4   Add 1 mL acetate buffer (6.3.3) and check the pH is about 5.2 $\pm$
          0.3. Adjust the pH to about 5.2 with acetic acid if necessary.
9.5   Add 50 μL *Helix pomatia* juice (6.2.1) and incubate overnight at
          50°C in a water bath or oven.
Steps 9.6 to 9.11 are optional and can be used for urines from adult
cattle.
9.6   Transfer the hydrolysed urines to rotary evaporation flasks.
9.7   Add 25 mL methanol. Evaporate the methanol using a rotary
          evaporator and a water bath at about 45°C.
9.8   Concentrate the aqueous phase to about 3 mL.
9.9   Transfer the aqueous phase to a test tube with a pasteur pipette
          and rinse out the flask twice with 5 mL phosphate buffer (6.3.4).
9.10   Centrifuge at 3500 rpm for about 10 min. A precipitate should
          form on the tube.
9.11   Check and adjust the pH to 6.0 ± 0.3 if necessary. Use all the
          clear aqueous phase for step 9.13.

9.12   If steps 9.6 to 9.11 were not carried out add 4 mL phosphate
            buffer (6.3.4) to the hydrolysate, adjust the pH to 6.0 (final
            volume to 15 mL.
9.13   Column extraction;
9.13.1   Place the columns on the Vac-Elut system and successively rinse
            with; 2 mL methanol; 2 mL water (6.2.3); 2 mL phosphate buffer
            (6.3.4).
9.13.2   Transfer the clear extracts (9.11 or 9.12) with a pasteur pipette
            to the top of the column and allow to drain slowly using slight
            negative (ca.12 cm Hg) pressure.
9.13.3   Rinse the columns using negative pressure of about 40 cm Hg with
            1 mL 1M acetic acid (6.2.8) and allow to dry before rinsing with
            6 mL methanol by applying a strong vacuum.
9.13.4   Place the ethyl acetate / ammonium hydroxide solution (6.3.5) in
            an ultra-sonic bath to agitate the mixture during step 9.13.3.
9.13.5   Elute the analytes with 6 mL the ethyl acetate / ammonium
            hydroxide solution (6.3.5)
9.14   Evaporate the eluate with nitrogen using an evaporation system
            and a heating block at 40 ± 5°C.
9.15   Dissolve the residue in 200 µL methanol with vigorous vortexing.
9.16   Transfer the solution to a reaction vial.
9.17   Dissolve and transfer to the reaction vial any remaining residue
            with a further 100 µL methanol and vortexing.
9.18   Evaporate the methanol to dryness using a heating block at 40° ±
            5°C.
9.19   Derivatisation
9.19.1   Add 50 µL BSTFA (6.2.9) and vortex.
9.19.2   Place vials in heating block at 75°C ± 5°C for 90 min.
9.19.3   Transfer the vials to a heating block at 40° ± 5°C. Allow the
            vials and block to cool to room temperature (25°C) then evaporate
            to dryness with nitrogen.
9.19.4   Add 25 µL toluene (6.2.10) and vortex vigorously.
9.19.5   The vials may be stored in a refrigerator at +4°C.
9.20   Inject 2 µL of 9.19.5 into the GC-MS.

9.21   The GC-MS is run in the positive chemical ionisation mode seeking four major characteristic ions for each suspected ß-agonist. The major ions and the retention times of the derivatives of the ß-agonists are shown in table 1.

Table 1.

ß-agonist	N	RT (min)	(M+H)	(M-15)	(M-89)	Other	Adducts
Tulobuterol	1	9.43	300	284	210		328
Mabuterol	1	10.61	383	367	293	363	411
Mapenterol	1	11.42	397	381	307	377	425
Terbutaline	3	12.29	442	426	352	356	470
Clenbuterol	1	12.56	349	333	259		377
Cimaterol	1	12.69	292	276	202		320 332
Cimbuterol	1	12.97	306	290	216		334 346
Salbutamol	3	13.03	456	440	366	394 369 350	
Cimaterol	2	13.41	364	348	274	292	392 404
Metoprolol (I.S)	1	13.49	340	324			
Clenpenterol	1	13.63	363	347	273		391
Cimbuterol	2	13.66	378	362	288	306	406 418
Hydroxymethyl-clenbuterol	2	15.30	437	421	347	313 387	465
Fenoterol	4	20.73	592	576	502	236 412 357	
Ractopamine	3	20.88	518	502	428	250 456	

N is the number of TMS groups. RT are the retention times recorded in an analysis at LDH, Nantes.

Adducts are ions induced by the gas which are useful to select.

Note. Experience shows that it is rarely possible to obtain sufficient information on at least four ions using this PCI mode of mass spectrometry. Therefore it is recommended that the spectra obtained using EI mode are also taken into account (for the method using the same extraction procedure and gas chromatographic conditions but with detection in the EI mode see method Sg 2.1).

10.0   INTERPRETATION OF RESULTS

10.1   Validity of Analysis; The criteria set out in EC Decision 256
          must be fulfilled especially the following;-

10.1.1   The relative retention times for the TMS derivatives of the
          standard analytes in the appropriate matrix and the suspected ß-
          agonist must be the same.
10.1.2   The relative intensities of the selected ions to the base peak
          must be same as in the assay of spiked blank urines and of
          standards.
10.1.3   The ions for the internal standard (metoprolol-monoTMS) **must** be
          present at the correct retention time.
10.1.4   The analysis of the blank urine containing the internal standard
          must show NO evidence of carry-over of ß-agonists from the GC-MS
          system. This is a check for contamination of the system.

11.   SPECIAL CASES

12.   NOTES ON PROCEDURE.

The retention times (RT) of the TMS derivatives differ slightly from those
in the screening method.

13.   QUALITY CONTROLS

See section 8 of manual detailing the RMs for the ß-agonists.

14.   TEST REPORT

15.   LIST OF ABBREVIATIONS

A full list of abbreviations is given in Annex I, Section 12

16.   FLOW DIAGRAM

```
          hydrolysis
   URINE -----------> METHANOL PRECIPITATION--------> EXTRACT by SPE Chrom.
                                                                   |
                                                                   |
                                                                   |
                    (PCI mode)                                     |
   INTERPRET RESULTS <----------- GC-MS <------------ TMS DERIVATIVES
                    (methane)
```

Cy 3.1. SULPHONAMIDES - CONFIRMATION OF SULPHONAMIDES BY GAS CHROMATOGRAPHY-MASS SPECTROMETRY

WARNING AND SAFETY PRECAUTIONS

SAFETY

1. Organic solvents - all organic solvents must be treated as potentially hazardous and all procedures using them must be performed in a fume cupboard.
2. Ammonia   - use only in a fume cupboard and wear safety glasses.
3. Homogenising   - perform in a fume cupboard to avoid aerosols.
4. Dry ice   - wear thick hide gloves and face shield. Dry ice   can cause burns and frostbite if in contact with the skin.
5. Diazomethane

ALL REACTIONS INVOLVING THE PREPARATION AND USE OF DIAZOMETHANE MUST BE CARRIED OUT IN A FUME CUPBOARD. PROTECTIVE CLOTHING MUST BE WORN.

DO NOT USE EQUIPMENT WITH GROUND GLASS JOINTS - THERE IS A POTENTIAL EXPLOSION HAZARD!

You should ensure that you and anyone else in the room are aware of the potential explosion hazards associated with diazomethane. All diazomethane generated MUST be destroyed immediately if it is not being used for direct methylation. This is achieved by bubbling through dilute HCl. All glassware used should be rinsed in HCl before it leaves the fume cupboard.

FIRST AID

1. Solvents, acids and alkalis in contact with skin - wash with copious amounts of cold water. Splashes in the eye - irrigate with water and seek medical attention immediately.
2. Cuts - seek assistance of first aider immediately.
3. Burns and frostbite - run affected part under cold water (burns) or tepid water (frostbite) for 10 minutes and seek medical attention.

1.   INTRODUCTION

<u>Purpose</u>
The confirmation of the presence of sulphonamides in samples taken from farm animals in compliance with the Residues Directive 86/469/EEC.

<u>Background</u>
Sulphonamides are antimicrobial compounds, which have been developed to combat disease caused by viruses, bacteria, protozoa or fungi. Used in sub-therapeutic doses, they may also exhibit a growth promoting action and so are added to feedstuffs to increase productivity.

Residues of these substances may reach the consumer, but as some can induce hypersensitivity reactions in consumers and one is a suspected carcinogen, the tolerance level of these substances in food for human consumption has been set at 0.1 ppm by the CVMP. The monitoring of sulphonamide residues in meat is carried out to ensure that withdrawal periods are being observed and that residues do not reach the consumer.

Cy 3.1/1

Residue levels are monitored in tissues taken at slaughter under the National Surveillance Scheme for Residues in Meat. From 1 January 1989 this monitoring was carried out in compliance with the Residues Directive (86/469/EEC). In the UK scheme kidney has been chosen as the tissue for analysis.

The samples are initially screened by TLC or ELISA (refer to SOP for the method). The CVL, UK confirms positive samples by either an HPLC method or by this GC-MS method.

1.   SCOPE

This method of analysis describes the determination of the total content of sulphadimidine in pig kidney.

2.   FIELD OF APPLICATION.

The method is described to be used for porcine kidney. The detection limit, for sulphadimidine is 100 ug/kg or litre of sample.

3.   REFERENCES.

Commission Decision, 93/256/EEC, laying down the methods for detecting residues of substances having a hormonal or thyrostatic action. [OJ. Nº L.118, 14.4.93. pp 64-74]

2052/VI/84 File 6.11 II-4, Scientific Veterinary Committee, Working Group - "Reference Methods for Residues", General Criteria for the establishment of Reference Methods for the Detection of Residues.

ISO Standard 78/2-1982 Layout for standards - Part 2: Standard for Chemical Analysis

MAFF (1987) Working Party on Veterinary Residues in Animal Products. Food Surveillance Paper No. 22.

Takatsuki, E and Kikuchi, T., (1990), Gas chromatographic-mass spectrometric determination of six sulfonamide residues in egg and animal tissues. J.A.O.A.C. _73_, 886-892

Simpson, R.M., Suhre, F.B. and Shafer, J.w. (1985), Quantitative gas chromatographic-mass spectrometric assay of five sulfonamide residues in animal tissue. J.A.O.A.C. _68_, 23-26

Matusik, J.E., Sternal, R.S., Barnes, C.J. Sphon, J.A. (1990) Confirmation of identity by gas chromatography/tandem mass spectrometry of sulfathiazole, sulfamethazine, sulfachloropyridazine, and sulfademethoxine from bovine or swine liver extracts after quantisation by gas chromatography/electron capture detection.

4.   DEFINITIONS.

Sulphadimidine content is taken to mean the amount of sulphadimidine in kidney determined according to the described method and expressed as ug sulphadimidine per kg test sample.

5.0   PRINCIPLE

Dried extracts of kidney or muscle, cleaned up by a Bond-Elut method, are methylated with diazomethane and the methylated extracts are subjected to analysis by gas chromatography-mass spectrometry (GC-MS).

6.   MATERIALS

6.1.   Chemicals

6.1.1. Diazald   Aldrich Chemical Co Ltd
6.1.2. Potassium hydroxide   AR grade
6.1.3. Diethyl ether   Distol grade
6.1.4. Ethyl digol (carbitol)   Technical grade, BDH
6.1.5. Hydrochloric acid   AR grade
6.1.6. Methanol   Distol grade
6.1.7. Acetone   Distol grade

6.2.   Standards

Solid sulphonamides may be obtained from Sigma. A mixed standard of concentration = 1 mg/mL of each sulphonamide in methanol should be prepared using available sulphonamides. At present CVL are using: sulphamethazine, sulphamerazine, sulphanilamide, sulphapyridine, sulphathiazole, sulphadiazine, sulphaguanidine, sulphachloropyridazine, sulphadimethoxine and sulphaquinoxaline.
Working standards of concentrations = 0.1 ug/mL, 1 ug/mL, 10 ug/mL and 100 ug/mL should be prepared by dilution from the stock.

7.   EQUIPMENT

7.1.   Mini diazald apparatus (Aldrich Chemical Co Ltd)
7.2.   Separating funnel with teflon stopcock 125 mL
7.3.   Centrifuge tubes
7.4.   Water bath
7.5.   Manifold supplying oxygen-free nitrogen
7.6.   Mass spectrometer; Finnigan MAT, coupled to a gas chromatograph
        and linked to an INCOS data system

8.   SAMPLES AND SAMPLING PROCEDURE.

N.B. Attention is drawn to section 6.3.1 and ISO document 78/2-1982 and the following notes derived from Annex II of 2052/VI/84-EN.

8.1. Nature of the Sample; Samples shall be such as to enable the detection of residues in meat as defined in Directive 64/433/EEC. Failing this biological fluids or faeces may constitute the samples for the detection of residues.

8.2. Size of Sample; The size of the sample must be large enough to allow the reference method to be carried out and to allow repeat analysis where required. In this method for sulphadimidine the sizes shall not be less than 20 g kidney.

9.0.   PROCEDURE

9.1.   Sample preparation

Samples are extracted via a Bond-Elut method and the extracts taken to dryness. Mixed standards of varying concentrations are also taken to dryness. Both standards and samples are resuspended in 1 mL of methanol.

9.1.1.   Weigh 2.5 g thawed and chopped sample into a 30 mL tube.

9.1.2.   Add 6 mL of 0.1M acetic acid:acetone mixture (1:1 v/v) and add 12 mL ethyl acetate. Homogenise for 1 minute and centrifuge at 2500 rpm for 15 minutes.

9.1.3.   Transfer supernatant to another 30 mL tube and repeat Step 2 on the tissue pellet. Combine supernatants and place tubes in a rack.

9.1.4.   Place rack into cardice box until aqueous layer is completely frozen (at least 15 minutes).

9.1.5.   Decant ethyl acetate into another 30 mL tube ready for clean-up.

9.1.6.   Using vacuum apparatus prepare NH_2 Bond Elut column by washing with 1 column volume of hexane. Prepare SCX Bond Elut column by washing with 1 column volume of hexane followed by two column volumes of 5% acetic acid in ethyl acetate. (**N.B.** Do **NOT** let SCX column run dry.) Assemble the columns in tandem.

9.1.7.   Transfer the ethyl acetate extract to the reservoir and draw it through the assembly by vacuum.

9.1.8.   Wash the assembly with 2 column volumes of methanol (ca 6 mL).

9.1.9.1.   Close the vacuum tap and discard the NH_2 column and reservoir.

9.1.10.   Wash the SCX column with 2 column volumes of water followed by 4 column volumes of methanol. (**N.B.** Do **NOT** let SCX column run dry.)

9.1.11.   Remove column from assembly, attach to Luer syringe and elute sulphadimidine with 3 mL of 25% ammonia in methanol into 2 dram vial, using positive pressure.

9.1.12.   Evaporate eluate under N_2 at 45-50°C in a water bath. Dissolve residue in 0.5 mL acetone and transfer with a Pasteur pipette to another vial. Wash with a further 0.5 mL acetone and combine washes. Eluate can then be stored overnight at -20°C if needed.

9.1.13.   Evaporate eluate under N_2 at 45-50°C in a water bath. Dissolve residue in 1 mL methanol.

9.2.   Derivatisation

DO NOT CARRY OUT THIS METHYLATION UNLESS YOU HAVE BEEN TRAINED TO DO SO. READ THE SECTION ON SAFETY AND FOLLOW THE ADVICE GIVEN CAREFULLY.

9.2.1.   Prepare the following reagents:
            (a)   2 g diazald in 20 mL diethyl ether.
            (b)   3 g potassium hydroxide in 3 mL distilled water added to 10 mL ethyl digol.
            (c)   10% hydrochloric acid, 100 mL.

9.2.2.   Set up the Mini-diazald kit according to the maker's instructions.

9.2.3.   Until you are ready to methylate the samples, the diazomethane generated must be passed through the 10% HCl, which will neutralise it. Ensure that the kit is set up for this.

9.2.4.   Place reagent (b) (KOH in H_2O + ethyl digol) in the reaction vessel.

9.2.5.   Place a separatory funnel over the reaction vessel. Reagent (a) (diazald in ether) is placed in this funnel.

9.2.6.   Warm the reaction vessel, by placing in a water bath at 50-60°C.

Slowly and carefully add the diazald solution over a period of
approximately 20 minutes. Once the reaction has started, the
diazomethane is bubbled through the sample and standards until
the solution is coloured yellow. Whenever the diazomethane is
not bubbling through a sample or standard it is important that it
is passed through the HCl to neutralise it.

9.2.7.   Once all of the standards and samples have been derivatised,
check that the diazomethane generated is being passed through the
HCl solution, and allow the reaction to continue until all of the
reagents have been used up.

9.2.8.   Concentrate the derivatives to dryness under nitrogen. Resuspend
in 100 μL acetone.

9.3.   GC-MS Analysis

9.3.1.1. The GC parameters are

COLUMN: J&W fused silica capillary column, SE-54, 15 m x 0.25 mm.
INJECTIONS: 0.5 μL manual injections.
TEMPERATURES: Interface: 270°C;   Injector: 260°C
OVEN TEMPERATURES:

from temp (°C)	to temp (°C)	rate (°C/min)	time (min)	total time (min)
210	210	-	2.0	2.0
210	260	5	-	12.0
260	260	-	4.0	16.0

CARRIER GAS: Helium; flow rate = 1 cm^3/min
injector pressure = 10 psi.

9.3.1.2.
Using an OV-1 column and injecting a mixture of methylated sulphonamides
(10 ng) CVL recorded the following retention times in minutes.

Sulphanilamide, 5.3; Sulphapyridine, 8.8; Sulphathiazole, 9.0;
Sulphadiazine, 9.9; Sulphamerazine, 10.8; Sulphadimidine, 11.8;
Sulphaguanidine, 12.1; Sulphamethizole, 15.2;
Sulphadimethoxine, 15.7; Sulphamethoxypyridazine, 19.7

9.3.2 The mass spectrometry parameters are

IONISER:
   Mode: EI positive ion
   Temperature: 150°C
MANIFOLD TEMPERATURE: 90 (± 5) °C
ELECTRON MULTIPLIER: 1.4 kV
ELECTRON ENERGY: 70 electron volts.
Other parameters should be set up by adjusting the instrument controls to
give the optimum peak height and shape for a suitable calibration compound.
The CVL uses perfluorotributylamine (PFTBA).

9.3.3.   Operate the MS in EI mode and scan between m/z = 50 and 500.
9.3.4.   Analyst the mixed standard (10 ug/100 uL) and identify the peaks
by comparison with those previously set up and stored in a
library. The individual sulphonamides are separated by the GC,
enabling identification on the basis of retention time as well as

9.3.5.   Analyst the remaining samples and standards. It is advisable to:
           (a)   Analyst standards in order of increasing concentration.
           (b)   Inject hexane between each injection.

10.0.   RESULTS

The presence of a sulphonamide in a sample is confirmed if the GC-MS data satisfies the following criteria:

1.   The peak in the sample has the same GC retention time as that in the standard.
2.   The ions present in the mass spectrum of the sample GC peak are identical to those in the mass spectrum of the standard.
3.   The ratios of the ions to one another must be the same as those in the standard.
           The limit of detection of this method for sulphadimidine is 100 μg per kg of tissue.

11.   SPECIAL CASES.

12.   NOTES ON PROCEDURE.

13.   SAMPLE CONTROLS

The quality control sample was obtained from a sample previously analyzed and found to contain sulphadimidine above the maximum residue limit (MRL).

The blank sample was obtained from a sample previously analyzed and found to contain no sulphadimidine. Fortify (spike) with 100 μL of 2.5 μg mL sulphadimidine standard.

14.   TEST REPORT

15.   LIST OF ABBREVIATIONS.

See abbreviations in Annex I, Section 12, of Manual.

16.   FLOW DIAGRAM

```
     SAMPLE  --------> Homogenise------> Bond-Elut extract ----¬
                                                               ¦
                                                               ¦
                                                               ¦
     Calculate results <--------  GC-MS  <--------- Derivatise
```

Cy 3.2. SULPHADIMIDINE - CONFIRMATION AND DETERMINATION OF SULPHADIMIDINE IN PIG KIDNEY OR DIAPHRAGM MUSCLE TISSUE BY HIGH PERFORMANCE LIQUID CHROMATOGRAPHY.

<u>SAFETY</u>
Personal safety. Normal laboratory protective clothing and equipment should be worn.

1.0.   INTRODUCTION
A method is described by which the content of sulphadimidine in pig kidney or diaphragm muscle tissue may be confirmed. This method which is used officially in Northern Ireland is different from the HPLC method (see Cy 3.3) used at the Central Veterinary Laboratory, UK

Sulphadimidine, otherwise known as sulphamethazine is one of a group of antimicrobials called sulphonamides. Its use is widespread in animal production and it is most commonly fed to pigs in their ration at 100 g per tonne. Residues at or above the violative level have been reported in many countries.

2.   SCOPE AND FIELD OF APPLICATION.

This method of analysis describes the determination of the total content of Sulphadimidine in pig kidney or diaphragm muscle tissue.

The detection limit, defined as three times the noise level of the blank determination, is 0.05 mg per kg of kidney or muscle sample for Sulphadimidine.

Twelve kidney or muscle samples including two spiked samples can be analysed in a working day.

3.   REFERENCES.

Commission Decision, 93/256/EEC, laying down the methods for detecting residues of substances having a hormonal or thyrostatic action. [OJ. № L.118, 14.4.93. pp 64-74]

ISO Standard 78/2-1982 Layout for standards - Part 2: Standard for Chemical Analysis

Method based on Standard Operating Procedure SOP B10 17 V.1, (1988) for the confirmatory determination of sulphamethazine in porcine tissue by HPLC;- Veterinary Sciences Division, Stoney Road, Stormont, BELFAST BT4 3SD

Aerts, M.M.L., Beek, W.M.J. and Brinkman, U.A.Th. (1988). Monitoring of Veterinary Drug Residues by a combination of continuous flow techniques and column-switching HPLC. I. Sulphonamides in egg, meat and milk using post-column derivatization with dimethylaminobenzaldehyde. J. Chromat. <u>435</u>, 97-112.

4.   DEFINITIONS.

Sulphadimidine content is taken to mean the amount of Sulphadimidine in the substance in question, regardless of the chemical form, determined according to the described method and expressed as ug Sulphadimidine per kg of test sample.

Cy 3.2/1

5.   PRINCIPLE

The methods comprises 5 stages;-

- Homogenisation of pig kidney samples in buffer

- Extraction of Sulphadimidine with organic solvents

- Partition of Sulphadimidine between hexane and aqueous methanol/acetic
  acid.

- End point determination with HPLC with post column derivatisation.

- The amount of Sulphadimidine is calculated by interpolation from a
standard curve and taking into account the recovery of Sulphadimidine,
especially from tissue samples.

6.0   MATERIALS

N.B.:   The reagents for which examples of their source are quoted are
known to be satisfactory, nevertheless reagents from other sources may be
equally suitable.

6.1   Reagents
6.1.1   Chloroform (Rathburn Chemicals Ltd)
6.1.2   Methanol (HPLC Grade, Rathburn Chemicals Ltd)
6.1.3   Acetone (Rathburn Chemicals Ltd)
6.1.4   Hexane (Rathburn Chemicals Ltd)
6.1.5   Deionised water prepared using equipment 7.16.
6.1.6   N, N-Dimethyl-Aminobenzaldehyde - Ehrlichs reagent (Sigma
        Chemical Co, Cat No D8904).
6.1.7   Glacial Acetic acid (BDH Lab. Supplies, Cat. No. 27013).
6.1.8   Sulphamethazine crystalline sodium salt (Sigma Chemical Co., PO
        Box 14508 St Louis, MO63178 USA, Cat No S-55637).

6.2   Solutions
6.2.1   50% Methanol (6.1.2) v/v deionised water (6.1.5)
6.2.2   50% methanol in 2% acetic acid. Mix 125 mL methanol with 5 mL
        glacial acetic acid in a 250 mL graduated flask. Make up to the
        mark with water and mix.
6.2.3   N, N-Dimethyl-Aminobenzaldehyde Reagent
        Acetic Acid (6.1.7)   125 mL
        Methanol (6.1.2)   75 mL
        Deionised water (6.1.5)   50 mL
        N, N-Dimethyl-Aminobenzaldehyde (6.1.6)   3.75 g
        Before adding the N, N-Dimethylbenzaldehyde degas the solution
        using the equipment described in (7.4) for 2 minutes,
6.2.4   2% Acetic Acid
        Acetic Acid (6.1.7)   10 mL
        Deionised water (6.1.5)   490 mL
6.2.5   HPLC Mobile Phase
        2% Acetic acid (6.2.4)   325 mL
        Methanol (6.1.2)   175 mL
        (degas for 2 minutes (7.4)
6.2.6   Wash solution. Add 200 mL of water to 800 mL methanol in a 1 L
        measuring cylinder. Mix and degas as in 6.2.3.
6.2.7   Mix equal volumes of chloroform and acetone with stirring.

6.3   Standards
6.3.1   Stock standard
          Dissolve an accurately weighed (7.2) quantity of sulphamethazine
          (6.1.8) in Methanol (6.1.2) to give a solution of 1 mg to
          sulphamethazine per mL using a 100 ml volumetric flask (7.12).
          Store at +4°C. (7.5).
6.3.2.1   Intermediate standards. 100 μg per mL. Dilute the 1 mL stock
          standard to 10 mL with methanol. Use a volumetric flask.
6.3.2.2   Intermediate standards. 10 μg per mL. Dilute the 1 mL stock
          standard to 100 mL with methanol. Use a volumetric flask.
6.3.2.3   Working standard. 1 μg per mL.
          Take 1 mL of intermediate standard ((6.3.2.1) and make up to 100
          mL with 50% Methanol in 2% acetic acid (6.2.2). Prepare daily and
          store at +4°C.

7.0   EQUIPMENT

7.1   Balance top-pan (Sartorius, Gottingen, Germany model L610D).
7.2   Balance analytical (Sartorius, Gottingen, Germany model R160P).
7.3   Magnetic Stirrer (Gallenkamp model 300).
7.4   Degassing apparatus.
7.5   Refrigerator +4°C (Williams Refrigeration Ltd, Kings Lynn, UK).
7.6   Fume cupboards (Nordia, Lab Design, Walthamstow, London, E17 6AB.
7.7   Test tubes, 10 mL round bottomed with ground glass stoppers.
7.8   Round bottomed flasks, 150 mL
7.9   Polyethylene bottles, 125 mL, with wide mouth
7.10   Graduated glass pipettes, 10 mL and 25 mL (FSA Lab Supplies, Cat
          Nos G519 and G520).
7.11   Measuring cylinders, 250 mL and 1 L (FSA Lab Supplies)
7.12   10 mL and 100 mL volumetric flask (FSA Lab Supplies).
7.13   Pasteur pipettes
7.14   Chromacol microvials, 200 μL.
7.15   Water pump
7.16   Millipore RO60 reverse osmosis and milli Q deionised water
          system. (Millipore SA, 67120 Molsheim, France, Cat Nos
          ZFRONCO6and PFOO671/U respectively).
7.17   Silversun heavy duty homogeniser
7.18   Centrifuge, Sorvall RT 6000 refrigerated.
7.19   Filtering equipment, Buchner funnel, Hartley pattern with PTFE
          perforated disc.
7.20   Filter paper, Whatman glass GF/C microfibre filters (7.0 cm)
7.21   Ultrasonic bath, Ultrasonics Ltd/Decon FS 200

7.22   HPLC System
7.22.1   Waters type 501 pump
7.22.2   Waters Model 455LC Spectrophotometer set at 450 nm
7.22.3   Lloyd Instrument CR 650 pen recorder
7.22.4   Whatman Particil 50DS - 3 column (25 cm x 4.6 mm i.d.)
7.22.5   Hitachi AS-2000 autosampler fitted with 50 μL loop
7.22.6   Post column equipment. Reaction coil 10 ft length of Teflon
          Tubing (0.023 ins i.d.). Low dead volume T-piece mixing chamber

8.   SAMPLES AND SAMPLING PROCEDURE.

N.B. Attention is drawn to section 6.3.1 and to ISO document 78/2-1982 and
also the following notes derived from Annex II of 2052/VI/84-EN and EEC
93/256.

8.1. Nature of the Sample; Samples shall be such as to enable the detection of residues in meat as defined in Directive 64/433/EEC. Failing this biological fluids or faeces may constitute the samples for the detection of residues.

8.2. Size of Sample; The size of the sample must be large enough to allow the method to be carried out and to allow repeat analysis where required.

8.3. The samples must be taken and packed in such a way as to allow proper identification in the laboratory.

8.4. The method of packing, preservation and transport must maintain the integrity of the sample and not prejudice the result of the examination. Samples for the analysis of thyreostatic substances must be stored and transported at temperatures below -18°C.

9.0	PROCEDURE
9.1	All samples are prepared singly.
9.2	Weigh into 125 mL polyethylene bottle (7.9) 5 g $\pm$ 0.02 g of fresh tissue.
9.3	Controls are prepared using 3 x 5 g negative tissue and adding 1. nothing 2. 100 µL of control solution (6.3.2.2) 3. 200 µL of control solution (6.3.2.2)
9.4	To all bottles add 50 mL of chloroform/acetone mixture (1:1, v/v), (6.2.7)
9.5	Cap and homogenise at full speed for approximately one minute (7.17).
9.6	Filter through Whatman GF/C glass microfibre filters using a water pump.
9.7	To all bottles add 10 mL of chloroform/acetone mixture. (6.2.7). Wash and filter as in 9.6.
9.8	Combine the filtrates and transfer to a 100 mL pear-shaped flask. Remove solvent by rotary evaporation at 30°C.
9.8	Add 2 mL 50% methanol in 2% acetic acid and 6 mL hexane to the residue. Swirl the flask <u>gently</u> to dissolve, and to partition the fats into the hexane. Do not shake or emulsions will be formed.
9.9	Transfer into 10 mL test tubes (7.7) and centrifuge at 2000 rpm for 10 min. Discard the top layer and transfer a 200 µL aliquot of the bottom layer to the HPLC vials (7.14). The samples are now ready to be analysed by HPLC.
9.10	HPLC
9.10.1	Ensure wavelength monitor is set at 450 nm (7.22.2).
9.10.2	The column is run at room temperature.
9.10.3	Equilibrate the system by running the mobile phase (6.2.5) through at 1 mL per min for 30 min. Introduce the post-column reagent at a rate of 0.5 mL per min for a further 30 min.
9.10.4	Calibrate the system by injecting 50 µL of the previously prepared working standard (6.3.2.3) until a constant height of 110 $\pm$ 10 mm is obtained.
9.10.5	Inject 50 µL of each extract (9.9). A 1 µg per mL working standard (6.3.2.3) is run after every fourth sample. Each sample takes 10 min to run and the retention time of the sulphadimidine is 8 min.

9.10.6   If a peak having a retention time similar to the standards is
          seen in the sample, mix equal volumes of an appropriate standard
          and the sample and re-chromatograph to check for co-elution.
9.10.7   After the last injection, allow 80% (v/v) methanol/water to run
          through the system at 0.5 mL per min overnight. Store the column
          in 80% methanol/water when not in use.

10.0   CALCULATION OF RESULTS

Calculate the concentration of sulphadimidine in the samples by the
equation ;

$$C(s) = \frac{S(h) \times C(Std)}{Std(h)}$$

where   C(s) is sample concentration in mg per kg
          S(h) is the peak height of the sample
          Std(h) is the peak height of the standard
          C(Std) is the conc. in mg per kg that the standard is equivalent
          to. In this extraction the working standard of 1 mg per L is
          equivalent to 0.4 mg per kg (C(Std)).

10.2 Validation Data.

10.2.1 Liver

Blank samples from untreated animals were spiked at zero, 0.2 and 0.4 mg
per kg sulphadimidine. The assay was performed on three consecutive days.
The recoveries were in percentages

Day	Kidney (0.2 mg/kg) Mean SD CV	Kidney (0.4 mg/kg) Mean SD CV	Muscle (0.2 mg/kg) Mean SD CV	Muscle 0.4 (mg/kg) Mean SD CV
1	76 ± 6.7 8.8	84 ± 6.0 7.2	86 ± 3.3 3.9	83 ± 4.5 5.4
2	79 ± 8.7 10.9	84 ± 10.8 12.7	82 ± 7.8 9.5	77 ± 2.9 3.7
3	84 ± 8.1 9.7	83 ± 6.4 7.7	77 ± 3.9 5.1	76 ± 3.9 5.1
ALL	80 ± 7.8 9.8	84 ± 7.7 9.2	82 ± 5.0 6.2	79 ± 3.8 4.7

11.0   SPECIAL CASES

12.0   NOTES ON PROCEDURES

The retention times of other sulphonamides were evaluated in the HPLC
system and were,

Sulphonamide	Retention time (min)
Sulphadimidine	8.4
Sulphaguanidine	4.1
Sulphanilamide	4.2
Sulphathiazole	5.9
Sulphadiazine	6.0
Sulphapyridine	6.2
Sulphamethoxazole	10.5
Sulphadoxine	12.0
Sulphadimethoxine	23.8
Sulphaquinoxaline	29.3

13.0   QUALITY CONTROLS.

The RM for pig tissues are in the final stages of preparation and
certification. They were prepared at VRL, Belfast.

14.0   TEST REPORT. To give the indications necessary for the
identification of the sample, the reference to the method employed, the
results and the form in which these are expressed, any particular points
observed in the course of the test and any operations not specified in the
method or regarded as optional which might affect the results.

15.   LIST OF ABBREVIATIONS

A full list of abbreviations is given in Annex I, Section 12

16.   FLOW DIAGRAM

```
                homogenise
TISSUE   --------------------> SOLVENT EXTRACT ------> PARTITION
                                                            ¦
                                                            ¦
                                                            ¦
                                                            ¦
                                                            V
                   CALCULATE RESULTS  <----------- HPLC
```

**Cy 3.3.   SULPHADIMIDINE - HPLC ANALYSIS OF SULPHADIMIDINE IN PORCINE
KIDNEY**

WARNING AND SAFETY PRECAUTIONS

SAFETY
1.   Organic solvents - all organic solvents must be treated as
      potentially   hazardous and all procedures using them must be
      performed in a fume cupboard.
2.   Ammonia - use only in a fume cupboard and wear safety glasses.
3.   Homogenising - perform in a fume cupboard to avoid aerosols.
4.   Dry ice - wear thick hide gloves and face shield. Dry ice
      can cause burns and frostbite if in contact with the skin.

FIRST AID
1.   Solvents, acids and alkalis in contact with skin - wash with
      copious amounts of cold water. Splashes in the eye - irrigate
      with water and seek medical attention immediately.
2.   Cuts - seek assistance of first aider immediately.
3.   Burns and frostbite - run affected part under cold water (burns)
      or tepid water (frostbite) for 10 minutes and seek medical
      attention.

0.   INTRODUCTION

Sulphadimidine (sulphamethazine) is an antibiotic widely used
prophylactically and as a growth promoter in pig production.

To minimise risks from residues in the human diet, withdrawal periods are
set. High residue levels may occur if these periods are not adhered to.
Residue levels are monitored in tissues taken at slaughter and carried out
in compliance with the Residues Directive (86/469/EEC). In the UK scheme
kidney has been chosen as the tissue for analysis.

The samples are initially screened by TLC or ELISA. The CVL, UK confirms
positive samples by this HPLC method and by a GC-MS method.

1.   SCOPE

This method of analysis describes the determination of the total content of
Sulphadimidine in pig kidney.

2.   FIELD OF APPLICATION.

The method is described to be used for porcine kidney. The minimum limit
of determination for Sulphadimidine is 10 μg per kg of kidney.

3.   REFERENCES.

Commission Decision, 93/256/EEC, laying down the methods for detecting
residues of substances having a hormonal or thyrostatic action. [OJ. №
L.118, 14.4.93. pp 64-74]

2052/VI/84 File 6.11 II-4, Scientific Veterinary Committee, Working
Group - "Reference Methods for Residues", General Criteria for the
establishment of Reference Methods for the Detection of Residues.

ISO Standard 78/2-1982 Layout for standards - Part 2: Standard for Chemical
Analysis

MAFF (1987) Working Party on Veterinary Residues in Animal Products. Food
Surveillance Paper No. 22.

MAFF, CVL, Standard Operating Procedure No 15, HPLC Analysis of
Sulphadimidine in Porcine Kidney.

see also;
Aerts, M.M.L., Beek, W.M.J. and Brinkman, U.A.Th., (1988), Monitoring of
veterinary drug residues by a combination of continuous flow techniques and
column-switching HPLC. I. Sulphonamides in egg, meat and milk using post-
column derivatization with dimethylaminobenzaldehyde. J. Chrom., <u>435</u>, 97-
112

4.   DEFINITIONS.

Sulphadimidine content is taken to mean the amount of sulphadimidine in
kidney determined according to the described method and expressed as μg
sulphadimidine per kg test sample.

5.   PRINCIPLE.

Samples are extracted using acidified ethyl acetate. Co-extractives are
removed using solid phase extraction columns (Bond-Elut amino (NH_2) and
cation exchange (SCX)). Sulphadimidine is eluted with ammoniated methanol
and quantified by reverse phase high performance liquid chromatography
(HPLC) with UV detection.

6.   MATERIALS

6.1.   Chemicals

6.1.1.   Acetone   HPLC Grade (BDH)
6.1.2   Ethyl acetate   HPLC Grade (FSA)
6.1.3.   Hexane   HPLC Grade (FSA)
6.1.4.   Methanol   HPLC Grade (BDH)
6.1.5.   Ammonia solution   Specific gravity 0.88; approx 35% (FSA)
6.1.6.   Acetonitrile   HPLC Grade (BDH)
6.1.7.   Glacial acetic acid   AR Grade (BDH), $0.1M$ (0.57 mL
                                  made up to 100 mL with deionised water)
6.1.8   Ammonium acetate solution   AR Grade (BDH), $0.0124M$ (770 mg
                                  made up to 1 litre deionised with
water)
6.1.9.   Sulphadimidine   Crystalline (Sigma Chemicals Ltd)
3.1.10. Solid carbon dioxide Cardice (dry ice) (Distillers Co)

6.1.11. Solutions
6.1.11.1 5% Acetic acid in ethyl acetate;- 5 mL acetic acid made up to
         100 mL with ethyl acetate
6.1.11.2 25% Ammonia in methanol;- 25 mL ammonia made up to 100 mL
         with methanol
6.1.12. Mobile Phase $0.01M$ ammonium acetate/methanol/acetonitrile
         85/7.5/7.5; v/v/v
6.1.13   Sulphadimidine Standards

6.1.13.1 Stock Standard; 1 mg/mL sulphadimidine in acetone. Store
         at -20°C. Stable for at least 4 months.
6.1.13.2 Intermediate Standards. Dilute stock standard with acetone to
         make 100 μg/mL standard. At monthly intervals, dilute 100 μg/mL
         with acetone to make 10 μg/mL standard.
6.1.13.3 Working Standards. On day of use, take 10 μg/mL standard. Take
         aliquots (12.5, 25, 50, 75 ul) from this, evaporate and
         redissolve in 500 μL mobile phase for HPLC (i.e. 20 μL
         injections containing 5, 10, 20, 30 ng respectively).

7.   EQUIPMENT

7.1.   Glassware
7.1.1   Centrifuge tubes, 30 mL, round bottomed with ground glass
         stoppers
7.1.2   Measuring cylinders, 500, 50 mL
7.1.3   Volumetric flasks, 100, 50, 10 mL
7.1.4   Graduated pipettes, 10 mL
7.1.5   Glass vials with caps, 2 dram
7.1.6   Syringes, 100 ul, 25 μL (Rheodyne)
7.1.7   Luer-syringe, 5 mL (disposable)
7.1.8   Pasteur pipettes

7.2   Apparatus
7.2.1.   Homogenizer (Silverson heavy duty laboratory mixer emulsifier
         (sealed unit model))
7.2.2.   Centrifuge (Mistral 6L set to 4-5°C)
7.2.3.   Insulated dry ice box
7.2.4.   Bond Elut reservoirs, 25 mL capacity
7.2.5.   Bond Elut adapters (Jones Chromatography)
7.2.6.   Bond Elut cartridges, Amino (NH_2) and cation exchange (SCX) (500
         mg/2.8 mL capacity)
7.2.7.   Filtering equipment containing 0.45 um filter (Millipore -
         Waters)
7.2.8.   Water bath set at 45-50°C
7.2.9.   SPE-ED Mate 30 Vacuum Apparatus (Lab Impex Ltd)
7.2.10. Nitrogen manifold
7.2.11. HPLC equipment
Waters M-45 pump with Kratos Spectroflow 733 absorbance detector set at 266
nm and Linseis type LS4 flat bed recorder or equivalent. Waters 4 u C_{18}
Novapak column (15 x 0.46 cm) with 2 cm disposable LC-18 Pelliguard
cartridge guard column (Supelco) Rheodyne injector (7125) fitted with 20 μL
loop.

8.   SAMPLES AND SAMPLING PROCEDURE.

N.B. Attention is drawn to section 6.3.1 and ISO document 78/2-1982 and
the following notes derived from Annex II of 2052/VI/84-EN.

8.1. Nature of the Sample; Samples shall be such as to enable the
detection of residues in meat as defined in Directive 64/433/EEC. Failing
this biological fluids or faeces may constitute the samples for the
detection of residues.

8.2. Size of Sample; The size of the sample must be large enough to allow
the reference method to be carried out and to allow repeat analysis where

required.

In this method for sulphadimidine the sizes shall not be less than 20 g
kidney.

9.   PROCEDURE
9.1.   Weigh 2.5 g thawed and chopped sample into a 30 mL tube.
9.2.   Add 6 mL of 0.1M acetic acid:acetone mixture (1:1 v/v) and add 12
            mL ethyl acetate. Homogenise for 1 minute and centrifuge at 2500
            rpm for 15 minutes.
9.3.   Transfer supernatant to another 30 mL tube and repeat step 9.2 on
            the tissue pellet. Combine supernatants and place tubes in a
            rack.
9.4.   Place rack into cardice box until aqueous layer is completely
            frozen (at least 15 minutes).
9.5.   Decant ethyl acetate into another 30 mL tube ready for clean-up.
9.6.   Using vacuum apparatus prepare NH_2 Bond Elut column by washing
            with 1 column volume of hexane. Prepare SCX Bond Elut column by
            washing with 1 column volume of hexane followed by two column
            volumes of 5% acetic acid in ethyl acetate. (**N.B.** Do **NOT** let SCX
            column run dry.) Assemble the columns in tandem.
9.7.   Transfer the ethyl acetate extract to the reservoir and draw it
            through the assembly by vacuum.
9.8.   Wash the assembly with 2 column volumes of methanol (ca 6 mL).
9.9.   Close the vacuum tap and discard the NH_2 column and reservoir.
9.10.   Wash the SCX column with 2 column volumes of water followed by 4
            column volumes of methanol. (**N.B.** Do **NOT** let SCX column run
            dry.)
9.11.   Remove column from assembly, attach to Luer syringe and elute
            sulphadimidine with 3 mL of 25% ammonia in methanol into 2 dram
            vial, using positive pressure.
9.12.   Evaporate eluate under N_2 at 45-50°C in a water bath. Dissolve
            residue in 0.5 mL acetone and transfer with a Pasteur pipette to
            another vial. Wash with a further 0.5 mL acetone and combine
            washes. Eluate can then be stored overnight at -20°C if needed.
9.13.   Evaporate to dryness and redissolve in 200 µL of acetone. Take
            an aliquot of 100 ul, evaporate and redissolve in 500 µL of
            mobile phase for HPLC.
9.14.   HPLC is performed at room temperature. Equilibrate the system by
            running mobile phase through at 1 mL/min for about 90 min before
            commencing analysis.
9.15.   Calibrate the system by injecting 20 µL of each of the previously
            prepared HPLC standards made up in mobile phase.
9.16.   The extract dissolved in mobile phase is injected. Appropriate
            working standards are run after every fifth sample. Each sample
            takes about 12 minutes to run and retention time (T_R) of
            sulphadimidine is about 7 minutes.
9.17.   If a peak having a T_R similar to the standards is seen in the
            sample, mix equal volumes of an appropriate standard and the
            sample. Inject the mixture to check for co-chromatography.
9.18.   After the last injection, allow methanol to run through the
            system (0.2 mL/min) overnight. Store column in methanol when not
            in use.

10.   CALCULATION OF RESULTS

A calibration curve is constructed of peak height against concentration for a range of standards from 5 to 30 ng. The quantity of sulphadimidine in each sample injection is then calculated from the measured peak height. This figure is then corrected for injection volume and mean % recovery (calculated from spiked samples) to give a concentration in mg/kg (ppm). The standard injection of 20 μL is equivalent to 0.05 g of extracted sample.

$$\% \text{ recovery} = \frac{\text{amount of sulphadimidine found}}{\text{amount of sulphadimidine added}} \times 100$$

Concentration of sulphadimidine in sample (mg/kg) =

$$\frac{\text{ng sulphadimidine (from calibration curve)}}{1000} \times \frac{1}{0.05} \times \frac{100}{\% \text{ recovery}}$$

For samples containing sulphadimidine at concentrations beyond the range of the standard curve, a dilution of the extract is prepared and chromatographed, and the appropriate volumetric correction is applied.

SENSITIVITY
The limit of determination of sulphadimidine by this method is 0.01 mg/kg. Recovery of added sulphadimidine at 0.1 mg/kg is in excess of 80%.

11.   SPECIAL CASES.

12.   NOTES ON PROCEDURE.

13.   SAMPLE CONTROLS
It is convenient to analyze 11 tissue samples plus 1 quality control sample* and 2 blank spike samples** in each batch.

* The quality control sample was obtained from a sample previously analyzed
  and found to contain sulphadimidine above the maximum residue limit (MRL).
**The blank sample was obtained from a sample previously analyzed and found
  to contain no sulphadimidine. Fortify (spike) with 100 μL of 2.5 μg mL
  sulphadimidine standard.

14.   TEST REPORT
15.   LIST OF ABBREVIATIONS.
See abbreviations in Annex I, Section 12 of Manual.
16.   FLOW DIAGRAM

```
          acidified ethyl acetate                  decant
KIDNEY --------------------------> FREEZE ------------> ETHYL ACETATE
                                                        EXTRACT      ---->


                    elute                       elute
----> NH2-BOND-ELUT ------------> SCX-BOND-ELUT ------> Ammonia/MeOH ----->
           COLUMN                      COLUMN

----> DRY ----> HPLC Mobile -------> HPLC ----------> CALCULATE RESULTS
```

Cy 3.4. SULPHADIMIDINE. DETERMINATION OF SULPHADIMIDINE IN REFERENCE MATERIAL AND FRESH TISSUES BY HIGH PERFORMANCE LIQUID CHROMATOGRAPHY.

<u>SAFETY</u>

Personal safety. Normal laboratory protective clothing and equipment should be worn.

1.0.   INTRODUCTION

A method is described by which the content of sulphadimidine in reference material and fresh tissues may be estimated.

Sulphadimidine, otherwise known as Sulphamethazine is one of a group of antimicrobials called sulphonamides. Its use is widespread in animal production and it is most commonly fed to pigs in their ration at 100 g per tonne. Residues at or above the violative level have been reported in many countries.

2.   SCOPE AND FIELD OF APPLICATION.

This method of analysis describes the determination of the total content of Sulphadimidine in foodstuffs and samples of animal origin.

The method can be used for muscle, liver, kidney and fat. The detection limit, defined as three times the standard deviation of the blank determination, is 50 µg per kg of sample for Sulphadimidine.

3.   REFERENCES.

Commission Decision, 93/256/EEC, laying down the methods for detecting residues of substances having a hormonal or thyrostatic action.

ISO Standard 78/2-1982 Layout for standards - Part 2: Standard for Chemical Analysis

Method based on Standard Operating Procedure described by;- Veterinary Sciences Division, Stoney Road, Stormont, BELFAST BT4 3SD

Aerts, M.M.L., Beek, W.M.J. and Brinkman, U.A.Th. (1988). Monitoring of Veterinary Drug Residues by a combination of continuous flow techniques and column-switching HPLC. I. Sulphonamides in egg, meat and milk using post-column derivatization with dimethylaminobenaldehyde. J. Chromat. <u>435</u>, 97-112.

4.   DEFINITIONS.

Sulphadimidine content is taken to mean the amount of Sulphadimidine in the substance in question, regardless of the chemical form, determined according to the described method and expressed as µg Sulphadimidine per kg of test sample.

5.   PRINCIPLE

The methods comprises 5 stages;-

- Homogenisation of tissue samples in 10 mL dichloromethane or dispersing
  lyophilised tissue in buffer
- Extraction of Sulphadimidine with organic solvents
- Purification of Sulphadimidine by SPE
- End point determination with HPLC
- The amount of Sulphadimidine is calculated by interpolation from a
  standard curve and taking into account the recovery of Sulphadimidine,
  especially from tissue samples.

6.0   MATERIALS

N.B.:   The reagents for which examples of their source are quoted are
known to be satisfactory, nevertheless reagents from other sources may be
equally suitable.

6.1   Reagents
6.1.1   Dichloromethane (HPLC Grade, Rathburn Chemicals Ltd, Walkerburn,
         Scotland),
6.1.2   Methanol (HPLC Grade, Rathburn Chemicals Ltd)
6.1.3   Silica gel (SiOH) disposable extraction columns - 6 mL (Bakerbond
         SPE, 7086-06, J.T. Baker Inc., Philipsburg, NJ 08865 USA).
6.1.4   Sulphamethazine crystalline (Sigma Chemical Co, PO Box 14508 St
         Louis, MO63178 USA, Cat No S-6256).
6.1.5   Deionised water (7.9).
6.1.6   Sodium carbonate anhydrous 'Analar' (BDH Lab. Supplies, Poole,
         Dorset, Cat No 102404H).
6.1.7   Sodium hydrogen carbonate 'Analar' (BDH Lab Supplies, Cat No
         102474V).
6.1.8   N, N-Dimethyl-Aminobenzaldehyde - Ehrlichs reagent (Sigma
         Chemical Co, Cat No D2004).
6.1.9   Acetic acid GPR (BDH Lab. Supplies, Cat. No. 27013).

6.2   Solutions
6.2.1   Buffer, pH 10.0
         0.2 M sodium carbonate (6.1.7) 27.5 mL
         0.2 M sodium hydrogen carbonate (6.1.8) 22.5 mL
         Deionised water (7.9) 150 mL
6.6.2   50% Methanol (6.1.2) v/v deionised water (7.9)
6.2.3   N, N-Dimethyl-Aminobenzaldehyde Reagent
         Acetic Acid (6.1.10)   125 mL
         Methanol (6.1.2)   75 mL
         Deionised water (7.9)   50 mL
         N, N-Dimethyl-Aminobenzaldehyde (6.1.9)   3.75 g
         Before adding the N, N-Dimethylbenzaldehyde degas the solution
         using the equipment described in (7.12) for 2 minutes,
6.2.4   2% Acetic Acid
         Acetic Acid (6.1.10)   10 mL
         Deionised water (7.9)   490 mL
6.2.5   HPLC Mobile Phase
         2% Acetic acid (6.2.4)   325 mL
         Methanol (6.1.2)   175 mL
         (degas for 2 minutes (7.12))

6.3	Standards
6.3.1	Intermediate standard

6.3   Standards
6.3.1   Intermediate standard
        Dissolve an accurately weighed (7.2) quantity of sulphamethazine
        (6.1.5) in methanol (6.1.2) to give a solution of 1 mg to
        sulphamethazine per mL using a 100 ml volumetric flask (7.27).
        Store at +4°C. (7.5).
6.3.2   Working standards.
        Diluting in 50% Methanol (6.2.2) prepare standard working
        solutions of 20, 40, 80 ng/50 μL in 100 ml volumetric flasks
        (7.27). Store a +4°C.
6.3.3   Control solutions
        Diluting in Methanol (6.1.2) prepare control solutions of 12.5
        μg/mL (6.3.31) and 25 μg/mL (6.3.32).   When 50 μL of these
        solutions are added to negative samples they are equivalent to
        250 ng.g and 500 ng/g respectively in the final extract.

7.0   EQUIPMENT

7.1   Balance top-pan (Sartorius, Gottingen, Germany model L610D).
7.2   Balance analytical (Sartorius, Gottingen, Germany model R160P).
7.3   Magnetic Stirrer (Gallenkamp model 300).
7.4   Vortex mixer (SMI model 2601).
7.5   Refrigerator +4°C (Williams Refrigeration Ltd, Kings Lynn, UK)
7.6   Fume cupboards (Nordia, Lab Design, Walthamstow,London, E17 6AB.
7.7   Multi sample concentrator for tubes (Techne, Jencons Scientific
        Ltd, Leighton Buzzard, Beds, England DB3).
7.8   Semi-automatic pipettes with disposable tips: 5 - 40 μL,
        40 - 200 μL, 200 - 1000 μL and 1 - 5 ml volumes (eg Finnpipettes,
        Jencons Scientific Ltd, Cherrycourt Way Ind Estate, Leighton
        Buzzard, Beds, England).
7.9   Millipore RO60 reverse osmosis and milli Q deionised water
        system. (Millipore SA, 67120 Molsheim, France, Cat Nos ZFRONCO60
        and PF00671/U respectively).
7.10   End over end mixer (Luckham Ltd, Burgess Hill, Sussex, England,
        model TM/1).
7.11   Baker solid phase extraction system. (J.T. Baker Inc.
        Philipsburg NJ 08865 USA).
7.12   Cylinder of helium gas filled to 200 bar max at 15°C (BOC Ltd,
        10 Priestley Road, Guilford, Surrey SI No 1046).
7.13   HPLC Controller 2152 (LKB, Pharmacia Ltd, Pharmacia LKB
        Biotechnology Division, Midsummer Boulevard, Central Milton
        Keynes, Bucks MK9 3HP).
7.14   HPLC Pump 2150 X2 (LKB).
7.15   Variable wavelength monitor 2151 set at 450 nm wavelength (LKB).
7.16   Integrator (model HP3396A, Hewlett-Packard, Avondale Division,
        Route 41, Avondale, PA, USA).
7.17   Column Oven (Jones Chromatography, Collic Road, Llanbrodach, Mid
        Glamorgan CF8 3QQ Wales).
7.18   Microsorb C-18 (Octadecylsilane) 80-215-C5 column (15 cm x 4.6 mm
        ID) - Rainin Instrument Co Inc, Mack Road, Woburn, MA USA).
7.19   Reaction coil 10 ft length of Teflon Tubing (0.023 in. ID).
7.20   Low dead volume mixing chamber (LKB).
7.21   Rheodyne injector (Model 7125), Rheodyne Inc, PO Box 996, Cotati,
        California 94931 USA).
7.22   Glass tubes 75 mm by 10 mm (FSA Laboratory Supplies, Cat No
        G002/73, Bishop Meadow Road, Loughborough, Leics, LE11 ORG).
7.23   Glass tubes 125 mm by 16 mm (FSA Lab Supplies, Cat No G002/81).

7.24   Glass universal bottles and lids, capacity 29.5 mL (FSA Lab
         Supplies, Cat No BM/4).
7.25   Graduated glass pipettes, 10 mL and 25 mL (FSA Lab. Supplies, Cat
         Nos G519 and G520).
7.26   Measuring cylinders, 100 mL and 500 mL (FSA Lab. Supplies, Cat
         Nos 3200/10 and 3200/14).
7.27   100 mL volumetric flask (FSA Lab Supplies, Cat No BJ138).
7.28   Piped Nitrogen gas supply.

8.   SAMPLES AND SAMPLING PROCEDURE.

N.B. Attention is drawn to section 6.3.1 and to ISO document 78/2-1982 and
also the following notes derived from Annex II of 2052/VI/84-EN.

8.1. Nature of the Sample; Samples shall be such as to enable the
detection of residues in meat as defined in Directive 64/433/EEC. Failing
this biological fluids or faeces may constitute the samples for the
detection of residues.

8.2. Size of Sample; The size of the sample must be large enough to allow
the method to be carried out and to allow repeat analyses where required.

8.3. The samples must be taken and packed in such a way as to allow proper
identification in the laboratory.

8.4. The method of packing, preservation and transport must maintain the
integrity of the sample and not prejudice the result of the examination.
Samples for the analysis of thyreostatic substances must be stored and
transported at temperatures below -18^{0}C.

9.0   PROCEDURE

9.1   All samples are prepared singly.
9.2   Weigh into glass universals (7.24) a quantity of lyophilised
         tissue equivalent to 2.5 g $\pm$ 0.01 of fresh tissue (approximately
         0.60 g).
9.3   Controls are prepared from negative tissue and 50 μL of each
         control solution (6.3.31 and 6.3.32).
9.4   To all universals add 2 mL of carbonate/bicarbonate buffer
         (6.2.1).
9.5   Cap and vortex each universal for approximately one minute (7.4).
9.6   To all universals add 15 mL dichloromethane (6.1.1).
9.7   Mix all universals end over end for 20 minutes at approximately
         60 rpm (7.10).
9.8   Pour dichloromethane from universals into clean universals and
         cap (7.14).
9.9   Remove 12 mL from each universal and transfer into test tubes
         (7.23). If it is not possible to remove 12 mL, remove as much as
         possible. The calculation at the end must be modified
         accordingly.
9.10   Using the Baker solid phase extraction system (7.11) and the
         silica gel columns (6.1.4) condition the columns with 6 cm3 of
         dichloromethane (6.1.1) but do not allow the columns to dry
         before the samples are added.
9.11   To each column add 12 mL dichloromethane from each sample (9.9)
         and pass through the column at approximately 5 mL/minute.

9.12   Wash the columns with a further 6 mL of dichloromethane (6.1.1)
           and air dry the columns for 10 minutes at a vacuum pressure of 10
           psi.
9.13   Elute the sample from each column with 3 mL of methanol (6.1.2)
           passed slowly through the column over a 20 minute period.
           Collect the eluate in test tubes (7.22).
9.14   Evaporate the eluate using the multi sample concentrator (7.7).
9.15   Resuspend residue in 1 mL 50:50 v:v methanol/deionised
           water(6.2.2). The samples are now ready to be analyzed by HPLC.
9.16   HPLC
9.16.1   Ensure wavelength monitor is set at 450 nm (7.15).
9.16.2   Turn the column oven to 40°C and allow to heat for 30 minutes
           (7.17).
9.16.3   Set one pump (pump A) at a flow rate of 1 mL per min and the
           other pump (B) at a flow rate of 0.5 mL per min.
9.16.4   Pass methanol (6.1.2), which has been degassed with helium for 2
           min, through both pumps for 5 min.
9.16.5   Equilibrate the system by passing both the mobile phase (6.2.5)
           via pump A and the N,N-dimethyl-aminobenzaldehyde reagent (6.2.3)
           via pump B through the column (7.18), mixing chamber (7.20),
           reaction coil (7.19) and wavelength monitor (7.15) for 30 min.
9.16.6   Calibrate the system by injecting 50 µL of the prepared working
           standards (6.3.2) using the Rheodyne injector (7.21).
9.16.7   Inject 50 µL of each extract (9.15). Each sample takes about 10
           min to run and the retention time of sulphadimidine is
           approximately 4 min.
9.16.8   After the last injection allow methanol to run through the system
           overnight.

10.0   CALCULATION OF RESULTS

10.1   From the height of the peaks produced by the standards the height,
which is equivalent to 1 ng per 50 µL, can be calculated by dividing the
total height of the peak by the value of the standard.

e.g. For the 40 ng per 50 µL standard; 1 ng per 50 µL = $\dfrac{\text{height of peak}}{40}$

The amount of sulphadimidine in the samples (9.15) can then be calculated
by dividing their peak height by the height obtained from the standards
equivalent to 1 ng per 50 µL. This gives a result in ng per 50 µL. This
can be converted to ng per mL or ng per g as required.

10.2 Validation Data.
10.2.1 Liver
Lyophilised liver samples (equiv. to 2.5 g liver) from untreated animals
were spiked with 0.625 µg sulphadimidine. The recovery was 91.3% ± 7.5%
(CV = 8.2%), N = 6
Six randomly selected lyophilised liver samples from a batch of incurred
Reference Material were assayed on three different days. The results are
multiplied by a fictitious factors (<4) to avoid undue influence on future
collaborative studies organised by MAT.

	µg per kg	CV (%)
First day	2018 ± 124	6.1
Second day	2040 ± 138	6.8
Third day	1868 ± 50	2.7

Mean for daily measurement (interassay) 1976 ± 96 µg per kg; CV = 4.7%

10.2.2 Kidney

Lyophilised kidney samples (equiv. to 2.5 g kidney) from untreated animals
were spiked with 0.625 µg sulphadimidine. The recovery was 83.1% ± 3.6%
(CV = 4.3%), N = 6
Six randomly selected lyophilised kidney samples from a batch of incurred
Reference Material were assayed on three different days.

The results are multiplied by a fictitious factors (<4) to avoid undue
influence on future collaborative studies organised by MAT.

	µg per kg	CV (%)
First day	1266 ± 45	3.6
Second day	1320 ± 24	1.8
Third day	1257 ± 54	4.3

Mean for daily measurement (interassay)   1281 ± 35 µg per kg; CV = 2.7%

10.2.3 Muscle

Lyophilised muscle samples (equiv. to 2.5 g muscle) from untreated animals
were spiked with 0.625 µg sulphadimidine. The recovery was 80.7% ± 13.3%
(CV = 16.4%), N = 6
Six randomly selected lyophilised muscle samples from a batch of incurred
Reference Material were assayed on three different days. The results are
multiplied by a fictitious factors (<4) to avoid undue influence on future
collaborative studies organised by MAT.

	µg per kg	CV (%)
First day	1400 ± 43	3.0
Second day	1414 ± 48	3.4
Third day	1193 ± 36	3.0

Mean for daily measurement (interassay)   1336 ± 124 µg per kg; CV = 9.3%

11.0   SPECIAL CASES

12.0   NOTES ON PROCEDURES

Sulphadimidine is not stable in fresh or frozen tissues. The rate of post-
mortem metabolism can be reduced by storage at low temperatures, however
the response is variable and cannot be predicted. In the reference
materials stability has been achieved by adding merthiolate to achieve a
final concentration of 0.013% and removing available water by double freeze
drying. At this concentration merthiolate has no effect on the HPLC
analytical procedure however it will interfere with immuno- and
microbiological assay procedures. Freeze drying results in a fine powder
which must be rehydrated before extractions are performed. For this
purpose the bicarbonate buffer is preferred and increases the extraction
efficiency. There have not been studies on the stability of the
reconstituted tissue powder or extract.

13.0   QUALITY CONTROLS.

RMs for sulphadimidine have been prepared for pig muscle, liver and kidney
and are undergoing the intercomparison and certification studies (see
section 8).

14.0   TEST REPORT.

To give the indications necessary for the identification of the sample, the reference to the method employed, the results and the form in which these are expressed, any particular points observed in the course of the test and any operations not specified in the method or regarded as optional which might affect the results.

15.   LIST OF ABBREVIATIONS

A full list of abbreviations is given in Annex I, Section 12

16.   FLOW DIAGRAM

```
TISSUE              homogenise                                      elute
                    -----------------------> SOLVENT EXTRACT ------> SPE ---------
LYOPHILLISATE       disperse                                              !
                                                                         !
                                                                         !
                                                                         v
                                 CALCULATE RESULTS  <----------- HPLC
```

Cy 3.5. CHLORAMPHENICOL - CONFIRMATION OF CHLORAMPHENICOL IN MEAT, MILK, EGGS AND URINE BY GAS CHROMATOGRAPHY-MASS SPECTROMETRY.

WARNING AND SAFETY PRECAUTIONS

0.   INTRODUCTION

Chloramphenicol (CAP) is a bacteriostatic with a broad spectrum of activity, frequently used for therapeutic and prophylolactic purposes in veterinary medicine. In several countries the use of CAP is prohibited in laying hens and lactating cattle. MRLs in meat products are set by many countries between zero and 10 µg per kg.

1.   SCOPE

The use of CAP is restricted throughout the EEC. To ensure that farmers are not continuing to use chloramphenicol in laying hens or lactating cattle, and to control the use in meat producing animals samples are collected on farms and at slaughterhouses and screened for the presence of this compound using a number of techniques (see Section 4). Whenever there is a positive screening result, this must be confirmed. This work is carried out in compliance with the Residues Directive (86/469/EEC).

2.   FIELD OF APPLICATION.

This method is used for confirmation of the presence of chloramphenicol in meat, eggs and urine. With appropriate adaption the method is also suitable for milk. The detection limit is 0.1 µg/litre or kg of matrix for Chloramphenicol.

3.   REFERENCES.

Commission Decision, 93/256/EEC, laying down the methods for detecting residues of substances having a hormonal or thyrostatic action. [OJ. № L.118, 14.4.93. pp 64-74]

2052/VI/84 File 6.11 II-4, Scientific Veterinary Committee, Working Group - "Reference Methods for Residues", General Criteria for the establishment of Reference Methods for the Detection of Residues.

ISO Standard 78/2-1982 Layout for standards - Part 2: Standard for Chemical Analysis

Development and validation of a gas chromatographic spectrometric procedure for the quantitation and identification of residues of chloramphenicol. Van Ginkel, L.A., van Rossum, H.J., Zoontjes, P.W., van Blitterswijk, H., Ellen, G., van der Heeft, E., de Jong, A.P.J.M. and Zomer, G. (1990), Anal. Chim. Acta. 237,, 61-69.

Eine Radioimmunologische Bestimmung von Chloramphenicol-Rückständen in Muskulatur, Milch und Eiern. Arnold. D., Berg, D. van, Biertz, A.K., Mallick, U and Somogyi, A (1984), Arch. Lebensmittelhyg. 35, 131-136.

Reference Standards for residue analysis of chloramphenicol in meat and milk: A critical study. Balizs, G. and Arnold, D. (1989), Chromatographia, 27, 489-493.

Trace analysis of chloramphenicol residues in Eggs, Milk and Meat:
Comparison of gas chromatography and radioimmunoassay. Arnold, D. and
Somogyi, A. (1985), J.A.O.A.C., 68, 984-990

EEC Document: 2406/VI/85-EN File 6.21 II-4 "Draft Reference Method for the
detection of residues of chloramphenicol in meat."

4.   DEFINITIONS.

Chloramphenicol content is taken to mean the amount of Chloramphenicol in
the substance in question, regardless of the chemical form, determined
according to the described method and expressed as µg Chloramphenicol per
kg or litre of test sample.

5.   PRINCIPLE.

The method of analysis comprises six stages:

Urine   (1)   Hydrolysis of the urine.
                        (2)   Extrelut column extraction
                        (3)   Sep-Pak C18 column purification.
Muscle and eggs   (1)   Homogenisation
                        (2)   Extract into ethyl acetate (EtAc)
                        (3)   Sep-Pak Si column purification
                        (4)   HPLC purification
                        (5)   Derivatisation.
                        (6)   Analysis by gas chromatography/mass
                              spectrometry (GC/MS).

Note (6): Chloramphenicol can be analyzed with mass spectrometry using
either electron impact (EI) or electron capture negative ion chemical
ionisation (ECNICI). As a rule ECNICI ionisation result in a 5 to 10 times
more sensitive detection.

After appropriate defatting, milk can be extracted as urine.

6.   MATERIALS

6.1.   Chemicals and reagents

6.1.1.   Reference compounds.

The following standard compounds are used.
Chloramphenicol, Cas No. 56-75-7; $C_{11}H_{12}Cl_2N_2O_5$, Mol. Wt. 323.1;
(Boehringer-Mannheim, NL, Art No. 634433)

6.1.2.   Internal standard $^{37}Cl_2$-chloramphenicol synthesised at RIVM.

6.1.3.   Ethanol (Merck, art. no. 983).
6.1.4.   Methanol (Merck, art. no. 9623).
6.1.5.   Isooctane (Merck, art. no. 4727).
6.1.6.   Acetonitrile (Merck, art. no. 30).
6.1.7.   Dichloromethane (Merck, art. no. 6050).
6.1.8.   Hydrochloric acid (Merck, art. no. 317).
6.1.9.   Ethyl acetate (Merck, art. no. 9623).
6.1.10.   Acetic acid (Merck, art. no. 63).

6.1.11.   Sodium acetate (Merck, art. no. 6268).
6.1.12.   Sodium sulphate (Merck art. no., 6643).
6.1.13.   Extrelut[R] (Merck, art. no. 11737; refills art. no. 11738)
6.1.14.   Acetate buffer 2.0 mol/L, pH 5.2.
          Mix 25.2 g acetic acid (6.1.10) with 600 mL water, add 129.5 g
          sodium acetate (6.1.11.). Adjust the pH at 5.2 ± 0.1 and add
          water to a final volume of 1000 mL.
6.1.15.   HPLC-eluting buffer.
          Mixture of ethanol/isooctane, 3:97 v/v
6.1.16.   Disodium hydrogen phosphate (Merck, art. no. 6586).
6.1.17.   Potassium dihydrogen phosphate (Merck, art. no. 4873).
6.1.18.   Solid phase extraction solvent mixtures
6.1.18.1 Methanol:water, mixture 10:90 v/v, mix 10 ml of methanol with 90
          ml of water
6.1.18.2 Methanol:water, mixture 45:55 v/v, mix 45 ml of methanol with 55
          ml of water
6.1.18.3 Acetonitrile:water, mixture 20:80 v/v, mix 20 ml of acetonitrile
          with 80 ml of water
6.1.19.   Stock solutions of (internal) standards containing 1 g/L in
          ethanol, stored at -20°C in the dark.
6.1.20.   Working solutions of (internal) standards containing 0.01 g/L in
          ethanol, stored at +4°C for a maximum period of 2 weeks.
          Smallest volume pipetted out of the stock solution is 0,1 mL.
6.1.21.   Derivatization reagent: N,O- 613 (trimethylsilyl)
          trifluoracetamine (BSTFA) with 1% TMS (Pierce, art. no. 38832).
6.1.22.   Beta-glucuronidase/sulfatase, Sigma G-0876 (Brunschwig Chemie,
          Amsterdam, NL)
6.1.23.   Solid phase extraction cartridge (Sep-Pak, C18) (Water-Millipore,
          art. no. 51910)
6.1.24.   Solid phase extraction cartridge (Sep-Pak, Silica) (Waters-
          Millipore, art. no 51900)

7.   EQUIPMENT

7.1.   Glass roundbottomed flasks, 150 mL (Corex, art. no. 8422-A).
7.2.   Glass Pasteur capillary pipettes.
7.3.   Automatic pipettes (Gilson P20, P200, P1000 and P5000)   .
7.4.   Refrigerated centrifuge (RC-3, Sorvall).
7.5.   Bench-lop centrifuge (GLC-4, Sorvall).
7.6.   Centrifuge tubes, glass, (55 mm x 11.5 mm) (Renes, RB55)
7.7.   Electric water bath with thermostat adjustable to 50 ± 2°C and 37
          ± 2°C (GFL, Salm & Kipp) with nitrogen facility.
7.8.   Vortex (Vortex-genic, Wilton & Co).
7.9.   HPLC-system
7.9.1.   Standard isocratic HPLC equipment is suitable for extract
          purification.
7.9.1.1. HPLC pump, model 6000 A (Waters/Millipore).
7.9.1.2. Automatic injection system Wisp (Waters/Millipore).
7.9.1.3. Fixed wavelength UV-detector (254 nm) Model 440
          (Waters/Millipore).
7.9.1.4. Guard column, type Chromguard (Chrompack 028185)
7.9.1.5. HPLC column (150 mm x 4.6 mm) packed with Lichrosorb Diol 5 μm
          (Merck).
7.10.   Glass derivatization vials (chromacol 250 (A)) with screw caps
          (chromacol 85c) and septa (chromacol 8-ST15).
7.11.   Incubator 60°C (Selvis).

7.12.   Heating module for derivatization vials (Pierce no. 18790) with
          nitrogen facility.
7.13.   Glass injection vials (Chrompack, art. no. 10201) with glass
          inserts (Chrompack, art. no. 10381).
7.14.   Aluminium caps (Chrompack, art. no. 10210).
7.15.   GC-MS equipment, system for EI-ionisation
7.15.1.   Gas chromatograph (Hewlett Packard, type 5890).
7.15.2.   Automatic injection (Hewlett Packard, type 7637A).
7.15.3.   Mass selective detection (Hewlett Packard, type 5970).
7.15.4.   Workstation (Hewlett Packard, type 59970).
7.15.5.   Printer (Hewlett Packard, ink jet).
7.15.6.   GC-column, fused silica permaband SE-52, 25 m x 0.25 mm ID, film
          thickness 0.25 µm (Machery-Nagel, art. no. 723054).
7.16.   GC-MS equipment, system for chemical ionisation.
7.16.1.   Gas chromatograph (Finnigan type 9610, San Jose, CA).
7.16.2.   Mass spectrometer (Finnigan 4500 quadrupole)
7.16.3.   GC-column, fused silica CP-Sil-19CB (25 m x 4.4 mm i.d., film
          thickness 0.25 um (chrompack Middelburg, NL).
7.17.   Rotavapor with water bath at 40 ± 2°C (Rotavapor).
7.18.   Moulinette homogeniser
7.19.   Ultra-Turrax homogeniser

8.   SAMPLES AND SAMPLING PROCEDURE.

N.B. Attention is drawn to section 6.3.1 and ISO document 78/2-1982 and
the following notes derived from Annex II of 2052/VI/84-EN and EEC 93/256

8.1. Nature of the Sample; Samples shall be such as to enable the
detection of residues in meat as defined in Directive 64/433/EEC. Failing
this biological fluids (in this method bile) or faeces may constitute the
samples for the detection of residues.

8.2. Size of Sample; The size of the sample must be large enough to allow
the reference method to be carried out and to allow repeat analysis where
required.

This method for Chloramphenicol uses the following amounts for a single
determination.

Meat 10 g,   Urine 10 mL, egg 10 g, milk 10 mL.

8.3. The samples must be taken and packed in such a way as to allow proper
identification in the laboratory.

8.4. The method of packing, preservation and transport must maintain the
integrity of the sample and not prejudice the result of the examination.

Samples for the analysis of CAP must be stored and transported at
temperatures below -18°C.

9.   PROCEDURE

9.1.   URINE

9.1.1.   <u>Hydrolysis</u>

To 10 mL urine add acetic acid (6.1.10) to adjust pH to 5.2. Add 0.5 mL of

2 mol per L acetate buffer (6.1.14.), pH 5.2, and 20 µL of glucuronidase
(6.1.22) in a 20 mL universal bottle and incubate 2 hours at 37°C.
The procedure for addition of the internal standard is given in 9.7.

9.1.2.   Extrelut Clean-up

Prepare an Extrelut column (6.1.13) according to the maker's instructions.

Add the cooled urine/buffer mix together with a further 2 mL water and
allow to absorb onto the column for 15 minutes. CAP is extracted from the
absorbed urine with 2 X 25 mL ethyl acetate.

Reduce the ethyl acetate to dryness under reduced pressure at 50°C. A
small residue is normally left after drying. Resuspend the extract in 2 mL
of methanol and transfer to a glass tube containing 5 mL of water. Two
additional volumes of methanol are used to complete the transfer. The
volume of the combined methanol/water is reduced to 4 mL under a stream of
nitrogen in a water bath at 50°C.

9.1.3.   Sep-Pak C18 Purification

The Sep-Pak cartridges (6.1.23) are prepared by washing twice with 2 mL of
methanol (6.1.4) and 5 mL of water. Add the extract and wash with 5 mL of
water, and 5 mL methanol:water::10:90 V/V (6.1.18.1). The CAP is eluted
with 5 mL methanol:water::45:55 V/V (6.1.18.2). The extract is reduced to
dryness under a stream of nitrogen in a water bath at 50°C and is ready for
HPLC purification.

9.2.   MILK

After proper defatting an extract can be prepared a described for urine.

9.3.   MUSCLE AND EGGS.

9.3.1   Extraction

If available, 200 g of muscle or eggs are homogenised in a Moulinette
homogeniser (7.18).   10 g of the homogenate is accurately weighed into 250
mL centrifuge tube (7.6) and 100 mL ethyl acetate (6.1.9) and 30 g sodium
sulphate (6.1.12) are added and the mixture further homogenised for 1
minute in an Ultra-Turrax homogeniser (7.19). The tubes are centrifuged
for 30 minutes at 1800 g. 75 mL of the supernatant is transferred to a
round bottomed 150 mL flask (7.1) and the solvent is evaporated under
reduced pressure at 50°C (7.17).
The addition of the internal standard is given in 9.7.

9.3.2.   Sep-Pak Clean Up

A Sep-pak silica cartridge (6.1.24) is pretreated with 5 mL
acetonitrile:water:::20:80 V/V (6.1.18.3) and 5 mL dichloromethane (6.1.7).
The cartridge is flushed with nitrogen. The residue of the extract is
dissolved in 5 mL dichloromethane (6.1.7) and applied to the cartridge.
The transfer is completed by washing the flask with two further 5 mL
volumes of dichloromethane. The cartridge is flushed with nitrogen until
all the dichloromethane is removed.

CAP is eluted with 5 mL acetonitrile/water 20:80 V/V. The eluate is

extracted three times with 1 mL ethyl acetate. The combined extract is
washed with 1 mL water and evaporated to dryness under a stream of nitrogen
in a water bath at 50°C and is ready for HPLC purification.

9.4.   HPLC Purification.

The dry residue is dissolved in 0.3 mL eluent (6.1.15). An aliquot of 0.25
mL is injected into the HPLC and the CAP fraction collected over a one
minute time period, starting 0.5 minute before the elution of CAP. The
fraction is evaporated to dryness under a stream of nitrogen in a water
bath at 50°C and is ready for derivatisation.

9.5.   Derivatisation

The dry extract (9.4) is transferred with absolute ethanol to a
derivatisation vial (7.10) and derivatised with 0.1 mL BSTFA/1% TMCS
(6.1.21.) by heating for 1 hour at 60°C. The reagent is evaporated with a
stream of nitrogen at 50°C and the residue dissolved in 25 µL isooctane.

Concurrently run chloramphenicol standards through the derivatisation
steps.

9.6.   GC-MS Analysis , chemical ionisation.

For the determination and identification of residues of CAP with mass
spectrometry, either electron capture negative ion chemical ionisation
(ECNICI) or electron impact (EI) ionisation can be used

9.6.1   GC-ECNICI(MS)

The GC-MS system (7.16) was used with: A CP-Sil-19CB fused Silica capillary
column, Helium as carrier gas at a column head pressure of 1.1×10^5 Pa,
Splitless injections at an injection port temperature of 260°C,
ballistically increasing the oven temperature from its initial temperature
of 150°C to 270°C 1 minute after injection, GC and separator oven at 260
and 270°C respectively, source temperature of 140°C, filament emission
current 200 uA, methane as reagent gas with an ion-source pressure of 50
Pa, the electron energy optimized between 70 and 90 eV, dwell time of 0.052
s. Analysis is performed in the SIM mode recording the abundances of the
ions at m/z = 376, 378, 466, 468, 470 (internal standard)

9.6.2   GC-EI(MS)

The GC-MS system (7.16) was used with: A SE-52 fused Silica capillary
column, Helium as carrier gas at a column head pressure of 1×10^5, dwell
time 0.05 s, Analysis is performed in the SIM mode recording the abundance
of the ions at m/z/ 225, 242, 361 and 451.

9.7.   Procedure for Spiking (Quantitation and recovery)

9.7.1   Test samples of 10 g or 10 mL of the homogenate are spiked with
          0.1 mL solution of the internal standard (6.1.2).   The amount of
          added CAP corresponds with approximately half the maximum
          concentration expected. The test sample is mixed thoroughly and
          stood for 30 min at room temperature or overnight at 4°C.

Cy 3.5/6

10.   CALCULATION OF RESULTS

The presence of chloramphenicol in a sample is confirmed if the GC-MS data agree with the following criteria: (see also Section 5 of Manual)

1. The peak has the same retention time on GC as the standards.

2. All the selected ions are present in the mass spectrum of that peak after subtraction of the background.

3.   <u>GC-ECNICI(MS)</u>. The selected ions are present in the same ratio to one another as seen in the standard. Effectively the following criteria are used; the ratio A468/466 (r_1) has to be within 10% of the theoretical value of 0.76, the ratio A378/376 (r_2) has to be within 10% of the theoretical value 0.70 and the ratio A376/A466 (r_3) has to be within 10% of the corresponding standard, experimentally determined under the same conditions as for the sample.

3.   <u>GC-EI(MS)</u>. The selected ions are present in the same ratio to one another as seen in the standard. Effectively the following criteria are used; the ratios A242/225 (r_1), A361/225 (r_2) and A451/A225 (r_3) have to be within 10% of the corresponding standard, experimentally determined under the same conditions as for the sample.

If chloramphenicol is present in a sample and satisfies the above criteria, then an estimate of the quantity present may be calculated;
For quantification (ECNICI(MS)) the ratio A466/Ac470 is calculated in which Ac470 is the corrected value of A470 according to:
 Ac470 = A470 - 0.184 A466.
This correction is necessary since the chlorine isotope peak of ion m/z 466 contributes to the response at m/z 470. Linearity over the range from 0 - 20 µg per kg or L is good (r = 0.9992, intercept not deviating significantly from zero).
For quantification after EI(MS) a similar procedure can be followed.

Limit of detection: 0.1 µg per L of urine or milk and 0.1 µg per kg meat or egg.

10.1.   PRECISION

Repeatability and reproducibility were calculated at RIVM and determined for urine in three separate experiments, five replicates each time (GC-MS method)

The values were;-

Concentration (ug per L)	within assay variability CV	between assay CV
2.83	8.0%	8.7%
12.0	2.3%	9.9%

11.   SPECIAL CASES

12.   NOTES ON PROCEDURE

13.   QUALITY CONTROL.   STANDARDS AND REFERENCE MATERIALS.

RMs will be available under the BCR programme for meat, milk and eggs (see Section 8 of manual).

The internal standard is $^{37}Cl_2$-CAP

Note; D^5-CAP is used by BGA as internal standard.

14.   TEST REPORT.
To give the indications necessary for the identification of the sample, the reference to the method employed, the results and the form in which these are expressed, any particular points observed in the course of the test and any operations not specified in the method or regarded as optional which might affect the results.

15.   LIST OF ABBREVIATIONS
A list of the most important abbreviations is given in Annex I section 12.

16.   FLOW DIAGRAM.


```
        enzyme hydrolysis                           EtAc  eluate
  URINE --------------------> EXTRELUT COLUMN --------------> DRY --->


                                                elute
  ----> Water/MeOH  -----------> SEP-PAK C18 ------> Water/MeOH -----> HPLC
                                 COLUMN


or
.......................................................................
                 homogenise/EtAc                        elute
  MUSCLE, EGGS  -----------------> DRY ---> SEP-PAK Si ----------------->
                                                       Acetonitrile/water


  ----->Extract into EtAc --------> DRY ------> HPLC
.......................................................................

                 EtOH/isooctane
  -----> HPLC CLEAN UP ---------------> DERIVATISE WITH BSTFA/TMCS -->


  ----> GCMS OF TMS DERIVATIVES -----------------> CALCULATE RESULTS
```

Cy 3.6. CHLORAMPHENICOL - CONFIRMATION OF CHLORAMPHENICOL IN MEAT BY GAS CHROMATOGRAPHY-MASS SPECTROMETRY.

WARNING AND SAFETY PRECAUTIONS

0.   INTRODUCTION

Chloramphenicol (CAP) is a bacteriostatic with a broad spectrum of activity, frequently used for therapeutic and prophylolactic purposes in veterinary medicine. In several countries the use of CAP is prohibited in laying hens and lactating cattle. MRLs in meat products are set by many countries between zero and 10 µg per kg.

1.   SCOPE

The use of CAP is restricted throughout the EEC. This is a method for the quantitative determination and for the confirmation of the presence of CAP residues in meat samples. This work is carried out in compliance with the Residues Directive (86/469/EEC).

2.   FIELD OF APPLICATION.

This method is used for confirmation of the presence of chloramphenicol in meat at the quantitative determination of 10 µg per kg. The limit of detection is 1.0 µg per kg for chloramphenicol.

3.   REFERENCES.

Commission Decision, 93/256/EEC, laying down the methods for detecting residues of substances having a hormonal or thyrostatic action. [OJ. № L.118, 14.4.93. pp 64-74]

2052/VI/84 File 6.11 II-4, Scientific Veterinary Committee, Working Group - "Reference Methods for Residues", General Criteria for the establishment of Reference Methods for the Detection of Residues.

EEC Document: 2406/VI/85-EN File 6.21 II-4 "Draft Reference Method for the detection of residues of chloramphenicol in meat."

ISO Standard 78/2-1982 Layout for standards - Part 2: Standard for Chemical Analysis

Arnold. D., Berg, D. van, Boertz, A.K., Mallick, U and Somogyi, A., (1984),Eine Radioimmunologische Bestimmung von Chloramphenicol-Rückständen in Muskulatur, Milch und Eiern. Arch. Lebensmittelhyg. 35, 131-136.

Arnold, D. and Somogyi, A. (1985), Trace analysis of chloramphenicol residues in Eggs, Milk and Meat: Comparison of gas chromatography and radioimmunoassay. J.A.O.A.C., 68, 984-990

Balizs, G. and Arnold, D. (1989), Reference Standards for residue analysis of chloramphenicol in meat and milk: A critical study. Chromatographia, 27, 489-493.

Van Ginkel, L.A., van Rossum, H.J., Zoontjes, P.W., van Blitterswijk, H., Ellen, G., van der Heeft, E., de Jong, A.P.J.M. and Zomer, G. (1990), Development and validation of a gas chromatographic spectrometric procedure

for the quantitation and identification of residues of chloramphenicol.
Anal. Chim. Acta. $\underline{237}$,, 61-69.

4.   DEFINITIONS.

Chloramphenicol content is taken to mean the amount of Chloramphenicol in
the matrix in question, regardless of the chemical form, determined
according to the described method and expressed as μg Chloramphenicol per
kg of test sample.

5.   PRINCIPLE.

The method of analysis comprises six stages:

        (1)   Homogenisation
        (2)   Extract into ethyl acetate (EtAc)
        (3)   Sep-Pak C18 reverse phase column purification
        (4)   Extract with ethyl acetate
        (5)   Derivatisation.
        (6)   Analysis by gas chromatography/mass spectrometry (GC/MS).

6.   MATERIALS

During the analysis, unless otherwise stated use only reagents of
recognised analytical grade and only distilled water or water of equivalent
purity.

6.1.1.   Chloramphenicol, Cas No. 56-75-7; $C_{11}H_{12}Cl_2N_2O_5$, Mol. Wt.
          323.1;(Sigma C-0378)) or Sigma drug standard solution, 1 mg per
          mL (C-9028)
6.1.2.   Chloramphenicol - meta isomer donated by Parke Davis, Freiburg,
          Germany
6.1.3.   Internal standard - deuterated chloramphenicol (98%) CAP-ring-D_4-
          benzyl--D_1 (Promochem GmbH, Wesel, Germany).
6.1.4.   Pyridine - dried   (Merck 7463)
6.1.5.   Hexamethyldisilazine (Baker 8788)
6.1.6.   Chlorotrimethylsilane (Aldrich C7,285-4)
6.1.7.   Methanol p.a. (Merck 6009)
6.1.8.   Chloroform p.a. (Merck 2445)
6.1.9.   Acetonitrile (Merck 3)
6.1.10   Ethylacetate p.a. (Merck 9623)
6.1.11   n-Hexane p.a. (Merck 4371)
6.1.12   Sodium chloride p.a. (Merck 6404)
6.1.13   Solid phase extraction cartridge (Sep-Pak, C18) (Water-Millipore,
          art. no. 51910)
6.1.14   Heptacosafluorotributylamine (Fluka 77299)
6.1.15   Methyl iodide for synthesis (Merck 806064)
6.1.16   Nitrogen (Linde)
6.1.17.   Ethanol abs. p.a. (Merck 983)

6.2.   Solutions.

6.2.1.   Solutions of standards, concentration and storage.
6.2.1.1. It is recommended to use a commercially available standard
          solution (6.1.1), 1 mg per mL; transfer 600 μL to a 100 mL
          volumetric flask and make up to volume with ethanol (6.1.17).

This stock solution can be stored for six months at +4°C.

6.2.1.2. Transfer 1 ml stock solution (6.2.1.1) (10 μg per mL) to a 10 mL volumetric flask and make up volume with ethanol. For a calibration curve ranging from 240 pg to 1200 pg CAP (equivalent to 4 to 20 μg per kg meat) per 2 μL injection take 20 to 100 μL, derivatise and dissolve in 1000 μL n-hexane. The standard solution should be prepared monthly, stored at +4°C and silylated daily for the analysis.

6.2.1.3. CAP internal standard solution. (D_5-CAP).

Take 5 mL of the D_5-CAP stock solution (10 mg per 100 mL ethanol and make up to 100 mL with ethanol (Solution I). Transfer 10 mL of solution I to a volumetric flask and make up to 100 mL with ethanol (Solution II). Add 60 μL solution II to the sample (equivalent to 30 ng per 3 g meat).

These solutions can be stored for six months at +4°C.

6.2.2. Silylating reagent. Mix pyridine (9 parts), hexamethyldisilazine (3 parts) and chlorotrimethylsilazine (1 part).

7.   EQUIPMENT

7.1   Mincer or other device for mincing meat
7.2   Vortex mixer
7.3   Centrifuge (e.g Sorvall, USA)
7.4   Sample concentrator with heating block
7.5   Speed-vac concentrator (Savant Instruments, Hicksville, N.Y., USA)
7.6   UNIVAPO 150H (UniEquipe, Martinsried, Germany)
7.7   Dispensets - 3 mL and 5 mL (Brand, Germany)
7.8   Pipettes - 20 μL, 200 μL, 1000 μL
7.9   Tubes - 15 mL, 113 mm x 17 mm
7.10   Tubes 25 mL, 100 mm x 24 mm
7.11   GC-micro sample vials -200 μL (Chrompack, Netherlands)
7.12   5 mL syringe (Hamilton)
7.13   5 μL syringe (SGE, Australia)
7.14   GC-MS System
7.14.1.   GC - HP 5890 with direct capillary interface (Hewlett-Packard)
7.14.2.   MS - SSQ 710 (Finnigan MAT, San Jose, Ca., USA)

8.   SAMPLES AND SAMPLING PROCEDURE.

N.B. Attention is drawn to section 6.3.1 and ISO document 78/2-1982 and the following notes derived from Annex II of 2052/VI/84-EN.

8.1.   Nature of the Sample; Samples shall be such as to enable the detection of residues in meat as defined in Directive 64/433/EEC.
8.2.   Size of Sample; The size of the sample must be large enough to allow the reference method to be carried out and to allow repeat analysis where required. Not less than 200 g should be collected.
          This method for Chloramphenicol uses 3 g of meat for a single determination.

8.3.   The samples must be taken and packed in such a way as to allow proper identification in the laboratory.

8.4.   The method of packing, preservation and transport must maintain

the integrity of the sample and not prejudice the result of the
examination.

Samples for the analysis of CAP must be stored and transported at
temperatures below -18°C.

9.   PROCEDURE

9.1.   Sample Clean-up

         Take a coherent part of muscle tissue and mince at 0°C to 4°C.
         In the case of frozen meat add the excess liquid, produced when
         the meat is thawed, quantitatively to the minced meat and mix
         well. The sample can now be stored at 0°C to 4°C for analysis
         within 48 hours. For prolonged storage, freeze aliquots at < -
         20°C preferably at -80°C to ensure stability.

9.1.2   First Extraction

9.1.2.1 Weigh 3 g of minced tissue in a centrifuge tube (7.9) and add the
         internal standard (30 ng D_5-CAP or meta-isomer per 100 μL
         ethanol).
9.1.2.2 Add 8 mL acetonitrile - 4% aqueous sodium chloride (1:1, v/v) and
         mix well
9.1.2.3 Centrifuge 10 min at 4000 x g.
9.1.2.4 Decant supernatant liquid into a centrifuge tube (7.10)
9.1.2.5 Add 5 mL n-hexane, mix well, centrifuge 5 min at 1700 x g.
9.1.2.6 Discard upper layer
9.1.2.7 Repeat the hexane extraction (9.1.2.5 - 9.1.2.6)
9.1.2.8 Add 5 mL ethyl acetate (water saturated) to lower aqueous phase,
         mix, centrifuge 5 min at 1700 x g.
9.1.2.9 Take off upper layer
9.1.2.10 Repeat the ethyl acetate extraction (9.1.2.8 - 9.1.2.9)
9.1.2.11 Evaporate collected organic phase (9.1.2.9) to dryness
9.1.2.12 Dissolve dry residue in 3 mL acetonitrile:water (5:95, v/v)

9.1.3.   Sep-Pak C18 Purification

The Sep-Pak cartridges (6.1.13) are prepared by washing sequentially with 5
mL of methanol (6.1.7), 5 mL of chloroform (6.1.8), 5 mL methanol and 10 mL
water. Add the extract and wash with 5 mL acetonitrile:water::5:95 v/v.
The CAP is eluted with 3 mL acetonitrile:water::50:50 v/v.

9.1.4.   Second Extraction

9.1.4.1 Extract the CAP from the eluted fluid with 5 mL ethyl acetate
         (water saturated), and centrifuge at 1700 x g.
9.1.4.2 Take off the upper layer.
9.1.4.3 Repeat the ethyl acetate extraction (9.1.4.1 - 9.1.4.2)
9.1.4.4. Evaporate the combined collected organic phase to dryness.

9.1.5.   Silylation

9.1.5.1 Add 50 μL silylating agent (6.2.2) to the sample and standard.
9.1.5.2 Evaporate immediately under a gentle stream of dry nitrogen.
9.1.5.3 Dissolve immediately in 1000 μL n-hexane (6.1.11).

9.2   Instrumental Conditions.

GC Column   DB5, 26 m x 0.25 mm i.d.
                                   0.1 um stationary phase thickness.
Carrier Gas   Helium 5.0
Flow Rate   ca. 40 mL per min
Injection System   split/splitless
                                           splitless time, 1 minute

Injection volume   1 μL
Injector Temperature   280°C
Temperature Programme   70°C to 250°C (25°C per min), final temp. for
                                   8 min.
Transfer line   270°C
Retention times.   CAP meta-isomer 9.12 min
                                   CAP and deut. CAP 9.26 min

9.2.2   MS Parameters
Operating in Negative CI mode.

Ion source parameters   Source temp. 100°C
                                  Emission current; 300 uA
                                  Electron energy; 50 eV
Reactant Gas   Ammonia
       pressure   3 x 10^{-6} torr
Calibration   Perfluorotributylamine (FC 43)
                                  masses 169, 283, 414, 514, 557, 595, 633

Resolution Parameters   Resolution; 300
Dwell time   100 msec per ion
Dynode   20 kV

Ions to be measured   Para-CAP; <u>466</u> 468 470 378 376
                                  Meta-CAP; <u>466</u> 468 470
                                  deut-CAP; <u>471</u> 473 475

10.   CALCULATION OF RESULTS

The presence of chloramphenicol in a sample is confirmed if the GC-MS data
agree with the following criteria: (see also Section 5 of Manual)

1. The peak has the same retention time on GC as the standards.

2. All the selected ions are present in the mass spectrum of that peak
after subtraction of the background.

3. The selected ions are present in the same ratio to one another as seen
in the standard.
If chloramphenicol is present in a sample and satisfies the above criteria,
then the quantity present may be calculated;
For quantification the results are calculated using the ratio of the peak
areas of CAP and the internal standard. The quality of the standard curve
is judged by linear regression.

10.1.   PRECISION

The method was validated by comparison to the results obtained with
  (I)   pig muscle incurred with CAP and prepared as reference material
           at BGA.
  (II)   two independent methods; RIA and GC with ECD.

           Results for incurred samples.

           RIA   9.45 µg per kg; n = 44[*]
           GC with ECD   9.92 µg per kg; n = 10
           GC-NCI-MS   9.53 µg per kg; n = 8

           [*] value is corrected by a random factor

11.   SPECIAL CASES

12.   NOTES ON PROCEDURE

13.   QUALITY CONTROL.   STANDARDS AND REFERENCE MATERIALS.

RMs will be available under the BCR programme for meat, milk and eggs (see
Section 8 of manual).

D^5-CAP is used by BGA as internal standard.

Note; The internal standard used at RIVM is $^{37}Cl_2$-CAP

14. TEST REPORT.
To give the indications necessary for the identification of the sample, the
reference to the method employed, the results and the form in which these
are expressed, any particular points observed in the course of the test and
any operations not specified in the method or regarded as optional which
might affect the results.

15.   LIST OF ABBREVIATIONS
A list of the most important abbreviations is given in Annex I section 12.

16.   FLOW DIAGRAM.

              homogenise   elute
  MUSCLE ------------------> SOLVENT EXTRACTION -----> SEP-PAK C18 ------>

  EXTRACT WITH ETHYL ACETATE ----------> DERIVATISE AS TMS ETHERS ----->

  GC-MS (NCI) -------> CALCULATE RESULTS

Cy 3.7.   CHLORAMPHENICOL - HPLC ANALYSIS OF CHLORAMPHENICOL IN MILK.

WARNING AND SAFETY PRECAUTIONS

SAFETY
Organic solvents - all organic solvents must be treated as potentially
hazardous and all procedures using them must be performed in a fume
cupboard.

0.   INTRODUCTION

Chloramphenicol (CAP) is a bacteriostatic with a broad spectrum of
activity, frequently used for therapeutic and prophylolactic purposes in
veterinary medicine. The EEC, through the CVMP, specifically does not
recommend the use of CAP in laying hens and lactating cattle (see section
2).

1.   SCOPE

The use of CAP is restricted throughout the EEC. To ensure that farmers
are not continuing to use chloramphenicol in laying hens or lactating
cattle, and to control the use in meat producing animals samples are
collected on farms and at slaughterhouses and screened for the presence of
this compound using a number of techniques (see Section 4). Whenever there
is a positive screening result, this must be confirmed.

2.   FIELD OF APPLICATION.

This method is used for confirmation of the presence of chloramphenicol in
milk. The detection limit with UHT sterilised milk is <1 µg/litre or kg of
matrix for Chloramphenicol.

3.   REFERENCES.

Commission Decision, 93/256/EEC, laying down the methods for detecting
residues of substances having a hormonal or thyrostatic action. [OJ. №
L.118, 14.4.93. pp 64-74]

ISO Standard 78/2-1982 Layout for standards - Part 2: Standard for Chemical
Analysis

ISO Standard 5725 (1986)

Determination of chloramphenicol in milk by high performance liquid
chromatography. CNEVA, Lab. des Medicaments Veterinaires, Fougeres,
Document no. UCM/90/04

4.   DEFINITIONS.

Chloramphenicol content is taken to mean the amount of chloramphenicol in
milk determined according to the described method and expressed as µg
chloramphenicol per L test sample.

5. PRINCIPLE.

The method comprises three stages
 - Samples of milk are extracted using ethyl acetate.

- purification of the extract with a mixture of chloroform-hexane
- quantification by high performance liquid chromatography (HPLC) on silica coated column type C-18 with UV detection at 278 nm.

6.   MATERIALS

6.1.   <u>Chemicals</u>

6.1.1   Ethyl acetate, Analytical grade (Merck 9623) distilled in a rotary evaporator (7.2.6) before use
6.1.2   Methanol, Analytical grade (Merck 6009)
6.1.3   Chloroform, Analytical grade (Merck 2445)
6.1.4   Hexane, Analytical grade for analysis (Merck 4367)
6.1.5   Acetonitrile, HPLC grade (Prolabo 20059326)
6.1.6   37% HCl, analytical grade (Merck 317). Make 5 mol per L solution.
6.1.7   Di-ammonium hydrogenphosphate (Merck 1207): prepare 0.005 mol per L solution, (0.66 g per L)
6.1.8   Demineralised water, resistivity above 18 MΩ.cm, filtered on active carbon and a 0.45 um filter.
6.1.9   Chloramphenicol >99% pure, Crystalline (Sigma Chemicals Ltd)
6.1.10   Control milk free of any trace of CAP.

6.1.11.   <u>Solutions</u>   see 6.1.6., 6.1.7.

6.1.13.   <u>Chloramphenicol Standards</u>

6.1.13.1 Standard solution; 500 μg/mL chloramphenicol in methanol. Store at 4°C. Stable for at least three months.
6.1.13.2 Intermediate Standards; Dilute stock standard with water (6.1.8) to make 5 and 50 μg per mL solutions. Store at 4°C. Stable for maximum period of 2 weeks.
6.1.13.3 Working Standards   On day of use, dilute intermediate solutions with water to give a set of 9 standards with concentrations in ng per mL equal to 10, 25, 50, 100, 125, 250, 500, 1250, 2500.

7.   EQUIPMENT

7.1.   Glassware
7.1.1   Graduated pipettes, 1 mL, 5 mL and 25 mL
7.1.2   50 mL glass centrifuge tubes with screw caps.
7.1.3   5 mL glass haemolysis tubes.
7.1.4   Round bottomed stoppered flasks, 25 mL or 50 mL.
7.1.5   Volumetric stoppered flasks, 20 mL, 25 mL, 50 mL and 100 mL
7.1.6   Silicone stoppers, type Rhodorsil[R] which fit the centrifuge and haemolysis tubes.
7.1.7   Polyethylene stoppers to fit stoppered glassware
7.1.8   Glass pipettes

7.2.   Apparatus
7.2.1   Rubber pear-shaped sucking up system type PROLABO "Propipette", fittable to glass pipettes.
7.2.2   Automatic pipettes, 100 μL, 1000 ul and 5000 μL (type Gilson "Pipetman")
7.2.3   5 to 25 mL automatic dispenser, type BRAND "Dispensette".

Cy 3.7/2

7.2.4.   Stirrer for tubes, type HEIDOLPH "Top-mix"
7.2.5.   Rotary stirrer with rotating plates, type HEIDOLPH "Reax 2"
7.2.6.   Rotary evaporator, type BUCHLI, linked to vacuum pump.
7.2.7.   Agitation water bath, type BIOBLOCK "Polytest 20"
7.2.8.   Analytical balance
7.2.9.   Refrigerated centrifuge, type JOUAN E 96, set at 15°C
7.2.10.   Ultrasonic water bath, type BIOBLOCK B72 401
7.2.11.   HPLC equipment
          Kratos spectroflow 400 pump with Kratos Spectroflow 773
          absorbance detector set at 278 nm with Spectra-Physics SP 4290
          integrator. Waters 4 um C-18 Novapak column (150 x 3.9 mm).
          Rheodyne injector (7125) fitted with 200 µL loop.
7.2.12   250 µL Glass syringe for chromatography, type HAMILTON
7.2.13.   Filtering equipment, Containing 0.45 um filter (Millipore -
          Waters)

8.   SAMPLES AND SAMPLING PROCEDURE.

N.B. Attention is drawn to section 6.3.1 and ISO document 78/2-1982 and
the following notes derived from Annex II of 2052/VI/84-EN and eec 93/256.

8.1. Nature of the Sample; Samples of milk shall be such as to enable the
detection of residues.

8.2. Size of Sample; The size of the sample must be large enough to allow
the reference method to be carried out and to allow repeat analysis where
required.

In this method for chloramphenicol the sizes shall not be less than 30 mL
milk.

8.3. The milk must be cooled after collection and stored at $\leq$ -20°C
pending analysis.

9.   PROCEDURE

9.1.   Thaw the milk sample in a water bath at 30°C.
9.2.   Homogenise the milk sample so as to blend if necessary the cream
          with the milk.
9.3.   Transfer 5 mL milk into a 50 mL centrifuge tube with an automatic
          pipette.
9.4.   Add 50 µL 5 mol/L HCl solution (6.1.6) and stir for 10 sec.
9.5.   Add 25 mL distilled ethyl acetate (6.1.1) using an automatic
          dispenser (7.2.3) and plug the tube with a silicone stopper.
9.6.   Place the tubes between the plates of the rotary stirrer (7.2.5),
          perpendicularly to the axis of rotation of the plates. Stir for
          10 min. at 40 rpm.
9.7.   Centrifuge for 5 min at 2400 g.
9.8.   Transfer 20 mL of the organic phase with a 25 mL glass pipette
          (7.1.1) into 25 mL or 50 mL round bottomed flask (7.1.4).
9.9.   Evaporate to dryness using a rotary evaporator at 30°C.
9.10.   Resuspend the oily residue in 1.6 mL mixture of hexane:chloroform
          (1:1 v/v) using an automatic pipette (7.2.2).
9.11.   Stir for 15 sec (7.2.4) at the highest speed.
9.12.   Add 0.8 mL water with an automatic pipette.
9.13.   Plug with a polyethylene stopper and stir for 5 min at 35 rpm
          with the rotary stirrer (7.2.5) placing the flasks horizontally

	so that their axles are parallel to rotation of the plates.
9.14.	Transfer the content of the flask into an haemolysis tube and plug it (7.1.6).
9.15.	Centrifuge for 10 min at 3300 g.
9.16.	Take 250 µL supernatant with a syringe (7.2.12) and inject into the chromatographic system.
9.17.	Spiking
9.17.1	Transfer 4.9 mL control milk into 5 centrifuge tubes (7.1.2) with an automatic pipette.
9.17.2	Add 0.1 mL of each of the standard solutions containing 100, 250, 500, 1250 and 2500 ng per mL so as to obtain 5 samples of milk respectively spiked at 2, 5, 10, 25 and 50 ng per mL.
9.17.3	Stir the mixtures and allow to stand for 15 min.
9.17.4	Carry out the extraction steps 9.4 to 9.16.
9.18.	HPLC
9.18.1	Mobile phase is acetonitrile, 0.005 mol/L ammonium hydrogen phosphate (18:82, v/v).
9.18.2	Flow rate 1 mL per min.
9.18.3	Wavelength 278 nm
9.18.4.	The retention of CAP is about 10 min.

10. CALCULATION OF RESULTS

10.1 Inject the working standards containing 10, 25, 50, 125 and 250 ng per mL, equivalent to 2, 5, 10, 25 and 50 ng per mL milk. Derive the calibration curve and check the linearity of the detector response.

10.2 Calculate the recovery from the results obtained for the spiked extracts (see 9.17). The mean recovery is reported in the range 93.2 ± 4.7% for the concentrations ranging 2 to 50 ng per mL.

10.3 Calculate the concentration of CAP present in the samples to be analyzed using the calibration curve and taking into account the recovery and the possible dilution.

$$C = \frac{A \times Ce \times 0.8 \times 25}{Ae \times 5 \times 20} = \frac{A \times Ce}{Ae \times 5}$$

where A is area or height of CAP in the sample
Ae is area or height of CAP in the standard
Ce is the concentration of the standard

10.4. Specificity; The chromatograms corresponding to the extracts of milk used to determine the limit of detection (see Section 5, 1.1.10) do not reveal significant interference at the retention time of CAP.

10.5 Accuracy; The accuracy was measured from whole UHT milk samples spiked to 2, 5, 10, 25 and 50 ng per mL with four replicates for each concentration. The results are shown in table 1.

Table 1; Accuracy of the method.

Theoretical Conc, (ng/mL)	Found (ng/mL)	SD (ng/mL)	CV (%)	Recovery (%)
2	2.01	0.09	4.46	100.3
5	4.62	0.21	4.42	92.5
10	9.35	0.08	0.82	93.6
25	22.71	0.05	0.24	90.9
50	44.45	0.55	1.23	88.9

10.6 Limits of detection and quantification.

10.6.1 The limit of detection was assessed on 30 either whole or half skimmed UHT sterilized milk samples. It is equal to the mean quantity measured on the control samples to which is added three times the standard deviation of the mean.
In experiments at CNEVA this was equal to 0.292 + (3 x 0.136) = 0.7 ng per mL.

10.6.2. The limit of quantification assessed using the same samples as in 10.6.1, was the mean value plus 10 times the SD, i.e. 1.66 ng per mL.

10.7. Linearity; The regression line was calculated from the samples analyzed in 10.1. At CNEVA this value was e.g. Y = 0.885X + 0.355, r = 0.9998

10.8. Precision. Precision data were obtained at CNEVA in a study using 3 operators and 4 levels of concentrations, 5,10,25 and 50 ng per mL (the 2 ng per mL concentration was not studied because some detectors may not reach the required level of sensitivity). Each level of concentration was assayed in quadruplicate by each operator.   The results of repeatability and reproducibility were calculated according to ISO standard 5725 (1986) and are given in table 2.

Table 2. Precision data

Level	Theor conc. (ng/mL)	mean conc. found (ng/mL)	range (ng/mL)	repeatability Sr	CVr(%)	r	reproducibility SR	CVR(%)	R
1	5	4.83	4.50 - 5.11	0.089	1.86	0.054	0.228	4.71	0.645
2	10	8.89	8.35 - 9.43	0.281	3.16	0.794	0.397	4.46	1.123
3	25	23.50	22.05 - 24.80	0.337	1.44	0.959	1.078	4.59	3.051
4	50	44.34	42.08 - 46.13	1.151	2.60	3.258	1.169	2.64	3.309

For each concentration level, for repeatability the SD is Sr, the CV is CVr, and the repeatability is r; for reproducibility the SD is SR, the CV is CVR and the reproducibility is R.

R and r are the values below which the difference between two results of a single trial, obtained for conditions of repeatability (r) and reproducibility (R) can be expected to occur with a 95% probability.

Note; The CVr range is 1.44% - 3.16% which is well below the limits (15% at 10 ng per g) for CVs set out in the Criteria document in section 5.

11.   SPECIAL CASES.

12.   NOTES ON PROCEDURE.

13.   SAMPLE CONTROLS.   Note that most of the working solutions are
only used for validation purposes.

14.   TEST REPORT

15.   LIST OF ABBREVIATIONS.

See abbreviations in Annex I, Section 12 of Manual.

16.   FLOW DIAGRAM

  MILK ----------->   SOLVENT EXTRACT (EtAc) ------> EXTRACT
(CHCl$_3$/HEXANE)

  ----------> EXTRACT WITH WATER -------->   HPLC

Cy 3.8.   TETRACYCLINES - DETERMINATION BY HPLC OF TETRACYCLINES AT RESIDUE LEVELS IN ANIMAL TISSUES.

WARNING AND SAFETY PRECAUTIONS

0.   INTRODUCTION

Tetracylines are a group of antibiotics including tetracycline, chlortetracycline, and oxytetracycline which are used therapeutically and prophylactically in animal husbandry. Residues of these substances are often found in animals especially pigs. The residues are sometimes at violative levels. The provisional MRLs set in the EEC for tetracylines is 10-600 µg per kg meat and 100 µg per L of milk.

1.   SCOPE

This method of analysis describes the determination of the total content of tetracycline, chlortetracycline and oxytetracycline in samples of animal origin.

2.   FIELD OF APPLICATION.

The method can be used for muscle, kidney and milk. The limit of determination following the validation of the method is 10 µg/kg or litre of sample for tetracyclines.

3.   REFERENCES.

Commission Decision, 93/256/EEC, laying down the methods for detecting residues of substances having a hormonal or thyrostatic action. [OJ. № L.118, 14.4.93. pp 64-74]

2052/VI/84 File 6.11 II-4, Scientific Veterinary Committee, Working Group - "Reference Methods for Residues", General Criteria for the establishment of Reference Methods for the Detection of Residues.

ISO Standard 78/2-1982 Layout for standards - Part 2: Standard for Chemical Analysis

MAFF, 1989, Determination of tetracyclines at residue levels in animal tissues. Food Science Laboratory, Colney Lane, Norwich, UK Standard Operating Procedure.

Farrington, W.H.H., Tarbin, J., Bygrave, J. and Shearer, G. (1991). Analysis of trace residues of tetracyclines in animal tissues using metal chelate affinity chromatography/HPLC.   Food Addit. & Contamin. <u>8</u>, 55-64

4.   DEFINITIONS.

Tetracyclines content is taken to mean the amount of tetracyclines in the substance in question, regardless of the chemical form, determined according to the described method and expressed as µg or mg tetracyclines per kg or litre of test sample.

5.   PRINCIPLE

The methods comprises 6 stages;-

- Homogenisation of tissue samples in buffer or diluting milk in buffer
- Extraction on chelating Sepharose column
- Extraction on XAD-2 resin column
- Addition of 5% mercapto-propionic acid as an antioxidant
- End point determination with HPLC by UV detection at 350 nm.
- The amount of tetracyclines is calculated by interpolation from a
standard curve and taking into account the recovery of tetracyclines,
especially from tissue samples.

6.   CHEMICALS

6.1.1   Succinic anhydride (BDH)
6.1.2   Sodium hydroxide (BDH)
6.1.3   EDTA (BDH)
6.1.4   Methanol, redistilled (BDH)
6.1.5   Ethanol (Burroughs Ltd)
6.1.6   Acetonitrile (Romil)
6.1.7   Oxalic acid (BDH)
6.1.8   Chelating Sepharose, fast flow in 20% ethanol (Pharmacia)
6.1.9   Amberlite XAD-2 (BDH)
6.1.10   Copper sulphate
6.1.11   ß-mercaptopropionic acid

6.2.   Solutions and Buffers.
6.2.1   Succinate Buffer pH 4.0;   5 g succinic anhydride dissolved in
         900 mL water adjusted to pH 4.0 with 0.1M NaOH and made up to 1 L
         water.
6.2.2   EDTA:Succinate buffer; The succinate buffer, (6.2.1), containing
         37.2 g EDTA per L.
6.2.3   HPLC Mobile Phase;   0.01M oxalic acid:acetonitrile 1:1 v/v
6.2.4   Copper sulphate solution;   0.5 g per L water
6.2.5   ß-mercaptopropionic acid;   50 g per L Methanol

6.3   Column Preparations.
6.3.1   Chelating Sepharose;   5 mL chelating sepharose was thoroughly
         mixed and placed in 200 mm x 20 mm i.d. glass column. Excess
         liquid was run off. Aqueous copper sulphate (6.2.4), 20 mL, was
         passed through the column, followed by succinate buffer (6.2.1).
         After use the columns can be stored in 20% aqueous ethanol at 4°C
         and may be reused 15 times.
6.3.2   Amberlite XAD-2; The resin was washed with acetone, methanol and
         water. Glass columns 200 mm x 20 mm i.d. were packed to a bed
         height of 10 cm with aqueous slurry.
         After use the columns can be regenerated by washing with acetone,
         methanol and water.

6.4.   Standards

6.4.1   Tetracycline (T 3258), chlortetracycline (C 4881) and
         oxytetracycline (O 5750) were obtained from Sigma Chemical Co.
6.4.2.   Stock standards; 1 mg per mL tetracycline in methanol. Store at
         4°C and make fresh weekly.
6.4.3   Intermediate standards; Dilute 1 mL stock to 100 mL with

6.4.4   distilled water. Store at 4°C and make fresh weekly.
Working standards; Dilute 1 mL intermediate standard to 10 mL with distilled water. Final concentration is 1 ng per ul. Make fresh daily.

6.5.   Spiking Procedure
Using the working standards (6.4.4) spike 10 g sample with 100 ul and 500 ul standard solution. Allow to stand for 15 minutes.

7.   EQUIPMENT

7.1	Centrifuge tubes 250 mL and 50 mL capacity.
7.2	Glass columns 200 mm x 20 mm i.d. fitted with sintered glass frit and stopcock
7.3	Glass filter funnel 250 mL
7.4.	Conical flasks 250 mL
7.5	Pear shaped flasks 50 mL
7.6	Round bottomed flasks 250 mL
7.7.	Filter paper (Whatman) 541
7.8	Ultra-Turrax Homogeniser
7.9	Mixer (Vortex)
7.10	Rotary evaporator - Buchli with water bath at 40°C
7.11	HPLC-LKB 2150 pump

Column; Chromsep (Chrompack) cartridge column assembly packed with Lichrosorb RP8 with integral (10 mm x 2.1 mm i.d.) guard column packed with pellicular (30-40 um) reverse phase.
Mobile phase was pumped at 0.4 mL per min.
UV detection was at 350 nm (0.005 AUFS) (Severn, SA6510) and the chromatogram recorded and integrated using an electronic integrator (Spectra Physics 4290). 10 μL samples were injected using a Waters Wisp 712.

8.   SAMPLES AND SAMPLING PROCEDURE.

N.B. Attention is drawn to section 6.3.1 and ISO document 78/2-1982 and the following notes derived from Annex II of 2052/VI/84-EN.

8.1. Nature of the Sample; Samples shall be such as to enable the detection of residues in meat, as defined in Directive 64/433/EEC and also in milk.

8.2. Size of Sample; The size of the sample must be large enough to allow the reference method to be carried out and to allow repeat analysis where required.

In this method for tetracyclines the sizes shall not be less than
50 g muscle, kidney;   50 mL milk

 8.3. The samples must be taken and packed in such a way as to allow proper identification in the laboratory.
8.4. The method of packing, preservation and transport must maintain the integrity of the sample and not prejudice the result of the examination.

Samples for the analysis of tetracyclines must be stored and transported at temperatures below -18°C.

9.   PROCEDURE

9.1.   10 g milk or finely sliced tissue and 40 mL succinate buffer were
            placed in an ultrasonic bath (3 min) homogenised (2 min) and
            centrifuged (5 min) at 12,000 r.c.f.
9.2   Supernatant was filtered through Whatman 541 filter paper.
9.3   The stages 9.1 and 9.2 were repeated using the sediment instead
            of tissue.
9.4.   The stages 9.1 and 9.2 were again repeated using the sediment
            instead of tissue and with only 20 mL buffer.
9.5   The combined filtrates were loaded onto the prepared chelating
            Sepharose column which was subsequently washed with water (10
            mL), methanol (30 mL) and water (2 x 10 mL).   The flow should
            not exceed 4 mL per min.
9.6   The tetracylines were eluted with EDTA-succinate buffer (40 mL)
            followed by a further 10 mL of this buffer. Flow ca. 4 ml per
            min.
9.7   The combined eluates were loaded directly onto the XAD-2 column.
9.8   The column was washed with water (2 x 100 mL) and eluted with
            redistilled methanol (100 mL at 4 mL per min).
9.9   The methanol was reduced to a small volume by rotary evaporation
            and the residue transferred to a pear shaped flask with
            redistilled methanol (3 x 2 mL)
9.10   5% ß-mercaptopropionic acid (0.1 mL) was added and the methanol
            removed by rotary evaporation.
9.11   The residue was dissolved in the HPLC mobile phase (500 µL) with
            vortexing and ultrasonication before transfer to a WISP vial.
9.12   HPLC was performed using 10 ul.

10. CALCULATION OF RESULTS
10.1. A calibration curve is constructed of peak height against
concentration for a range of standards from 1 to 20 ng. The quantity of
each of the tetracylines in each sample injection is then calculated from
the measured peak height. This figure is then corrected for injection
volume and mean % recovery (calculated from spiked samples) to give a
concentration in mg/kg (ppm). The standard injection of 10 ul is
equivalent to 0.2 g of extracted sample.

Retention times are normally of the order; oxytetracyline, 6 min,
tetracycline, 8 min, chlortetracycline 10 min.

$$\% \text{ recovery} = \frac{\text{amount of tetracycline found x 100}}{\text{amount of Spike added}}$$

Concentration of tetracycline in sample (mg/kg) =

$$\frac{\text{µg tetracycline (from calibration curve)}}{1000} \times \frac{1}{0.05} \times \frac{100}{\% \text{ recovery}}$$

For samples containing tetracyclines at concentrations beyond the range of
the standard curve, a dilution of the extract is prepared and
chromatographed, and the appropriate volumetric correction is applied.

10.2.   SENSITIVITY
The minimum limit of determination of tetracyclines by this method is
0.01 mg/kg.

10.3.   RECOVERIES
Recoveries determined at MAFF, Norwich (mean ± SD) of added tetracyclines
to twelve pig kidneys were;-

Spike	Oxytetracyline	Tetracycline	Chlortetracycline
0.01 mg per kg	80 ± 7	72 ± 7	87 ± 15
0.05 mg per kg	75 ± 7	63 ± 6	73 ± 8

11.   SPECIAL CASES.

12.   NOTES ON PROCEDURE.

13.   SAMPLE CONTROLS

It is convenient to analyze 5 or 7 tissue samples plus 1 spiked quality
control blank sample in each batch. The sample numbers depend on the
centrifuge head capacity.

*The blank sample was obtained from a sample previously analyzed and found
to contain no tetracyclines.

14.   TEST REPORT

15.   LIST OF ABBREVIATIONS.
See abbreviations in Annex I, Section 12 of Manual.

16.   FLOW DIAGRAM

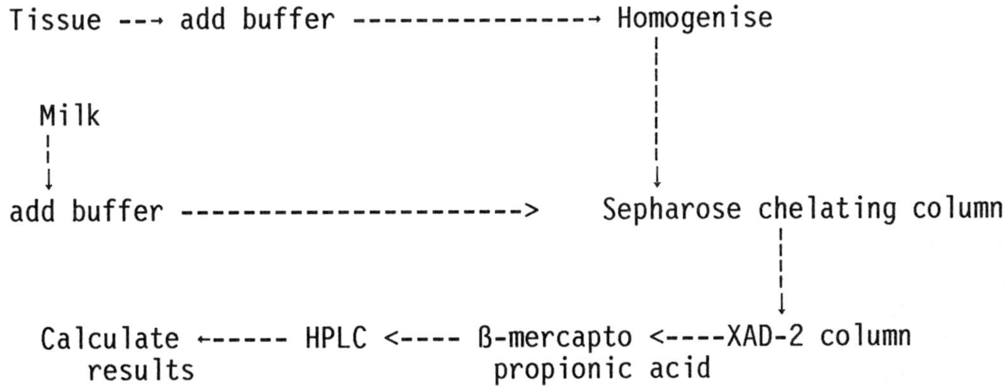

Cy 3.9.   NITROFURANS - HPLC ANALYSIS WITH A DIALYSIS METHOD FOR DETERMINING RESIDUES OF NITROFURANS IN EGGS, MILK AND MEAT.

WARNING AND SAFETY PRECAUTIONS

SAFETY
Organic solvents - all organic solvents must be treated as potentially hazardous and all procedures using them must be performed in a fume cupboard.

0.   INTRODUCTION

Nitrofurans (here furazolidone, nitrofurazone, nitrofurantoin and furaltadone) are antibacterial agents used in pigs and poultry.

1.   SCOPE

This work is carried out in compliance with the Residues Directive (86/469/EEC).

2.   FIELD OF APPLICATION.

This method is used for determining the presence of nitrofurans in eggs, meat or milk. The method is operated at RIKILT in the Netherlands, as a routine monitoring method analyzing about 30 samples per day. It can be used as a confirmatory method. The limits of determinations range from 1-10 µg per kg of matrix for Nitrofurans.

3.   REFERENCES.

Commission Decision, 93/256/EEC, laying down the methods for detecting residues of substances having a hormonal or thyrostatic action. [OJ. № L.118, 14.4.93. pp 64-74]

2052/VI/84 File 6.11 II-4, Scientific Veterinary Committee, Working Group - "Reference Methods for Residues", General Criteria for the establishment of Reference Methods for the Detection of Residues.

ISO Standard 78/2-1982 Layout for standards - Part 2: Standard for Chemical Analysis

ISO Standard 5725 (1986)

Aerts, M.M.L., Beek,W.M.J. and Brinkman, U.A.Th., (1990), On-line combination of dialysis and column-switching liquid chromatography as a fully automated sample preparation technique for biological samples. Determination of nitrofuran residues in edible products. J.Chromatogr. <u>500</u>, 453-468

4.   DEFINITIONS.

Nitrofurans content is taken to mean the amount of nitrofurans in eggs, milk or meat determined according to the described method and expressed as µg nitrofurans per kg test sample.

5.   PRINCIPLE.

The method comprises four stages all carried out in the absence of daylight
or white light.

- Samples of decreamed-milk are mixed in saline. Meat and eggs are
  homogenised in saline
- Centrifugation
- purification of the supernatant extract by dialysis
- quantification by high performance liquid chromatography (HPLC) with UV
  detection at 365 nm.

6.   MATERIALS

6.1.   <u>Chemicals</u>

6.1.1   Sodium chloride
6.1.2   Methanol, Analytical grade
6.1.3   Acetone, Analytical grade
6.1.4   Acetonitrile, HPLC grade
6.1.5   Sodium azide
6.1.6.   Sodium acetate
6.1.7.   Glacial acetic acid
6.1.8.   Demineralised water, filtered on Milli-Q purification system
           (Millipore, Milford, USA)

6.2.   <u>Solutions</u>
6.2.1.   0.9% NaCl in water (6.1.8).
6.2.2.   1% sodium azide in water (6.1.8.)
6.2.3.   10% sodium azide in water (6.1.8.)
6.2.4.   0.1M sodium acetate - acetic acid buffer; pH 5.0.
6.2.5.   HPLC eluent; Mix 800 mL of acetate buffer (6.2.4) with 200 mL
           acetonitrile (6.1.4.)

6.3.   <u>Nitrofuran Standards</u>

        Furazolidone, nitrofurazone, nitrofurantoin and furaltadone were
        obtained from Sigma, USA.

6.3.1.   Standard solution;   100 µg/mL nitrofurans in acetone:methanol,
           1:1 v/v.
           Store at 4°C in the dark. Stable for maximum period of at least
           one month.

6.3.2.   Working Standards are 10 µg nitrofuran per mL saline (6.2.1).
           They should be prepared fresh daily.

7.   EQUIPMENT

7.1.   Glassware
7.1.1   Graduated pipettes,
7.1.2   Glass centrifuge tubes
7.1.3   Glass test tubes to take 6 mL samples.
7.1.4   Normal laboratory glassware

7.2.   Apparatus
7.2.1.   Automatic pipettes,

7.2.2.   Analytical balance
7.2.3.   Refrigerated centrifuge
7.2.4.   Refrigerator at <-18°C
7.2.5.   Vibromixer
7.3. Dialysis Equipment

An autosampler-dialysis module is a modified Gilson ASTED system consisting
of a Model 231 autosampling injector, two Model 401 diluters equipped with
5 mL and 1 mL syringes and two poly(methyl methacrylate) flat-plate
dialyser blocks and fitted with a Cuprophan membrane (10,000-15,000 Daltons
cut-off) having donor volumes of 100 µL and 370 µL and acceptor volumes of
175 µL and 650 µL, respectively.

The selection and arrangement of the blocks depends on the volume of
material available for analysis.

7.4   HPLC equipment

A constant pulseless-flow pump (Gilson Medical Electronics, Model 302/5),
with a Kratos Spectroflow 783 absorbance detector set at 365 nm, 0.001
a.u.f.s., a rise time of 5 sec and an automatic six-port valve (Model 7010,
Rheodyne, USA) mounted either on a switching-valve module (Must, Spark,
Emmen, NL) or on an autosampling injector (Model 231, Gilson).
Chromatographic peaks are recorded with an integrator (Chromatopac C-R2A,
Shimadzu, Japan) or a Kipp DD-U1 recorder. All timed events are controlled
by the ASTED controller. The precolumn used is 60 mm x 4.6 mm i.d. column
fitted with 20 um frits and containing 37-50 um Bondapak C_{18}/Corasil
(Millipore). The column is a 250 mm x 4.6 mm i.d. column containing 5 um
Hypersil ODS (Chrompack, Middelburg, NL). The flow rate of the eluent
(6.2.5) was 1 mL per min.

7.5.   Homogeniser, Model 400 Stomacher laboratory blender, (Lameris,
           NL)
7.6.   Light sealed room lit by yellow light.

8.   SAMPLES AND SAMPLING PROCEDURE.

N.B. Attention is drawn to section 6.3.1 and ISO document 78/2-1982 and
the following notes derived from Annex II of 2052/VI/84-EN.

8.1. Nature of the Sample; Samples of meat, milk and eggs shall be such
as to enable the detection of residues. Only samples which are not spoiled
by bacteria may be examined.

8.2. Size of Sample; The size of the sample must be large enough to allow
the reference method to be carried out and to allow repeat analysis where
required.

8.3. The samples must be cooled after collection and stored at $\leq$ -20°C
pending analysis.

9.   PROCEDURE

9.1.   Thaw the sample.
9.2.   Raw milk - samples are decreamed by centrifugation (10 min, 2000
           g) and subsequent freezing (15 min at -20°C). An aliquot (10 mL)

9.3.   is diluted with 10 mL of saline solution (6.2.1) and 2 mL of 1% sodium azide (6.2.2).

9.3.   Meat - 10 g of homogenised meat is blended for 3 min in a Stomacher (7.5) with 30 mL saline (6.2.1). After centrifugation (2000 g), 20 mL of the clear upper phase are isolated and mixed with 2 mL 1% sodium azide (6.2.2).

9.4.   Eggs - 10 g of homogenised whole egg is diluted with 10 mL saline (6.2.1) and 3 mL of 10% sodium azide solution (6.2.3).

9.5.   Dialysis - Aliquots of diluted solutions 9.2, 9.3 or 9.4 are injected into the dialysis module. The maximum of about 4 mL of sample can be introduced either as a continuously flowing injection or divided into multiple pulsed injections. During the dialysis the dialyser acceptor stream (water) is continuously transported with a second, 1 mL syringe, diluter and successive 1 mL volumes of the dialysate are led to the trace enrichment column. After application of the total dialysate, the enrichment column can be flushed with acceptor stream solvent and, after switching of the automatic six-port valve, back-flushed to he analytical column with the HPLC eluent (6.2.5).

[Note;   The dialyser donor and acceptor channels are then flushed with water (6.1.8.), the six port valve returned to its original position and the enrichment column is regenerated with water.]

9.5.1   Configuration of Dialysis Blocks.
RIKILT uses a pulsed dialysis mode in which two dialyser blocks are fitted in series having donor volumes of 2 x 370 µL and acceptor volumes of 2 x 650 µL. A 4 mL sample is injected as five 750 µL pulses and one 250 µL pulse. The final pulse consisted of 500 µL of the already dialysed fifth pulse and the remaining 250 µL sample extract. The first five samples are statically dialysed for 3 min at an acceptor flow-rate of 0.36 mL per min, giving a dialyser efficiency of about 30%. The final pulse is dialysed for 9 min at the same acceptor flow-rate. Using this prolonged dialysis time, the last 2 mL of acceptor solvent are essentially free from matrix components, and can be used to flush the precolumn. The total acceptor volume that is led over the precolumn is about 8.6 mL. After application of this volume, the precolumn is backflushed for about 5 min with HPLC eluent (6.2.5) and the enriched analytes are separated on the analytical column.

9.6.   Blank samples and spiked blank samples are run as quality controls and to provide a standard curve. The spiked samples are prepared by injecting 1 - 100 µL of aqueous standard solutions (6.1.13.2) into the raw samples.

10.   CALCULATION OF RESULTS

10.1   Derive the calibration curve using the results for the spiked blank samples (9.6) and check the linearity of the detector response.

10.2   The mean recoveries observed at RIKILT are measured for spiked (5 µg per kg) samples compared with the same spikes in saline. The results are shown in table 1.

Table 1. Limits of Determination (LD) and Recoveries.

| Drug | Meat (veal, chicken) | | | Eggs | | |
	LD (ug/kg)	Recovery %	CV%	LD (ug/kg)	Recovery %	CV%
Nitrofurazone	2	76	1.7	1	85	4.1
Nitrofurantoin	2	75	2.6	1	76	2.0
Furazolidone	2	89	2.2	1	88	4.8
Furaltadone	5	86	4.0	3	86	6.5

(data from Aerts et al., 1990.)

10.3 Calculate the concentration of nitrofuran present in the samples to be analyzed using the calibration curve obtained for spiked blank samples and taking into account the possible dilution.

10.4. Specificity; The chromatograms corresponding to the extracts of blank samples of eggs,milk and meat do not reveal significant interference at the retention time of the four nitrofurans. Furthermore the most common used antimicrobials and cocccidiostats do not interfere.

10.5 Limits of detection and determination.

(ug/kg)

| | Limit of detection (ug/kg) | | Limit of determination (ug/kg) | |
	eggs	meat	eggs	meat
Nitrofurazone	0.5	1.0	1	2
Nitrofurantoin	0.5	1.0	1	2
Furazolidone	0.5	1.0	1	2
Furaltadone	1.5	2.5	3	5

(Data from H. Keukens, RIKILT)

10.6. Precision. The CVs for the recoveries of spikes from eggs, milk and meat are shown in table 1.

11. SPECIAL CASES.
12. NOTES ON PROCEDURE.

NITROFURANS DECOMPOSE IN WHITE/DAY LIGHT. IT IS ESSENTIAL THAT ALL PROCEDURES ARE CARRIED OUT IN THE ABSENCE OF DAYLIGHT AND WHITE LIGHT.

13. SAMPLE CONTROLS
14. TEST REPORT
15. LIST OF ABBREVIATIONS.

See abbreviations in Annex I, Section 12 of Manual.

16. FLOW DIAGRAM

MILK, EGGS, MEAT ----------->   SALINE EXTRACT ------> DIALYSIS

-------->   HPLC -------> CALCULATE RESULTS

Cy 4.1. BENZIMIDAZOLES - DETERMINATION OF BENZIMIDAZOLES AT RESIDUE LEVELS IN ANIMAL TISSUES AND MILK.

WARNING AND SAFETY PRECAUTIONS

0.   INTRODUCTION

The benzimidazoles are a group of substances with the common benzimidazole structure, they include Oxfendazole, Fenbendazole, Cambendazole, Thiabendazole, and Albendazole. Febantel is a pro-drug which is rapidly cyclised in the animal to benzimidazole type compounds. Benzimidazoles are anthelmintics used for the protection and cure of internal worm parasites in food producing animals. Benzimidazoles are administered orally as solutions, suspensions or pellets.
The MRL set in the EEC for Benzimidazoles are listed in section 2.

1.   SCOPE

This method of analysis describes the determination of the content of Benzimidazoles in samples of animal origin.

2.   FIELD OF APPLICATION.

The method was developed for monitoring milk and liver tissue. The limit of determination following validation of the method is 0.02 mg/kg of sample or 0.02 mg per L milk for Benzimidazoles.

3.   REFERENCES.

Commission Decision, 93/256/EEC, laying down the methods for detecting residues of substances having a hormonal or thyrostatic action. [OJ. № L.118, 14.4.93. pp 64-74]

ISO Standard 78/2-1982 Layout for standards - Part 2: Standard for Chemical Analysis

MAFF, 1989, Determination of Benzimidazoles at residue levels in animal tissues and milk. Food Science Laboratory, Colney Lane, Norwich. Standard Operating Procedure.

Marti, A.M., Mooser, A.E. and Koch, H. (1990), Determination of benzimidazoles anthelmintics in meat samples. J. Chromatogr. _498_, 145-157

4.   DEFINITIONS.

Benzimidazoles content is taken to mean the amount of Benzimidazoles in the substance in question, regardless of the chemical form, determined according to the described method and expressed as µg or mg Benzimidazoles per kg or L of test sample.

5.   PRINCIPLE

The methods comprises 6 stages;-

- Homogenisation of tissue samples in buffer
- Extraction with organic solvent
- Clean-up on solid phase Silica column.

- Extraction on reverse phase C18 column
- End point determination with HPLC by fluorescent UV detection (see note on GC-MS verification)
- The amount of Benzimidazoles is calculated by interpolation from a standard curve and taking into account the recovery of Benzimidazoles, especially from tissue samples.

Note; In the method developed at the Swiss Federal Veterinary Office, Berne, by Marti et al, (1990), positive results obtained by HPLC were verified using GC-MS after forming the methyl or pentaflourobenzyl derivatives of the benzimidazoles.

6.   CHEMICALS

6.1.1   Chloroform (BDH)
6.1.2   Acetone (BDH)
6.1.3   Sodium hydroxide 0.1N AVS (BDH)
6.1.4   Methanol, redistilled (BDH)
6.1.5   Acetic anhydride (Sigma)
6.1.6   Acetonitrile HPLC Grade (Romil)
6.1.7   Ethyl acetate (May & Baker)
6.1.8   Hexane (BDH)
6.1.9   Toluene (BDH)
6.1.10   Potassium dihydrogen orthophoshate (BDH)
6.1.11   Ammonium carbonate (BDH)

6.2.   Solutions
6.2.1   0.25M phosphate buffer, pH 7.0 ; 34 g potassium dihydrogen orthophoshate was dissolved in 900 mL water. The pH was adjusted to 7.0 with 0.1M sodium hydroxide and the volume made up to 1 L.
6.2.2.   0.1M ammonium carbonate; 15.7 g of ammonium carbonate was dissolved in 1 L water.
6.2.3   60% hexane in chloroform; Mix 60 mL of hexane and 40 mL chloroform.
6.2.4.   HPLC Mobile Phase; 400 mL methanol was added to 600 mL 0.1M ammonium carbonate. The solution was mixed and passed through a "Durapore " filter, assisted by vacuum. The mobile phase was degassed using ultrasonication and with reduced pressure.

6.3.   Standards
         Benzimidazoles reference standards were -
6.3.1.   Thiabendazole (Merck, Sharpe and Dohme Ltd.)
6.3.2.   Albendazole (Smith, Kline and French)
6.3.3.   Oxfendazole (Syntex)
6.3.4.   Cambendazole (Merck, Sharpe and Dohme Ltd.)
6.3.5.   Stock standards; 5 mg Benzimidazoles in 100 mL methanol. Store at 4°C and make fresh monthly.
6.3.6   Working standards;
6.3.6.1 Dilute 1 mL stock to 100 mL with methanol. Final concentration is 0.5 μg per mL. Store at 4°C and make fresh weekly.
6.3.6.2 Dilute 0.5 mL stock to 100 mL with methanol. Final concentration is 0.25 μg per mL. Make fresh weekly
6.5.   Spiking Procedure

         Using separately the working standards (6.3.6.1 & 6.3.6.2) spike 5 g sample with 1 mL of solution. Allow to stand for 15 minutes.

7.   EQUIPMENT

7.1   Centrifuges tubes 100 mL capacity, plastic.
7.2   Glass filter funnel - 77 mm diameter
7.3   All glass filter holder, 47 mm - Millipore.
7.4.   Glass sample bottles, 5 mL & 25 mL
7.5   Pear shaped flasks   50 mL and 100 mL
7.6   Glass reactivials 3 mL with PTFE lined screw caps.
7.7.   Glass syringes, 1 mL and 10 mL
7.8   Ultra-Turrax Homogeniser
7.9   Mixer (Vortex)
7.10   Rotary evaporator - Buchli with water bath at 40°C
7.11.   Vials, low volume for autosampler
7.12.   Syringes 1 mL plastic disposable
7.13.   Centrifuge - IEC Centra-7R or equivalent
7.14.   Ultrasonic bath- L&R 140S or equivalent
7.15.   Adjustable pipettes 5 mL
7.16.   Filter paper, 15 cm, phase separation - Whatman PS-1
7.17.   Membrane filter holder - Millipore Swinney Stainless, 13 mm
7.18.   Membrane filters, 13 mm and 47 mm - Millipore Ltd.
7.19.   Solid Phase Extraction
7.19.1.   Vacuum Manifold - Vac-Elut
7.19.2.   C18/500 mg cartridges - Bond-Elut, Jones Chromatography Ltd.
7.19.3.   Silica 500 mg cartridges - Bond-Elut, Jones Chromatography Ltd.
7.19.4.   Cartridge taps - Jones Chromatography Ltd.
7.19.5.   Reservoirs 50 mL for cartridges - Jones Chromatography Ltd.

7.20   HPLC   LKB 2150 pump
          Column; 20 cm x 3 mm i.d. Chromsep (Chrompack) cartridge column
          assembly packed with Chromspher C8 with integral (10 mm x 2.1 mm
          i.d.) guard column packed with pellicular (30-40 um) reverse
          phase.
          Mobile phase was pumped at 0.4 mL per min.
          The fluorescence detector was a Perkin Elmer LS4 with the
          excitation wavelength 312 nm, slit width 10 nm, and the emission
          wavelength at 355 nm, slit width 10 nm.
          The chromatogram was recorded and integrated using an electronic
          integrator (Spectra Physics 4290). 20 µL samples were injected
          using a Waters Wisp 712.

8.   SAMPLES AND SAMPLING PROCEDURE.

N.B. Attention is drawn to section 6.3.1 and ISO document 78/2-1982 and
the following notes derived from Annex II of 2052/VI/84-EN.

8.1. Nature of the Sample; Samples shall be such as to enable the
detection of residues in meat, as defined in Directive 64/433/EEC and also
in milk.

8.2. Size of Sample; The size of the sample must be large enough to allow
the reference method to be carried out and to allow repeat analysis where
required.
 8.3. The samples must be taken and packed in such a way as to allow
proper identification in the laboratory.

8.4. The method of packing, preservation and transport must maintain the
integrity of the sample and not prejudice the result of the examination.

Cy 4.1/3

Samples for the analysis of Benzimidazoles must be stored and transported at temperatures below -18°C.

9.   PROCEDURE

9.1.   5 g finely sliced tissue or 5 mL milk and 15 mL acetonitrile were placed into a centrifuge tube.
9.2.   25 mL ethyl acetate were added and the mixture was homogenised (4 min) and centrifuged (5 min) at 2,500 rpm.
9.3   The supernatant was filtered through the phase separating paper containing sodium sulphate, into a 100 mL pear shaped flask.
9.4   Steps 9.2 and 9.3 were repeated.
9.5.   The pooled filtrates were reduced to about 1 mL by rotary evaporation (7.10).
9.6.   The residue was transferred to a pre-conditioned Bond-Elut Silica cartridge using 3 x 2 mL 60% hexane in chloroform.
         The Silica Bond-Elut columns were conditioned by drawing through 5 mL 60% hexane in chloroform.acetonitrile.
9.7.   The cartridge was allowed to dry and then washed through with 2 mL toluene and air dried.
9.8.   The benzimidazoles were eluted with 10 mL acetone.
9.9.   The acetone was removed by rotary evaporation and the residue transferred in 10% methanol in water (3 x 2 mL).
9.10.   After allowing the column to dry the benzimidazoles were eluted with 10 mL acetonitrile into glass sample bottles (7.4).
9.11   The eluate was transferred to a 50 mL pear-shaped flask using 2 x 2 mL acetonitrile rinses.
9.12   The organic phase was evaporated to dryness using a rotary evaporator with a water bath set at 40°C.
9.13   The residue was redissolved in 1 mL HPLC mobile phase.
9.14   Standards for Calibration Curve.
         The standard additions are done at this stage (9.7) for the preparation of a standard curve over the range 0 - 5 µg per kg.
9.15   HPLC was performed using 20 µL.

10.   CALCULATION OF RESULTS

10.1. A calibration curve, 0 - 5 µg, is constructed of peak height against concentration for a range of standards. The quantity of each of the Benzimidazoles in each sample injection is then calculated from the measured peak height. This figure is then corrected for injection volume and mean % recovery (calculated from spiked samples) to give a concentration in mg/kg (ppm). The standard injection of 20 µL is equivalent to 100 mg or mL of extracted sample.

$$\% \text{ recovery} = \frac{\text{amount of Benzimidazoles found}}{\text{amount of Spike added}} \times 100$$

Concentration of Benzimidazoles in sample (mg/kg) =

$$\frac{\text{µg Benzimidazoles (from calibration curve)}}{1000} \times \frac{1}{0.05} \times \frac{100}{\% \text{ recovery}}$$

For samples containing Benzimidazoles at concentrations beyond the range of the standard curve, a dilution of the extract is prepared and chromatographed,
and the appropriate volumetric correction is applied.

10.2.   SENSITIVITY
The minimum limit of determination of Benzimidazoles by this method is
0.02 mg/kg for all four benzimidazoles in all tissue types.

10.3.   QUALITY ASSURANCE PROCEDURES.
10.3.1. Validation;   Batches of up to six blank samples are spiked at the
0.05 or 0.1 mg per kg level for all the four benzimidazoles and extractions
are performed on each of three consecutive days. Each batch comprised the
following samples;-
2 blanks; 2 standard additions at 0.05 mg per kg;
2 standard additions at 0.1 mg per kg; 6 spikes at 0.05 or 0.1 mg per kg.

Recovery of the analyte should fall within 60-90%. CV values should fall
within the range 5-15% for inter and intra batch precision.

10.3.2. Examples of quality assurance data obtained at MAFF, Norwich.

MILK;
Recovery of benzimidazoles from milk measured at level of 10 µg per L in 3
samples on day 1, 5 samples on day 2 and 4 samples on day 3

Albendazole sulphone,   77 ± 3% CV=4%,   Thiabendazole,   53 ± 6%   CV=11%
Oxfendazole,   70 ± 4% CV=6%,   Cambendazole,   52 ± 6%   CV=12%

LIVER;
Recovery of benzimidazoles from liver measured at level of 20 µg per kg in
6 samples per day for 3 consecutive days.

Albendazole sulphone,   90 ± 10% CV=11%,   Thiabendazole,   77 ± 5%   CV=7%
Oxfendazole,   71 ± 9%   CV=13%,   Cambendazole,   82 ± 13%   CV=13%

11.   SPECIAL CASES.
In samples in which a positive is suspected, further confirmatory evidence
may be obtained by comparison of the stopped-flow analysis of the emission
spectra of the suspect peaks.
For bovine milk samples thiabendazole is not excreted as the parent drug
and can be used as an internal standard.

12.   NOTES ON PROCEDURE.
It is convenient to analyze up to ten samples per batch per day with HPLC
overnight. A batch would include unknowns, plus spiked quality control
samples.

13.   SAMPLE CONTROLS
The blank samples were obtained from a sample previously analyzed and found
 to contain no Benzimidazoles.

14.   TEST REPORT

15.   LIST OF ABBREVIATIONS.
See abbreviations in Annex I, section 12 of Manual.

16.   FLOW DIAGRAM
     Tissue --→ add ethyl acetate---------→ Homogenise ------> Si column
                                                                   |
                                                                   |
                                                                   ↓
                    Calculate results <---- HPLC <------- C18 column

Cy 4.2. LASALOCID - DETERMINATION OF LASALOCID AT RESIDUE LEVELS IN POULTRY MUSCLE AND POULTRY EGGS.

WARNING AND SAFETY PRECAUTIONS

0.   INTRODUCTION

Lasalocid is an ionophore antibiotic that is used as a growth promoter in cattle and as a coccidiostat in poultry.

1.   SCOPE

This method of analysis describes the determination of the total content of Lasalocid in samples of poultry origin.

2.   FIELD OF APPLICATION.

The method can be used for poultry muscle and poultry eggs. The limit of determination following validation of the method when confirmed by stop-flow analysis of the emission spectra is 10 µg/kg of sample for Lasalocid.

3.   REFERENCES.

Commission Decision, 93/256/EEC, laying down the methods for detecting residues of substances having a hormonal or thyrostatic action. [OJ. № L.118, 14.4.93. pp 64-74]

2052/VI/84 File 6.11 II-4, Scientific Veterinary Committee, Working Group - "Reference Methods for Residues", General Criteria for the establishment of Reference Methods for the Detection of Residues.

ISO Standard 78/2-1982 Layout for standards - Part 2: Standard for Chemical Analysis

MAFF, 1989, Determination of Lasalocid at residue levels in poultry muscle and eggs. Food Science Laboratory, Colney Lane, Norwich. Standard Operating Procedure.

4.   DEFINITIONS.

Lasalocid content is taken to mean the amount of Lasalocid in the substance in question, regardless of the chemical form, determined according to the described method and expressed as µg or mg Lasalocid per kg of test sample.

5.   PRINCIPLE

The methods comprises 6 stages;-

- Homogenisation of tissue samples in buffer
- Extraction with organic solvent
- Extraction on Solid phase Silica column
- End point determination with HPLC by fluorescent UV detection
- The amount of Lasalocid is calculated by interpolation from a standard curve and taking into account the recovery of Lasalocid, especially from tissue samples.

6.   CHEMICALS

6.1.1   Chloroform - redistilled (May & Baker)
6.1.2   Carbon Tetrachloride - Glass distilled grade (Rathburn)
6.1.3   Sodium chloride (BDH)
6.1.4   Methanol, redistilled (FSA)
6.1.5   Sodium sulphate anhydrous (BDH)
6.1.6   Acetonitrile (Rathburn HPLC Grade)
6.1.7   Hexane (Rathburn)
6.1.8   1,1,3,3-tetramethylguanidine - redistilled (Aldrich)

6.2.   Solutions
6.2.1   Saturated sodium chloride;- Sodium chloride dissolved in water to
          saturation.
6.2.2.   5% methanol in chloroform;- 5 mL methanol made to 100 mL with
          chloroform
6.2.3.   HPLC Mobile Phase; 5 mL 1,1,3,3-tetramethylguanidine diluted to
          1 L with acetonitrile.

6.3.   Standards
6.3.1   Lasalocid reference standard was obtained from Sigma Chem Co.
6.3.2.   Stock standards; 50 mg Lasalocid in 250 mL methanol. Store at
          4°C and make fresh monthly.
6.3.3   Intermediate standards; Dilute 1 mL stock to 10 mL with
          methanol. Store at 4°C and make fresh daily.
6.3.4   Working standards;
6.3.4.1   Dilute 0.2 mL intermediate standard to 10 mL with HPLC mobile
          phase. Final concentration is 0.4 µg per mL. Make fresh daily.
6.3.4.2   Dilute 1 mL working standard (6.3.4.1) to 10 mL with HPLC mobile
          phase. Final concentration is 0.04 µg per mL. Make fresh daily.

6.5.   Spiking Procedure
          Using the working standards (6.3.4) spike 5 g sample with 50 ul
          and 125 ul standard solution. Allow to stand for 15 minutes.

7.   EQUIPMENT

7.1   Centrifuges tubes 100 mL capacity
7.2   Separating funnels, 250 mL capacity
7.3   All glass filter holder, 47 mm - Millipore.
7.4.   Test tubes - 125 x 16 mm (to fit vacuum Manifold)
7.5   Pear shaped flasks 25 mL
7.6   Round bottomed flasks, 250 mL capacity
7.7.   Glass pipettes, 1 mL and 10 mL graduated
7.8   Ultra-Turrax Homogeniser
7.9   Mixer (Vortex)
7.10   Rotary evaporator - Buchli with water bath at 50°C
7.11.   Vials 2 mL and 0.3 mL volume for autosampler
7.12.   Disposable syringes 1 mL capacity
7.13.   Centrifuge - IEC Centra-7R or equivalent
7.14.   Ultrasonic bath- L&R 140S or equivalent
7.15.   Adjustable pipettes 200 µL and 1000 µL
7.16.   Multiport nitrogen evaporator with heater block (40°C) for
          reactivials.
7.17.   Membrane filter holder - Millipore Swinney Stainless, 13 mm
7.18.   Membrane filters, 13 mm and 47 mm - Millipore Ltd.
7.19.   Filter paper 15 cm, type PS-1 Whatman
7.20.   Solid Phase Extraction
7.20.1.   Vacuum Manifold - Spe-ed mate 30 (Applied Separations)

7.20.2. Bond-Elut Silica cartridges, 500 mg/2.8 mL - (Jones
         Chromatography Ltd.)
7.20.3   Bond-Elut adaptors (Jones Chromatography Ltd.)
7.20.4   Bond-Elut Reservoirs 75 mL for cartridges - (Jones Chromatography
         Ltd.)
7.20.5   The columns were washed with 5 mL hexane before use.

7.21   HPLC-Waters 590 pump
         Column; 10 cm x 4.6 mm i.d. packed with Hypercarb 7 μm (porous
         Graphite Carbon) (Shandon)
         Mobile phase was pumped at 0.5 mL per min.
         The fluorescence detector was a Philips PU 4027 with the
         excitation wavelength 310 nm and the emission wavelength at 420
         nm.
         The chromatogram was recorded and integrated using an electronic
         integrator (Spectra Physics 4400). 25 μL samples were injected
         using a Waters Wisp 712.
         The column and mobile phase were maintained at 35°C using a Jones
         model 7962 oven.

8.   SAMPLES AND SAMPLING PROCEDURE.

N.B. Attention is drawn to section 6.3.1 and to ISO document 78/2-1982 and
also the following notes derived from Annex II of 2052/VI/84-EN and EEC
93/256.

8.1. Nature of the Sample; Samples shall be such as to enable the
detection of residues in meat, as defined in Directive 64/433/EEC and also
in milk.

8.2. Size of Sample; The size of the sample must be large enough to allow
the reference method to be carried out and to allow repeat analysis where
required.

8.3. The samples must be taken and packed in such a way as to allow proper
identification in the laboratory.

8.4. The method of packing, preservation and transport must maintain the
integrity of the sample and not prejudice the result of the examination.

Samples for the analysis of Lasalocid must be stored and transported at
temperatures below -18°C.

Samples for analysis of muscle should be obtained by removing thin slices
from the frozen tissue. The bulk sample should not be allowed to thaw.

9.   PROCEDURE

9.1.   2 g finely sliced tissue or homogenised egg were homogenised in
         25 mL acetonitrile. The homogenate was placed in an ultrasonic
         bath (5 min) and centrifuged (5 min) at 3,000 rpm.
9.2   The supernatant was transferred to 250 mL separating funnel.
9.3   The residue was reextracted with 25 mL acetonitrile and the
         supernatants combined in the separating funnel.
9.3   The supernatant was shaken for one minute with 50 mL carbon
         tetrachloride and 20 mL saturated sodium chloride.
9.4   The lower organic phase was filtered through anhydrous sodium

sulphate and Whatman PS-1 paper into 250 mL round bottomed flask.

9.5.   The filtrate was evaporated to dryness by rotary evaporation (7.10)

9.6   The residue was transferred quantitatively to a Silica Cartridge using 3 x 2 mL hexane.

9.3   The C8 Bond-Elut columns were conditioned by drawing through 5 mL acetonitrile followed by 5 mL aqueous acetonitrile/triethylamine mixture (6.2.1).

9.5   The column was washed with 5 mL chloroform

9.6   The lasalocid was eluted with 10 mL 5% methanol in chloroform.

9.7.   The eluate was transferred to a 25 mL pear-shaped flask and evaporated to dryness by rotary evaporation (7.10).

9.8.   The residue was redissolved in 0.5 mL HPLC mobile phase by Vortex mixing (15 sec) and ultrasonication (3 minutes).

9.9.   The extract was transferred to a 1 mL disposable syringe and filtered through a Millipore HVLP 0.45 μm disc into an HPLC vial.

9.10.   Standards for Calibration Curve.
        The standard additions are done at this stage (9.7) for the preparation of a standard curve over the range 0 - 100 μg per kg. Each point is done in triplicate.

9.14   HPLC was performed using 25 μL.

10.   CALCULATION OF RESULTS

10.1.   A calibration curve is constructed of peak height against concentration for a range of standards. The quantity of each of the Lasalocids in each sample injection is then calculated from the measured peak height. This figure is corrected for injection volume and mean % recovery (calculated from spiked samples) to give a concentration in mg/kg (ppm). The standard injection of 25 μL is equivalent to 100 mg of extracted sample.

$$\% \text{ recovery} = \frac{\text{amount of Lasalocid found}}{\text{amount of Spike added}} \times 100$$

Concentration of Lasalocid in sample (mg/kg) =

$$\frac{\mu\text{g Lasalocid (from calibration curve)}}{1000} \times \frac{1}{0.05} \times \frac{100}{\% \text{ recovery}}$$

For samples containing Lasalocids at concentrations beyond the range of the standard curve, a dilution of the extract is prepared and chromatographed, and the appropriate volumetric correction is applied.

10.2.   SENSITIVITY
The minimum limit of determination of Lasalocids by this method is 10 μg/kg when confirmed by stop-flow analysis of the emission spectra.

10.3.   QUALITY ASSURANCE PROCEDURES.

10.3.1. Validation; Batches of up to eight blank samples are spiked at the 10 or 100 μg per kg level and extractions are performed on each of three consecutive days. Each batch should include blanks and spiked samples.

Recovery of the analyte in the 100 µg per kg spike should fall within the range 65-90%. CV values should be less than 15% for inter and intra batch precision.

11.   SPECIAL CASES.

In samples in which a positive is suspected, further confirmatory evidence may be obtained by comparison of the stopped-flow analysis of the emission spectra of the suspect peaks.

12.   NOTES ON PROCEDURE.

13.   SAMPLE CONTROLS

It is convenient to analyze 16-20 samples per batch per day. A batch would include 9-13 unknowns, plus spiked quality control samples.

The blank samples were obtained from a sample previously analyzed and found to contain no Lasalocid.

14.   TEST REPORT

15.   LIST OF ABBREVIATIONS.
See abbreviations in Annex I, section 12 of Manual.

16.   FLOW DIAGRAM

```
   Tissue --→ add acetonitrile----------→ Homogenise ------> solvent
                                                             extract
                                                                |
                                                                |
                                                                |
                                                                |
                                                                ↓
   Calculate <---- HPLC <------- Filter <------------- Sep-pak Si column
        results
```

Cy 4.3.   CARBADOX AS QCA - DETERMINATION BY GC-MS OF QUINOXALINE CARBOXYLIC ACID (QCA) IN LIVER TISSUE.

WARNING AND SAFETY PRECAUTIONS

SAFETY
1.   Organic solvents - all organic solvents must be treated as potentially hazardous and all procedures using them must be performed in a fume cupboard.
2.   Ammonia - use only in a fume cupboard and wear safety glasses.
3.   Homogenising - perform in a fume cupboard to avoid aerosols.
4.   Dry ice - wear thick hide gloves and face shield. Dry ice can cause burns and frostbite if in contact with the skin.
5.   Do not carry out the methylation using diazomethane unless you have been trained to do so.

ALL REACTIONS INVOLVING THE PREPARATION AND USE OF DIAZOMETHANE MUST BE CARRIED OUT IN A FUME CUPBOARD. PROTECTIVE CLOTHING MUST BE WORN.

DO NOT USE EQUIPMENT WITH GROUND GLASS JOINTS - THERE IS A POTENTIAL EXPLOSION HAZARD!

You should ensure that you and anyone else in the room are aware of the potential explosion hazards associated with diazomethane. All diazomethane generated MUST be destroyed immediately if it is not being used for direct methylation. This is achieved by bubbling through dilute HCl. All glassware used should be rinsed in HCl before it leaves the fume cupboard.

FIRST AID
1.   Solvents, acids and alkalis in contact with skin - wash with copious amounts of cold water. Splashes in the eye - irrigate with water and seek medical attention immediately.
2.   Cuts - seek assistance of first aider immediately.
3.   Burns and frostbite - run affected part under cold water (burns) or tepid water (frostbite) for 10 minutes and seek medical attention.

0.   INTRODUCTION

Purpose
The confirmation of the presence of QCA in samples taken from farm animals in compliance with the Residues Directive 86/469/EEC.

Background
Carbadox is an animal drug used to increase the rate of weight gain, improve feed efficiency and control swine dysentery and bacterial enteritis. Carbadox is a suspected carcinogen but is itself not normally found as a residue in edible tissues. The major metabolite quinoxaline-2-carboxylic acid (QCA) is found as a residue and may also be produced as an artefact during the assay for QCA. QCA is not a carcinogen.

1.   SCOPE

This method of analysis in use at CVL, UK, describes the determination of the total content of QCA in pig liver.

2.   FIELD OF APPLICATION.

The method is described to be used for porcine liver. The detection limit
has not yet been defined.

3.   REFERENCES.

Commission Decision, 93/256/EEC, laying down the methods for detecting
residues of substances having a hormonal or thyrostatic action. [OJ. №
L.118, 14.4.93. pp 64-74]

2052/VI/84 File 6.11 II-4, Scientific Veterinary Committee, Working
Group - "Reference Methods for Residues", General Criteria for the
establishment of Reference Methods for the Detection of Residues.

ISO Standard 78/2-1982 Layout for standards - Part 2: Standard for Chemical
Analysis

Standard operating procedure - Central Vet Lab., UK. Confirmation of a
metabolite of Carbadox in tissues by GC-MS. (1988)

4.   DEFINITIONS.

QCA content is taken to mean the amount of QCA in liver determined
according to the described method and expressed as µg QCA per kg test
sample.

5.0   PRINCIPLE

Dried extracts of liver cleaned up by an ion-exchange system are methylated
with diazomethane and the methylated extracts are subjected to analysis by
gas chromatography-mass spectrometry (GC-MS) by selected ion monitoring.

6.   MATERIALS

6.1.   <u>Chemicals</u>

6.1.1.   Diazald   Aldrich Chemical Co Ltd
6.1.2.   Potassium hydroxide   AR grade
6.1.3.   Sodium hydroxide 3*M*   BDH
6.1.4.   Ethyl digol (carbitol)   Technical grade, BDH
6.1.5.   Hydrochloric acid 1M   AR grade May & Baker
6.1.6.   Methanol   Distol grade, Fisons
6.1.7.   Acetone   Distol grade, Fisons
6.1.8   Ethyl acetate   Distol Grade, Fisons
6.1.9.   Chloroform   Distol Grade, Fisons
6.1.10   Hexane   Distol Grade, Rathburns
6.1.11   Perfluorotributylamine (PFTBA)   Finnigan MAT
6.1.12   Macroporous cation resin (AF MP-50), AR grade, Bio-Rad
6.1.13   Citric acid buffer, pH 6, 0.5*M*; Adjust pH of 100 mL citric acid
          to pH 6 with 5*M* sodium hydroxide. Make up to 200 mL with water
          and readjust pH to 6.

6.2.   <u>Standards</u>

Solid QCA may be obtained from Pfizer.
A standard of concentration = 1 mg/mL of QCA in methanol should be prepared

using available QCA.
Working standards of concentrations = 0.01 µg/mL, 0.1 µg/mL, 1 µg/mL,
5 µg/mL, 10 µg/mL should be prepared by dilution from the stock.

7.   <u>Equipment</u>

7.1.   Mini diazald apparatus (Aldrich Chemical Co Ltd)
7.2.   Separating funnels with teflon stopcock 100 mL, 250 mL
7.3.   Stoppered centrifuge tubes, 10 mL
7.4.   Boiling Water bath
7.5.   Buchner funnel and Whatman No 1 filter paper.
7.6   Glass chromatography column, 10.5 mm diameter
7.7   Ice bath
7.8   Round bottomed flask, 250 mL
7.9.   Rotary evaporator
7.10.   Mass spectrometer, Finnigan MAT, coupled to a gas chromatograph
          and linked to an INCOS data system
7.11   Preparation of Resin and Ion-exchange column;
          Set up a Buchner funnel with a filter paper and filter flask
          attached to suction. Place 100 g resin (6.1.12) in the funnel.
          Wash the resin with a) 1 L methanol, b) 1 L water, c) 500 mL 1M
          HCl.
          Stir the resin and maintain a moderate filter rate.
          Store the filter cake in a capped amber jar.

          Mix 7 g washed resin with 1M HCl and transfer to a chromatography
          column. Pack the resin to a height of 100 mm and maintain the
          level of HCl just above the resin bed.

8.   SAMPLES AND SAMPLING PROCEDURE.

N.B. Attention is drawn to section 6.3.1 and ISO document 78/2-1982 and
the following notes derived from Annex II of 2052/VI/84-EN.

8.1. Nature of the Sample; Samples shall be such as to enable the
detection of residues in meat as defined in Directive 64/433/EEC. Failing
this biological fluids or faeces may constitute the samples for the
detection of residues.

8.2. Size of Sample; The size of the sample must be large enough to allow
the reference method to be carried out and to allow repeat analysis where
required.

In this method for QCA the sizes shall not be less than 20 g liver .

9.0.   PROCEDURE

9.1.   <u>Sample preparation</u>
9.1.1.   5 g thawed sample is minced and placed into a 50 mL centrifuge
          tube.
9.1.2.   10 mL of 3M sodium hydroxide is added, the tube stoppered lightly
          and placed in a boiling water bath for 30 minutes.
9.1.3.   After cooling the hydrolysate in an ice bath the pH is adjusted
          to < 1 using 4 mL conc. HCl. 15 mL ethyl acetate is added and
          the mixture shaken for 20 seconds before centrifuging at 1500 rpm
          to clarify the organic phase.
9.1.4   The ethyl acetate phase is transferred with a Pasteur pipette to

Cy 4.3/3

	a 100 mL separating funnel.
9.1.5	The aqueous phase is re-extracted with 2 additional 15 mL of ethyl acetate as above and the ethyl acetate phases combined.
9.1.6	5 mL citric acid buffer (6.1.13) is added and the mixture shaken for 1 minute. After allowing the lower phase to clarify the aqueous phase is run into a beaker. This step is repeated twice with further 5 mL portions of buffer. The combined aqueous phases are acidified with 2 mL conc. HCl.
9.1.7.	The acidified extract is transferred to the ion-exchange column (7.11) and the column drained to the top of the bed. The resin is washed with 40 mL 1M HCl and the eluent discarded. A 250 mL separating funnel is placed beneath the column and the column eluted with 75 mL 10% methanol in water (v/v) until the column is dry.
9.1.8.	1 mL conc HCl is added to the eluate. The eluate is extracted with 3 x 50 mL chloroform into a round bottomed flask. The chloroform extract is evaporated to dryness using a rotary evaporator at 45-50°C. The residue is transferred to a 10 mL centrifuge tube with 10 mL methanol. The volume is reduced to 1 mL under a stream of nitrogen at 45-50°C.
9.2.	Derivatisation

DO NOT CARRY OUT THIS METHYLATION UNLESS YOU HAVE BEEN TRAINED TO DO SO. READ THE SECTION ON SAFETY AND FOLLOW THE ADVICE GIVEN CAREFULLY.

9.2.1.	The following reagents are prepared:	
	(a)	2 g diazald in 20 mL diethyl ether.
	(b)	3 g potassium hydroxide in 3 mL distilled water added to 10 mL ethyl digol.
	(c)	10% hydrochloric acid, 100 mL.
9.2.2.	The Mini-diazald kit is set up according to the maker's instructions.	
9.2.3.	Until ready to methylate the samples, the diazomethane generated must be passed through the 10% HCl, which will neutralise it. Ensure that the kit is set up for this.	
9.2.4.	Reagent (b) (KOH in H_2O + ethyl digol) is placed in the reaction vessel.	
9.2.5.	A separating funnel is positioned over the reaction vessel. Reagent (a) (diazald in ether) is placed in this funnel.	
9.2.6.	The reaction vessel is placed in a water bath at 50-60°C and the diazald solution added slowly and carefully over a period of approximately 20 minutes. Once the reaction has started, the diazomethane is bubbled through the sample and standards until the solution is coloured yellow. Whenever the diazomethane is not bubbling through a sample or standard it is important that it is passed through the HCl to neutralise it.	
9.2.7.	Once all of the standards and samples have been derivatised, the diazomethane generated is passed through the HCl solution, and the reaction continued until all of the reagents have been used up.	
9.2.8.	The derivatives are taken to dryness under nitrogen and resuspended in 100 μl hexane.	
9.2.9	At the same time a series of standards at different concentrations should be run through the derivatization stages.	

9.3.   GC-MS Analysis
9.3.1.   The GC parameters are

COLUMN: J&W fused silica capillary column, SE-54, 15 m x 0.25 mm.
INJECTIONS: 0.5 μl manual injections.
TEMPERATURES: Interface: 270°C
               Injector: 260°C
OVEN TEMPERATURES:

from temp (°C)	to temp (°C)	rate (°C/min)	time (min)	total time (min)
55	55	-	1.0	1.0
55	240	20	9.2	10.2
240	240	-	10.0	20.2

CARRIER GAS: Helium
         flow rate   = 1 mL/min
         injector pressure = 10 psi.

9.3.2 The mass spectrometry parameters are
IONISER:
     Mode: EI positive ion
     Temperature: 150°C
MANIFOLD TEMPERATURE: 90 (± 5) °C
ELECTRON MULTIPLIER: 1.2 kV
ELECTRON ENERGY: 70 electron volts.

Other parameters should be set up by adjusting the instrument controls to give the optimum peak height and shape for a suitable calibration compound. The CVL uses perfluorotributylamine (PFTBA).

9.3.3.   The MS is operated in EI mode and scanned between m/z = 50 and 400.

9.3.4.   The following are analyzed;
          a) hexane
          b) 10 μg per mL derivatised QCA standard in a volume of 100 μL
          1000 scans were collected. After 4 minutes the filament is turned off.
9.3.5   The QCA derivative peak elutes between 6-7 minutes after injection. This peak is examined and the exact masses to 3 decimal places were found for at least the ions
                m/z = 102, 130, 158, 188
9.3.6   These ions are used to set up or modify and then create a multiple ion detection (MID) scan list.
9.3.7   Hexane is rerun through the system to check that there is no carry over of QCA derivative.
9.3.8.   The remaining samples and standards are analyzed using 0.5 μL. It is advisable to:
          a) Analyze 1 μg of QCA derivative first to ensure that the MID is set up correctly. This is followed by hexane.
          b) Analyze standards in order of increasing concentration.
          c) Switch the filament on 100 scans before the QCA derivative elutes from the column and switch it off 100 scans afterwards.
          d) Inject hexane between each injection.

10.0   RESULTS

The presence of a QCA in a sample is confirmed if the GC-MS data satisfy
the following criteria:
1.   The peak in the sample has the same GC retention time as that in
          the standard.
2.   The ions present in the mass spectrum of the sample GC peak are
          identical to those in the mass spectrum of the standard.
3.   The ratios of the ions to one another are the same as those in
          the standard.
          The limit of detection for this method has not yet been assessed.

11.   SPECIAL CASES.

12.   NOTES ON PROCEDURE.

13.   SAMPLE CONTROLS

The blank sample was obtained from a sample previously analyzed and found
to contain no QCA.

14.   TEST REPORT

15.   LIST OF ABBREVIATIONS.

See abbreviations in Annex I, section 12 of Manual.

16.   FLOW DIAGRAM

```
     SAMPLE   --------> Homogenise------> alkaline digestion ----¬
                                                                 ¦
                                                                 ↓
        derivatise <------- ion-exchange column <--- solvent extraction
                   ¦
                   ↓
          GC-MS ------>  Calculate results
```

Cy 4.4 IVERMECTIN - DETERMINATION OF IVERMECTIN AT RESIDUE LEVELS IN ANIMAL TISSUES.

WARNING AND SAFETY PRECAUTIONS

0.   INTRODUCTION

Ivermectin is a potent endo- and ectoparasitic agent with a broad spectrum of activity in several animal species including cattle, sheep, pigs, horses and humans. Ivermectin may be administered orally, parentally or as a pour on preparation. The dose is usually in the range 0.2 - 0.6 mg/kg body weight (B.W.).

The MRL set in the EEC for Ivermectins is 15 µg per kg liver and 0 µg per L of milk.

1.   SCOPE

This method of analysis describes the determination of the total content of Ivermectin in samples of animal origin.

2.   FIELD OF APPLICATION.

The method can be used for bovine muscle and bovine and porcine kidney. The limit of determination following the validation of the method is 2 µg/kg of sample for Ivermectin.

3.   REFERENCES.

Commission Decision, 93/256/EEC, laying down the methods for detecting residues of substances having a hormonal or thyrostatic action. [OJ. № L.118, 14.4.93. pp 64-74]

2052/VI/84 File 6.11 II-4, Scientific Veterinary Committee, Working Group - "Reference Methods for Residues", General Criteria for the establishment of Reference Methods for the Detection of Residues.

ISO Standard 78/2-1982 Layout for standards - Part 2: Standard for Chemical Analysis

MAFF, 1989, Determination of Ivermectin at residue levels in animal tissues. Food Science Laboratory, Colney Lane, Norwich. Standard Operating Procedure.

Nordlander, I. and Johnsson, H. (1990). Determination of Ivermectin residues in swine tissues - An improved clean-up procedure using solid phase extraction. Food Addit. Contamin. 7, 79-82

Tway, P.C., Wood, J.S. and Downing, G.V. (1981) Determination of ivermectin in cattle and sheep tissues using high performance liquid chromatography with fluorescence detection. J.Agric. Food Chem. 29, 1059-1063

4.   DEFINITIONS.

Ivermectin content is taken to mean the amount of Ivermectin in the substance in question, regardless of the chemical form, determined according to the described method and expressed as µg or mg Ivermectin per kg of test sample.

5.   PRINCIPLE

The methods comprises 6 stages;-
-        Homogenisation of tissue samples in buffer
-        Extraction with organic solvent
-        Extraction on reverse phase C8 column
-        Derivatisation
-        Clean-up on solid phase column.
-        End point determination with HPLC by fluorescent UV detection
-        The amount of Ivermectin is calculated by interpolation from a
         standard curve and taking into account the recovery of
         Ivermectin, especially from tissue samples.

6. CHEMICALS

6.1.1   Chloroform (BDH)
6.1.2   Triethylamine (Sigma)
6.1.3   Methylimidazole (Sigma)
6.1.4   Methanol, redistilled (BDH)
6.1.5   Acetic anhydride (Sigma)
6.1.6   Acetonitrile (Romil)
6.1.7   Dimethylformamide (Sigma)

6.2. Solutions
6.2.1   Aqueous acetonitrile with triethylamine; 1 mL triethylamine is
          added to 300 mL acetonitrile and made up to 1 L with water.
6.2.2.   Derivatisation mixture; Mix methylimidazole, acetic anhydride
          and dimethylformamide in the ratio 2:6:9 v/v. Prepare
          immediately before use. Use 100 µL per derivatisation.
6.2.3.   HPLC Mobile Phase; 30 mL methanol was added to 970 mL water,
          mixed and passed through a Durapore " filter, assisted by vacuum.
          The mobile phase was degassed using ultrasonication and with
          reduced pressure.

6.3.   Standards
6.3.1   Ivermectin reference standards were obtained from Merck, Sharpe
          and Dohme Ltd.
6.3.2.   Stock standards; 10 mg Ivermectin in 100 mL methanol. Store at
          4°C and make fresh fortnightly.
6.3.3   Intermediate standards; Dilute 4 mL stock to 100 mL with
          methanol. Store at 4°C and make fresh fortnightly.
6.3.4   Working standards; Dilute 5 mL intermediate standard to 100 mL
          with methanol. Final concentration is 0.2 ng per ul. Make fresh
          daily.

6.5.   Spiking Procedure
          Using the working standards (6.3.4) spike 5 g sample with 50 ul
          and 125 ul standard solution. Allow to stand for 15 minutes.

7.   EQUIPMENT

7.1   Centrifuges tubes 50 mL capacity, plastic.
7.2   100 mL glass beakers
7.3   All glass filter holder, 47 mm - Millipore.
7.4.   Glass sample bottles, 25 mL
7.5   Pear shaped flasks 50 mL
7.6   Glass reactivials 3 mL with PTFE lined screw caps.

7.7.   Glass syringes, 1 mL and 10 mL
7.8   Ultra-Turrax Homogeniser
7.9   Mixer (Vortex)
7.10   Rotary evaporator - Buchli with water bath at 40°C
7.11.   Vials low volume for autosampler
7.12.   Glass vials 2 mL
7.13.   Centrifuge - MSE High Speed 18 or equivalent
7.14.   Ultrasonic bath- L&R 140S or equivalent
7.15.   Adjustable pipettes 200 µL and 1000 µL
7.16.   Multiport nitrogen evaporator with heater block (40°C) for
           reactivials.
7.17.   Membrane filter holder - Millipore Swinney Stainless, 13 mm
7.18.   Membrane filters, 13 mm and 47 mm - Millipore Ltd.
7.19.   Solid Phase Extraction
7.19.1.   Vacuum Manifold - Vac-Elut
7.19.2.   C8/500 mg cartridges - Bond-Elut, Jones Chromatography Ltd.
7.19.3.   Silica cartridges - Sep-pak, Waters Associates.
7.19.4.   Cartridge taps - Jones Chromatography Ltd.
7.19.5.   Reservoirs 50 mL for cartridges - Jones Chromatography Ltd.

7.20   HPLC-LKB 2150 pump
           Column; 10 cm x 3 mm i.d. Chromsep (Chrompack) cartridge column
           assembly packed with 5 um Hypersil CDS with integral (10 mm x 2.1
           mm i.d.) guard column packed with pellicular (30-40 um) reverse
           phase.
           Mobile phase was pumped at 0.4 mL per min.
           The fluorescence detector was a Perkin Elmer LS4 with the
           excitation wavelength 364 nm, slit width 10 nm, and the emission
           wavelength at 470 nm, slit width 10 nm. The scale expansion was
           4.0 units.
           The chromatogram was recorded and integrated using an electronic
           integrator (Spectra Physics 4290). 25 µL samples were injected
           using a Waters Wisp 712.

8.   SAMPLES AND SAMPLING PROCEDURE.

N.B. Attention is drawn to section 6.3.1 and ISO document 78/2-1982 and
the following notes derived from Annex II of 2052/VI/84-EN.

8.1. Nature of the Sample; Samples shall be such as to enable the
detection of residues in meat, as defined in Directive 64/433/EEC and also
in milk.

8.2. Size of Sample; The size of the sample must be large enough to allow
the reference method to be carried out and to allow repeat analysis where
required.

In this method for Ivermectins the sizes shall not be less than 30 g
muscle, kidney

 8.3. The samples must be taken and packed in such a way as to allow
proper identification in the laboratory.

8.4. The method of packing, preservation and transport must maintain the
integrity of the sample and not prejudice the result of the examination.
Samples for the analysis of Ivermectins must be stored and transported at
temperatures below -18°C.

Cy 4.4/3

9.   PROCEDURE

9.1.   5 g finely sliced tissue and 15 mL acetonitrile were placed in an
        ultrasonic bath (3 min) homogenised (2 min) and centrifuged (5
        min) at 5,000 rpm.
9.2   The Supernatant was transferred to beaker containing 40 mL water
        and 0.05 mL triethylamine. The contents were mixed by stirring.
9.3   The C8 Bond-Elut columns were conditioned by drawing through 5 mL
        acetonitrile followed by 5 mL aqueous acetonitrile/triethylamine
        mixture (6.2.1).
9.4.   The extract was transferred to the Bond-Elut column which was
        fitted with a tap and a reservoir. After allowing the column to
        drain but not dry the column was eluted with 5 mL acetonitrile
        into glass sample bottles (7.4).
9.5   The eluate was transferred to a 50 mL pear-shaped flask using 2 x
        2 mL acetonitrile rinses.
9.6   The organic phase was evaporated to dryness using a rotary
        evaporator with a water bath set at 40°C.
9.7   The residue was redissolved in 1 mL methanol.
9.8.   Standards for Calibration Curve.
        The standard additions are done at this stage (9.7) for the
        preparation of a standard curve over the range 0 - 5 µg per kg.

Vol. Working Standard (6.3.4) µL	Vol. Methanol µL	Equiv. Conc. Ivermectin µg per kg
0	1000	0
25	975	1
50	950	2
75	925	3
100	900	4
125	875	5

9.9   A 500 µL aliquot of extract (9.7) was transferred to a
        reactivial. Samples may be stored at -20°C at this point.
        Otherwise remove methanol by evaporating to dryness under a
        stream of nitrogen.
9.10   100 µL derivatisation mixture (6.2.2.) was added. The vial was
        capped tightly and the contents gently swirled. The reactivials
        were placed in an oven at 95°C for 1 hour.
9.11   After cooling the vials the contents were transferred
        quantitatively with 3-4 mL chloroform to a 10 mL glass syringe
        attached to a silica Sep-pak cartridge (7.19.3). The sample was
        passed through the cartridge and the eluate collected in a 50 mL
        pear-shaped flask. A further 9 mL chloroform was passed through
        the cartridge and the eluate also collected in the pear-shaped
        flask.
9.12   The chloroform was removed by rotary evaporation at 40°C.
9.13.   The viscous residue was taken up in 0.50 mL methanol and filtered
        through a 0.45 um Millipore filter attached to a 1 mL syringe.
        The sample was collected in a glass autosampler vial (7.11).
9.14   HPLC was performed using 25 µL.

10.   CALCULATION OF RESULTS

10.1. A calibration curve is constructed of peak height against
concentration for a range of standards The quantity of each of the
Ivermectins in each sample injection is then calculated from the measured

peak height. This figure is then corrected for injection volume and mean %
recovery (calculated from spiked samples) to give a concentration in mg/kg
(ppm). The standard injection of 25 µL is equivalent to 0.25 g of
extracted sample.

The retention time of ivermectin is approximately 7 minutes.

$$\% \text{ recovery} = \frac{\text{amount of Ivermectin found}}{\text{amount of Spike added}} \times 100$$

Concentration of Ivermectin in sample (mg/kg) =

$$\frac{\text{µg Ivermectin (from calibration curve)}}{1000} \times \frac{1}{0.05} \times \frac{100}{\% \text{ recovery}}$$

For samples containing Ivermectins at concentrations beyond the range of
the standard curve, a dilution of the extract is prepared and
chromatographed, and the appropriate volumetric correction is applied.

10.2.   SENSITIVITY
The minimum limit of determination of Ivermectins by this method is
0.002 mg/kg.

10.3.   QUALITY ASSURANCE PROCEDURES.
10.3.1. Validation;   Batches of up to six blank samples are spiked at the
2 or 5 µg per kg level and extractions are performed on each of three
consecutive days. Each batch comprised the following samples;-

        2 blanks
        2 standard additions at 2 µg per kg
        2 standard additions at 5 µg per kg
        6 spikes at 2 or 5 µg per kg.
Recovery of the analyte should fall within 70-110%. Cv values should fall
within the range 5-15% for inter and intra batch precision.

11.   SPECIAL CASES.
12.   NOTES ON PROCEDURE.
13.   SAMPLE CONTROLS
It is convenient to analyze 16-20 samples per batch per day. A batch would
include 9-13 unknowns, plus spiked quality control samples.
The blank samples were obtained from a sample previously analyzed and found
to contain no Ivermectin.

14.   TEST REPORT
15.   LIST OF ABBREVIATIONS.
See abbreviations in Annex I, Section 12 of Manual.

16.   FLOW DIAGRAM

    Tissue --→ add acetonitrile----------→ Homogenise ------> C8 column
                                                                 ¦
                                                                 ↓
    Calculate <----- HPLC <------- Sep-pak Si column <------ Derivatise
        results

Cy 4.5. TRANQUILLIZERS AND CARAZOLOL - AN HPLC METHOD WITH ON-LINE UV SPECTRUM IDENTIFICATION AND OFF-LINE TLC CONFIRMATION FOR RESIDUES IN PIG KIDNEYS.

WARNING AND SAFETY PRECAUTIONS

SAFETY
Organic solvents - all organic solvents must be treated as potentially hazardous and all procedures using them must be performed in a fume cupboard.

0.   INTRODUCTION

Tranquillizers and the ß-blocker carazolol are used to aid the management of stress in many veterinary practices. Of particular interest for residues is the treatment of pigs to prevent mortality and loss of meat quality during transport to the slaughterhouse. The time between drug administration and slaughter is usually not more than a few hours and this can result in high residues in the edible tissues.

1.   SCOPE

The use of many of the tranquillizers and carazolol varies throughout the EEC. To ensure that farmers are not using these drugs in non-approved situations and to control the use in meat producing animals samples of kidneys are taken at slaughterhouses and screened for the presence of these compounds using a number of techniques (see Section 4). Whenever there is a positive screening result, this must be confirmed.   This work is carried out in compliance with the Residues Directive (86/469/EEC).

2.   FIELD OF APPLICATION.

This method is used for confirmation of the presence of six tranquillizers and carazolol in pig kidney. The limits of identification ranges from 1 to 2.5 ug per kg kidney for the tranquillizers and carazolol. Azaperone forms a major metabolite, azaperol, and the two compounds appear together as residues.

3.   REFERENCES.

Commission Decision, 93/256/EEC, laying down the methods for detecting residues of substances having a hormonal or thyrostatic action. [OJ. № L.118, 14.4.93. pp 64-74]

2052/VI/84 File 6.11 II-4, Scientific Veterinary Committee, Working Group - "Reference Methods for Residues", General Criteria for the establishment of Reference Methods for the Detection of Residues.

ISO Standard 78/2-1982 Layout for standards - Part 2: Standard for Chemical Analysis

ISO Standard 5725 (1986)

Van Ginkel, L.A.. Schwillens, P.L.W.J. and Olling, M., (1989), Liquid chromatographic method with on-line UV spectrum identification and off-line thin-layer chromatographic confirmation for the detection of tranquillizers and carazolol in pig kidneys. Anal. Chim. Acta. <u>225</u>, 137-146

Haagsma, N., Bathelt, E.R. and Engelsma, J.W. (1988), Thin-layer
chromatographic method for the tranquillizers azaperone, propiopromazine
and carazolol in pig tissues. J.Chrom. 436, 73-79.

4.   DEFINITIONS.

Tranquillizers and carazolol content is taken to mean the amount of
tranquillizers and carazolol in kidney determined according to the
described method and expressed as ug tranquillizers or carazolol per kg
test sample.

5.   PRINCIPLE.

The method comprises four stages

-       Samples of kidney are extracted from an alkaline homogenate using
        diethylether.
-       clean-up with silica-based diol cartridges
-       analysis and fractionation of eluate with HPLC using a diode-
        array detector
-       confirmation of tranquillizers and carazolol by TLC of selected
        HPLC fractions.

6.   MATERIALS

6.1.   <u>Chemicals</u>

Note: The chemicals were all of analytical grade and obtained from Merck
unless stated otherwise.

6.1.1   Ethyl acetate
6.1.2   Ethanol
6.1.3   Chloroform
6.1.4   Hexane
6.1.5   Acetonitrile, HPLC grade
6.1.6   Sodium hydroxide
6.1.7   Diethyl ether
6.1.8   Anhydrous sodium sulphate
6.1.9   Light petroleum, B.Pt. 40-60°C
6.1.10   Conc. sulphuric acid
6.1.11   Ammonium acetate
6.1.12   Acetone
6.1.13.   Dichloromethane
6.1.14.   Ammonia
6.1.15.   Bismuth(III) nitrate
6.1.16.   Glacial acetic acid
6.1.17.   Potassium iodide
6.1.18.   Vanillin
6.1.19.   85% Phosphoric acid

6.2   <u>Solutions</u>
6.2.1.   Acetonitrile : water (80:20 v/v)
6.2.2.   Acetonitrile : water (60:40 v/v)
6.2.3   Acetonitrile : water (60:40 v/v) containing 0.1 mol per L
            ammonium acetate
6.2.4.   Acetonitrile : water : 1 mol per L ammonium acetate
            (44.5:54.5:1, v/v/v)

6.2.5.   TLC solvents
6.2.5.1. Mobile phase I; acetone : dichloromethane : 25% ammonia
          (40:60:1, v/v/v)
6.2.5.2 Mobile phase II; acetone : 25% ammonia (100:0.1, v/v)
6.2.5.3. Mobile phase III; acetone
6.2.6.   Colour reagents for TLC.
6.2.6.1. Dragendorff reagent; Mix a solution of 0.8 g bismuth(III)
          nitrate in 10 mL glacial acetic acid and 40 mL distilled water
          with a solution containing 8 g potassium iodide in 20 mL
          distilled water. Store this solution in the dark and prepare the
          working reagent fresh by mixing 6 mL of the above-described
          solution with 12 mL glacial acetic acid, 100 mL ethanol (96% v/v)
          and 100 mL diethyl ether.
6.2.6.2 Vanillin-Phosphoric acid reagent; dissolve 3 g vanillin in 100 mL
          ethanol (96% v/v) and subsequently add, with stirring, 75 mL of
          85% phosphoric acid, 50 mL distilled water and 50 mL diethyl
          ether.
6.2.6.3. Sulphuric acid reagent; Add 20 mL concentrated sulphuric acid to
          100 mL ethanol (96% v/v), cool the mixture and add 20 mL of
          diethyl ether.

6.3.   STANDARDS; Azaperone and Haloperidol (Janssen Pharmaceutica);
          acepromazine (Clin Midy); Chlorpromazine (Sigma); Propiopromazine
          and xylazine (Bayer).
6.3.1.   Fraction I was a solution in chloroform of azaperone and azaperol
          at concentrations 2 ug per L
6.3.2.   Fraction II was a solution in chloroform of carazolol,
          haloperidol and xylazine at concentrations 1 ug per L
6.3.3.   Fraction III was a solution in chloroform of acepromazine,
          propiopromazine and chlorpromazine at concentrations 1 ug per L

7.   EQUIPMENT

7.1.   Glassware
          The normal range of minor laboratory glassware is needed.

7.2.   Apparatus
7.2.1.   Ultra-Turrax homogeniser
7.2.2.   Rotary evaporator, type Buchli linked to vacuum pump.
7.2.3.   water bath at 95°C
7.2.4.   water bath at 45°C with nitrogen dispensing tubes for evaporating
          solvents.
7.2.5.   Glass syringes for chromatography, type HAMILTON
7.2.6   Silica based diol based cartridges (Baker 70-9403) washed with 3
          mL ethanol and 3 mL diethyl ether before applying extract.
7.2.7.   Baker 10 SPE system

7.3.   HPLC equipment
The system consisted of an LKB 2150 pump with LKB 2152 controller, an LKB
2212 fraction collector, a Hewlett Packard 1040A diode-array detector, a
Chromguard replacement column and holder as a reversed-phase pre-column (10
mm x 3 mm i.d.) and an analytical column (150 mm x 4.6 mm i.d.)packed with
SAS-Hypersil (5 um) (Shandon), and solvent 6.2.4. as the eluent at a flow
rate of 2 mL per min. The eluent was monitored at 235 nm and collected as
three separate fractions so as to contain azaperone and azaperol in
fraction one, carazolol, xylazine and haloperidol in fraction two and
azopromazine, propiopromazine and chlorpromazine in the third fraction.

7.4.   TLC equipment. e.g. tanks, sprayers, applicators
7.4.1   TLC plates, type HPTLC-Fertigplatten Kieselgel-60 (Merck).
          Purchased as 20 cm x 20 cm and cut into four plates of 5 cm x 5
          cm.
7.4.2.   Oven at 70°C or 120°C for TLC plates

8. SAMPLES AND SAMPLING PROCEDURE.

N.B.   Attention is drawn to section 6.3.1 and ISO document 78/2-1982 and
the following notes derived from Annex II of 2052/VI/84-EN.

8.1.   Nature of the Sample; Samples of kidneys shall be such as to enable
the detection of residues.
8.2.   Size of Sample; The size of the sample must be large enough to allow
the reference method to be carried out and to allow repeat analysis where
required.
8.3.   The kidney must be cooled after collection and stored at $\leq$ -20°C
pending analysis.

9.   PROCEDURE

9.1.   Thaw the kidneys and remove parts of the marrow.
9.2.   Homogenise 50 g of the remaining material in an Ultra-Turrax
          homogeniser.
9.3.   To 20 g homogenate add 4 mL of 5 mol per L NaOH.
9.4.   For the quality controls add a mixture of standards to kidneys
          from pigs untreated with Tranquillizers and carazolol (control
          pigs - blank samples). Allow to stand for at least 30 min at
          room temperature or at +4°C overnight.
9.5.   The resulting suspensions was incubated for 1 hour at 95°C in a
          water bath.
9.6.   Cool to room temperature and extract with 70 mL diethyl ether.
9.7.   Add 10 g anhydrous sodium sulphate and filter.
9.8.   Add 20 mL light petroleum (6.1.9).
9.9.   Solid Phase Extraction.
9.9.1   Add crude extract to column (7.2.6) with the aid of a 50 mL
          funnel.
9.9.2   Wash with 3 mL diethyl ether, 3 mL ethanol, 1 ml acetonitrile :
          water (80:20 v/v) (6.2.1), 3 mL acetonitrile : water (60:40
          v/v) (6.2.2).
9.9.3   The cartridges are eluted with 1.5 mL of acetonitrile : water
          (60 :40 v/v) containing 0.1 mol per L ammonium acetate. The
          eluate is collected in a glass tube containing 0.025 mL of 5 mol
          per L NaOH.
9.10.   The solvent was evaporated after the addition of 1 mL acetone.
9.11.   The dry residue is dissolved in 0.1 mL water and extracted with
          2.5 mL hexane. The hexane extract is evaporated to dryness and
          redissolved in 0.07 mL of HPLC eluent (6.2.4).
9.12.   HPLC. 0.055 mL of extract 9.11 was injected into the HPLC
          system.
          3 tubes containing 0.05 mL of 5 mol per L NaOH are used to
          collect the fractions as outlined in 7.3.
9.13.   The volume of the fractions is reduced under a stream of nitrogen
          to half the original volume.
9.14.   The fractions were extracted with 2 x 2 mL diethyl ether. After
          drying with 0.5 g of anhydrous sodium sulphate the ether is
          evaporated to dryness.

9.15.   0.4 mL of ethanol is added to the extracts which may be stored in
          the dark at -20°C until TLC analysis.
9.16.   TLC. The detection systems are based on the work of Haagsma et.,
          (1988)
9.16.1   The extracts 9.15. are evaporated to dryness, dissolved in 0.05
          mL chloroform and 0.015 mL spotted onto two separate TLC plates
          (a & B) for each fraction. 0.005 mL of the corresponding
          standards (6.3) were spotted onto plate B.
9.16.2   The extract from fraction one (see 7.3) is run in mobile phase I
          (6.2.5.1), dried, developed in mobile phase III (6.2.5.3), dried
          and dipped for a few seconds in Dragendorff reagent (6.2.6.1).
          After drying for 2-5 min the spots of azaperone and azaperol
          become visible. If the detectability was insufficient, the
          following procedure is followed: Heat the plates for 5 min at
          70°C, cool to room temperature and place in the vanillin-
          phosphoric acid solution. After drying for 10 min inspect the
          plates at 365 nm on a transilluminator. The tranquillizers
          become visible as red spots. Heating the plates for 5 min at
          70°C accelerates this process.
9.16.3   The extract from fraction two is treated in the same way, except
          that instead of mobile phase III, mobile phase II(6.2.5.2) is
          used. However for the detection of carazolol, heating after
          treatment with the vanillin-phosphoric acid is essential.
          Sometimes heating at 120°C for 5 min is needed.
9.16.4.   The extracts from fraction three are developed in mobile phase
          I,dried, developed in mobile phase II, dried again and heated for
          1 min at 120°C. The plates are dipped in the sulphuric acid
          reagent (6.2.6.3) for a few seconds and heated for 4 min at
          120°C. After cooling the plates are placed in Dragendorff
          reagent for a few seconds and then dried. The tranquillizers
          become visible as dark brown spots.

10.   CALCULATION OF RESULTS
10.1   The limit of detection for the tranquillizers and carazolol on
          HPLC measured at 235 nm was determined using the criteria in
          section 5 of this manual, i.e. the limit of detection was the
          mean of the measured content of a representative blank plus three
          time the standard deviation of the mean.

          The limit of identification based on the diode-array detection
          system was defined as: the maximum absorption wavelength in the
          spectrum of the analyte should be the same as that of the
          standard material within a margin determined by the resolution of
          the detection system; for diode-array detection this is typically
          within ± 2 nm; and the spectrum of the analyte should not be
          different from that of the standard material for those parts of
          the spectrum with a relative absorbance >10% of the absorbance of
          the standard material; this criterium is met when the same maxima
          are present and at no point is the difference between the two
          spectra more than 10% of the absorbance of the standard material.

          The values for the limits of detection by both HPLC and TLC and
          the limits of identification by HPLC diode-array are given in
          table 1 taken from the paper by Van Ginkel et al., (1989).

Table 1.

Compound	Limit of Detection (ug per kg)		Limit of Identification (ug per kg)	Recovery n = 6	
	HPLC	TLC		%	SD (%)
Azaperol	<1	1	2.5	64	4.4
Azaperone	<1	1	2.5	60	2.3
Carazolol	<1	0.3	1	56	7.5
Xylazine	2.5	3	10	31	7.0
Haloperidol	2.5	6	10	59	6.0
Acepromazine	5	0.3	10	55	3.9
Propiopromazine	5	0.3	10	61	11
Chlorpromazine	10	0.3	25	59	11

10.2.   RECOVERIES;
The recoveries of tranquillizers and carazolol from spiked samples at concentration ranges 1-5 times the limit of detection was reported by Van Ginkel et al., (1989)(see table 1). The recoveries are calculated from their relative UV absorbances. These values correspond to the actual recovery in the HPLC fractions and are not corrected for aliquot factors. With the exception of xylazine all recoveries are between 55 and 64%. The lower recovery of xylazine is caused by incomplete elution from the SPE cartridge.

11.   SPECIAL CASES.

12.   NOTES ON PROCEDURE.

13.   SAMPLE CONTROLS

14.   TEST REPORT

15.   LIST OF ABBREVIATIONS.
See abbreviations in Annex I, Section 12 of Manual.

16.   FLOW DIAGRAM

Homogenise kidney -----> alkaline digest -----> extract with diethyl ether

-------> SPE clean-up -------> HPLC ------> TLC -----> Results.

Cy 4.6. TRANQUILLIZERS - IDENTIFICATION USING GC-MS CONFIRMATION FOR RESIDUES OF TRANQUILLIZERS IN PIG KIDNEYS.

WARNING AND SAFETY PRECAUTIONS

SAFETY
Organic solvents - all organic solvents must be treated as potentially hazardous and all procedures using them must be performed in a fume cupboard.
Dilute the concentrated sulphuric with care.

0.   INTRODUCTION

Tranquillizers and the ß-blocker carazolol are used to aid the management of stress in many veterinary practices. Of particular interest for residues is the treatment of pigs to prevent mortality and loss of meat quality during transport to the slaughterhouse. The time between drug administration and slaughter is usually not more than a few hours and this can result in high residues in the edible tissues.

1.   SCOPE

The use of many of the tranquillizers and carazolol varies throughout the EEC. To ensure that farmers are not using these drugs in non-approved situations and to control the use in meat producing animals samples of kidneys are taken at slaughterhouses and screened for the presence of these compounds using a number of techniques (see Section 4) and method Sg 4.1. Whenever there is a positive screening result, this must be confirmed. This work is carried out in compliance with the Residues Directive (86/469/EEC).

2.   FIELD OF APPLICATION.

This method is used for confirmation of the presence of five tranquillizers in pig kidney. The limits of identification are 50 ug per kg kidney for the tranquillizers. Azaperone forms a major metabolite, azaperol, and the two compounds appear together as residues. The method is operated at RIKILT-DLO in the Netherlands.

3.   REFERENCES.

Commission Decision, 93/256/EEC, laying down the methods for detecting residues of substances having a hormonal or thyrostatic action. [OJ. Nº L.118, 14.4.93. pp 64-74]

2052/VI/84 File 6.11 II-4, Scientific Veterinary Committee, Working Group - "Reference Methods for Residues", General Criteria for the establishment of Reference Methods for the Detection of Residues.

ISO Standard 78/2-1982 Layout for standards - Part 2: Standard for Chemical Analysis

ISO Standard 5725 (1986)

Hoogland, H., Beek, W.M.J., Keukens, H.J. and Aerts, M.M.L. (1991), Confirmation of tranquillizers in porcine kidney by GC-MS. Archiv. für Lebensm. 42, 79-83

Keukens, H.J. and Aerts, M.M.L., (1989), Determination of residues of carazolol and a number of tranquillizers in swine kidney by high-performance liquid chromatography with ultraviolet and fluorescence detection. J.Chromatog. _464_, 149-161

Van Ginkel, L.A.. Schwillens, P.L.W.J. and Olling, M., (1989), Liquid chromatographic method with on-line UV spectrum identification and off-line thin-layer chromatographic confirmation for the detection of tranquillizers and carazolol in pig kidneys. Anal. Chim. Acta. _225_, 137-146

4.   DEFINITIONS.

Tranquillizers content is taken to mean the amount of tranquillizers in kidney determined according to the described method and expressed as ug tranquillizers per kg test sample.

5.   PRINCIPLE.

The method comprises four stages

- Samples of kidney are extracted with acetonitrile
- clean-up with Sep-Pak C18 cartridges
- solvent/solvent partition
- confirmation of tranquillizers by GC-MS of selected HPLC fractions.

6.   MATERIALS

6.1.   Chemicals

Note: The chemicals were all of analytical grade and obtained from Merck unless stated otherwise. Reagents of similar quality may be used from other sources.

6.1.1   Acetone (Merck-14)
6.1.2   Methanol (Merck-6009)
6.1.3   25% ammonia solution (Merck-5432)
6.1.4   n-Hexane (Merck-714)
6.1.5   Acetonitrile, HPLC grade (Merck-3)
6.1.6   Sodium chloride (Merck-6404)
6.1.7   Acetic acid (Merck-63)
6.1.8   Anhydrous sodium acetate (Merck-6268)
6.1.9   Conc. sulphuric acid (Merck-714)
6.1.10   Sodium hydroxide
6.1.11   Tert-butyl methyl ether
6.1.12   Ethyl acetate (Uvasol grade) (Merck-863)

6.2   Solutions

6.2.1   Sodium chloride solution; Dissolve 100 g sodium chloride in
          water and make up to 1 L.
6.2.2   Sulphuric acid solution, 0.01 - 0.05M; Mix 28 mL of sulphuric
          acid (6.1.9) in a beaker with 500 mL water. Allow the solution
          to reach room temperature. Transfer 20 to 100 mL of this
          solution to 250 mL water in a 1 L beaker. Fill the beaker with
          more water.
6.2.3   Acidic Acetonitrile : Add 1 mL of 0.05M sulphuric acid solution
          (6.2.2) to 100 mL acetonitrile.

6.2.4   0.5*M* sodium hydroxide. Dissolve 20 g sodium hydroxide in 600 mL water and make up to 1 L with water.

6.3.   Standards; Acepromazine, Azaperol and Haloperidol (RIVM) Chlorpromazine hydrochloride, Propionylpromazine and xylazine (Sigma). Azaperone; (Janssen Pharm - Beerse, Belgium)

6.3.1.   Stock Standards. Weigh accurately 10 ± 1 mg of each individual standard (6.3) into a 100 mL graduated flask. Make up to 100 mL with methanol. The solution is stored in the dark at 4-8°C and is stable for up to one year.

6.3.2.   Working Standards. Pipette 1 mL of stock standard for acepromazine and haloperidol, chlorpromazine hydrochloride, propionylpromazine and azaperone into a 100 mL graduated flask and make up to 100 mL with sulphuric acid solution, 0.01 - 0.05*M*, (6.2.2). The concentration of each standard is 1 mg per L.

6.3.3.   Working Standard for azaperone and azaperol; Pipette 1 mL of stock standard for azaperol and azaperone into a 100 mL graduated flask and make up to 100 mL with 0.01*M* sulphuric acid solution, (6.2.2). Transfer 20 mL of this solution into another 100 mL graduated flask and make up to 100 mL with sulphuric acid solution, 0.01*M*, (6.2.2). The concentration of each standard is 0.2 mg per L.

6.3.4   Internal standard for GC-MS. Make up a solution of 2 ng per μL of 2,3,4-2,4',5'-hexachlorobiphenyl (PCB) (Promochem, Wesel, Germany) in ethyl acetate (6.1.12).

6.4   Control Samples; Certified blank samples of pig kidneys should be spiked with the standards at concentrations of 20 and 50 μg per kg. Do this by pipetting 100 or 250 μL of the working standard 6.3.2 and/or 6.3.3 into an 80 mL centrifuge tube containing 5 g homogenised sample and allow to stand for 10 min. before extraction.

7.   EQUIPMENT

7.1   Analytical balances
7.2   Normal laboratory glassware including graduated volumetric flasks, 100 mL capacity
7.3   Centrifuge (MSE-Coolspin)
7.3.1   Polypropylene centrifuge tubes, capacity 80 mL
7.4   Ultrasonic bath
7.5   Sep-Pak C18 cartridges (Waters art. 51910)
7.6   Heating block with thermostat and evaporation system with nitrogen (Pierce Reacti Therm Module № 18790 and Pierce Reacti Vap № 18780)
7.7   Vibromixer
7.8   Food Processor (Moulinette)
7.9   Syringes, 50 mL (Terumo)
7.10   pH meter
7.11   GC-MS
7.11.1   GC-MS is Hewlett Packard HP-MSD equipped with a HP5890A gas chromatograph, a model HP5970B mass selective detector, a model HP7673A autosampler and a model HP59970C chemstation.
7.11.2   Conditions
         GC column   ; Fused silica capillary column, 25 x 0.22 mm. i.d. coated with 0.12 μm layer of CP Sil-5
         Carrier gas   ; Helium, linear velocity, 30 cm per sec

Cy 4.6/3

Split   :   20 mL per min, opened 4 min after injection
Septum flush   :   3 mL per min, opened 4 min after injection
T-injector   :   260°C
Injection   :   5 µL splitless
T-oven   :   80-260°C; rate 10°C per min;
                      initial hold 2 min; final hold 2 min.
MS interface   :   direct coupling of column to ion source
T interface   :   260°C
Mass range   :   m/z 40-800
Ion source   :   Electron impact (EI), 70 eV
t-measuring   :   50 ms

8. SAMPLES AND SAMPLING PROCEDURE.

N.B. Attention is drawn to section 6.3.1 and to ISO document 78/2-1982 and also the following notes derived from Annex II of 2052/VI/84-EN.

8.1.   Nature of the Sample; Samples shall be such as to enable the detection of residues in meat as defined in Directive 64/433/EEC.

8.2.   Size of Sample; The size of the sample must be large enough to allow the method to be carried out and to allow repeat analysis where required.

8.3.   The samples must be taken and packed in such a way as to allow proper identification in the laboratory.

8.4.   The method of packing, preservation and transport must maintain the integrity of the sample and not prejudice the result of the examination.
          Samples for the analysis of tranquillizers must be stored and transported at temperatures below -18°C.

9.0   PROCEDURE
9.1   Homogenise the kidney sample in a food processor (7.8)
9.2   Weigh 10 g of the homogenised sample into an 80 mL centrifuge tube (7.3.1).
9.3   Pipette 20 mL acetonitrile into the tube. During the addition the sample is mixed gently on a Vibromixer. Increase the speed to 1500 rpm for 45 sec. Transfer the tubes to an ultrasonic bath for 2 min. Centrifuge for 5 min at 4000 g.
9.4   Clean up with Sep-Pak cartridges;
9.4.1   Activate the cartridges (7.5) with 5 mL methanol and 5 mL water.
9.4.2   Drain the cartridges using a syringe (7.9).
9.4.3   Add 50 mL 10% sodium chloride solution (6.2.1) and 7.5 mL supernatant from the sample extract (9.3) together, mix and flush through the column.
9.4.4   Pass through the column 1 mL 0.01M sulphuric acid (6.2.2) and then 2 mL of air.
9.4.5   Prepare calibrated 10 mL test tubes by washing with ammonia solution (6.1.3), water, methanol and acetone.
9.4.6   Elute the analytes with 2 mL acidic acetonitrile solution (6.2.3) into the prepared test tubes (9.4.5).
9.5   Reduce the volume of the eluate to 300 µL by evaporation with nitrogen on a heating block at 70°C. Do not dry.
9.6   Add immediately 1 mL n-hexane. Mix for 30 sec on a Vibromixer at

9.7 700 rpm and centrifuge at 2000 g for 5 min.
9.7 Discard the hexane fraction and repeat step 9.6. and discard the hexane fraction.
9.8 Adjust the pH to 10 by the addition of 150 μL of 0.5M sodium hydroxide.
9.9 After gentle mixing add 1 mL tert-butyl methyl ether. Vortex for 30 sec. Centrifuge. Transfer the upper organic phase into a 4 mL vial.
9.10 Repeat 9.9 two times.
9.11 Evaporate the combined organic phases to dryness using a stream of nitrogen and at 30°C.
9.12 Dissolve the residue in 25 μL of the PCB internal standard solution (6.3.4) with Vortex mixing.
9.13 Inject 5 μL into the GC-MS system.
9.14 With each series of samples standard solutions of the standards of interest over the range 0 - 10 ng per μL were analyzed.

10.0 CALCULATION OF RESULTS
10.1 The MS spectra were evaluated according to the criteria in EC 93/256 (see section 5). The reproducibility for four ions is good for all the tranquillizers except xylazine and haloperidol and also carazolol. These latter compounds have to be excluded from the test.
10.2 Data on repeatability of retention times.
  The retention times in minutes and their percentage coefficients of variation (in parenthesis) for 10 analyses were;-
  PCB 138 (IS), 16.125 (1.5%); xylazine, 12.731 (4.2%); chlorpromazine, 17.593 (2.0%); azaperone, 19.152 (2.3%); acepromazine, 19.238 (1.3%); azaperol, 19.599 (2.6%); propionylpromazine, 19.817 (2.0%); haloperidol, 20.993 (2.5%)
10.3 Repeatability of Ion intensity. n = 10, CV in parenthesis Concentration is 5 ng per μL.

Analyte	Base Peak	Ion m/z (CV%)	Ion m/z (CV%)	Ion m/z (CV%)
PCB 138 (IS)	360			
Xylazine	205	220 (19.0)[u]	177 (13.8)[u]	145 (16.0)[u]
Chlorpromazine	318	272 (1.1)	86 (3.3)	233 (2.6)
Azaperone	107	233 (3.6)	165 (3.6)	309 (4.6)
Acepromazine	326	280 (0.9)	241 (4.2)	197 (7.0)
Azaperol	107	235 (7.0)	121 (4.2)	222 (5.9)
Propionylpromazine	340	294 (3.8)	255 (3.3)	197 (5.0)
Haloperidol	224	237 (6.0)[u]	123 (12.2)[u]	206 (11.7)[u]

Superscript u means result does not meet criteria in EC 93/256.
Ions are in order of intensity.
Data in 10.2 and 10.3 are from Hoogland et al, (1991).

All four ions can be reliably detected at concentrations of 50 μg per kg kidney.

10.4   Recoveries; No data available.
The percentage recoveries must be in the following ranges;
Carazolol, 84-113; xylazine, 24-80; azaperone, 74-124; haloperidol, 75-115;
acepromazine, 78-124; propionylpromazine, 77-113; chlorpromazine, 58-128.

11.   SPECIAL CASES.
Interference; The presence of the compounds; promazine, diazepam,
oxazepam, amitryptyline, lorazepam, prochlorperazine, nefofam, cyclizine,
perphenazine and hydroxizine in kidney samples did _not_ interfere with the
SIM analysis of the compounds investigated.

12.   NOTES ON PROCEDURE.

The analytes are unstable in light. Keep all samples in the dark and work
only under an amber light.

13.   SAMPLE CONTROLS

14.   TEST REPORT

15.   LIST OF ABBREVIATIONS.
See abbreviations in Annex I, Section 12 of Manual.

16.   FLOW DIAGRAM

Homogenise kidney -----> extract with acetonitrile -----> C18 Sep-Pak
                                                                   |
                                                                   |
                                                                   ↓
Identify & Quantify <------- GC-MS <-------- Solvent/solvent partition
                                 (EI-mode)

**7.0 THE CONCENTRATION OF RESIDUES OF VETERINARY DRUGS AND LEVELS OF
NATURALLY OCCURRING STEROIDS IN FARM ANIMALS.**

This section provides information on the residues and in the case of
naturally occurring substances found in farm animals the physiological
levels of substances of interest in the control of residues in farm animals
and their products.

Part 7.1. is a copy of report produced for the EEC by Professor Hoffmann,
Veterinary Faculty, University of Giessen, Germany. None of the data is
changed but the report has been edited to conform with the style of the
manual.

For the purposes of the report by Hoffmann, naturally occurring steroids
are considered to be testosterone, epitestosterone, oestradiol-17α,
oestradiol-17ß, oestrone and progesterone. 19-nortestosterone is covered
in section 7.2. as a xenobiotic compound but it has to be noted that this
compound occurs naturally in pigs and horses.

Part 7.2. gives information on the residues of some key xenobiotic
substances of special interest for residue control. It is planned to
expand this section in future editions. The drugs covered so far are

7.2.1.	ANABOLIC AGENTS
7.2.1.1.	TRENBOLONE
7.2.1.2	ZERANOL
7.2.1.3	STILBENES, DES, HEX, DE
7.2.1.4.	19-NORTESTOSTERONE
7.2.2.	ANTIBIOTICS
7.2.2.1	SULPHONAMIDES, (Sulphadimidine, sulphathiazole)
7.2.2.2.	ß-LACTAMS (Benzylpenicillin, penicillin-V)
7.2.2.3.	CHLORAMPHENICOL
7.2.3.	ANTHELMINTHICS AND PARASITICIDES
7.2.3.1.	BENZIMIDAZOLES (Albendazole, Febantel, Fenbendazole, Flubendazole, Oxfendazole, Thiabendazole, Triclabendazole)
7.2.3.2.	IVERMECTIN
7.2.3.3.	CLOSANTEL
7.2.4.	ß-AGONISTS

7.1. LEVELS OF NATURALLY OCCURRING SEX STEROIDS IN EDIBLE BOVINE TISSUES

Reference Levels of naturally occurring hormones; report of Professor
B.Hoffmann as requested with letter of October 6, 1987, Directorate-General
for Agriculture, VI/B/II.2; and submitted to the Scientific Veterinary
Committee.

1.   SCOPE OF THE REPORT

Among the mechanisms controlling physiology and pathophysiology of higher
organisms autocrine, paracrine and endocrine regulatory factors are of
utmost importance. Hence their presence in all edible animal and plant
products has to be expected.

With this paper it is intended to present information on the occurrence of
endogenous sex hormones in edible animal tissues and products. Reference
will only be made to those data which have been obtained by applying
adequate methodology according to presently accepted reliability criteria.
Where possible suggestions will be made for upper tissue concentration
which might serve as preliminary aids to discriminating between treated and
untreated animals.

2.   INTRODUCTION

Endogenous sex hormones are defined as substance of steroidal nature
produced by the male and female gonad. However, other endocrine active
organs like the placenta or adrenal gland may similarly produce these
compounds in respectable amounts. Characteristic of the female animal is
the production of oestrogens (C18-steroids) and of progesterone
(C21-steroid), while sex steroid production in the male animal is
characterized by the release of testosterone (C19-steroid) from the testis.
In the female oestradiol-17ß is the main product coming from the ovary
while other oestrogens, like for example oestrone and oestrone-sulphate,
represent the main oestrogens coming from the placenta.

It should be noted that differences between males and females in respect to
the production of sex hormones are not qualitative but quantitative and
that within sexes production rates and hence tissue levels vary depending
on age and physiological status of the animal (16).

When reviewing the literature it becomes evident that the only animal
species investigated in some detail is cattle. Thus all data presented in
this report refer to this species.

All the data presented have been obtained by competitive protein binding
analysis; in most studies, however, highly specific antisera were used,
while only few papers refer to the use of receptor proteins. It should
further be noted that prior to protein binding analysis additional
extraction and purification steps had been included, like high performance
liquid chromatography, thin layer chromatography or column chromatography.
As stated above the data quoted have been obtained with validated methods.

3.   CONCENTRATIONS IN EDIBLE PRODUCTS

3.1   TESTOSTERONE

The levels of free, unconjugated testosterone determined in various tissues
of veal calves, heifers, pregnant cattle and slaughter bulls are summarized
in Table 1. Obviously highest levels are found in slaughter bulls with
fatty tissue showing maximal concentrations; in the other animals highest
concentrations were determined in the kidney. Levels of conjugated
testosterone, expressed as percent of total testosterone, are presented in
Table 2. Conjugated testosterone is very low in muscle while it dominates
in the liver and is about equal to the percentage of free testosterone in
the kidney.
The cumulation of testosterone in fat of bulls can be explained by the
ongoing and rather continuous production of testosterone (about 50mg/24h)
and the lipophilic properties of this steroid. The cumulation of
testosterone in kidneys of the other animals examined may be due to the
presence of specific testosterone binding sites. In female veal calves
testosterone is of ovarian and adrenal origin (16).

Based on the levels determined for free testosterone Table 3 shows the
ranking of organs and tissues in cattle subpopulations. The fact, that
testosterone is highest in fat of slaughter bulls is well demonstrated.

Testosterone has also been determined in milk of cattle with lower levels
at oestrus (50pg/ml) compared to the luteal phase of the cycle (122pg/ml)
(1). The ratio of free to conjugated testosterone has been determined to be
1:1 (3). Also the presence of 5a-androstane-3,17-dione (1ng/ml) and some of
its isomers has been shown in milk (2).

3.2   PROGESTERONE

Tissue levels of progesterone for female cattle are given in Table 4. The
ongoing progesterone production during pregnancy expresses itself in the
relatively high levels measurable in pregnant cattle. The accumulation of
progesterone in fatty tissue of all types of cattle examined is explained
by the lipophilic properties of this steroid hormone. Hence also in milk
and in milk products progesterone levels are correlated with the percentage
of fat as shown in Table 5.

In milk itself progesterone levels relate to the stage of oestrous cycle,
with minimal concentrations at oestrus and highest levels during the luteal
phase and pregnancy (see Table 5).

3.3   OESTROGENS

Tables 6 - 9 show data for oestradiol-17ß, oestrone and total oestrogens.
The term "total oestrogens" refers to the application of an assay using an
antiserum with a high cross reactivity between oestrone, oestradiol-17a and
oestradiol-17ß; other oestrogens are less cross reactive.

The levels for oestradiol-17ß are presented in Table 6. Lowest levels have
been determined in steers, followed by veal calves and heifers; highest
levels were found in pregnant cattle (as a result of placental oestrogen

production). The concentrations determined in pregnant cattle increase with
the length of pregnancy and are highest in liver followed by kidney, fat
and muscle. The low levels observed in steers show no significant
differences between the various tissues examined.

Table 7 gives the data established for oestrone . Since oestrone is the
primary product of placental oestrogen production there is a dramatic
increase during pregnancy with highest levels measurable in fat.

Total oestrogens have been determined in tissues of 6 female and 17 male
veal calves. The results are presented in Table 8 and figure 1. There are
striking differences between the concentrations determined in liver and
kidney, compared to muscle.

Figure 1. Total oestrogens in Calves.

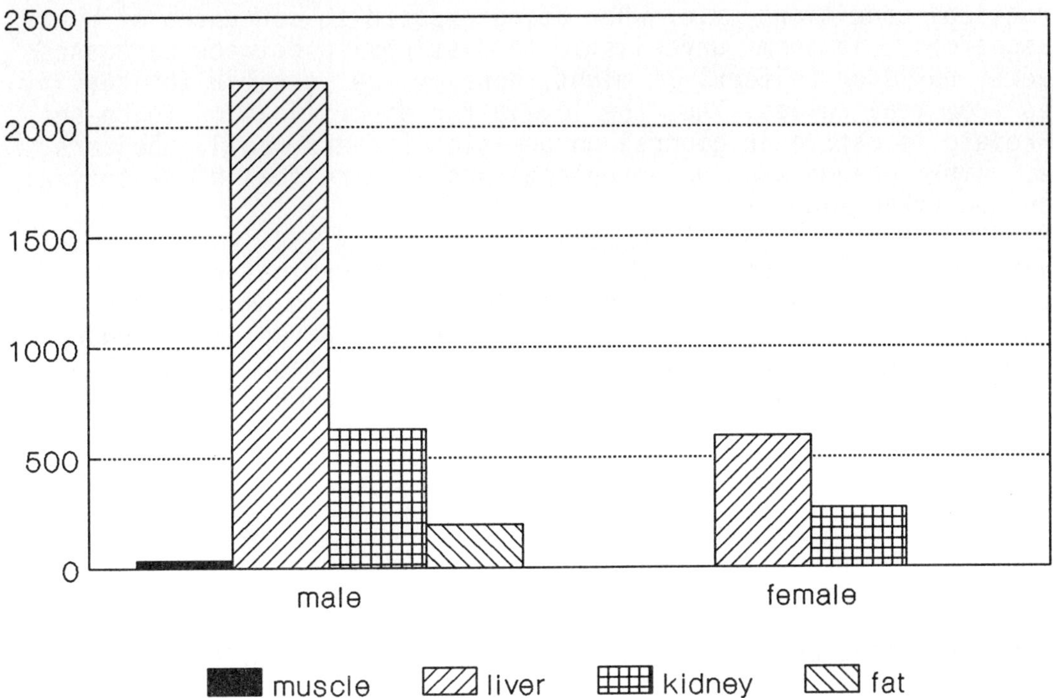

Oestrogen concentrations in milk have also been determined. Total
oestrogens (0.64 - 2.14 ng per mL) were highest in milk sampled in the five
day period immediately before parturition and fall below 0.2 ng per mL
after one day post-partum (13), the levels obtained during other stages of
the reproductive phase are presented in Table 9. Obviously there are only
small variations in oestradiol-17ß and oestrone concentrations, however, as
determined between days 205 and 209 of pregnancy, oestrone sulphate levels
are somewhat higher than oestradiol-17ß (13).

4.   TENTATIVE RECOMMENDATIONS FOR PRELIMINARY LEVELS AS AIDS TO
DISCRIMINATE BETWEEN TREATED AND UNTREATED CATTLE

To our present knowledge up to now distinctions between untreated animals
and those treated with oestradiol-17ß, testosterone or progesterone can
only be made on a quantitative and not a qualitative basis. This statement
is based on the fact that the three steroids mentioned above
(oestradiol-17ß, testosterone, progesterone) will enter the same metabolic
pathways, regardless of whether they are of endogenous or exogenous origin.
Thus, treated animals can only be identified if their tissue levels
significantly exceed those of untreated animals; if such a situation is
detected it further has to be verified that the particular animal showing
this levels was clinically sound and that no reproductive problems, such as
cystic ovaries or tumours of sex hormone producing organs had been present
at slaughter.

Under practical conditions, i.e. when being exposed to carcasses or parts
of carcasses only, it seems unrealistic to distinguish between carcasses
from steers, bulls or heifers. It might, however, be possible to identify
carcasses from veal calves. Thus the levels for discrimination to be set
have to relate to cattle in general on one side (steers, bulls, heifers,
and cows, either pregnant or non-pregnant) and - where feasible - to veal
calves on the other side.

When trying to establish preliminary levels for discrimination the in some
respects limited data base has to be considered. Thus in order to account
for the biological variation and following generally accepted procedures, 3
standard-deviations (SD) were added to the calculated mean values. The
resulting figures were further rounded up to an even number by allowing for
another correction around 10%.

4.1   TESTOSTERONE

4.1.1   Female, sexually immature veal calves

By applying the above mentioned procedure the following figures were
obtained from the data presented for 5 female veal calves:

Tissue	Metabolites estimated	Mean value plus 3 SD (ng / g)	rounded up to
Muscle	free testosterone	0.06	0.07
Liver	free and conj. testosterone (3:7)	0.31	0.35
Kidney	free and conj. testosterone (1:1)	1.17	1.30
Fat	free testosterone	0.53	0.60

4.1.2   Cattle including male veal calves

No special data for male veal calves are available. However, as has been
shown from determining testosterone in plasma, testicular function is well
expressed even right after parturition and many bull calves may have
entered the process of puberty at the time of slaughter. Hence they have to
be considered with the other types of cattle. There in respect to the
classification of carcasses, preliminary levels for discrimination have to
be delineated from the bull.

Tissue	Metabolites estimated	Mean Value plus 3SD	rounded up to (ng / g)
Muscle	free testosterone	2.97	3.20
Liver	free and conj. testosterone (3:7)	6.55	7.00
Kidney	free and conj. testosterone (1:1)	18.63	20.00
Fat	free testosterone	37.00	40.00

4.2 PROGESTERONE

4.2.1 Sexually immature male and female veal calves

Since it can be assumed that ovarian progesterone production has not yet started in female veal calves going to slaughter, the available data for 5(4) male veal calves can be taken to set preliminary levels of discrimination for the whole group of veal calves.

Tissue	Metabolite estimated	Mean value plus 3 SD	rounded up to (ng / g)
Muscle	progesterone	0.51	0.55
Liver	progesterone	0.60	0.70
Kidney	progesterone	1.09	1.20
Fat	progesterone	13.30	15.00

4.2.2 C a t t l e

With respect to the frequent slaughtering of pregnant cattle, levels of discrimination must be based on the progesterone concentration determined in tissues obtained from this type of animal.
The figures given below (preliminary levels of discrimination) are derived from 3 animals for muscle, liver and kidney and 10 animals for fat.

Tissue	Metabolite estimated	Mean value plus 3 SD	rounded up to (ng / g)
Muscle	progesterone	29.90	32.00
Liver	progesterone	7.53	8.50
Kidney	progesterone	11.77	13.00
Fat	progesterone	656.40	700.00

4.3 OESTROGENS

As is obvious from Tables 6, 7, and 8 the data obtained so far for oestrogens are less coherent than those obtained for testosterone and progesterone. This may be due to slight methodological differences between the various laboratories particularly in relation to purification steps or other types of antisera used. The most homogeneous pool has been obtained for oestrone, which is a major metabolite of oestrogen metabolism in cattle (16). Thus it is suggested to use oestrone as the marker compound for distinction between treated and untreated animals

It must further be assumed, that liver and kidney particularly contain conjugated oestrone. However, no data in relation to the occurrence of this steroid in tissue of untreated cattle have been reported.

Hence for the time being only free oestrone can be used as a marker compound; yet it is strongly recommended to carry out extra work to allow the inclusion of conjugated oestrone and to possibly establish a firm data base for oestradiol-17ß.

4.3.1 Sexually immature male and female veal calves

Tissue	Metabolite estimated	Mean value plus 3 SD (ng / g)	rounded up to
Muscle	oestrone	0.19	0.20
Liver	oestrone	0.47	0.50
Kidney	oestrone	0.16	0.20
Fat	oestrone	0.53	0.60

4.3.2 C a t t l e

In respect to the frequent slaughtering of pregnant cattle, levels of discrimination must be based on the oestrone concentration determined in tissues obtained form this type of animal.

Tissue	Metabolite estimated	Mean Value plus 3 SD (ng / g)	rounded up to
Muscle	oestrone	1.24	1.30
Liver	oestrone	0.38	0.40
Kidney	oestrone	0.77	0.90
Fat	oestrone	8.42	9.00

REFERENCES

(1)   Hoffmann, B.; Rattenberger, E. (1977) Testosterone concentration in tissue from veal calves, bulls and heifers and in milk-samples.   J. Anim. Sci._46_, 635-641

(2) Darling, J.A.B.; Laing, A.M.; Harkness, R.A. (1974) A survey of the steroids in cow's milk. J. Endocr._62_, 291-297

(3) Hoffmann, B. (1977) Vorkommen und Bedeutung von Hormonen in der Milch. Milchwissenschaft _32_, 477-482

(4) Heinritzi, K.H. (1974) Entwicklung von Methoden zur Bestimmung von Östron, Östradiol-17ß und Progesteron in verschiedenen Geweben vom Kalb und deren Anwendung im Rahmen von Rückstandsuntersuchungen. Diss. vet. med. TÜ München

(5) Kushinsky, S. (1983) Safety aspects of the use of cattle implants containing natural steroids. Int. Symp. Safety Anim. Drug Residues, Berlin

(6) Hoffmann, B.; Hamburger, R.; Karg, H. (1975) Naturliche Vorkommen von Progesteron in handelsublichen Milchprodukten. Z. Lebensm. Unters. Forsch. 158, 257-259

(7) Ginther, O.J.; Nuti, L.C.; Garcia, M.C.; Wentworth, B.C.; Tyler, W.J. (1976) Factors affecting progesterone concentration in cow's milk and dairy products. J. Anim. Sci. 42, 155-159

(8) Hoffmann, B.; Karg, H.; Heinritzi, K.H.; Behr, E.H.; Rattenberger, E. (1975) Moderne Verfahren der Östrogenbestimmung und deren Anwendung fur die Rückstandsproblematik. Mitt. Gebiete Lebensm. Hyg. 66, 20-37

(9) Henricks, D.M. (1980) Assay of naturally occurring estrogens in bovine tissues. Steroids in Anim. Production, Intern. Symp. Warsaw, 161-170

(10) Meyer, H.H.D. (1983) Neue Methode zur Bestimmung von Steroidoestrogenen im Gewebe. Wien. tierärztl. Mschr. 6/7, 243-244

(11) Meyer, H.H.D.; Rapp, M.; Landwehr, M. (1985) Analytische Erfassung und Bewertung natürlicher Steroidöstrogene im eßbaren Gewebe und Galle unbehandelter und mit dem Östradiolpräparat "Compudose" behandelter Mastkälber. Arch. Lebensmittelhyg. 36, 5-8

(12) Henricks, D.M.; Gray, St.; Hoover, J.L.B. (1983) Residue levels of endogenous levels in beef tissues. Proc. Symp. OIE Anabol. Anim. Prod., Paris, 233-248

(13) Monk, E.L.; Erb, R.E.; Mollett, T.A. (1975) Relationships between immunoreactive estrone and estradiol in milk, blood, and urine of dairy cows. J. Dairy Sci. 58, 34-40

(14) Hoffmann, B. (1978) Use of radioimmunoassay for monitoring hormonal residues in edible animal products. J. Assoc. Anal. Chem. 61, 1263-1273

(15) Foote, R.H.; Oltenacu, A.B.; Kummerfeld, H.L.; Smith, R.D.; Riek, P.M.; Braun, R.K. (1979) Milk progesterone as a diagnostic aid. Br. vet. J. 135, 551-558

(16) Hoffmann, B.; Evers, P. (1986) Anabolic agents with sex hormone-like activities - problems of residues. Academic Press Inc. 1986, pp. 111-146

(17) Hoffmann, B. (1983) Natural occurrence of steroid hormone in food producing animals. Proc. Symp. OIE Anabol. Prod., Paris, 215-231

Table 1: Levels of free endogenous testosterone in edible animal tissues (ng/kg mean ± SD).

	muscle	liver	kidney	fat
female veal calves (1)	16 ± 13 n = 5	39 ± 18 n = 5	256 ± 110 n = 5	178 ± 118 n = 5
heifers (1)	92 ± 29 n = 5	193 ± 101 n = 5	595 ± 650 n = 5	250 ± 64 n = 5
(2)	20 ± 7 n = 15	13 ± 2 n = 10	189 ± 92 n = 15	26 ± 7 n = 35

pregnant cattle

	muscle	liver	kidney	fat
day 120 (5)	302 ± 163 n = 15	39 ± 13 n = 8	1930 ± 453 n = 5	406 ± 101 n = 7
day 180 (5)	343 ± 117 n = 11	121 ± 19 n = 11	3505 ± 1537 n = 6	751 ± 174 n = 11
day 240 (5)	418 ± 180 n = 4	274 ± 69 n = 4	4014 ± 2269 n = 4	694 ± 231 n = 4
bull (1)	776 ±730 n = 4	749 ± 405 n = 4	2738 ± 2192 n = 3	10950 ± 8683 n = 5
(1)	294 ± 319 n = 4			

Values in parentheses are number of animals.

Table. 2:   Conjugated testosterone as % of total testosterone in tissues of 2 female veal calves and slaughter bulls (1)

Animal	% of conj. testosterone		
	muscle	liver	kidney
Female veal calves	below detection level	74 70	38 44
Bulls	17 below detection level	76 80	35 40

Table 3:   Ranking of organ and tissue concentration according
            to the presence of free testosterone in cattle sub-
            populations (1)

| | ranking factor and tissues | | | |
Animal	muscle	liver	kidney	fat
Female veal calf	1	2.4	16.0	11.1
Heifer	1	2.1	6.5	2.7
Slaughter bull	1	1.4	5.2	20.5

Table 4: Levels of free endogenous progesterone in edible animal tissues
(ng/kg mean ± SD).

	muscle	liver	kidney	fat
veal calves calves (4)	247 ± 87 n = 5	269 ± 110 n = 5	456 ± 211 n = 5	
(14)				5800 ± 2500 n = 4
heifers (14)				16700 ± 16800 n = 5
steer (5)	270 ± 330 n = 16	260 ± 70 n = 17	170 ± 140 n = 18	2480 ± 1610 n = 21
pregnant cattle (5)	10100 ± 6600 n = 3	3420 ± 1370 n = 3	6190 ± 1860 n = 3	239000 ± 116000 n = 3
(14)				336000 ± 106700 n = 10

The values in parentheses are the reference numbers, n is the number of
animals.

Table 5: Levels of free endogenous progesterone in milk and milk products
(ug/l mean ± SD).

Product	fat %	[6]	[7]	[15]
Skim milk	0.1	1.4	4.6 ± 0.4 (12) 2.1 ± 0.6 (4)	0.17 ± 0.04^{e} (10) 0.84 ± 1.0^{cl} (10) 1.1 ± 0.1^{p} (10)
Buttermilk	1.0	6.5	4.7 ± 0.8 (?)	
Homogenised	1.5	6.0		
Heated milk	3.5	11.8		
Normal milk	3.5	12.5	11.3 ± 0.6 (12) 9.5 ± 0.5 (4)	0.92 ± 0.19^{e} (8) 23.1 ± 3.6^{cl} (8) 35.7 ± 5.6^{p} (8)
Milk powder	25	98.4		
Cream	32	43	58.7 ± 5.3 (12) 72.7 ± 5.8 (4)	
Butter	82	300	133 ± 5 (?)	
Butter fat			13 ± 14^{e} (?) 360 ± 110^{cl} (?) 360 ± 110^{p} (?)	

The values in [ ] are reference numbers, those in ( ) are the number of
animals.
e is oestrus, cl is luteal phase, p is pregnancy.

Table 6: Levels of free endogenous oestradiol-17ß in edible animal tissues (ng/kg mean ± SD).

	muscle	liver	kidney	fat
veal calves (8)	113 ± 143 n = 5	73 ± 163 n = 5	11 ± 10 n = 5	129 ± 57 n = 5
heifers (9)	12 ± 18 n = 9	38 ± 2 n = 9	40 ± 4 n = 9	10 ± 3[a] n = 8 8 ± 1[b] n = 6
(5)	6 ± 9 n = 15	2 ± 1 n = 10	3 ± 3 n = 15	13 ± 14 n = 35
pregnant cattle				
day 120 (5)	16 ± 12 n = 8	58 ± 50 n = 8	127 ± 46 n = 5	31 ± 13 n = 7
day 180 (5)	27 ± 14 n = 11	380 ± 280 n = 11	230 ± 100 n = 6	72 ± 37 n = 11
day 240 (5)	33 ± 16 n = 4	1027 ± 365 n = 4	274 ± 85 n = 4	68 ± 35 n = 4
month 4 (8)	860 n = 1			
month 9 (8)	370 n = 1			
months 1-3 (9)				5 ± 1 n = 3
months 3-6 (9)				22 ± 9 n = 4
months 6-9 (9)				163 ± 74 n = 5
steer (9)	14 ± 1 n = 14	12 ± 1 n = 14	13 ± 1 n = 14	10 n = 1
(9)	6 [max 13] n = 43	4 [max 9] n = 43	7 [max14] n = 43	7 [max 21] n = 43
(5)	1 ± 0.3 n = 16	1 ± 0.4 n = 18	2 ± 2 n = 18	2 ± 1 n = 21

Values in ( ) are the reference numbers,n is number of animals.
a is follicular phase of cycle; b is luteal phase.

Table 7: Levels of free endogenous oestrone in edible animal tissues (ng/kg mean ± SD).

	muscle	liver	kidney	fat
veal calves (8)	75 ± 38 n = 5	204 ± 88 n = 5	47 ± 38 n = 5	275 ± 84 n = 5
heifers (9)				40 ± 12[a] n = 8
				48 ± 24[b] n = 6
(5)	3 ± 1 n = 15	2 ± 1 n = 10	1 ± 1 n = 15	11 ± 6 n = 35
(12)	31 ± 4 n = 8	23 ± 3 n = 8	14 ± 2 n = 8	28 ± 3 n = 8
pregnant cattle				
day 120 (5)	203 ± 170 n = 8	30 ± 33 n = 8	84 ± 2(?) n = 5	780 ± 641 n = 7
day 180 (5)	482 ± 301 n = 11	115 ± 83 n = 11	166 ± 94 n = 6	2717 ± 1259 n = 11
day 240 (5)	523 ± 240 n = 4	145 ± 56 n = 4	142 ± 41 n = 4	2765 ± 1497 n = 4
month 4 (8)	120 n = 1			
months 1-3 (12)	13 ± 3 n = 5	25 ± 8 n = 5	10 ± 4 n = 5	18 ± 3 n = 5
(9)				40 ± 25 n = 3
months 3-6 (12)	186 ± 13 n = 9	125 ± 26 n = 9	262 ± 67 n = 9	462 ± 55 n = 9
(9)				964 ± 353 n = 4
months 6-9 (12)	208 ± 53 n = 9	252 ± 43 n = 9	550 ± 72 n = 9	3687 ± 549 n = 9
(9)				3874 ± 1516 n = 16
steer (9)	5 [max 11] n = 192	9 [max 14] n = 192	8 [max 15] n = 192	11 [max 26] n = 192
(5)	2 ± 0.7 n = 16	0.7 ± 0.2 n = 18	1 ± 0.5 n = 18	8 ± 5 n = 21
bull (12)	15 ± 2 n = 7	13 ± 1 n = 7	3 ± 0.4 n = 7	36 ± 5 n = 7

Values in ( ) are the reference numbers, n is number of animals.
a is follicular phase of cycle; b is luteal phase.

Tab. 8:   Levels of total oestrogens in tissues of veal calves (pg/g; ± SD)

	muscle	liver	kidney	fat
Female veal calves	1.8 ± 1.5	600 ± 339	270 ± 227	-
Male veal calves	35 ± 23	2200 ± 1300	630 ± 310	198 ± 177

Table. 9:   Oestradiol-17ß and oestrone concentrations milk (pg/ml, mean ± SE)

	oestradiol-17ß	oestrone
Oestrus	84 ± 41 n = 6	58 ± 6 n = 6
Cl-phase	29 ± 4 n = 6	45 ± 7 n = 6
pregnancy day 55-81	85 ± 9 n = 5	57 ± 20 n = 5
day 107-145	52 ± 14 n = 4	35 ± 13 n = 4
day 205-209	48 ± 21 n = 4	97 ± 21 n = 4

7.2.1.   ANABOLIC AGENTS
7.2.1.1.   TRENBOLONE
7.2.1.2   ZERANOL
7.2.1.3   STILBENES, DES, HEX, DE
7.2.1.4.   19-NORTESTOSTERONE

7.2.2.   ANTIBIOTICS
7.2.2.1   SULPHONAMIDES, (Sulphadimidine, sulphathiazole)
7.2.2.2.   ß-LACTAMS (Benzylpenicillin, penicillin-V)
7.2.2.3.   CHLORAMPHENICOL

7.2.3.   ANTHELMINTHICS AND PARASITICIDES
7.2.3.1.   BENZIMIDAZOLES (Albendazole, Febantel, Fenbendazole,
             Flubendazole, Oxfendazole, Thiabendazole, Triclabendazole)
7.2.3.2.   IVERMECTIN
7.2.3.3.   CLOSANTEL

7.2.4.   ß-AGONISTS (Clenbuterol, Salbutamol)

This section provides information on the levels of residues of some of the
veterinary drugs.   Importance is given to situations where the
concentrations of residues are those which are found when the drugs are
used according to recommended doses for good veterinary practice in those
situations where the drug is licensed.   In countries where the drugs are
specifically prohibited the information may be useful in providing a guide
to the concentrations of residues which might be encountered if the drugs
are used illegally.   There is also information on residues of substances
which have been used in high dosage and at shorter than recommended
withdrawal times.

Many drugs and particulary antimicrobials are administered in the feed or
drinking water. The resultant absorption from the enteric system is
partly dependant on the size of the molecule. Thus with large M.Wt
compounds (> 500 daltons) they are not readily absorbed. This results in
the drug being most active in the gut and not much use for systemic
activity. Also there is not much of a residue problem for the tissues
since most of the drug is eliminated through the faeces or the bile.

With drugs of M.Wt. < 500 daltons then they are absorbed and can exert a
whole animal antimicrobial therapeutic effect and also cause residues in
all the tissues. The residues are excreted in the urine as well as the
faeces.

Thus there are few residue problems with most of the high molecular weight
antimicrobial feed additives, and problems occur, especially in pigs, with
the low M.Wt. drugs namely, sulphonamides, tetracylines and penicillins.

7.2.1. RESIDUES OF XENOBIOTIC ANABOLIC AGENTS.

During the period 1970 to the early 1980's when anabolic agents were being
widely used in several countries a large amount of scientific data was
collected on the levels of residues found in animals. Much of the original
information was for the stilbene compounds and later for trenbolone,
zeranol and 19-nortestosterone. Since the introduction by way of the EEC
Directive 85/649 of a complete ban on the use of xenobiotic anabolic agents
as growth promoters there has been a number of incidences where not only
the compounds mentioned above but also several other anabolic agents e.g.
MPA, MGA, EE_2, boldenone, MT, and the ß-agonists, have been used illegally.
Methods were developed to detect these substances and to determine the
concentrations of residues which occur in animals treated with the drugs.

A general guide (based on published results) to the concentrations of
residues which might be found following the use of anabolic agents in
cattle and sheep is shown in table 1. There will be concentrations outside
of these ranges which will be lower with either the use of very low doses
or very long periods between sampling and treatment or high if very large
doses are used e.g. > 1 gramme, and sampled within a few days of drug
administration.

Table 1. Concentrations of Anabolic Agents in Food-producing Animals.

Tissue/sample	Concentration range µg per kg or L
Site of administration	10^5 - 10^8
Muscle	0.05 - 0.5
Liver	0.1 - 5
Kidney	0.05 - 2
Fat	0.05 - 1
Urine	0.2 - 100
Bile	1 - 1000
Faeces	1 - 500
Blood	0.01 - 0.5

7.2.1.1. TRENBOLONE

Trenbolone is the active component of the veterinary preparation containing
trenbolone acetate. It is a steroid with a structure similar to other C_{18}-
androgens. In ruminants trenbolone is metabolised from the 17ß-OH to the
17α-OH form namely, epi-trenbolone.
The use of trenbolone is prohibited within the EEC but is allowed in other
countries including the USA. Some typical residue levels are shown in
table 2.

Table 2. RESIDUES OF IMPLANTS OF TRENBOLONE ACETATE OUTSIDE INJECTION SITE (µg per kg or µg per L).

SPECIES	DOSE (mg)	DAYS POST DOSE	MUSCLE	LIVER	KIDNEY	FAT	BILE	URINE	Ref.
COW	300	10	0.13ß	0.30ß					1
				0.32α					
		30	0.17ß	0.45ß					1
				0.40α					
		60	0.03ß	0.16ß					1
				0.22α					
COW	300	63		1.7α			10.9α	0.13	2
STEER	300	63	0.30	0.39	0.11	0.24			3
	140E	63	0.25	0.21	0.06	0.18			3
	300Z	60	0.06ß	0.09ß	0.21ß	0.10ß			4
	300Z	60	0.03	0.08	0.25	0.07			4
STEER	200E	60	0.23	0.05		0.08			6
CALF	140E	78	0.19	0.47	0.19	0.44			5
CALF	140E	70	0.13	0.52		0.39			6
	1400E	70	0.80	3.45		2.58			6

RESIDUES AT IMPLANT SITE.

ANIMAL	DOSE (mg)	DAYS post dose	WEIGHT (mg TBA)	% DOSE	Ref.
STEER	140	100	8.4	6	7
	300	150	54	18	7

α is residue of αTB, ß is residue of ßTB, all other conc. are unresolved mixture of both isomers. E is TBA in admixture with 20-40 mg E_2-ß
Z is zeranol implanted in same animal.

REFERENCES.
1. Heitzman, R.J. (1986) Unpublished results of residue study in cattle.

2. Heitzman, R.J., Little, W. & Russell, K.R. (1984). Efficacy and the assessment of hazards of residues following the use of trenbolone acetate (Finaplix) in cull dairy cows. Proc. Brit, Soc. Anim. Prod. Winter mtg, paper No. 131.

3. Heitzman, R.J. and Harwood, D.J. (1977). Residue levels of trenbolone and oestradiol-17ß in plasma and tissues of steers implanted with anabolic steroid preparations. Br. vet. J., _133_, 564-571

4. O'Keefe, M., (1984), Trenbolone levels in tissues of trenbolone acetate-implanted steers: Radioimmunoassay determination using different antisera. Br. vet J. _140_, 592-599

5. Heitzman, R.J., Oettel, G. and Hoffmann, B. (1976). The determination by radioimmunoassay of residues of an anabolic steroid in tissues of calves treated with a combined preparation of trenbolone acetate and oestradiol-

17ß. J.Endocr. <u>69</u>, 10-11P.

6. Hoffmann, B, (1978) Use of radioimmunoassay for monitoring hormonal residues in edible animal tissues. J.A.O.A.C. <u>61</u>, 1263-1273

7. See Dixon, S.N. and Heitzman, R.J. (1983). In "Anabolic Agents in Animal Production" OIE Symposium, Paris, Ed. E.Meissonier, Soreograph, Paris pp 381-391.

7.2.1.2. ZERANOL

The use of zeranol is prohibited within the EEC but is allowed in some countries including the USA. Typical residue levels are shown in table 3.

Table 3. RESIDUES OF IMPLANTS OF ZERANOL OUTSIDE INJECTION SITE (μg per kg or μg per L).

SPECIES	DOSE (mg)	DAYS POST DOSE	MUSCLE	LIVER	KIDNEY	FAT	BILE	URINE	FAECES	Ref.
STEER	36	7	0	0.37		0	14	6	3	1
		14	0.28	0.63		0.11	22	5	5	
		30	0	0.71		0.03	16	3	3	
		70	0	0.1	0.03	0	5	1	0.7	
		>90	0	0	0	0	2.5	<1	<0.5	
	36	67	0.01	0.35	0.08	0.06	-	-	-	2
SHEEP	12	2						7		3
		14						2-19		
		42						25-78		
		70						10		

RESIDUES AT IMPLANT SITE.

ANIMAL	IMPLANT	DOSE (mg)	DAYS post dose	WEIGHT (mg Z)	% DOSE	Ref.
STEER	^{3}H-Z	72	65	11	15	4
	^{3}H-Z	72	125	8.6	12	

REFERENCES.
1. Dixon, S.N., Russell, K.L., Heitzman, R.J. and Mallinson, C.B. (1986), Radioimmunoassay of the anabolic agent zeranol. V. Residues of zeranol in the edible tissues, urine, faeces, and bile of steers treated with Ralgro. J. vet. Pharmacol. Therap. <u>9</u>, 353-358

2. O'Keefe, M. (1984), Tissue levels of the anabolic agents, trenbolone and zeranol, determined by radioimmunoassay. Proc. Symposium on the Analysis of Steroids. Szeged, Hungary. 225-229

3. Dixon, S.N. and Russell, (1983), Radioimmunoassay of the anabolic agent zeranol. II. Zeranol concentrations in urine of sheep and cattle implanted with zeranol (Ralgro). J. vet. Pharmacol. Therap. <u>6</u>, 173-179.

4. Sharp, G.D. and Dyer, I.A. (1972), Zearalenol metabolism in steers. J.Anim. Sci, <u>34</u>, 176-179

7.2.1.3. THE STILBENES, DES, HEX AND DE.

The stilbenes were used legally for more than 20 years, especially in the USA and the UK. Drug disposition studies using radiolabelled DES provide information on the maximum concentrations of residues in animals which were either fed, implanted or injected with DES. Residue data is also provided where residues were measured in situations where the stilbenes were administered both legally and where misuse of the drugs was simulated.

Table 4. RESIDUES OF IMPLANTS OF DES AND HEX OUTSIDE INJECTION SITE (μg per kg or μg per L).

SPECIES	DRUG	ROUTE /DOSE (mg)	DAYS POST DOSE	MUSCLE	LIVER	KIDNEY	FAT	BILE	URINE	FAECES	Ref
SHEEP	DES*	0,3-100	7	<1	<1	<1	<1				1
STEER	DES*	0, 20	1	0.09	3.9	3.7		119			2
			10	0.04	0.08	0.09		0.08			
STEER	DES*	I, 28	30	0.03	0.4	0.3	0.2	13			3,4
			120	0.03	0.7	0.5	0.1	5			
CALF	DES	Inj,100	4	0.09	0.3	0.8	<0.05				5
CALF	DES -DP	Inj,200	7	0.54	18.9	8.9	8.3				5
CALF	DES -DP	Inj,150	28	0.21	2.3	1.5					5
CALF	DES -DP	Inj,150	90	0.05	0.2	0.2					5
CALF	DES -DP	Inj,200	1-50						>10	>10	6
STEER	HEX	I, 60	90	0.03	0.1	0.5		3.2	0.2	2.4	7,8
SHEEP	HEX	I, 15	60	0.08	1.0	3.0	<0.05		4.9		8
POULTRY	HEX	I, 12	44	0.5	6.2		1.3				9

DES* is radiolabelled DES and values are for total residues.
DES-DP is DES-dipropionate.

The following points are relevant;
- Data is only available for residues of DES and HEX.
- Oral administration of DES results in high residues if samples are taken within one or two days of the last treatment.
- Implantation or injection of stilbenes is readily detected in faeces, bile or urine.
- Residues in muscle or fat are extremely low and difficult to detect but residues are detectable in liver and kidney.
- High concentrations of parent drug may be found at the injection sites.

REFERENCES;
1. Aschbacher, P.W., (1972), Metabolism of ^{14}C-diethylstilbestrol in sheep. J.Anim. Sci., _35_, 1031-1035

2. Aschbacher, P.W. and Thacker, E.J. (1974), Metabolic fate of oral diethylstilbestrol in steers. J. Anim. Sci., _39_,1185-1192

3. Aschbacher, P.W. et al (1975), Metabolic fate diethylstilbestrol
implanted in the ears of steers. J. Anim. Sci. _40_, 530-538

4. Rumsey, T.S., et al. (1975), Fate of radiocarbon in beef steers
implanted with ^{14}C-diethylstilbestrol. J. Anim. Sci., _40_, 550-560

5. Hoffmann, B. (1983), In "Gesundheitsaspekte von Anabolikaruckstanden in
Fleischwaren", WHO Regional Office for Europe, ICP/FSP 002(1) 1272I, p17
6. Karg, H., Meyer, H.H.D., Vogt, K., Landwehr, M., Hoffmann, B. and
Schopper, D., (1984), In "Manipulation of growth in farm animals", Eds.
J.F. Roche and D. O'Callaghan, Martius Nijhoff, pp. 34-60

7. Harwood, D.J., Heitzman, R.J. and Jouquey, A. (1980), A
radioimmunoassay method for the measurement of residues of the anabolic
agent, hexoestrol in tissues of cattle and sheep. J. vet, Pharmacol.
Therap., _3_, 245-254

8. Heitzman, R.J. and Harwood, D.J. (1983), The radioimmunoassay (RIA) of
hexoestrol residues in faeces, tissues and body fluids of bulls and steers.
Vet. Rec., _112_, 120-123

9. Herriman, I.D., Harwood,D.J., Blandford, T. and Lindsay, D., (1982),
Distribution of hexoestrol residues in caponised chickens. Vet. Rec., _111_,
435-436.

See also for methods; Covey, T.R., Silvestre, D., Hoffman, M.K. and Henion,
J.D. (1988), A GCMS screening, confirmation and quantification method for
oestrogenic compounds. Biomed. & Environ. MS. _15_, 45-46.

7.2.1.4.   19-NORTESTOSTERONE

Structure and Metabolites (Cattle)

19-nortestosterone
(NT)
epi-19-nortestosterone
(epi-NT)
5α-oestrane-3ß,17α-diol

NT is an androgenic steroid with an anabolic to androgenic activity ratio
greater than that of testosterone.

Metabolism

Cattle - The major metabolite is epi-19-nortestosterone (the 17α-ol).
Minor metabolites are 19-norepiandrosterone and 5α-oestrane-3ß,17α-diol.
All the metabolites and the parent compound are mostly in the conjugated

form in urine, bile, kidney and liver.

Pigs - 19-nortestosterone is a major metabolite in the urine of boars and also cryptorchid pigs (Vandenbroek et al., 1991). Epi-19-nortestosterone was not identified as a urinary metabolite (Debruyckere et al., 1990).

Horses - The major metabolites are 5α-oestrane-3β,17α-diol and 5α-oestrane-3β,17β-diol. There are several other minor metabolites including 19-norepiandrosterone.

Natural Occurrence

NT occurs naturally in male pigs (Maghuin-Rogister et al., 1988; Debruyckere et al., 1990) and stallions (Houghton et al, 1984; Benoit et al. 1985). The detection of epi-NT in urine of peripartum cows provided evidence of endogenous production of NT in late-pregnant cows (Vandenbroeck et al., 1991). More recent studies report that NT is endogenous in late-pregnant cows and new born calves (Meyer et al., 1992) and also in cows at other times during pregnancy (Meyer, private communication). NT was found in both uterine vein blood and jugular vein blood of peripartum cows. During the first few days after parturition the levels of NT fall below the detection limit of the assay (40 ng/L). Epi-19-nortestosterone (epi-NT) was readily detected in the urine of peripartum cows and new born calves (Meyer et al; 1992) and the result has been confirmed in other EC laboratories using the same urine samples from the pregnant cows at the Munich laboratory. Daeseleire et al., (1993) found no evidence of epi-NT in the urine of late pregnant cows.

Concentrations of NT and Metabolites in Farm Animals

Animal	Tissue	NT (μg/L or kg)	epi-NT (μg/L or kg)	Other metabs
Cow (late pregnant)	Urine Blood (Uterine) Blood (jugular vein)	+ve 0.6 - 4.4 0.2 - 0.9	up to 35	+ve
Calf (1-6d)	Urine		0.2 - 32	
Pig (Boar)	Urine	ca 300	-ve	
Horse (Stallion)	Urine	+ve	+ve	+ve

A study in Belgium (Daeseleire et al, 1992) examined the urine of one pregnant cow (gestation time not stated), three non-pregnant cows and six steers. There was no evidence of NT or epi-NT but the metabolite 5α-oestrane-3β,17α-diol was detected in the pregnant animal.

No measurements have been made of naturally occurring levels in bile although the metabolites of NT (e.g. epi-NT) should be easily detectable in bile if they are present in any other tissue or fluid.

<u>**Exogenous Nortestosterone**</u>

Nortestosterone (NT) is the active component of several veterinary
preparations containing nortestosterone esterified at the 17ß position
as either propionate, decanoate, laurate or phenylpropionate.

Haasnoot et al, (1989) measured the residues of both NT and epi-NT in the
urine of a male veal calf weighing 183 kg injected intramuscularly with 200
mg NT-laurate and 20 mg oestradiol-benzoate.   They recorded half lives of
2 days for NT and 15 days for epi-NT with the maximum concentrations in
urine about 7 days after treatment.

Most of the data in the literature refers to residues in urine but some
values are reported for other tissues.   Haasnoot et al. (1989) found high
concentrations of epi-NT in bile samples and the concentration (55 µg per
L) was much higher than that found in urine (3.1 µg per L) of the same
calf.   They also reported residues in meat of three calves treated with
NT-laurate (as above) and slaughtered 14 days after treatment. The
residues in µg per kg were;-

Calf	MUSCLE		LIVER		KIDNEY	
	NT	epi-NT	NT	epi-NT	NT	epi-NT
I	0.1 - 0.2	nd	0.1	0.8	0.5	0.5
II	0.1 - 0.2	nd	0.1	0.5	0.5	0.6
III	0.9 - 1.6	nd	<0.05	0.9	0.4	1.2

The residues of NT and epi-NT were measured in bile and urine samples of
treated calves (van Ginkel et al., 1989)(see figure 2).

Figure 2.

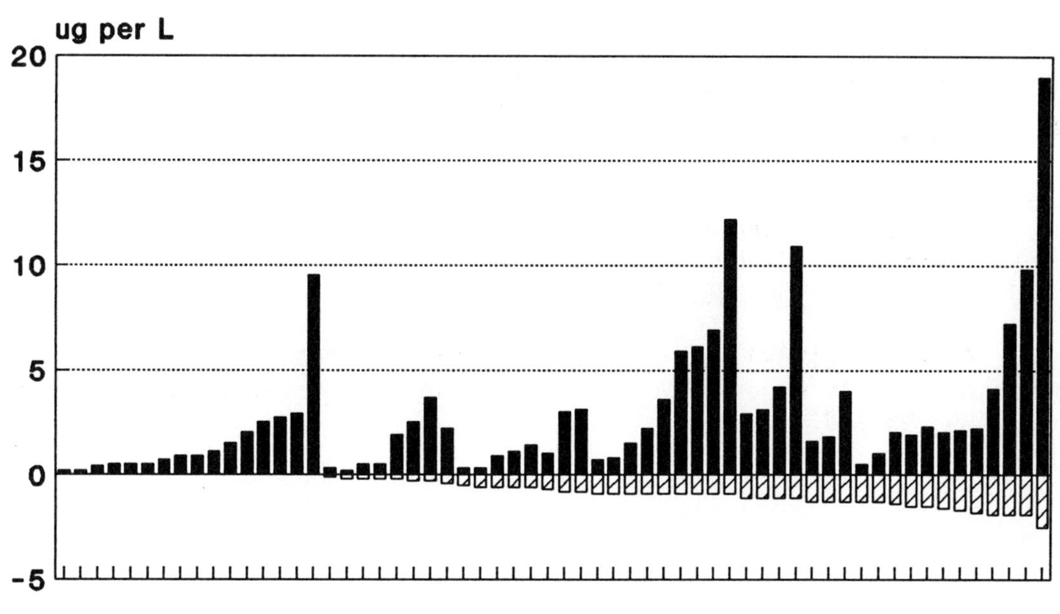

They reported that epi-NT was the most suitable substance to measure and
bile was better than urine because the concentrations were higher in bile
(6 - 18 μg per L). The ratio of NT to epi-NT in the urine of calves
treated with the drug varies between animals and time after treatment (see
figure 2). In most cases the concentration of epi-NT was greater than that
of NT.

REFERENCES

Benoit, E., Garnier, F., Courtot, D. and Delatour, P., (1985).
Radioimmunoassay of 19-nortestosterone. Evidence of its secretion by the
testes of the stallion. Ann. Rech. Vet. 16, 379-383.

Daeseleire, E., De Guesquière, A. and Van Peteghem. (1993). The metabolism
of 19-nortestosterone in urine of calves after oral intake and
intramuscular administration. Acta Clinica Chem. 275, 95-103

Debruyckere, G. Van Peteghem, C., DeBrabander, H.F. and Debackere, M.
(1990), Gas Chromatographic-Mass Spectrophotometric confirmation of 19-
nortestosterone in the urine of untreated boars - effect of the
administration of Laurabolin. Vet. Quart. 12, 246-250

Haasnoot, W., Schilt, R., Hamers, A.R.M. and Huf, F.A. (1989).
Determination of ß-19-nortestosterone and its metabolite α-19-
nortestosterone in biological samples at the sub parts per billion level by
HPLC with on-line immunoaffinity sample pretreatment. J. Chromatog. 489,
157-171

Houghton, E., Copsey, J., Dumasia, P.E., Haywood, P.E., Moss, M.S. and
Teale, P. (1984) Biomed. Mass Spectrom. 11, 96-

Maghuin-Rogister, G., Bosseloire, A., Gaspar, P., Dasnois, C. and Pelzer,
G. Identification de la 19-nortestosterone (nandrolone) dans l'urine de
verrats non castrés. (1988). Ann. Méd. Vét. 132, 437-440.

Meyer, H.H.D., Falckenberg, D., Janowski, T., Rapp, M., Rösel, E.F., Van
Look, L. and Karg, H. (1992). Evidence for the presence of endogenous 19-
nortestosterone in the cow peripartum and the neonatal calf. Acta
Endocrin. 126, 369-373.

Vandenbroeck, M., Van Vyncht, G., Gaspar, P., Dasnois, C., Delahaut, P.,
Pelzer, G., De Graeve, J. and Maghuin-Rogister, G. (1991), Identification
and characterization of 19-nortestosterone in urine of meat-producing
animals. J. Chromatog. 564, 405-412

Van Ginkel L.A. et al (1989), Effective monitoring of residues of
nortestosterone and its major metabolite in bovine urine and bile. J.
Chromatog. 489, 95-104.

7.2.2. RESIDUES OF ANTIMICROBIAL SUBSTANCES

Throughout the Community the common methods for screening for the presence
of antimicrobial substances are those based on the antimicrobial activity.
A widely used test for screening residues in meat and offal is the Four
Plate Test (Bogaerts and Wolf, 1980) and there are several suitable
screening tests available for milk (for Review see Bulletin of the
International Dairy Federation №258/1991). Because of the aspecific nature
of these screening methods more specific methods (e.g. the methods in
section 6) are needed to identify and quantify the antimicrobial residue.
The data given below was mostly derived from such specific methods.

7.2.2.1. SULPHONAMIDES

INTRODUCTION.

The sulphonamides are antibiotic substances used for therapeutic and
prophylactic purposes in all species of farm animals. The most commonly
used sulphonamide is sulphadimidine (sulphamethazine). The MRL for
sulphonamides used throughout the EEC is 0.1 mg of parent drug per kg
tissue. Residues are monitored by Member States and violations are often
detected especially in pigs.

There are many similarities in the metabolism and residue patterns of
sulphonamides and many of the analytical methods are common to the class of
drugs. Because the sulphonamides have been widely used for more than forty
years the information on residues was mostly not determined by the modern
and more acceptable techniques used today. One major study using C-14
radiolabelled sulphadimidine in pigs was commissioned by the Food and Drug
Administration, USA, (study No. 224-81-0007) and carried out in 1981. The
full report of the study was published in 1984, FDA 224-81-005. This
radiometric study of the residues provides the most comprehensive
information on sulphonamide residues. Radiometric studies using
sulphadimidine in other species or using sulphathiazole in any species have
not been reported.

The general metabolism of sulphonamides includes the acetylation of the
aromatic amino group in the reticuloendothelial cells of the liver and in
other tissues yields N-acetyl- derivatives, which are major metabolites of
sulphadimidine and sulphathiazole. The desamino-sulphonamides have also
been identified as residues of the parent drug in cattle (Woolley & Siegel,
1982) and may be the preferred route of metabolism in poultry (Kietzmann,
1981) but do not seem to be an important metabolic product in humans. The
desamino-metabolite is thought to be formed by bacteria in the gut
following oral administration of the drug. Because it is less polar than
the other metabolites the desamino-metabolite is cleared more slowly and
this possibly explains why desamino-sulphadimidine is present as a higher
percentage of the residues as withdrawal time increases. Small amounts
(<5% of total residues) of polar metabolites are produced but have not been
identified in most studies, but it is thought that they are produced by the
hydroxylation of the aromatic ring which may be further conjugated with
glucuronic acid. A complication is that residues of sulphadimidine in
liver and muscle of pigs are converted either chemically or enzymatically
to N-glucose-sulphadimidine during storage at -20 C. Thus the ratio of
sulphadimidine to N-glucose-sulphadimidine in pig meat will depend to some
extent on how long the meat is stored before eating.

RESIDUES OF SULPHADIMIDINE IN FARM ANIMALS AND TISSUES.

The data from six studies give information on residues of sulphadimidine in
edible tissues of pigs and sheep and also residues in milk and eggs. The
conditions of use are similar to those which might be observed in practice.

RESIDUES IN PIGS.

The radiometric study gives the only complete information on total residues
because all of the other analytical methods miss one or more of the
metabolites. Other studies (Ashworth et al, 1986; Samuelson et al., 1979)
are referenced at the end of this section.

RADIOMETRIC STUDY OF SULPHADIMIDINE IN PIGS.

Pigs were administered feed containing 110 mg sulphadimidine per ton and 76
µCi Carbon-14 labelled sulphadimidine (C^{14}-sulphadimidine) in a residue
depletion experiment. The nature and quantity of residues in tissues and
excreta were measured using combinations of radiometry with modern methods
of separation and identification.   The results showed that sulphadimidine
is converted in the live pig to three major metabolites, N-acetyl-
sulphadimidine, N-glucose-sulphadimidine and desamino-sulphadimidine.
Sulphadimidine was also converted to N-glucose-sulphadimidine in stored
deep frozen liver and muscle tissues. The major residues in all tissues
were a mixture of parent drug and the three metabolites. The
concentrations of residues were highest in the blood, GI tract plus
contents, liver and kidney and depleted in all tissues to levels below 0.1
mg per kg 10 days after drug withdrawal (see table 5).

TABLE 5. COMPARISON OF SULPHADIMIDINE RESIDUES AND TOTAL RESIDUES IN PIGS
AFTER WITHDRAWAL OF FEED CONTAINING C^{14}-SULPHADIMIDINE.

TISSUE	Withdrawal Time	TOTAL ^{14}C mg/kg	SULPHADIMIDINE mg/kg	%TOTAL
MUSCLE				
	8 hours	3.2	1.13	35
	2 days	0.93	0.31	33
	5 days	0.06	0.02	34
	10 days	0.004	0.0006	15
LIVER				
	8 hours	7.0	1.78	25
	2 days	2.4	0.50	21
	5 days	0.23	0.04	18
	10 days	0.06	0.004	8
KIDNEY				
	8 hours	9.3	4.38	46
	2 days	2.8	1.34	48
	5 days	0.18	0.07	40
	10 days	0.03	0.003	10
FAT				
	8 hours	1.2	0.29	24
	2 days	0.38	0.09	23
	5 days	0.02	0.002	12
	10 days	0.003	0.0001	5

Each value is the mean for three pigs .   Data from FDA 224-81-005 & USDA
SEA-12-14-3001-064 (1984)

RESIDUES OF SULPHADIMIDINE IN MILK

Lactating dairy cattle were administered therapeutic doses of
sulphadimidine by either the intravenous or intramammary routes and the
residues in the milk determined by an HPLC method, see table 6, (Boisseau,
1988).

TABLE 6. Residues of sulphadimidine in bovine milk treated with either an
i.v. injection of sulphadimidine-Na (100 mg per kg) or after 3
administrations of 200 mg sulphadimidine and 40 mg Trimethoprim in each
quarter.

TREATMENT

WITHDRAWAL TIME (DAYS)	TIME OF MILKING	Intravenous RESIDUES mg/L MEAN	SD	WT	Intramammary RESIDUES mg/L MEAN	SD
				1st inj -1 AM		
				2nd inj -1 PM	9.97	6.54
				3rd inj 0 AM	3.04	1.29
0.4	PM	24.6	5.1	0 PM	13.9	3.01
1	AM	5.74	1.32	1 AM	0.46	0.53
	PM	2.26	0.73	1 PM	0.17	0.16
2	AM	0.55	0.31	2 AM	0.08	0.05
	PM	0.22	0.12	2 PM	0.02	0.01
3	AM	0.12	0.07	3 AM	<0.01	
	PM	0.06	0.04	3 PM	<0.01	
4	AM	0.04	0.02	4 AM	ND	
	PM	0.03	0.02			
5	AM	0.03	0.02			
	PM	0.02	0.01	-	-	
6	AM	<0.01	-	-	-	
	PM	ND	ND			

The mean values are taken for five cows. ND is not detectable (<0.01 ppm)
Residues measured by HPLC method. Data provided by Boisseau, 1988.

The concentrations of sulphadimidine in whole eggs after oral
administration for 5 days at the dose of either 1 g or 2 g
sulphadimidine-Na per L in the drinking water of laying hens are shown in
figure 3.   After withdrawal of the drug for a period of 10 days the
concentrations of sulphadimidine were much less than 0.1 mg per kg.

Figure 3   RESIDUES OF SULPHADIMIDINE IN EGGS

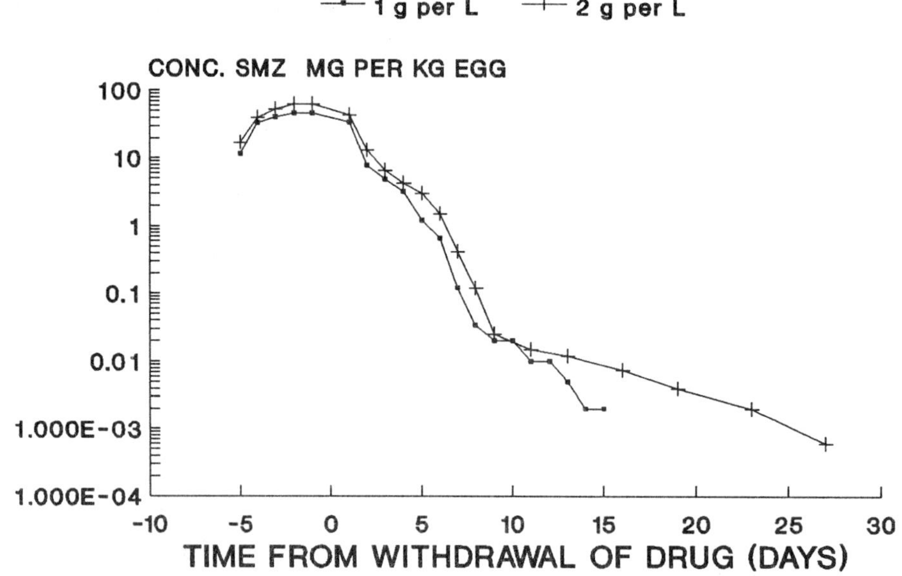

Each value is the mean (a) or maxima of 6 birds laying a total of 2 - 6
eggs per day.   Residues were measured by an HPLC method (Boisseau, 1988).

RESIDUES OF SULPHATHIAZOLE IN FARM ANIMALS AND TISSUES.

There is no definitive radiometric study and only one study where
sulphathiazole is administered orally in pig feed. Residues in tissues of
pigs (see table 7) fed 330 mg sulphathiazole per ton feed were highest in
liver (maximum 20 ppm) and kidney (maximum 74 ppm) 12 hours after
withdrawal of the drug. The concentrations declined very quickly and in
all tissues were <0.18 ppm 3 days after withdrawal and only detectable in
one muscle sample (0.01 ppm) after 10 days withdrawal time.   The residues
following large intravenous injections of sulphathiazole into both pigs
(Bourne et al.; 1978) and sheep (Bevill et al.; 1977b) produced very high
residues for the first few hours after administration but then the drug was
rapidly excreted and the residues were ca. 0-0.3 ppm 24 hours after dosing.

TABLE 7. RESIDUES OF SULPHATHIAZOLE IN PIG TISSUES AND URINE AFTER A THREE
DAILY ORAL DOSES OF SODIUM-SULPHATHIAZOLE AT 330 MG PER KG LIVE WEIGHT.

Withdrawal (days)	N	RESIDUES (mg per kg or L)				
		Muscle	liver	kidney	fat	urine
0.5	2	2.8	17	60	3.0	1405a
3	2	0.06	0.06	0.04	0.1	87.3a
5	3	0.03	0.01	0.06a	0.06	33.2a
7	3	0.11	0.02	0.04	0.13	-
10	3	0.00	0.00	0.00	0.00	6.0
12	3	0.00	0.00	0.00	0.00	-

N is number of pigs and values are the means except those marked "a" which
are results for only one pig. The values in parentheses are the maximum
values. Residues determined by method of Annino, (1961). (Righter et al.,
(1971).

REFERENCES.

Annino J. S., (1961), Sulphonamides, in Standard Methods of Clinical Chemistry, Ed by Sligson D.E., New York, Acad. Press, vol. 3, pp 200-206.

Ashworth, R.B., Epstein, R.L., Thomas, M.H., and Frobish, L.T. (1986), Sulfamethazine blood/tissue correlation study in swine.   Am. J. Vet. Res., 47, 2596-2603.

Bevill R.F., Koritz, G.D., Dittert, L.W. and Bourne, D.W.A. (1977b) J.Pharm. Sci. 66, 1297-1300

Boisseau, J. (1988) Data provided from studies at CNEVA, Fougeres, France.

Bourne, D.W.A., Dittert, L.W., Koritz, G.D. and Bevill, R.F. (1978), J. Pharmacokinetics Biopharm. 6, 123-134

FDA & USDA (1984), The Fate of Carbon-14 given to Swine as 14C-Sulfamethazine. USDA, SEA-12-14-3001-064, FDA-224-81-005

Righter, H.F., Worthington, J.M. and Mercer, H.D., (1971), Tissue residue depletion of sulfathiazole in swine.   J. Anim. Sci. 33, 797-798.

Samuelson, G., Whipple, D.M., Showalter, D.H., Jacobson, W.C. and Heath, G.E. (1979), Elimination of sulfamethazine residues in swine.   J.Am. Vet. Med.Ass, 175, 449-452.

7.2.2.2. RESIDUES OF ß-LACTAM ANTIBIOTICS, BENZYLPENICILLIN AND PENICILLIN V.

SUMMARY

Benzylpenicillin is one of the oldest and most widely used antibiotics. It is used to treat bacterial infections in all farm animals and is administered either orally or parentally. The drug is much used in the treatment of bovine mastitis and this use is a major concern for residues in milk.

RESIDUES IN MILK.

The persistence of residues in milk depends on the formulation and administration of the drug, but in the examples cited does not persist beyond five days after the end of treatment.   In many countries there are more than 50 separate preparations containing a penicillin for the treatment of bovine mastitis and each formulation produces a different residue pattern in milk. Since all preparations cannot be covered some studies recently done in France are cited (Moretain & Boisseau 1984, 1989) as illustrations of the residues in milk.

The residues of benzylpenicillin in milk following the administration of i.m. and intramammary injections of benzylpenicillin and/or procaine benzylpenicillin are shown in table 8. Above all they show that the persistence of the residues depends on the formulation of the commercial product.

Table 8. Residues (μg equiv to sodium benzylpenicillin/L) in milk

Milking Number	[.. INTRAMUSCULAR .....]				[.... INTRAMAMMARY ....]		
	A	B	C	D	E	F	G
-2	126	90	72	126	29100	174600	34800
-1	21	22	41	40	1590	109380	420
1	114	120	90	120	51650	173400	20520
2	23	34	38	29	3096	5556	184
3	7	16	20	11	329	331	15
4	2	5	8	13	48	26	1
5	nd	4	2	2	7	4	<1
6	nd	2	2	1	1	1	<1
7	nd	1	<1	<1	<1	<1	nd
8	nd	<1	nd	<1	<1	nd	nd
9	nd	nd	nd	nd	<1	nd	nd
10	nd	nd	nd	nd	nd	nd	nd

Each value is the mean of five animals.

Treatments;   Procaine benzylpenicillin (PBP),   benzylpenicillin (BP)
A is 40%BP, 60% PBP in aqueous solution.
B is PBP and dihydrostreptomycin in aqueous solution with
polyvinylpyrrolidone.
C is B plus lecithin.
D is B plus carboxymethylcellulose.
E is PBP plus neomycin sulphate in fatty alcohols and petrolatum.
F is PBP plus dihydrostreptomycin, polysorbate-80 and colloidal silica in
propylene glycolesters of saturated fatty acids.
G is PBP and glycerolmonostearate in peanut oil.

Penicillin dosage:
A, two injections i.m. of 16.8 mg/kg B.W. 24 hours apart.
B,C,D; two injections i.m. of 20 mg/kg B.W. 24 hours apart.
E; two administrations of 450 mg/quarter 24 hours apart
F; three administrations of 1 g/quarter after three consecutive milkings.
G; two administrations of 100 mg/quarter 24 hours apart.

Data from Moretain & Boisseau, 1984, 1989.

RESIDUES IN MEAT.

SUMMARY. Definitive studies of residues of benzylpenicillin in meat are
hard to find but there is evidence that benzylpenicillin therapy in meat
producing animals leaves residues in meat even though there is a rapid
absorbtion of the drug and fast clearance from the blood. Residues persist
in meat for at least 24 hours following parental administration. Because
procaine penicillin is absorbed more slowly the residues may persist
longer.

CATTLE

Guillot (1983) injected intramuscularly a cow weighing 450 kg with 250 μCi
14C-labelled benzylpenicillin at a dose of 6.7 mg/kg B.W. The cow was
sacrificed two hours after the injection and the radioactivity as
benzylpenicillin equivalents was measured by combustion analysis in a
number of tissues and fluids. The results are shown in table 9. Moats
(1984) injected intramuscularly a cow weighing 600 kg with benzylpenicillin
at a dose of 6 mg/kg B.W. The cow was slaughtered two hours after the
injection and the concentrations of benzylpenicillin in tissues and fluids
measured by both bioassay and HPLC. There is a lack of agreement most
probably the result of better more efficient extraction of benzylpenicillin
from cells using organic solvents. Moats found that about 90% of
benzylpenicillin was recovered from tissues during the HPLC assay.

Table 9. Residues in mg/kg of benzylpenicillin in bovine tissues and
fluids 2 hours after i.m. administration.

	[Guillot]	[...... Moats ....]	
Tissue	14C-activity	Bioassay	HPLC
Plasma or serum	2.7	0.79	0.95
Bile	117	nm	nm
Liver	14	0.58	22
Kidney	30a, 46b	0.55	6.1
Adrenals	2.4	nm	nm (4)
Muscle	0.37-0.76 (5)	0.03-0.05 (4)	0.06-0.18
Spleen	0.7	nm	nm
Tongue	0.8	nm	nm

nm is not measured; a is cortex; b is medulla. The numbers in brackets
are the number of different types of muscles examined.

McCracken et al. (1976) injected calves with 10 mg/kg B.W. benzylpenicillin
and slaughtered the animals 24 hours later. Residues of benzylpenicillin
were measured by bioassay and were >40 μg/kg in muscle and kidney and >40
μg/l in urine.

McCracken & O'Brien (1976) injected six calves twice i.m. with 3 mg/kg B.W.
benzylpenicillin 24 hours apart and sacrificed the animals 24 hours after
the last injection. The residues were declared positive when they
exceeded 40 μg/kg, the lower limit of detection of the bioassay. All
calves were positive in the following tissues; injection site (gluteus
muscle), the gluteus muscle opposite to the injection site, pectoral
muscle, diaphragm muscle, longissimus dorsi muscle, Masseter muscle,
kidney, liver, heart, serum. Positive results were also observed for urine
5/5, psoas muscle 5/6 and oblique muscle 3/6.

PIGS.

Penicillin V is a semi-synthetic penicillin. The residues pattern
illustrates the type of situation which may arise when penicillins are used
as in-feed additives. Forty pigs aged six weeks were fed feed for six
weeks containing 2 kg penicillin V per tonne feed. This dose is equivalent
to about 10 mg/kg B.W. The pigs were then fed drug free diet. Pigs were
sacrificed in groups of six at 0, 1, 5, 7 and 84 days after drug
withdrawal. The tissue residues were measured by a bioassay method with a
lower limit of detection of 50ug/kg.

No residues were detected at any sampling point for muscle, liver,skin and
fat. In the kidneys residues were detected in 3/6 pigs in the group
sacrificed at day 0 of drug withdrawal. The values of the positives was
54, 60 and 62 µg/kg which are only just above the limit of the assay. No
residues were found in kidneys sampled at later time points (FAO
Monograph, 36th JECFA 1990).

REFERENCES.

Guillot, Ph. (1983) "Etude Pharmacocinetique de la Penicillin G chez le
Bovin", University of Rennes.

McCracken, A., O'Brien, J.J. & Campbell, N. (1976) Antibiotic residues and
their recovery from animal tissues. J.Appl. Bact.<u>41</u>, 129-135.

McCracken, A. & O'Brien, J.J. (1976) Detection of antibiotic residues in
calf tissues. Res. Vet Sci., <u>21</u>, 240-241.

Moats, W.A. (1984) Determination of penicillin G and cloxacillin residues
in beef and pork tissue by high performance liquid chromatography.
J.Chrom. <u>317</u>, 311-318.

Moretain, J.P. & Boisseau, J. (1984) Excretion of penicillins in bovine
milk following intramuscular administration. Food Add. Contam. <u>1</u>, 349-358.

Moretain, J.P. & Boisseau, J. (1989) Excretion of penicillins and
cephalexin in bovine milk following intramammary administration. Food Add.
Contam. <u>6</u>, 79-90.

7.2.2.4. RESIDUES OF CHLORAMPHENICOL

RESIDUES IN EGGS.

Eggs from laying hens treated orally at a dose of 50 mg per kg BW every 12
hours for 3 days with a 10% solution of CAP contained residues of CAP of
8000 µg per kg at day 5 withdrawal period, 15 µg per kg at day 10 and 3 µg
per kg at day 15 in egg whites. Concentrations in the egg yokes were 1500
µg per kg at day 1, 8 µg per kg at day 5 and <1 µg per kg at day 7
(Boisseau, 1987).

RESIDUES IN CALVES

Calves were injected intravenously (i.v.) or intramuscularly (i.m.) with
CAP and residues determined in meat and at the injection site. A summary
of the results is shown in table 10.

Table 10. RESIDUES OF CAP (MG per KG) IN CALVES.

TREATMENT	WITHDRAWAL TIME (HOURS)	INJECTION SITE	MUSCLE SHOULDER	MUSCLE GLUTEAL
33 mg/kg BW	2	915	5.2	2.2
i.m.	6	663	6.1	7.3
	24	288	2.1	2.5
	48	11.6	0.5	0.5
	72	10.6	0.9	0.8 ?
66 mg/kg BW	2	2820	6.6	7.9
i.m.	4	1123	10.9	7.1
	24	389	7.3	8.2
	48	265	0.2	0.6
	72	12.8	0.7	0.6
66 mg/kg BW	2	75.9	68.2	74.4
i.v.	4	33.6	33.6	32.6
	24	0.3	0.2	0.4
	48	0.1	0.4	0.1

The values for the i.m. injections are the mean values for two animals,
the values for the i.v. data are for single animals (Epstein et al, 1986).

RESIDUES IN MILK

During the preparation of Reference materials (RMs see section 8)
containing CAP in milk samples it was necessary to follow the depletion of
CAP in the milk of two cows treated with two injections (15 hours apart) of
CAP at a dose of 20 mg per kg body weight (Preiß et al, 1993). The
depletion curves are shown in figure 4.

Figure 4. Depletion of CAP in cows.

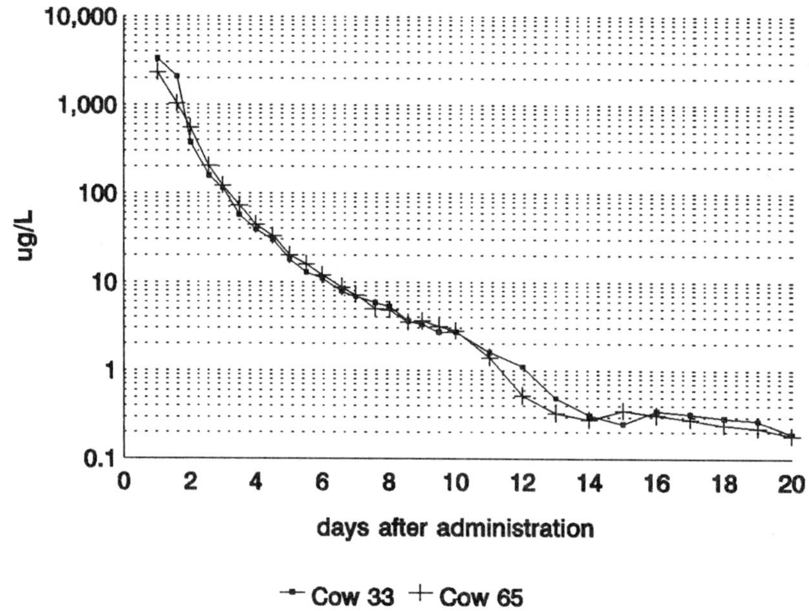

REFERENCES CAP

Boisseau, J (1987) Data from CNEVA submitted to FAO and published in FAO
Food and Nutrition Paper, No. 41. (1988) p. 3.

Epstein, r.l., Ashworth, R.B. and Simpson, R.M. (1986). Chloramphenicol
concentrations in calves. Am. J. Vet. Res. 47, 2075-2077.

Preiß, A., Balizs, G., Benesch-Girke, L. and Feier, U. (1993), Report of
BCR contract 5342/1/5/364/90/4-BCR-D(10). Chloramphenicol in milk. BGA,
Berlin.

7.2.3.   ANTHELMINTHICS AND PARASITICIDES

7.2.3.1.   BENZIMIDAZOLES

The benzimidazoles are characterised by a broad spectrum of anthelminthic
activity and low mammalian toxicity. They are not normally allowed for use
in lactating or pregnant animals. Among the benzimidazoles most widely
used in farm animals are albendazole, fenbendazole, oxfendazole and
thiabendazole. Also used is febantel, a pro-benzimidazole which readily
breaks down in the gut of the animal to form fenbendazole, oxfendazole and
their metabolites. The benzimidazoles are readily metabolised by oxidation
of the sulphur bridge to form the sulphone and sulphoxide derivatives and
these metabolites are normally major fractions of the residues.

7.2.3.1.1. ALBENDAZOLE

JECFA assessed Albendazole at their 34th meeting, 1989, and reported their
findings on the residues in FAO Food and Nutrition Paper 41/2 (1990).

The residue data clearly indicate that high (up to 30 mg per kg)
concentrations of total residues are present during the first few days
after administration of drug. These residues are readily extractable and
could be considered bioavailable. The total residues are highest in the
liver and kidney and fall gradually in cattle to about 1 mg per kg after 20
days withdrawal time. However by about day 10 most of the residues are not
extractable with ethyl acetate suggesting a large percentage of bound
residues of which less than 10% are bioavailable. The total residues in the
main edible tissues, muscle and fat are high on day 1 but fall very rapidly
to levels <0.1 mg per kg by day 4.

The parent drug, albendazole, is only found as a residue in edible tissues
during the first few days after drug administration and should not be
detected in farm animals treated according to the recommended withdrawal
periods observed for albendazole by most countries. Of the three main
metabolites, albendazole sulphone, albendazole sulphoxide and 2-amino-
albendazole sulphone, the metabolite 2-amino-albendazole sulphone can be
considered a good "Marker Residue" in liver tissue since it represents
about 18% of the total residues at withdrawal times extending beyond 4
days.

The levels of the marker residue, 2-amino-albendazole sulphone, under four
different conditions of use at a normal dosage are shown in table 11.

Table 11. Concentrations of 2-amino-albendazole sulphone in liver of
cattle treated with different formulations of albendazole at a single dose
of 10 mg per kg body weight.

Withdrawal Time (days)	Bolus	Suspension	Premix	Paste
	----------------(ug/kg)----------------			
12	364	nm	307	nm
16	227	nm	273	nm
20	146	131	201	148
24	146	113	137	100
28	115	78	101	81
32	79	52	86	64

Data from FAO Food and Nutrition Paper 41/2 (1990), pp 8.

7.2.3.1.2. FENBENDAZOLE, OXFENDAZOLE AND FEBANTEL.

Fenbendazole, oxfendazole and Febantel are considered together because they
have interconnected metabolism. Febantel is a pro-benzimidazole which
readily breaks down in the gut of the animal to form fenbendazole,
oxfendazole and their metabolites. The metabolites are formed by the
oxidation of the sulphur to the sulphone or sulphoxide and the loss of the
acetyl group to yield the amine. The main pathways are;-

    Febantel ---> Fenbendazole ---> Oxfendazole ---> Oxfendazole sulphone
                                (fenbendazole sulphone)

The MRLs set by the CVMP and the JECFA are the same for all three compounds
and expressed as the sum of the residues of fenbendazole, oxfendazole and
oxfendazole sulphone. They are 1000 mg per kg for liver and 10 mg per kg
for muscle, kidney, fat and milk. Using the recommended doses and
withdrawal times for all three drugs the MRLs should not be exceeded in
practice. It is noteworthy that the MRLs set by the CVMP are lower than
those suggested by JECFA (see section 2.2).

7.2.3.1.3. FLUBENDAZOLE.

Flubendazole is an anthelmintic for use in pigs and poultry. In both
species the major metabolite is (2-amino-1H-benzimidazol-5-yl)-4-
fluorophenyl-methanone. The highest concentrations of residues were found
in the liver and egg yolks. The residues persisted for at least 30 days in
pigs and for about two weeks in poultry (40th JECFA). The MRLs for
Flubendazole are given in table 1, section 2.

7.2.3.1.4. THIABENDAZOLE,

Thiabendazole is rapidly metabolised and excreted in all animal studies.
The major metabolite is 5-hydroxythiabendazole, usually found as its
glucuronide or sulphate ester. After oral dosing at the recommended rates
it was not possible to find residues in edible tissues of cattle, sheep and
pigs at withholding times of 3 and 7 days respectively (40th JECFA, 1992).

JECFA recommended MRLs for thiabendazole of 0.1 mg per kg for all edible
tissues of cattle, pigs and sheep and milk of cattle and goats. The marker
residue id the sum of the parent compound and 5-hydroxythiabendazole.

7.2.3.1.5. TRICLABENDAZOLE.

The absorption, metabolism, distribution and excretion of Triclabendazole
is qualitatively similar in cattle and sheep. A large proportion of the
residues in edible tissues are in the bound form. The 40th JECFA selected
the marker residue as 5-chloro-6-(2',3'-dichlorophenoxy)-benzimidazole-2-
one. This compound is formed when common fragments of Triclabendazole-
related residues are hydrolysed under alkaline conditions at 90-100^{0}C. The
MRL for this marker residue are given in table 1, Section 2.

7.2.3.2. IVERMECTIN

Ivermectin is a broad-spectrum antiparasitic drug against nematodes and
arthropods in food producing animals. It is a mixture of two homologous
compounds, H_2B1_a and H_2B1_b, derived from abermectin and differing by a

methylene group at C-26. Ivermectin was evaluated by the 36th and 40th
JECFA meeting and their report showed that there was full information on
the residues in all the species (cattle [not lactating], sheep and pigs)
for which use was recommended.

The drug is almost exclusively excreted in the faeces, with <1% eliminated
via the urine. The metabolism was similar in the ruminants but slightly
different from that in the pig. Very little residues are in the bound
form. The highest concentrations of residues are found in the liver and
fat and these tissues are the most suitable for residue control. The
parent drug accounts for a major proportion of the total residues and H_2B1_a
is a suitable marker residue. There are good HPLC methods for monitoring
the residues.

The depletion of the total residues of Ivermectin in liver and fat of
cattle, sheep and pigs is plotted in figure 5. The residues are below the
MRLs (see section 2) at 28 days withdrawal time.

Figure 5. Total Residues of Ivermectin in Liver and Fat.

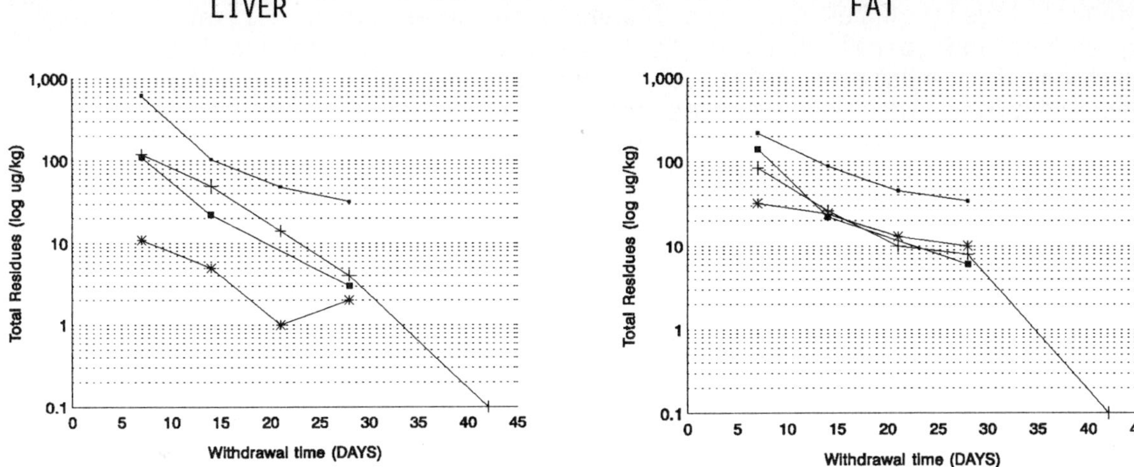

Intraruminal dose, 0.3 mg per kg BW; Cow -+-, Sheep -*-
Subcutaneous dose, 0.3 mg per kg BW; Cow -■-, 0.4 mg per kg BW; Pig -▮-

Graph drawn using data from 36th JECFA (WHO Technical Report Series, 799)
"Evaluation of certain veterinary drug residues in food." 1990.

7.2.3.3. CLOSANTEL

Closantel is an anthelminthic drug used in cattle and sheep. The residues
were evaluated at the 36th and 40th JECFA meetings. The residue depletion
patterns are similar in cattle and sheep with half-lives in tissues of 2-3
weeks. The residues are parent drug with the remaining residues being 3-
and 5- monoiodoclosantel. The highest concentrations of residues are found
in the kidney and fat with slightly lower levels in the muscle and liver.
The residues persist in most tissues for at least 42 days. JECFA
recommended MRLs (see section 2) which should be met if the recommended
treatments are used with withdrawal times of at least 28 days.

7.2.4. ß-AGONISTS

ß$_2$-agonist have a high affinity for the ß$_2$-adrenergic receptors such as occur in lung tissue and possess a lower affinity for the ß^1-receptors of other tissues. They are substituted phenylethanolamines that share some structural and pharmacological similarities with the catecholamines. When these compounds are included in the diet of growing animals, they promote lean tissue accretion and cause a marked reduction of fat deposition. In meat the percentage of protein is increased and that of fat reduced.

The list of ß-agonists which may be giving rise to residues in animals and animal feeds is increasing and the following substances have caused residue problems in many Member States;-
Clenbuterol, salbutamol, cimaterol, mabuterol, terbutaline, tulobuterol, carbuterol, mapenterol, clenpenterol, clenhexerol and cimbuterol. The last four were detected for the first time during 1991.

7.2.4.1. CLENBUTEROL.

Clenbuterol is possibly the most widely used ß-agonist in farm animals. The highest levels of residues are found in the eyes, lungs, liver, kidney, brain, thymus and spinal chord, with lower levels in muscle and fat. The disposition of clenbuterol relative to the concentrations in plasma for tissues and fluids of twelve calves treated orally with clenbuterol is shown in table 12. The dose and duration of the treatment and the time of slaughter during/after drug administration are not stated by Girault and Fourtillan, (1990).

Table12.

Tissue	clenbuterol	Tissue/Fluid	clenbuterol
Liver	5.2	Lung	7.8
Kidney	5.0	Thymus	2.2
Muscle	0.7 - 0.8	Spinal chord	1.8
Heart	1.8	Brain	2.7
Suet	0.3	Plasma	1
		Urine	9.5

Meyer (1991) states that the anabolic dosages of clenbuterol are 5 to 10-fold higher than the therapeutic doses for calves and these high doses will lead to accumulation of residues into most tissues. Calves were administered in the feed 10 µg clenbuterol per kg body weight daily for 21 days. The calves were slaughtered and the residues of clenbuterol measured in tissue samples as shown in table 13. An important observation is the high and persistent concentration of residues in the eyes. It is possible that this organ may be useful for screening farm animals for residues of ß-agonists.

Table 13.   Clenbuterol residues in calves (mean values in µg per kg) after feeding 10 µg clenbuterol per kg body weight daily for 21 days.

Tissue	Withdrawal time (days)		
	0	3.5	14
	(3)	(2)	(2)
Lungs	76	2.4	<0.08
Liver	39	1.6	0.6
Kidney	29	1.2	<0.08
Spleen	24	1.2	<0.08
Brain	12	0.4	<0.08
Masseter muscle	8.6	0.3	<0.08
Trapezius muscle	4.8	0.2	<0.08
Fat	4.4	0.3	0.2
Eye	118	58	15
Ovary	13	0.4	<0.08
Uterus	8.2	0.4	<0.08
Blood	1.1	0.05	<0.04
Urine	47	0.5	<0.05

The number of calves is shown in parenthesis.

Schilt et al (1991) measured the residues of clenbuterol in five week-old broilers fed at a rate of 1 mg drug per kg body weight for five days. Five broilers were slaughtered directly after the last feed containing drug and five more were killed 1 day later. Residues in the tissues were measured by IAC\SPE\ EIA and checked with HPLC. The results are shown in table 14.

Table 14.   Residues of clenbuterol (µg per kg) in broilers.

Time after withdrawing clenbuterol (days)	Meat	Liver	Kidney	Caecal contents	Gizzard
0	3	22	20	83	46
1	1	7	3	23	5

Clenbuterol is readily excreted into the urine.   Three cows were administered clenbuterol daily for 12 days as an additive to their morning feed. Urine, plasma and faeces were collected immediately after each feed and then 8 hours later during the period of administration and for 6 days after ceasing treatment. Each cow was administered a different daily dose, namely 2,5 or 10 µg clenbuterol per kg body weight. The results for the concentrations of clenbuterol in urine are shown in figure 6. In general the levels are much higher at 8 hours after feeding than at the time of feeding. When the drug is withdrawn there is a near exponential decline in the concentrations in each of the cows reaching the values for untreated control animals after 5 days withdrawal time (Delahaut et al., 1991).

The levels in the plasma and faeces were also measured in the above study and followed a somewhat similar pattern to the urine, except there was a much clearer relationship between the levels and dose. The highest levels (1.5 - 4 ng per ml plasma and ca 3 - 9 ng per g faeces) were observed in the animal given the highest dose and the lowest levels (<1 ng per ml or g) in the lowest dosed cow. All the levels declined to control values within 5 days of withdrawing the drug. (Delahaut et al. 1991)

Figure 6

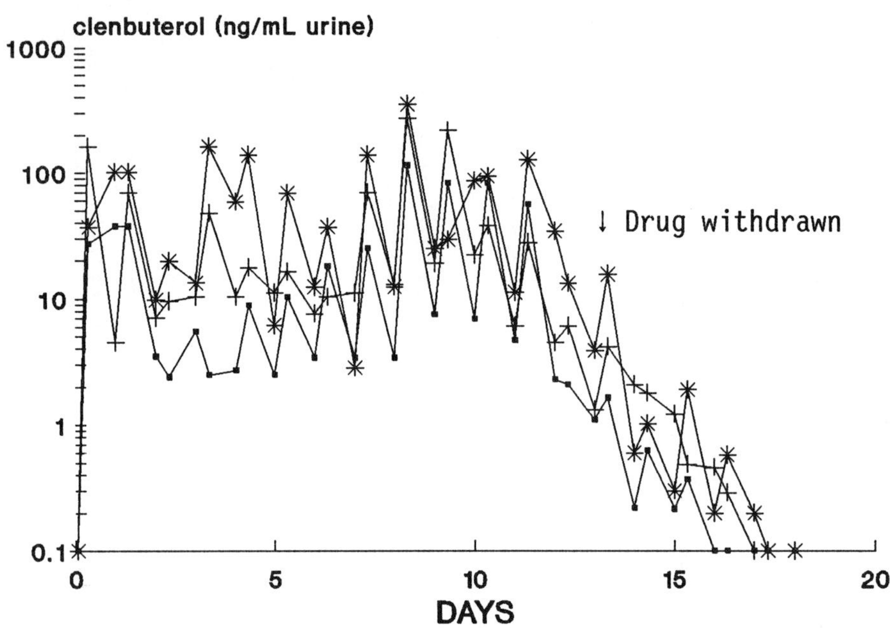

Legend; The clenbuterol was withdrawn on day 12, the treatments for each
cow were; in μg per kg body weight per day ; 2 (-■-); 5 (-+-); 10 (-*-).

7.2.4.2. SALBUTAMOL

Salbutamol enjoys a leading position in the sales of human medicines,
especially as a treatment for asthma. Residues of the drug have also been
found in farm animals. Only recently was it shown that salbutamol is
mostly in the conjugated form in the liver and therefore a hydrolysis step
is necessary to measure the residues.

Two calves were fed 32 mg of salbutamol hemisulphate twice daily for five
days and the concentration of salbutamol in the urine measured during after
the period of administration,see figure 7 (Van Ginkel et al., 1991).

Figure 7.

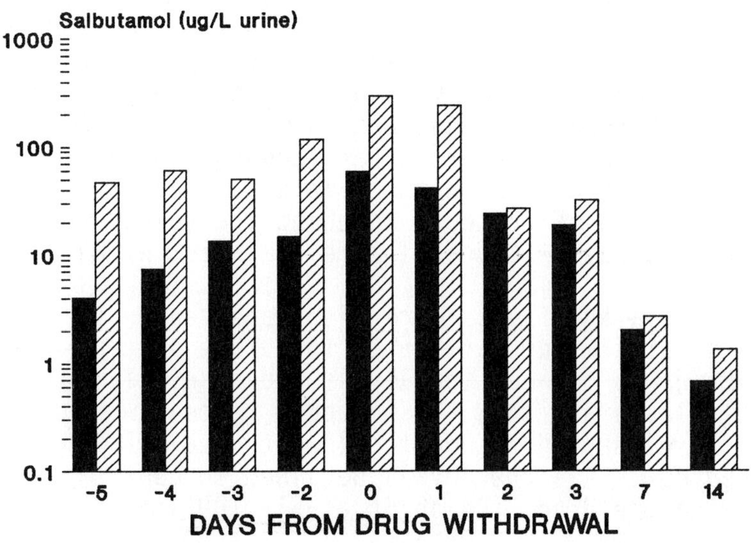

REFERENCES.

Delahaut, Ph., Dubois, M., Pri-Bar, I., Buchman. O., Degand, G. and Ectors. F. (1991), Development of a specific radioimmunoassay for the detection of clenbuterol residues in treated cattle.   Food Add. Contaminants. $\underline{8}$, 43-51

Ginkel, L.A.van, Stephany, R.W., Rossum, H.J. and Farla, J., (1991), Multiresidue test for ß-agonists in a variety of matrices. In Proceedings "New trends in veal calf production" (Eds: Metz, J.H.M. & Groenestein, C.M.) Wageningen, The Netherlands, ISBN 90-220-1016-3. pp 192-197.

Girault, J., and Fourtillan, J.B. (1990), Determination of clenbuterol in bovine plasma and tissues by gas chromatography-negative-ion chemical ionization mass-spectrometry. J. Chromatogr. $\underline{518}$, 41-52

Meyer, H.H.D., (1991), The illegal practice and resulting risks versus the controlled use of licensed drugs: views on the present situation in Germany. Annales de recherches veterinaires,$\underline{22}$, 299-304

Schilt, R., Hasnoot, W., Hamers, A.R.M. and van Bruchem, G.D. (1991), Screening methods for the determination of Beta(2)-agonists in urine and tissue samples. Proc 5th Congress of the European Assoc. Vet. Pharmacol & Therapeutics. Acta Vet Scand. Suppl. 87, 466-467

GENERAL REFERENCES

Bogaerts, R. and Wolf, F., (1980) A standardized method for the detection of residues of anti-bacterial substances in fresh meat. Fleischwirtsc. $\underline{60}$, 672-673.

Heitzman, R.J., (1986), Analytical methods for residues of veterinary drugs. In "Drug residues in animals", Ed. A. Rico, Academic Press, pp. 205-219

8. REFERENCE MATERIALS (RMs) AND SOURCES OF STANDARDS/REAGENTS.

8.1. MEASUREMENTS AND TESTING PROGRAMME (MAT) [previously The Community Bureau of Refererence (BCR)].

The Measurements and Testing Programme of the BCR is a research programme of the Commission of the European Communities having the broad aim of improving accuracy and measurement harmony in areas of concern at Community level. An overview of the activities of BCR was presented by Wagstaffe and Belliardo (1990).

The role of RMs in analytical chemistry is well established especially for the calibration and verification of the accuracy of methods (Griepink, 1990) and also in the biomedical sciences (Colinet, 1992) and the assay of biological materials (Marchandise (1987). The major problem facing the producers of RMs results from the virtually unlimited variety of analyses obtained in combining analytes, concentrations and matrices. More than 4000 methods of analysis have been counted in the field of food and agriculture and the choice of RMs depends on priority needs.

The priorities for the production of RMs for residues were established at a BCR meeting in April, 1989, and the resulting programme is outlined in table 8.I. The RMs will be stored by the CRLs and made available for the NRLs and commercially available by the BCR.

The production of RMs with the BCR programme expanded greatly and more than twenty are under preparation. In deciding the target values for the residues in the incurred lyophilised samples, the MAT/BCR takes into account the legislation from DGVI, the Maximum Residue Limits (MRL) set by DGIII (see section 2) and the quality of the analytical methods. Thus for those substances which are not allowed, RMs are prepared which are suitable for positive identification by the routine methods. For allowed drugs at least one of the RMs for a particular drug will have a target value close to the MRL.

The purpose of the RMs is to provide a unique collection of RMs for a particular veterinary drug analyte. They are expensive to produce and are limited in numbers (usually 200 - 500). Because they are Certified RMs (CRM) they should be by virtue of their <u>traceability the reference standard for measurements in the Community</u> and used only for specific problems and with careful consideration of the materials available.

Their use is recommended for;
1. Allocation to and use by the CRLs and NRLs to perform quality control measurements and to validate new methodology.

2. Controlling and validating the content and/or concentration of the same analyte in a comparable matrix in-house or so-called secondary materials. These secondary materials should be used on a regular basis as the internal quality control for the methods used to determine residues in tissues and fluids.
    They should also be used by the CRLs to fulfil their responsibilities under EC Decision 89/187 which includes the quality control of the NRLs through ring testing (proficiency testing schemes) of methods. These secondary materials can easily be prepared on the basis of the knowledge provided through the certified reference materials (CRMs) if the comparibility of the matrix characteristics are confirmed.

[Note; Essential information useful for the preparation of secondary
materials is given in the report which accompanies the CRMs (preparation of
materials, stability, homogeneity, storage, shipment and methodology for
characterization.]

8.2.   RMs FOR RESIDUE ANALYSIS.

8.2.1 REQUIREMENTS

1. Representative.
    -    incurred material, i.e. samples obtained from animals
         administered parent drug or contaminant. The sample will contain the
         total residues including all metabolites.
    -    prepared as lyophilised products which on reconstitution simulate as
         near as possible the samples obtained from animals.
    -    contain concentrations of residues applicable to control regulations
         and practice, i.e. levels close to the MRLs and the lower limits of
         detection (LLD) of the reference methods.
    -    available in appropriate matrices including muscle and urine.

2. Homogeneous.
    -    within the variability of the methods of analysis.
    -    within a single sample
    -    within a complete batch of RMs for a single analyte.

3. Stable.
    -    with respect to agreed time and temperature.
    -    ideal long term stability would be over 5 years at 4°C
    -    short term stability must include transport at ambient and
         other selected temperature.

4. Sterile.
    -    samples must be obtained from animals certified in good health and of
         known health history.
    -    samples may be made sterile by procedures which do not degrade the
         analyte or significantly alter the blank value (matrix effect).

8.3.   GENERAL SCHEME FOR PRODUCTION OF RMs

The RMs are produced in farm animals which are in good health and have a
known health history.

Scheme of production.
    -    Approved MAT/BCR project for selected residue/analyte
    -    Project proposals from EEC laboratories
    -    Appointed laboratory and investigators.
    -    Select animals and parent drug/contaminant
    -    Agreed target concentrations of residues
    -    Pilot study of stability of spiked analyte in animal samples
    -    Agreed dosage and route of administration
    -    Animal treatments including non-treated animals (blanks)
    -    Monitor residue levels in live animal
    -    Collect urine, faeces and blood from live animal
    -    Collect samples of fluids, faeces and tissues from slaughtered animal
    -    Determine concentration of analyte(s) in incurred and blank samples.
    -    Blend samples of incurred and blank material to achieve correct
         levels for RMs.

- Lyophilise small batch and measure concentration for content and to check for any losses due to lyophilisation.
- If levels are correct check independently by second laboratory.
- Sterilise and check stability
- Lyophilise main sample
- Fluids are dispensed into vials/ampoules and lyophilised and sealed under vacuum or an inert gas.
- Tissues are lyophilised as a large batch, the powder thoroughly mixed by tumbling and then dispensed to vials for sealing under an inert gas
- Sterilise
- Label
- Check homogeneity
- Check stability for one year at temperatures between -40°C and +37°C. and long term stability over 2 years at selected temperatures.
- Organise certification programme including ring testing of material in at least eight laboratories.
- Examine results and approve certification.
- CRMs and/or RMs available by information from BCR.

These procedures are described in a little more detail by Heitzman (1992), Heitzman et al. (1993), Marchandise and Colinet (1983), Maier et al. (1992) and in ISO/REMCO N263 (1992).

Table 8.I.   RMs AVAILABLE OR UNDER PRODUCTION in 1993

ANALYTE	MATRIX	SPECIES	WT[a] g	CONC ug/kg ug/L	SOURCE	START DATE	- STATUS
AMPICILLIN	Mk	cow	10	15-20	CNEVA	1993	On
BETA-AGONISTS							
SALBUTAMOL	U	calf	5	2-5	UNIV LIEGE	1991	On
CLENBUTEROL	U	calf	5	2-5	UNIV LIEGE	1991	On
CHLORAMPHENICOL	M	calf	25	10	BGA	1990	RC
	Eg	poultry	3	1	BGA	1990	RC
	Mk	cow	25	1	BGA	1990	RC
DIENOESTROL	U	steer	2	34 ± 7	RIVM	1990	C
	M	steer			RIVM	1989	RC
DIETHYLSTILBOESTROL	U	steer	2	12.8 ± 2.5	RIVM	1990	C
	M	steer			RIVM	1989	RC
NEOMYCIN	Mk	cow	10	3000	CNEVA	1993	On
HEXOESTROL	U	steer	2	13.3 ± 3.1	RIVM	1990	C
	M	steer			RIVM	1989	RC
19-NORTESTOSTERONE	U	calf	5	1-5	RIKILT	1990	RC
	M	calf	5	0.5-2	RIKILT	1990	On
OXYTETRACYCLINE	Mk	cow	10	300	CNEVA	1991	On
SULPHAMETHAZINE	M	pig	5	0.5 -1.0	VRL	1990	RC
	L	pig	5	0.75-1.5	VRL	1990	RC
	K	pig	5	0.75-1.5	VRL	1990	RC
TRENBOLONE	U	calf	5	1-5	RIVM	1989	On
ZERANOL	U	steer	5	5	NFC-DUBLIN	1991	On
	M	steer	10	2[b]	NFC-DUBLIN	1991	On
	L	steer	10	2	NFC-DUBLIN	1991	On

[a] = equivalent to weight of fresh sample. Cert = material certified.
[b] = spiked material
On = ongoing, RC = ready for certification, C = certified and available.

<u>ANALYTE</u>   <u>DIETHYLSTILBOESTROL (DES)</u>

<u>MATRIX</u>   Lyophilised bovine URINE

<u>Certification No</u>   EUR EN CRM 389

Summary: The animals used were certified in good health and had not
previously received veterinary drugs. The RM was prepared by lyophilising
a mixture of the urine from a steer injected intramuscularly with DES and
the urine from untreated steers. The latter was used to dilute the
incurred urine samples to the appropriate concentration of DES.   DES
occurs as a mixture of the <u>cis</u> and <u>trans</u> isomers. The total content of
both isomers and the content of the <u>trans</u> isomer were determined after
separation of the isomers by HPLC and determining the individual or summed
concentrations on GCMS. There was good agreement in the ring tests between
the values obtained for total DES by either the GCMS or RIA methods.

The vials contents are;
 - equivalent to 2 mL fresh urine
 - stored under nitrogen
 - stable at $\leq$ +20^{0}C

The results of the certification tests were:

        Mean concentration   12.8 μg total-DES per L fresh urine
        Mean concentration   7.7 μg trans-DES per L fresh urine
        Mean concentration   6.6 μg cis-DES per L fresh urine

        Standard Deviation   2.4 μg total-DES per L
        Standard Deviation   1.3 μg trans-DES per L
        Standard Deviation   1.1 μg cis-DES per L

        Number of Laboratories   7 (total-DES); 6 (trans-DES); 4 (cis-DES)

Date of certification by BCR; 1993

<u>Place of Manufacture</u>   AFRC; Inst. Animal Health, Compton, UK and RIVM,
Bilthoven, NL.

<u>Stored at;</u>   RIVM, Bilthoven, NL.

<u>Certified Blank Materials</u>
Lyophilised blank materials equivalent to 2 ml blank (control) urine were
prepared from untreated steers. The materials were prepared under the same
contract at the same institutes by the same personnel. The blank RMs are
stored at RIVM. The blanks are specific for the three stilbenes, DES,HEX
and DE.

ANALYTE   HEXOESTROL (HEX)

MATRIX   Lyophilised bovine URINE

Certification No   EUR EN CRM 391)

Summary: The animals used were certified in good health and had not
previously received veterinary drugs. The RM was prepared by lyophilising
a mixture of the urine from a steer injected intramuscularly with HEX and
the urine from untreated steers. The latter was used to dilute the
incurred urine samples to the appropriate concentration of HEX.   The
total content of HEX was determined after separation by HPLC and measuring
the concentration on GCMS. There was good agreement in the ring tests
between the values obtained for the content of HEX by either the GCMS or
RIA methods.

The vials contents are;
 - equivalent to 2 mL fresh urine
 - stored under nitrogen
 - stable at ≤ +20^{0}C

The results of the certification tests were:

      Mean concentration   13.3 µg HEX per L fresh urine

      Standard Deviation   3.0 µg per L

      Number of Laboratories   8

Date of certification by BCR; 1993

Place of Manufacture   AFRC; Inst. Animal Health, Compton, UK and RIVM,
Bilthoven, NL.

Stored at;   RIVM, Bilthoven, NL.

Certified Blank Materials
Lyophilised blank materials equivalent to 2 ml blank (control) urine were
prepared from untreated steers. The materials were prepared under the same
contract at the same institutes by the same personnel. The blank RMs are
stored at RIVM. The blanks are specific for the three stilbenes, DES,HEX
and DE.

<u>ANALYTE</u>   <u>DIENOESTROL (DE)</u>

<u>MATRIX</u>   Lyophilised bovine URINE

<u>Certification No</u>   EUR EN RM 390 (Indicative value)

Summary: The animals used were certified in good health and had not
previously received veterinary drugs. The RM was prepared by lyophilising
a mixture of the urine from a steer injected intramuscularly with DE and
the urine from untreated steers. The latter was used to dilute the
incurred urine samples to the appropriate concentration of DE.   The total
content of DE was determined after separation by HPLC and measuring the
concentration on GCMS. The ring tests showed poor comparison between the
GCMS method and the RIA methods.

The vials contents are;
 - equivalent to 2 mL fresh urine
 - stored under nitrogen
 - stable at ≤ +20^{0}C

The results of the certification tests were:

     Mean concentration   33.5 µg DE per L fresh urine

     Standard Deviation   6.1 µg per L

     Number of Laboratories   8

Date of certification by BCR; 1993 (Indicative value only)

<u>Place of Manufacture</u>   AFRC; Inst. Animal Health, Compton, UK and RIVM,
Bilthoven, NL.

<u>Stored at;</u>   RIVM, Bilthoven, NL.

<u>Certified Blank Materials</u>
Lyophilised blank materials equivalent to 2 ml blank (control) urine were
prepared from untreated steers. The materials were prepared under the same
contract at the same institutes by the same personnel. The blank RMs are
stored at RIVM. The blanks are specific for the three stilbenes, DES,HEX
and DE.

8/7

8.3 SOURCES OTHER THAN BCR

8.3.1 ANAREF COLLECTION IN THE BENELUX COUNTRIES.

The ANAREF project is a Benelux Public Health Reference Project involving
RIVM (Project 387914)and RIKILT, NL; IHE, Belgium; and Institute of Hygiene
and Public Health, Luxembourg.

The RMs prepared are listed in table 8.II.

Table 8.II.   RMs AVAILABLE OR UNDER PRODUCTION

ANALYTE	Code	MATRIX	SPECIES	WT[a] g	CONC µg/kg µg/L	No. Vials produced.	LAB
CHLORAMPHENICOL	88M0044	Ly-U	CATTLE	2	0	200	RIVM
	88M0045	Ly-U	CATTLE	2	5	200	RIVM
	87M1541	Ly-U	CATTLE	2	10	200	RIVM
	88M0046	Ly-U	CATTLE	2	20	200	RIVM
BLANKS		U	CATTLE	1	0		

20 sets of 4 x 25 different 1 ml samples - RIVM

TABLE 8.III.   PURE STANDARDS HELD AT RIVM

COMPOUND	RIVM Code No.	COMPOUND	RIVM Code No.
α-NT	87M0334	d3-NT	87M1252
Zearalenone	87M1036	α-Zearalenol	87M1037
Zearalenone	87M1038	Zeranol (Z)	87M1039
ß-Zearalenol	87M1040	Taleranol	87M1041
DES	88M1733	d6-DES	88M1734
d4-HEX	88M1768	DE	88M1736
d2-DE	88M1769		

The supply is limited and available only to approved laboratories against
payment. The standards are in 100 µg portions in amber glass ampoules,
sealed under nitrogen.
FTIR and GCMS (after derivatization) and data sheets are available.
(see reference Stephany, R.W., and Van Ginkel, L.A. (1989),

8.3.2
The two references below list a selection of reference materials and their
sources. There are some materials of animal origin although most of them
are residue free materials and very few contain residues of veterinary
drugs.

AOAC, (1990), Certified Reference Material. In AOAC, Official Methods of
Analysis. 1220-1221.

Roelandts, I., (1989), News on Reference Materials. Additional biological
reference materials. Spectrochimica, 44B, 985-988.

8.3.3 WHO INTERNATIONAL CHEMICAL REFERENCE SUBSTANCES.

This collection of reference drugs is held by the WHO Collaborating Centre
for Chemical Reference Substances at APOTEKSBOLAT AB, Centrallaboritoriet,
S-105 14, Stockholm, Sweden. They cost about $40 + $10 p&p per package.

The following drugs of veterinary interest are included in the list; for
those labelled with * Infrared spectra are available at a small charge.

	Substance	Size (mg)	Cat. №
	Ampicillin (anhydrous)	200	390001
	Ampicillin sodium	200	388002
*	Ampicillin trihydrate	200	274003
	Anhydrotetracycline hydrochloride	25	180096
	Bacitracin zinc	200	192174
*	Benzylpenicillin potassium	200	180099
	Benzylpenicillin sodium	200	280047
	Chloramphenicol	200	486004
	Chloramphenicol palmitate	1000	286072
	Chlortetracycline hydrochloride	200	187138
*	Cloxacillin sodium	200	274005
	Colecalciferol (Vitamin D_3)	500	190146
	Dapsone	100	183115
	Ethinyloestradiol	100	291016
*	Haloperidol	100	172063
	Methyltestosterone	100	167023
*	Metronidazole	100	183118
	Norethisterone	100	186132
	Norethisterone acetate	100	185123
	Oestradiol benzoate	100	167014
	Oestrone	100	279015
	Oxacillin sodium	200	382027
	Oxytetracycline dihydrate	200	189142
	Oxytetracycline hydrochloride	200	189141
	Prednisolone	100	389029
	Procaine hydrochloride	100	183119
	Progesterone	100	167033
	Propylthiouracil	100	185126
*	Sulphamethoxazole	100	179092
*	Sulphamethoxypyridazine	100	178079
	Sulphanilamide	100	179094
	Testosterone propionate	100	167036
	Tetracycline hydrochloride	200	180095
	Tolbutamide	100	179086
*	Trimethoprim	100	179093

8.4 COMMERCIAL SOURCES OF IMMUNOASSAY MATERIALS FOR VETERINARY DRUG
ANALYSES.

8.4.1 <u>EURO-DIAGNOSTICA B.V.</u> Wilmersdorf 24, P.O.Box 2820, 7303 GC
Apeldoom, The Netherlands.

The company market the following EIA kits;-
Beta-agonist kit for screening clenbuterol, salbutamol, mabuterol and
mapenterol directly in urine samples.
Chloramphenicol in urine (LOD 50 μg per L) and meat (LOD 10 μg per kg).

19-Nortestosterone in urine. The test also detects epi-19-nortestosterone
and 19-norandrostenedione.

8.4.2 <u>GENEGO</u>, 34170 Gorizia, Italy - This company market three multi-
analyte columns claiming a capacity of at least 20 ng or 100 ng (high
capacity column) per analyte. The products are -

    Multi-Prep I for DES, HEX, DE, Z, Taleranol ß-E$_2$, NT, T, MT, and TB
    Multi-Prep II for DES, HEX, DE, Z, NT, MT,T, TB and Taleranol
    Multi-Prep III for Clenbuterol, salbutamol, terbutaline, carbuterol
    and marbuterol all ß-agonists.

These columns are marketed as a complete kit, comprising the enzyme and the
buffer for the digestion of samples, extraction and washing buffers and
detailed instructions.

The company markets the following immunoassay kits for veterinary drug
residues;-
RIA   Stilbenes, Zeranol, Trenbolone.
ELISA   Zeranol, DES, 19-Nortestosterone, Progesterone,
           Chloramphenicol, Sulphadimidine, Penicillin-G.

      ß-agonists in serum, urine, liver, feeds, milk powders and
      milk. The kit is intended for the ß-agonists, with the lower
      limit of detection (LLD) in μg per L in parenthesis;
      clenbuterol (0.6), mabuterol (0.6), salbutamol (2), mapenterol
      (2) and terbutaline (3).

8.4.3 <u>LABORATORY OF HORMONOLOGY - MARLOIE</u>, Rue du Point de Jour, 8, B-
6900, Marloie, Belgium.

Antibodies are available against;
    testosterone*, oestradiol*, oestrone, androstenedione,
    dehydroepiandrosterone, cortisol, desoxycorticosterone, 17α-
    hydroxyprogesterone and progesterone, trenbolone*, zeranol,
    diethylstilboestrol, 19-nortestosterone*, methyltestosterone,
    ethinyloestradiol*, medroxyprogesterone acetate, dexamethasone

* either the 17α- or the 17ß- hydroxy compounds.

    ß-agonists (salbutamol, clenbuterol, mabuterol and others)

Gels for immunoaffinity chromatography are available (minimum quantity 1
mL) prepared from high affinity antisera and with a minimum capacity of 50
ng per mL for;

8/10

Anabolics; Nortestosterone, methyltestosterone, trenbolone,
        ethinyloestradiol, diethylstilboestrol
ß_2-agonists; Clenbuterol, Salbutamol (single or combined)
Antibiotics; Chloramphenicol, sulphadimidine
Enzyme conjugates; Salbutamol-horse radish peroxidase.

8.4.4 <u>RANDOX LABORATORIES LTD</u>, Ardmore, Diamond Road, Crumlin, Co. Antrim,
BT29 4QY, UK

Antisera are available against the following antigens;-
        Avoparcin-HSA, Chloramphenicol-HSA, Chloramphenicol-hemi-BTG,
        Cimaterol-BTG, Clenbuterol-HSA, DES-gluc-BTG, Dexamethazone-hemi-BTG,
        Flavomycin-BTG, Flavomycin-HSA, Hexoestrol-CPE-BTG, Hexoestrol-CPE-
        HSA, Hexoestrol-gluc-KLH, 19-Nortestosterone-3CMO-HSA, 19-
        Nortestosterone-17-hemi-HSA, Oestradiol-17α-hemi-HSA, Oestradiol-
        17α/ß-hemi-HSA, Progesterone-CMO-BSA, Progesterone-hemi-HSA, Mixed
        sulpha-HSA, Sulphadoxine-HSA, Sulphadiazine-HSA, Sulphadimidine-
        diazo-HSA, Sulphadimidine-HSA, Testosterone-3CMO-BSA, Testosterone-
        3CMO-HSA, Testosterone-17-hemi-HSA, Trenbolone-3CMO-HSA, Trenbolone-
        hemi-BTG, Tylosin-HBA-HSA, Tylosin-HSA, Zeranol-6CMO-HSA, Zeranol-
        16CPE-HSA, Zeranol-hemi-HSA.

The company markets the following ELISA kits;-
        Clenbuterol, 19-Nortestosterone, Testosterone, Trenbolone,
        Sulpha drugs.

Immunoaffinity columns for sale are;-
        Clenbuterol, Chloramphenicol,Dexamethazone,
        As Multi-columns;-
        Trenbolone and 19-Nortestosterone,
        Trenbolone, 19-Nortestosterone,testosterone and oestradiol.

8.4.5 <u>R-BIOPHARM GmbH</u>, Rößlerstraße 94, 6100 Darmstadt, Germany.
        UK agent, Digen Ltd, 28, Crown Road, Wheatley, Oxford, OX33 1UL.

The company markets ELISA kits (Ridascreen®-ELISA) for the following
veterinary drug residues;-
        Clenbuterol (ß-agonists), Acetylgestagenes, 17ß-oestradiol,
        Testosterone, 19-Nortestosterone, Ethinyloestradiol, Trenbolone,
        Diethylstilboestrol, Zeranol.
        Chloramphenicol, Sulphadimidine, Streptomycin, Tetracycline.

8.4.6 <u>RIEDEL-DE-HAEN</u> Aktiengeellschaft, Wunstorferstraße-40, D-3016
Seelze, Germany.

The company markets ELISA kits (Ridascreen®-ELISA) for the following
veterinary drug residues;-
        ß-agonists in serum and urine. The company claims that 40 samples
        can be screened in 2 hours. The kit is intended for the ß-agonists,
        with the lower limit of detection (LLD) in µg per L in parenthesis;
        clenbuterol (0.6), mabuterol (0.6), salbutamol (2), mapenterol (2)
        and terbutaline (3).

        DES in bovine urine, bile, liver, faeces and meat. LLD <1 ppb
        19-nortestosterone in urine, serum and meat. LLD 0.2 ppb
        Zeranol and taleranol in urine, serum and meat. LLD 0.37 ppb

Progesterone in plasma and meat. LLD 1 ppb
Trenbolone in urine, faeces, bile, liver & meat. LLD 0.1 ppb
Ethinyleostradiol in urine. LLD 0.2 μg per L.
Acetylgestegenes in fat. LLD 0.005 - 0.06 μg per kg
17ß-oestradiol in plasma. LLD 0.02 μg per L
Testosterone in plasma. LLD 0.02 μg per L.

8.4.7 <u>RHONE-POULENC DIAGNOSTICS LTD.</u> Montrose House, 187, George St.,
    Glasgow G1 1YT, Scotland.
This company supplies easy to use rapid EIA card tests for the antibiotics,
chloramphenicol, sulphadimidine, sulphamethoxine and gentamicin.

REFERENCES

Colinet, E.,(1992). Quality assurance in the field of biomedical analyses:
The role and contribution of the BCR program of the European Communities.
Microchem. J. <u>45</u>, 291-297.

Greipink, B., (1990), Fres. J. Anal. Chem. The role of CRM's in measurement
systems. <u>338</u>, 360-362.

Heitzman, R.J., Boenke, A. and Wagstaffe, P.J. (1993) Reference Materials
for Residues of Veterinary Substances occurring in Food-producing Animals
and their Products. In "Analysis of Veterinary Drugs in Food", Ed.
N.Haagsma, Wiley & Sons, UK, (in press).

Heitzman, R.J. (1993) The preparation of animal samples incurred with
residues of veterinary drugs. Fresenius J Anal. Chem. <u>345</u>, 207-208

ISO/REMCO N263. (1992). The international harmonised protocol for the
proficiency testing of (chemical) analytical laboratories. Nov. 1992,
prepared by M. Thompson & R. Wood.

Maier, E.A., Queauviller, Ph. and Griepink. B, (1992), Interlaboratory
Studies as a tool for many purposes: Proficiency testing, learning
exercises, quality control and certification of materials. Paper presented
at 12th International symposium on microchemical techniques, Cordoba,
September, 1992. Anal. Chim.Acta. (in press)

Marchandise, H. (1987). Accuracy in analyses of biological materials. Fres.
Z. Anal. Chem. <u>326</u>, 613-617.

Marchandise, H and Colinet, E. (1983), Assessment of methods of assigning
certified reference values to reference materials. Fres. Z. Anal. Chem.
<u>316</u>, 669-672.

Stephany, R.W., and Van Ginkel, L.A. (1989), Reference and quality
control materials for anabolic agents and veterinary drugs prepared by
RIVM, Status April 1st, 1989. RIVM report No. 387914 002.

Wagstaffe, P.W. and Belliardo, J.J. (1990). The BCR programme and
measurements for food and agriculture. Fres. J. Anal. Chem <u>338</u>, 469-472

9. CHEMICAL AND PHYSICAL DATA FOR RESIDUE SUBSTANCES.

INTRODUCTION.

The information about the availability and quality of the RMs and Reference
Compounds is given in section 8. This section provides additional chemical
and physical data about the analytes measured as probable residue
substances. Additional information may be found in The Merck Index, the
reports of the JECFA meetings, The Handbook of Chemistry and the RIKILT
reports 86.48 & 86.49

List;

Group
A I;   Boldenone, Chlorotestosterone, Dienoestrol (DEN),
              Diethylstilboestrol (DES), Ethinyloestradiol, Hexoestrol (HEX),
              Medroxyprogesterone acetate (MPA), Megestrol acetate,
              Melengestrol, Methyltestosterone (MT), 19-Nortestosterone
              (NT),
              Tapazole (TAP), Trenbolone (TB),
              2-Thiouracil (2-TU), Zeranol (Z),
A II;   17ß-Oestradiol (ßE$_2$), Progesterone (P), Testosterone (T),
A III,   Ampicillin, Benzylpenicillin, Chloramphenicol (CAP),
              Chlortetracycline, Dihydrostreptomycin, Furazolidone,
              Gentamicin, Neomycin, Nitrofurazone, Oxolinic acid,
              Oxytetracyline, Spiromycin, Sulphadimidine, Sulphaquinoxaline,
              Trimethoprim, Tylosin
B I;   Albendazole, Azaperone, Carazolol, Carbadox, Chlorpromazine,
              Cimaterol, Clenbuterol, Closantel, Dimetridazole, Febantel,
              Fenbendazole, Flubendazole, Haloperidol,
              Ipronidazole,Isometamidium chloride, Ivermectin, Lasalocid,
              Levamisole, Metronidazole, Monensin, Narasin, Nitroxynil,
              Oxfendazole, Propionylpromazine, Ractopamine, Ronidazole,
              Salbutamol, Salinomycin, Thiabendazole, Triclabendazole,
              Xylazine
B II;

Adequate peaks for Infra-red analysis.

Report 86.48 RIKILT
Adequate peaks are absorption maxima in the IR spectrum, 1800 -500 cm^{-1} of
a reference compound, that fulfil the following requirements.

1. A relative intensity of absorbance of not less than
   - 12.5% of the absorbance of the most intense peak , when both peaks are
       measured with respect to zero absorbance
   - or 5% of the absorbance of the most intense peak , when both peaks are
       measured with respect to their peak baseline

2. An intensity of absorbance of not less than
   - a specific molar absorbance of 40 with respect to zero absorbance
   - a specific molar absorbance of 20 with respect to the peak base line.

BOLDENONE

RM

Reference Compound.

Merck Index No. 1311   CAS No; 846-48-0

JECFA reference.

Analytical methods in Section 6; Cy 1.1, Cy 1.2

Species in which residues are most likely to occur; cattle, horses

Parent drug. boldenone

Therapeutic category. androgen, growth promoter

KEY Metabolites;

Structure.

Molecular Formula; $C_{19}H_{26}O_2$

Molecular Weight; 286.4

UV;

Melting Point; 164-166°C

Derivatives for GCMS;

Selected ions for identification in GCMS; TMS-enol-TMS

  EI TMS-enol-TMS, 430, 206, 415, 325, 299, 431

Selected peaks and relative intensity for identification by IR.

Source of compound for IR;
IAC column(s) developed or available .

4α-CHLORO-TESTOSTERONE

RM

Reference Compound;

Merck Index No. 2371   CAS No;   1093-58-9

JECFA reference.

Analytical methods in Section 6; Cy 1.2; Sg 1.2.

Species in which residues may occur; Cattle

Parent drug; 4α-chloro-testosterone or as an ester; e.g. acetate.

Therapeutic category; androgenic, growth promoter in cattle, sheep, pigs

Metabolites;

Structure;

Molecular Formula; $C_{19}H_{27}ClO_2$
Molecular Weight; 322.9

UV maximum at 256 nm in 95% ethanol
Melting Point; 188-190°C

Derivatives for GCMS; TMS-enol-TMS

Selected ions for identification in GCMS;

   EI, TMS-enol-TMS, 466, 468, 431, 451

Selected peaks for identification by IR;

IAC column(s) developed or available; ?

<u>**DIENOESTROL (DEN)**</u>

RM   Eur No. RM 390 for Urine; Muscle in preparation at RIVM, NL.

Reference Compound.   Yes, also deuterated-DEN

Merck Index No. 3085   CAS No; 84-17-3

JECFA reference.

Analytical methods in Section 6;   Cy 1.1; Cy 1.2; Cy 1.3; Cy 1.7;
                                   Sg 1.1; Sg 1.2.
Species in which residues are most likely to occur; calves, poultry

Parent drug. DEN

Therapeutic category. oestrogen, for endocrine control and as growth
promoter

KEY Metabolites;   none

Structure.

Molecular Formula; $C_{18}H_{18}O_2$

Molecular Weight;   266.3

UV;

Melting Point; 227-228°C

Derivatives for GCMS;   TMS, HFB and PFB

Selected ions for identification in GCMS;
    EI   TMS   <u>410</u>, 395, 381, 217, 193
    EI   HFB   658, 629, <u>445</u>, 341
    NI-CI   PFB$_2$ 445, 425
    EI   PFB$_2$ 626, 445, 249, 181
    PI-CI   ?   676, 480, 462

Selected peaks and relative intensity for identification by IR.
520, 30; 620, 52; 649, 16; 775, 45; 826, 55; 834, 56; 853, 51,
1102, 28; 1171, 53; 1205, 100; 1247, 57; 1333, 61; 1426, 34;
1513, 98; 1592, 36; 1606, 28; 1619, 18
Source of compound for IR; Sigma; Ref No; D-3253

IAC column(s) developed or available . Yes several

<u>**DIETHYLSTILBOESTROL (DES)**</u>

RM   Eur No. CRM 389 for Urine;   Muscle in preparation at RIVM, NL.

Reference Compound.   Yes, also deuterated-DES

Merck Index No. 3115   CAS No. 56-53-1

JECFA reference.

Analytical methods in Section 6;   Cy 1.1; Cy 1.2; Cy 1.3; Cy 1.7;
                                   Sg 1.1; Sg 1.2; Sg 1.3.
Species in which residues are most likely to occur;   calves, poultry

Parent drug. DES or as DES-dipropionate

Therapeutic category. oestrogen, for endocrine control and as growth
promoter

KEY Metabolites;   none

Structure.   Exists in the *cis* and *trans* forms

OH
HO
trans
HO
cis
OH

Molecular Formula; $C_{18}H_{20}O_2$

Molecular Weight; 268.3
UV;
Melting Point; 169-172°C

Derivatives for GCMS; TMS, HFB and PFB

Selected ions for identification in GCMS;
    EI   TMS   <u>412</u>, 387, 383, 397
    NI-CI   PFB$_2$ 447, 427
    EI   PFB$_2$ 628, 447, 238, 181
    PI-CI   HFB   661, 465, 464
    EI   HFB   660, 631, 447, <u>341</u>

Selected peaks and relative intensity for identification by IR.

586, 26; 646, 18; 721, 18; 805, 21; 831, 65; 851, 32; 1012, 13;
1114, 22; 1173, 86; 1204, 100; 1247, 63; 1282, 16; 1337, 35;
1427, 39; 1462, 15; 1514, 99; 1590, 28; 1609, 36
Source of compound for IR. Interpharm; Ref. No. P-4186

IAC column(s) developed or available . Yes several

<u>**ETHINYLOESTRADIOL**</u>

RM

Reference Compound;

Merck Index No. 3683   CAS No; 57-63-6

JECFA reference.

Species in which residues may occur; Calves, cattle, poultry, pigs

Analytical methods in Section 6; Cy 1.1; Cy 1.2; Cy 1.8; Sg 1.1; Sg 1.2.

Parent drug; Ethinyloestradiol

Therapeutic category; oestrogen, growth promoter

Metabolites; 17α-OH EE in ruminants

Structure;

Molecular Formula; $C_{20}H_{24}O_2$

Molecular Weight; 296.39

UV maximum in EtOH 281 nm

Melting Point; 182-184°C   EE-hemihydrate 141-146°C

Derivatives for GCMS;   HFB, TMS

Selected ions for identification in GCMS;
  EI HFB <u>474</u>, 459, 446, 353
  EI TMS <u>425</u>, 440, 300, 285

Selected peaks for identification by IR;

Source of compound for IR;

IAC column(s) developed or available; Gel available from Marloie.

9/6

<u>**HEXOESTROL (HEX)**</u>

RM   Eur No. CRM 391 for Urine;   Muscle in preparation at RIVM, NL.

Reference Compound.   Yes, also deuterated-HEX

Merck Index No. 4593   CAS No; 14188-82-0

JECFA reference.

Analytical methods in Section 6;   Cy 1.1; Cy 1.2; Cy 1.3; Cy 1.7;
                                   Sg 1.1; Sg 1.2.
Species in which residues are most likely to occur;   calves, poultry

Parent drug.   HEX

Therapeutic category. oestrogen, for endocrine control and as growth
promoter

KEY Metabolites;   none

Structure.

Molecular Formula; $C_{18}H_{22}O_2$

Molecular Weight; 270.4

UV;

Melting Point; 185-188°C

Derivatives for GCMS; TMS, HFB and PFB

Selected ions for identification in GCMS;
    EI   TMS   <u>207</u>, 414, 206, 399, 191, 179
    NI-CI PFB_2 449, 429   EI - 315, 181
    PI-CI HFB   680, 484, 466
    EI   HFB   332, <u>331</u>, 304, 303

Selected peaks and relative intensity for identification by IR.

510, 20;   574, 41;   646, 19;   716, 23;   804, 22;   830, 41;   847, 45;
1107, 17;   1174, 86;   1218, 63;   1440, 33;   1458, 22;   1516, 100;
1598, 30;   1613, 32;
Source of compound for IR;   INC;   Ref. No.; 15529

IAC column(s) developed or available . Yes several

MEDROXYPROGESTERONE

RM

Reference Compound;

Merck Index No. 5614   CAS No; 520-85-4

JECFA reference.

Species in which residues may occur; Calves, cattle, ewe sheep.

Analytical methods in Section 6; Cy 1.1; Cy 1.2; Sg 1.1; Sg 1.2

Parent drug; Medroxyprogesterone acetate (MPA)

Therapeutic category; Progestin, Growth promoter

Metabolites; 11 in urine, MPA not found in urine

Structure;

Molecular Formula; $C_{22}H_{32}O_3$ MPA $C_{24}H_{34}O_4$
Molecular Weight; 344.5   MPA 386.5

UV maximum in EtOH 241 nm   MPA maximum in EtOH at 240 nm
Melting Point; 220-223.5°C   MPA 207-209°C

Derivatives for GCMS;   MOX-TMS, MOX (MPA), TMS-enol-TMS

Selected ions for identification in GCMS;
   EI   MOX-TMS   474, 459, 443, 353
   EI   MOX (MPA) 415, 330, 312, 287
   EI   TMS-enol-TMS 560, 330, 315, 545, 455

Selected peaks for identification by IR;
  MP   597, 13; 871, 18; 1093, 13; 1123, 16; 1186, 17; 1233, 23;
       1271, 23; 1349, 24; 1448, 18; 1603, 32; 1664, 93; 1696, 100;

Source of compound for IR; Sigma; Ref. No.; M-6013

  MPA 965, 16; 1056, 13; 1080, 13; 1187, 15; 1253, 57; 1261, 58; 1365,
  29;   1607, 22; 1673, 83; 1717, 33; 1732, 100;

Source of compound for IR; Sigma; Ref. No. M-1629

IAC column(s) developed or available; no

MEGESTROL ACETATE

RM

Reference Compound;

Merck Index No. 5623   CAS No;   595-33-5

JECFA reference.

Analytical methods in Section 6; Cy 1.1; Cy 1.2; Sg 1.1; Sg 1.2.

Species in which residues may occur;   cattle

Parent drug; Megestrol acetate

Therapeutic category; Progestagen, Might be used as growth promoter

Metabolites;   megestrol

Structure;

Molecular Formula; $C_{24}H_{32}O_4$

Molecular Weight; 384.5

UV maximum at 287 nm in ethanol

Melting Point;   214-216°C

Derivatives for GCMS;   megestrol di-TMS

Selected ions for identification in GCMS;

   EI   diTMS   558, 453, 543, 353, 231

Selected peaks for identification by IR;

IAC column(s) developed or available;

<u>**MELENGESTROL**</u>

RM

Reference Compound;

Merck Index No. 5636 (melengestrol)   CAS No; 5633-18-1

JECFA reference.

Species in which residues may occur; Calves, cattle

Analytical methods in Section 6; Cy 1.1; Cy 1.2; Sg 1.1.

Parent drug; Melengestrol acetate (MPA)

Therapeutic category; Progestin, Used as growth promoter

Metabolites; melengestrol

Structure;

Molecular Formula; $C_{23}H_{30}O_3$ MGA $C_{25}H_{32}O_4$

Molecular Weight; 354.5   MGA 416.5

UV of MGA, maximum in EtOH at 287 nm

Melting Point; MPA 224-226°C

Derivatives for GCMS;   HFB (MGA)

Selected ions for identification in GCMS;
  EI   HFB - 477, 421, 381, 211

Selected peaks for identification by IR;

IAC column(s) developed or available; no

17α-METHYLTESTOSTERONE (MT)

RM

Reference Compound;

Merck Index No. 6000   CAS No; 58-18-4

JECFA reference.

Species in which residues may occur; Calves, cattle, pigs

Analytical methods in Section 6; Cy 1.1; Cy 1.2; Sg 1.1; Sg 1.2

Parent drug; 17α-methyltestosterone

Therapeutic category; androgenic, growth promoter

Metabolites;

Structure;

Molecular Formula; $C_{20}H_{30}O_2$

Molecular Weight; 302.4

UV maximum in EtOH about 241 nm

Melting Point; 161-166°C

Derivatives for GCMS; TMS, MOX-TMS, TMS-enol-TMS

Selected ions for identification in GCMS;

    EI   TMS   359, 317, 304, <u>284</u>
    EI   MOX-TMS   403, <u>313</u>, 298, 282
    EI   TMS-enol-TMS 446, 301, 431, 356

Selected peaks for identification by IR;
  873, 15; 950, 19; 1091, 17; 1156, 28; 1190, 13; 1234, 20; 1278, 14;
  1297, 14; 1374, 25; 1450, 18; 1611, 16; 1664; 100;

Source of compound for IR; Sigma; M-7252

IAC column(s) developed or available; Gel available from Marloie.

19-NORTESTOSTERONE (NT) (NANDROLONE)

RM   In preparation at RIKILT - bovine urine and muscle

Reference Compound

Merck Index No. 6211   CAS No. 434-22-0

JECFA reference.

Analytical methods in Section 6; Cy 1.1; Cy 1.2; Sg 1.1; Sg 1.2

Species in which residues may occur; calves, cattle, pigs, sheep, horses
Note; Occurs naturally in intact male horses and pigs, perinatal calves and
pregnant cows.

Parent drug; NT or one of several esters; propionate, decanoate, laurate,
              phenylpropionate

Therapeutic category; androgenic growth promoter, anabolic

Metabolites; 17αOH-NT (epi-nortestosterone)

Structure

Molecular Formula; $C_{18}H_{26}O_2$
Molecular Weight; 274.4

UV; maximum, 241 nm   Melting Point; 112°C and 124°C

Derivatives for GCMS; HFB, TMS, MOX-TMS, TFA, TMS-enol-TMS

Selected ions in GCMS αNT and βNT give identical m/z values
    EI-   HFB   666, 453, 306, 133
    EI   TMS   346, 331, 256, 215
    EI   MOX-TMS   375, 360, 344, 285
    EI   di-TMS   418, 403, 328, 287, 194
    EI   TFA   466, 353, 218, 206
    EI   TMS-eenol-TMS 418, 194, 403, 287, 182
Selected peaks and relative intensity for identification by IR.

NT; 885, 25; 967, 14; 1023, 19; 1052, 28; 1075, 24; 1133, 21;1206,31;
     1227, 14; 1259, 30; 1334, 21; 1412, 19; 1619, 27; 1666, 100;
Source of NT for IR; Sigma; Ref. No.; N-7252

17α-NT; 880, 18; 968, 16; 1051, 17; 1136, 13; 1211, 25; 1258, 18;
        1615, 31; 1643, 86; 1662, 100;
Source of αNT; Organon
IAC column(s) developed or available ; Yes. Gel from Marloie

TAPAZOLE (METHIMAZOLE)

RM In preparation in cattle urine and muscle

Reference Compound;

Merck Index No. 5844   CAS No; 60-56-0

JECFA reference.

Analytical method in Section 6; Cy 1.9; Sg 1.4

Species in which residues may occur; cattle

Parent drug; Tapazole

Therapeutic category; Thyreostatic

Metabolites;

Structure;

Molecular Formula; $C_4H_6N_2S$

Molecular Weight; 114.2

UV maximum in *0.1N* H_2SO_4 211, 251.5 nm

Melting Point; 146-148°C   Boiling point; 280°C (some decomp.)

Derivatives for GCMS; TMS

Selected ions for identification in GCMS;
    PI-CI
Selected peaks for identification by IR;

IAC column(s) developed or available; No

<u>**THIOURACIL (2-THIOURACIL)**</u>

RM   In preparation - cattle urine and muscle

Reference Compound;

Merck Index No. 9210   CAS No; 141-90-2

JECFA reference.

Analytical method in Section 6; Cy 1.9; Sg 1.4

Species in which residues may occur; cattle

Parent drug; Thiouracil

Therapeutic category; Thyreostatic and thyroid depressant

Metabolites;

Structure;

Molecular Formula; $C_4H_4N_2OS$

Molecular Weight; 128.2

UV

Melting Point; no definite point

Derivatives for GCMS; TMS

Selected ions for identification in GCMS;
        PI-CI 257, 273, 345
Selected peaks for identification by IR;

IAC column(s) developed or available;

<u>**TRENBOLONE (TB)**</u>

RM   In preparation calf muscle and urine.
Reference Compound ?

Merck Index No. 9402   CAS No.   10161-33-8

JECFA reference. 26th, 27th, 32nd and 34th Meetings

Analytical methods in Section 6; Cy 1.1; Cy 1.2; Cy 1.4; Sg 1.1; Sg 1.2

Species in which residues may occur; calves, cattle, sheep, pigs.

Parent drug   Trenbolone acetate

Therapeutic category, androgenic growth promoter

Metabolites; 17αOH-TB, 17βOH-TB (active ingredient), trendione

Structure,

Molecular Formula; $C_{18}H_{22}O_2$
Molecular Weight; 270.4
UV; Maximum at 239 and 340.5 nm
Melting Point; 186°C

Derivatives for GCMS; TMS, MOX-TMS   MOX (TBA)

Selected ions for identification in GCMS, α & ß isomers
        EI-PI TMS   <u>342</u>, 252, 237, 211
        EI   MOX-TMS   <u>371</u>, 281, 266, 253
    TBA EI   MOX   <u>341</u>, 298, 281, 266

Selected peaks for identification by IR.
 ßTB, 1017, 13; 1054, 17; 1075, 21; 1101, 25; 1199, 15; 1226, 25;
       1267, 16; 1288, 17; 1322, 15; 1346, 16; 1353, 15; 1379, 14
       1438, 15; 1569, 53; 1639, 100
Source of ßTB for IR; Roussel Uclaf; Ref. No.; 3E 0657

 αTB   762, 13; 795, 17; 852, 19; 937, 17; 1011, 22; 1028, 24;
       1088, 31; 1126, 13; 1150, 20; 1198, 27; 1229, 26; 1240, 27;
       1279, 25; 1310, 23; 1321, 18; 1346, 22; 1369, 20; 1391, 20;
       1435, 22; 1450, 16; 1578, 67; 1643, 100;
Source of αTB for IR; ?
 TBA   987, 16; 1023, 32; 1053, 35; 1096, 15; 1245, 100; 1375, 32;
       1439, 18; 1573, 32; 1660, 66; 1737, 83;
Source of TBA for IR; After extraction from Finaplix, Hoechst

IAC column(s) developed or available; Yes

ZERANOL (Z)

RM   in preparation - bovine urine, muscle, liver

Reference Compound

Merck Index No. 9923   CAS No; 7440-66-6

JECFA reference. 26th, 27th and 32nd meetings.

Analytical methods in Section 6; Cy 1.1; Cy 1.5; Cy 1.6; Sg 1.1; Sg 1.2.

Species in which residues may occur; calves, cattle, sheep, poultry

Parent drug   Zeranol

Therapeutic category; oestrogenic (mild) growth promoter

Metabolites, 7ßOH-Z, Zeralanone

Structure;

Molecular Formula; $C_{18}H_{26}O_5$

Molecular Weight; 322.4

UV; No useful absorbance

Melting Point; 181-183°C

Derivatives for GCMS, HFB, TMS

Selected ions for identification in GCMS
  EI-PI   HFB   536, 519, 296, 279
  EI   TMS   538, 523, _433_, 307, 379

Selected peaks for identification by IR.
 840, 16; 989, 24; 1075, 17; 1096, 41; 1167, 42; 1200, 37; 1259, 100;
1311, 58; 1353, 32; 1381, 21; 1464, 31; 1587, 43; 1615, 54; 1644, 70;

 Source of Zeranol for IR; International Mineral Corp. USA

IAC column(s) developed or available ; yes

OESTRADIOL-17ß (ßE$_2$)

RM

Reference Compound;

Merck Index No. 3648   CAS No;   50-28-2

JECFA reference.

Analytical methods in Section 6; Cy 1.1; Cy 1.2; Sg 1.1; Sg 1.2

Species in which residues may occur; Natural steroid

Parent drug; Oestradiol or an ester e.g E$_2$-benzoate

Therapeutic category; Oestrogenic, growth promoter

Metabolites; 17αOH-E$_2$, Oestrone

Structure;

Molecular Formula;
C$_{18}$H$_{24}$O$_2$
Molecular Weight; 272.4

UV maximum at 225, 280 nm
Melting Point; 173-179°C

Derivatives for GCMS; PFB/TMS, TMS

Selected ions for identification in GCMS;
  NI-CI   PFB/TMS   343
  EI   PFB   524, 393, 348, 253
  EI   TMS   416, 285, 231, 326
Selected peaks for identification by IR;

 ßE$_2$ 733, 29; 786, 30; 820, 56; 874, 51; 905, 16; 917, 24; 930, 34;
         962, 18; 1012, 55; 1021, 28; 1056, 83; 1102, 19; 1118, 22;
         1130, 30; 1156, 27; 1231, 78; 1250, 100; 1283, 69; 1302, 36;
         1320, 29; 1357, 44; 1382, 26; 1416, 27; 1449, 68; 1498, 74;
         1586, 47; 1610, 45;
Source of ßE$_2$ for IR; Merck; Ref. No.; 8984, Charge No. 9007942

 αE$_2$ 573, 18; 787, 28; 821, 27; 866, 40; 919, 51; 945, 27; 970, 35;
          994, 17; 1013, 30; 1036, 41; 1054, 31; 1074, 31; 1101, 21;
         1118, 16; 1154, 33; 1234, 100; 1253, 97; 1284, 78; 1352, 39;
         1379, 47; 1443, 75; 1500, 88; 1586, 31; 1610, 64;
Source of αE$_2$ for IR; Sigma; Ref. No.; E-8750
IAC column(s) developed or available; ?

<u>**PROGESTERONE**</u>

RM

Reference Compound;

Merck Index No. 7678   CAS No;   57-83-0

JECFA reference.

Analytical methods in Section 6; Cy 1.2;

Species in which residues may occur; Natural steroid

Parent drug; Progesterone

Therapeutic category; Progestagen, Growth promoter

Metabolites;

Structure;

Molecular Formula; $C_{21}H_{30}O_2$

Molecular Weight; 314.5

UV maximum at 240 nm

Melting Point; 127-131°C

Derivatives for GCMS;   TMS, TMS-enol-TMS

Selected ions for identification in GCMS;

      TMS   314, 272
   EI   TMS-enol-TMS   458, 353, 443

Selected peaks for identification by IR;
 871, 28; 948, 18; 1162, 25; 1204, 28; 1228, 26; 1237, 23; 1279, 18;
 1327, 19; 1358, 35; 1386, 22; 1439, 23; 1616, 35; 1663, 100;
 1699, 91

Source of P for IR; Sigma; Ref. No.; P-0130, Charge No. 13F-0838

IAC column(s) developed or available; probably

TESTOSTERONE

RM

Reference Compound;

Merck Index No. 9000   CAS No; 58-22-0

JECFA reference.

Analytical methods in Section 6; Cy 1.1; Cy 1.2; Sg 1.1; Sg 1.2.

Species in which residues may occur; Natural steroid

Parent drug; Testosterone or as an ester; e.g. acetate, propionate,
isocaproate, decanoate, undecanoate, phenylpropionate, benzoate

Therapeutic category; androgenic, growth promoter in cattle, sheep, pigs

Metabolites; 17αOH-T (αT) in liver, kidney, urine, bile, faeces

Structure;

Molecular Formula; $C_{19}H_{28}O_2$
Molecular Weight; 288.4

UV maximum at 238 nm
Melting Point; 155°C

Derivatives for GCMS; HFB, TMS, TMS-enol-TMS

Selected ions for identification in GCMS;

     EI, HFB, 680, 467, 355, 220
          TMS, 360, 270, 226, 345
     EI TMS-enol-TMS 432, 417, 301, 209

Selected peaks for identification by IR;
 ßT 870, 25; 943, 13; 957, 13; 1017, 16; 1056, 31; 1067, 31; 1114,
13; 1131, 14; 1199, 16; 1233, 29; 1277, 18; 1360, 19; 1378, 18;
1432, 20; 1470, 15; 1612, 29; 1658, 94; 1666, 100

Source of ßT for IR; Sigma; Ref. No.; T-1500; Charge No. 63F-0616

 αT 1189, 15; 1231, 16; 1276, 13; 1380, 14; 1432, 14; 1610, 25;
     1654, 100;

Source of αT for IR; Organon
IAC column(s) developed or available; ?

AMPICILLIN

RM   In preparation, milk and bovine muscle.

Reference Compound

Merck Index No. 612   CAS No; 69-53-4

JECFA reference.

Analytical method in Section 6; Sg 1.3.

Species in which residues may occur; all especially dairy cows,

Parent drug; anhydrous form, mono-, Sesqui- and tri-hydrates, Na & K salts

Therapeutic category; antibacterial

Metabolites;

Structure;

Molecular Formula; $C_{16}H_{19}N_3O_4S$

Molecular Weight;   349.4

UV

Melting Point; dec 202°C

Derivatives for GCMS

Selected ions for identification in GCMS

Selected peaks for identification by IR.

IAC column(s) developed or available

<u>**BENZYLPENICILLIN (PEN-G)**</u>

RM

Reference Compound

Merck Index No. 1149   CAS No; 61-33-6

JECFA reference. 36th meeting

Analytical method in Section 6; Sg 1.3

Species in which residues may occur; all

Parent drug; Pen-G, Na salt (Merck 1150), procaine penicillin

Therapeutic category; antibacterial

Metabolites;   penicilloic acid

Structure;

Molecular Formula; $C_{16}H_{18}N_2O_4S$

Molecular Weight; 334.4

UV maxima of Na salt in water at 252.5, 258.6, 264.4 nm

Melting Point; ?

Derivatives for GCMS

Selected ions for identification in GCMS

Selected peaks for identification by IR.

IAC column(s) developed or available

CHLORAMPHENICOL (CAP)

RM   in preparation   milk, eggs and calf muscle

Reference Compound;

Merck Index No.   2035   CAS No;   56-75-7

JECFA reference.   12th, 32nd, 44th meetings.

Analytical methods in Section 6; Cy 3.6; Cy 3.7; Sg 3.3.

Species in which residues may occur;   calf, cattle, pig?, poultry

Parent drug;   Chloramphenicol

Therapeutic category;   antimicrobial, not recommended by EEC (CVMP) in
laying hens and lactating cows

Metabolites

Structure

NO$_2$ —⟨benzene ring⟩— C(H)(OH) — C(H)(HN-COCHCl$_2$) — CH$_2$OH

Molecular Formula; $C_{11}H_{12}Cl_2N_2O_5$

Molecular Weight;   323.1

UV   maximum at 278 nm

Melting Point;   150.5-151.5°C

Derivatives for GCMS;   TMS

Selected ions for identification in GCMS
  TMS   NCI -   470, 468, 466, 378, 376   (reactant gas methane)
  TMS   EI -   224, 225, 242, 244, 246

Selected peaks for identification by IR.

IAC column(s) developed or available

CHLORTETRACYCLINE (CTC)

RM

Reference Compound

Merck Index No. 2170   CAS No;   57-62-5

JECFA reference.

Analytical method in Section 6; Cy 3.8; Sg 3.1

Species in which residues may occur; all especially pigs

Parent drug; CTC and CTC hydrochloride

Therapeutic category; antimicrobial

Metabolites

Structure

Molecular Formula; $C_{22}H_{23}ClN_2O_8$

Molecular Weight;478.9

UV maximum in 0.1N HCl, 230, 262.5, 367.5 nm; in 0.1N NaOH, 255, 285, 345 nm

Melting Point; 168-169°C

Derivatives for GCMS, parent

Selected ions for identification in GCMS, [M+1]$^+$

Thermospray, [M+1]$^+$, 479
Extensive fragmentation in EI-mode

Selected peaks for identification by IR.

IAC column(s) developed or available

<u>**DIHYDROSTREPTOMYCIN**</u>

RM   In preparation, milk

Reference Compound

Merck Index No. 3161   CAS No; 128-46-1

JECFA reference.

Analytical method in Section 6; Sg 3.1

Species in which residues may occur; all especially dairy cows

Parent drug; dihydrostreptomycin and as pantothenate (Merck No. 3162)

Therapeutic category; antibacterial

Metabolites;

Structure;

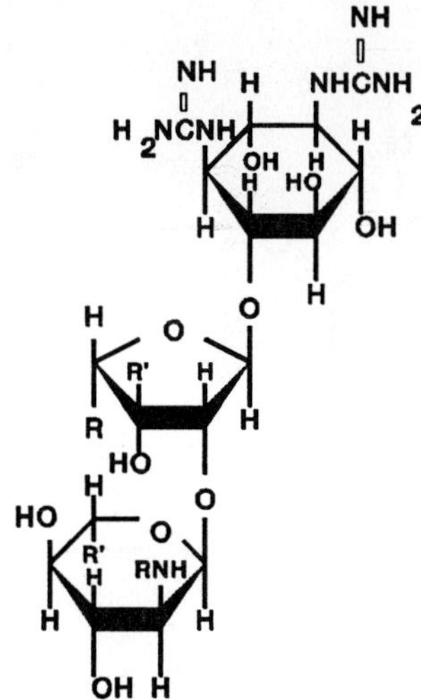

R $=$ CH$_3$

R^1 $=$ CH$_2$OH

Molecular Formula; $C_{21}H_{41}N_7O_{12}$

Molecular Weight; 583.6

UV

Melting Point; dec 255-256°C

Derivatives for GCMS

Selected ions for identification in GCMS

Selected peaks for identification by IR.

IAC column(s) developed or available; no

FURAZOLIDONE

RM

Reference Compound.

Merck Index No. 4175   CAS No; 67-45-8

JECFA reference. 40th Meeting

Analytical methods in Section 6; Cy 3.9; Sg 3.4.

Species in which residues are most likely to occur; All, especially pigs
and poultry

Parent drug. Furazolidone

Therapeutic category. Antibacterial; As in-feed antibiotic.

KEY Metabolites; Intensive metabolism, parent drug either absent or is
unstable in samples.

Structure.

Molecular Formula; $C_8H_7N_3O_5$

Molecular Weight; 225.2

UV; Maxima at 262 nm and 356 nm

Melting Point;   275°C

Derivatives for GCMS;

Selected ions for identification in GCMS;

Selected peaks and relative intensity for identification by IR.

Source of compound for IR;
IAC column(s) developed or available .

<u>**GENTAMICIN**</u>

Reference Compound.

Merck Index No. 4251   CAS Nos;1403-66-3

JECFA reference.

Analytical methods in Section 6; Sg 3.6

Species in which residues are most likely to occur;   ALL

Parent drug. Gentamicin mixture of three components; C_1, C_2, C_{1a}

Therapeutic category. Antibacterial

KEY Metabolites;

Structure.

Exists in four forms A,C_1, C_2, C_{1a}.

Molecular Formula;   A, $C_{18}H3_{26}N_4O_{10}$;
    C_1, $C_{21}H_{43}N_5O_7$; C_2, $C_{20}H_{41}N_5O_7$; C_{1a}, $C_{19}H_{39}N_5O_7$ (also known as D)

Molecular Weight; A, ;

UV;

Melting Point; A, 194-209°C;
C_1, 94-100°C; C_2, 107-124°C, C_{1a}, ?

Derivatives for GCMS;

Selected ions for identification in GCMS;

Selected peaks and relative intensity for identification by IR.

Source of compound for IR;

IAC column(s) developed or available .

<u>**NEOMYCIN**</u>

Reference Compound.

Merck Index No. 6300(B & C), 6238 (Neamine);   CAS Nos; A, 3947-65-7
                                                                     B & C; 1404-04-2

JECFA reference.

Analytical methods in Section 6;   Sg 3.6.

Species in which residues are most likely to occur;   ALL

Parent drug. Neomycin mixture of A (Neamine), B & C

Therapeutic category. Antibacterial

KEY Metabolites;

Structure.

Exists in three forms A (Neamine), B & C.

Molecular Formula;   A, $C_{12}H_{26}N_4O_6$;   B, $C_{23}H_{46}N_6O_{13}$; C, $C_{23}H_{46}N_6O_{13}$

Molecular Weight; A, 322.4;   B & C, 614.7

UV;

Melting Point; A, 225-226°C;

Derivatives for GCMS;

Selected ions for identification in GCMS;

Selected peaks and relative intensity for identification by IR.

Source of compound for IR;

IAC column(s) developed or available .

<u>**NITROFURAZONE**</u>

RM

Reference Compound.

Merck Index No. 6446   CAS No; 58-87-0

JECFA reference. 40th Meeting

Analytical methods in Section 6; Cy 3.9; Sg 3.4.

Species in which residues are most likely to occur; All especially pigs
and poultry.

Parent drug. Nitrofurazone

Therapeutic category. Antibacterial; Used as in-feed antibiotic.

KEY Metabolites; Extensive metabolism.

Structure.

$$O_2N \diagup O \diagdown CH=N-NHCONH_2$$

Molecular Formula; $C_6H_6N_4O_4$

Molecular Weight; 198.14

UV; Maxima at 264 nm and 367 nm

Melting Point; 236-240°C

Derivatives for GCMS;

Selected ions for identification in GCMS;

Selected peaks and relative intensity for identification by IR.

Source of compound for IR;
IAC column(s) developed or available .

<u>**OXOLINIC ACID**</u>

RM

Reference Compound.

Merck Index No. 6814   CAS No. 14698-29-4

JECFA reference.

Analytical method; see Takatsuki, K. (1991), J. Chromatog. <u>538</u>, 259-267
        Limit of detection 1µg per kg fish by GC-MS.
Species in which residues are most likely to occur; Farmed fish

Parent drug. Oxolinic acid

Therapeutic category. Antibiotic for treating diseases of fish.

KEY Metabolites;

Structure.

Molecular Formula; $C_{13}H_{11}NO_5$

Molecular Weight;   261

UV;

Melting Point; 314-316°C

Derivatives for GCMS; Reduction product

        after treatment with sodium tetraborate

Selected ions for identification in GCMS;

        204, 219, 176 Tatatsuki. K., J.Chrom. 1991, 538, 259-267

Selected peaks and relative intensity for identification by IR.
Source of compound for IR;
IAC column(s) developed or available . No

<u>**OXYTETRACYLINE (OTC)**</u>

RM

Reference Compound

Merck Index No. 6846   CAS No; 79-57-2

JECFA reference.

Analytical method in Section 6; Cy 3.8, Sg 3.1

Species in which residues may occur; all

Parent drug, OTC as dihydrate or hydrochloride

Therapeutic category; antimicrobial

Metabolites

Structure;

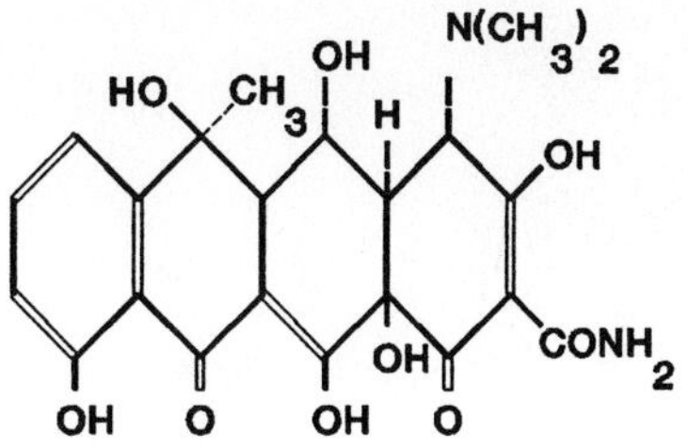

Molecular Formula; $C_{22}H_{24}N_2O_9$

Molecular Weight; 460.4

UV in pH 4.5 0.01M phosphate buffer - 249, 276, 353 nm

Melting Point; 181°C (decomp.)

Derivatives for GCMS; parent

Selected ions for identification in GCMS, $[M+1]^+$

CAD-MIKE using MS-MS in EI mode; $M^{+\cdot}$, 460. 442 416
Thermospray $[M+1]^+$, 461

Selected peaks for identification by IR.

IAC column(s) developed or available

<u>**SPIRAMYCIN**</u>

RM

Reference Compound.

Merck Index No. 8597   CAS No; 8025-81-8

JECFA reference. 12th & 38th meetings

Analytical methods in Section 6;

Species in which residues are most likely to occur; all

Parent drug. Spiramycin I, II & III

Therapeutic category. Antibacterial

KEY Metabolites; Neospiramycin (limited evidence)

Structure.

Molecular Formula; I, $C_{43}H_{74}N_2O_{14}$; II, $C_{45}H_{76}N_2O_{15}$; III, $C_{46}H_{78}N_2O_{15}$;

Molecular Weight; I, 843.1;   II, 885.2   III, 899.2

UV;

Melting Point;   I, 134-137°C;   II, 130-133°C;   III, 128-131°C

Derivatives for GCMS;

Selected ions for identification in GCMS;

Selected peaks and relative intensity for identification by IR.

Source of compound for IR;

IAC column(s) developed or available .

SULPHADIMIDINE (SULPHAMETHAZINE)

RM   IN PREPARATION - muscle, liver and urine of pig

Reference Compound;

Merck Index No. 8786   CAS No. 57-68-1

JECFA reference. 34th meeting

Analytical methods in Section 6; Cy 3.1; Cy 3.2; Cy 3.3; Cy 3.4; Sg 3.2

Species in which residues may occur; pigs, cattle, poultry

Parent drug; Sulfamethazine

Therapeutic category; antibacterial

Metabolites; N-acetyl-SMZ, N-glucose-SMZ, desamino-SMZ

Structure;

$$H_2N-\!\!\left\langle\ \right\rangle\!\!-SO_2NH-\!\!\left\langle\begin{array}{c}N\!=\!C-CH_3\\ \\N\!=\!C-CH_3\end{array}\right.$$

Molecular Formula; $C_{12}H_{14}N_4O_2S$

Molecular Weight; 278.3

UV; 241 nm in water, 243 & 257 nm in $0.01N$ NaOH, 241 & 297 in $0.01N$ HCl

Melting Point;176°C

Derivatives for GCMS; parent, methyl ester

Selected ions for identification in GCMS
Thermospray $[M+1]^+$ 279 (parent); $[M+1]^+$ 321 (N-4-acetyl-SMZ)

EI-? see; Siegert, K. (1985) Nachweis von Sulfonamiden und Antibiotica
mit Methoden der gekoppelten GCMS. Fleischwirtsch. <u>65</u>, 1496-1497

Selected peaks for identification by IR.

IAC column(s) developed or available; yes

SULPHAQUINOXALINE

RM

Reference Compound;

Merck Index No. 8815   CAS No;   59-40-5

JECFA reference.

Analytical method in Section 6; Cy 3.1; Sg 3.2.

Species in which residues may occur;

Parent drug; Sulphaquinoxaline

Therapeutic category; Antimicrobial

Metabolites;

Structure;

H_2N—⟨benzene ring⟩—SO_2NH—⟨quinoxaline ring with N, N⟩

Molecular Formula; $C_{14}H_{12}N_4O_2S$

Molecular Weight; 300.3

UV maximum, pH 6.6 in water 252 nm, 360 nm

Melting Point; 247-248°C

Derivatives for GCMS;

Selected ions for identification in GCMS;

Selected peaks for identification by IR;

IAC column(s) developed or available; ?

<u>**TRIMETHOPRIM**</u>

RM

Reference Compound;

Merck Index No. 9516   CAS No; 738-70-5

JECFA reference.

Analytical method in Section 6;

Species in which residues may occur; All

Parent drug; Trimethoprim

Therapeutic category; Antibacterial; usually mixed with a sulphonamide.

Metabolites;

Structure;

Molecular Formula; $C_{14}H_{18}N_4O_3$

Molecular Weight; 290.3

UV

Melting Point; 199-203°C

Derivatives for GCMS;

Selected ions for identification in GCMS;

Selected peaks for identification by IR;

IAC column(s) developed or available;   No

<u>**TYLOSIN**</u>

RM

Reference Compound.

Merck Index No. 9631   CAS No; 1401-69-0

JECFA reference. 12th & 38th meetings

Analytical methods in Section 6;

Species in which residues are most likely to occur; Cattle, pigs, poultry

Parent drug. Tylosin

Therapeutic category. Antibacterial

KEY Metabolites; Extensive metabolism

Structure.

Molecular Formula; $C_{46}H_{77}NO_{17}$

Molecular Weight; 916.1

UV; Maximum at 282 nm

Melting Point; 128-132°C

Derivatives for GCMS;

Selected ions for identification in GCMS;

Selected peaks and relative intensity for identification by IR.

Source of compound for IR;

IAC column(s) developed or available .

ALBENDAZOLE

RM

Reference Compound;

Merck Index No. 197   CAS No; 54965-21-8

JECFA reference. 34th meeting

Analytical method in Section 6; Cy 4.1;

Species in which residues may occur; cattle, sheep,

Parent drug; Albendazole

Therapeutic category; Anthelmintic

Metabolites; 2-amino-albendazole sulphone (Marker substance - JECFA)

Structure;

Molecular Formula; $C_{12}H_{15}N_3O_2S$

Molecular Weight;   265.3

Melting Point; 208-210°C   UV maximum 297 nm

Derivatives for GCMS; methyl or pentafluorobenzyl of albendazole
          t-butyldimethylsilyl of 2-amino-albendazole sulphone

Selected ions for identification in GCMS;
 Albendazole (ABZ); EI - 265, 236, 234, 233, 191, 190, 178
 ABZ-2-amino sulphone; EI - 239, 197, 196, 180, 148, 133, 132, 105
 Methyl- ABZ; EI - 293, 234, 192, 72, 59
 Pentafluorobenzyl-ABZ; EI - 625, 566, 444, 181
 Pentafluorobenzyl-ABZ; PICI - 654, 626, 446, 182, 181
 (Ref; Gyurik et al., (1981), Drug Metab. & Disposition, 9, 503-508)
  t-butyldimethylsilyl-2-amino-ABZ-sulphone; ? - 467, 410, 354, 189
 Ref; FAO Food and Nutrition Paper 41/2 (1990),

Selected peaks for identification by IR;
IAC column(s) developed or available; none

<u>**AZAPERONE**</u>

RM

Reference Compound;

Merck Index No. 903   CAS No; 1649-18-9

JECFA reference. 38th meeting

Analytical method in Section 6; Cy 4.5; Cy 4.6.; Sg 4.1

Species in which residues may occur; pigs

Parent drug; Azaperone

Therapeutic category; Tranquilizer

Metabolites; Azaperol

Structure;

$$F-\langle\text{phenyl}\rangle-COCH_2CH_2CH_2-N\langle\text{piperazine}\rangle N-\langle\text{pyridyl (N)}\rangle$$

Molecular Formula; $C_{19}H_{22}FN_3O$

Molecular Weight; 327.4

UV

Melting Point; 73-75°C

Derivatives for GCMS; Parent and azaperol.

Selected ions for identification in GCMS;
        Azaperone EI 107 (base peak), 233, 165, 309
        Azaperol   EI 107 (base peak), 235, 121, 222
Selected peaks for identification by IR;

IAC column(s) developed or available; no

<u>**CARAZOLOL**</u>

RM

Reference Compound;

Merck Index No. 1753   CAS No; 57775-83-2

JECFA reference. 38th meeting

Analytical method in Section 6; Cy 4.5; Cy 4.6; Sg 4.1

Species in which residues may occur; pigs, cattle

Parent drug; Carazolol

Therapeutic category; Tranquillizer, ß-andrenergic blocker

Metabolites; as glucuronide, lactate and acetate.

Structure;

Molecular Formula; $C_{18}H_{22}N_2O_2$

Molecular Weight; 298.4

UV maximum at 286 nm

Melting Point;135-138°C

Derivatives for GCMS;

Selected ions for identification in GCMS;

Selected peaks for identification by IR;

IAC column(s) developed or available; no

<u>**CARBADOX**</u>

RM

Reference Compound

Merck Index No. 1757   CAS No; 6804-07-5

JECFA reference. 36th meeting

Analytical method in Section 6; Cy 4.3 (as QCA);
                          Sg 4.2 (as QCA); Sg 4.3 (as Desoxycarbadox)

Species in which residues may occur; pigs, poultry?

Parent drug; Cardadox

Therapeutic category; antimicrobial

Metabolites; quinolinic acid (QCA), Desoxycarbadox.

Structure;

$CH=NNHCOOCH_3$

Molecular Formula; $C_{11}H_{10}N_4O_4$

Molecular Weight;   262.2

UV maximum in water 236, 251, 303, 366, 373 nm

Melting Point;239.5-240°C

Derivatives for GCMS; Prepare methyl ester of QCA

Selected ions for identification in GCMS
   EI QCA-methyl ester 188, 158, 130, 102

Selected peaks for identification by IR.

IAC column(s) developed or available

<u>**CHLORPROMAZINE**</u>

RM

Reference Compound;

Merck Index No. 2163   CAS No; 50-53-3

JECFA reference. 38th meeting

Analytical method in Section 6; Cy 4.5; Cy 4.6.; Sg 4.1.

Species in which residues may occur; pigs

Parent drug; Chlorpromazine

Therapeutic category; tranquillizer

Metabolites;

Structure;

Molecular Formula; $C_{17}H_{19}ClN_2S$

Molecular Weight; 318.9

UV

Boiling Point; 200-205°C

Derivatives for GCMS; parent

Selected ions for identification in GCMS;
      EI   318 (base peak), 272, 86, 233

Selected peaks for identification by IR;

IAC column(s) developed or available; no

<u>**CIMATEROL**</u>

RM

Reference Compound;   In preparation in bovine urine, pig muscle and liver

Merck Index No.   CAS No; 54239-37-1

JECFA reference.

Analytical method in Section 6; Cy 2.1; Cy 2.3;
                               Sg 2.1; Sg 2.2; Sg 2.3; Sg 2.4

Species in which residues may occur;   Cattle, pigs, chickens.

Parent drug; Cimaterol

Therapeutic category; B-agonist, bronchodilator, alters partition of
nutrients on favour of increased protein to fat ratios.

Metabolites; -CN grup oxidised to $-CONH_2$ or -COOH

Structure;

$$N\equiv C - \quad H_2N - \bigcirc - \overset{\overset{H}{|}}{\underset{\underset{OH}{|}}{C}} - \overset{\overset{H}{|}}{\underset{\underset{H}{|}}{C}} - \overset{\overset{H}{|}}{N} - \overset{\overset{CH_3}{|}}{\underset{\underset{CH_3}{|}}{C}} - H$$

Molecular Formula; $C_{12}H_{17}N_3O$

Molecular Weight;   219.3

UV

Melting Point;

Derivatives for GCMS;   Mono-TMS (M.W.= 291); Di-TMS (M.W.= 363)

Selected ions for identification in GCMS;
Mono-TMS EI   276, 234, 219, 186, 72
Di-TMS   EI   348, 291, 258, 72
Mono-TMS PI-CI   292, 276, 202

Selected peaks for identification by IR;

CLENBUTEROL

RM in preparation - calf urine

Reference Compound;   ? RIVM

Merck Index No. 2316   CAS No;   37148-27-9

JECFA reference.

Analytical methods in Section 6; Cy 2.1; Cy 2.2; Cy 2.3.
                                 Sg 2.1; Sg 2.2; Sg 2.3; Sg 2.4
Species in which residues may occur; pigs, calves, poultry

Parent drug; clenbuterol, clenbuterol hydrochloride

Therapeutic category; B-agonist, bronchodilator, tocolytic effects in
parturient cattle, aid in embryo transfer in cattle, alters partition of
nutrients on favour of increased protein to fat ratios.

Metabolites;

Structure;

Molecular Formula; $C_{12}H_{18}Cl_2N_2O$

Molecular Weight; 277.2

UV

Melting Point; 174-175.5^{0}C (hydrochloride)

Derivatives for GCMS; Mono-TMS (M.W.=348),
                cyclic 2(dimethyl)silamorpholine (D.M.S) (M.W.= 346)

Selected ions for identification in GCMS
 Mono-TMS   EI   333, 277, 262, 243, 187, 86
 Cyclic-DMS   346, 331, 283, 128, 100
 Mono-TMS   PI-CI   349, 333, 259
Selected peaks for identification by IR.

IAC column(s) developed or available ; yes

<u>**CLOSANTEL**</u>

RM

Reference Compound.

Merck Index No.   CAS No;

JECFA reference.   40th meeting

Analytical methods in Section 6;

Species in which residues are most likely to occur; Cattle and sheep

Parent drug. Closantel

Therapeutic category. Anthelminthic

KEY Metabolites; 3-monoiodoclosantel

Structure.

Molecular Formula; $C_{22}H_{14}Cl_2I_2N_2O_2$

Molecular Weight; 663.1

UV;

Melting Point; 215-235°C with decomposition

Derivatives for GCMS;

Selected ions for identification in GCMS;

Selected peaks and relative intensity for identification by IR.

Source of compound for IR;
IAC column(s) developed or available .

<u>**DIMETRIDAZOLE**</u>

RM

Reference Compound;

Merck Index No.   3262   CAS No; 551-92-8

JECFA reference. 34th meeting

Analytical method in Section 6;

Species in which residues may occur;

Parent drug; Dimetridazole

Therapeutic category;   Antiprotozoal; Control of histomoniasis in poultry
and swine dysentery caused by *Treponema hyodysenteriae*

Metabolites; extensive metabolism

Structure;

$$O_2N \overset{\displaystyle CH_3}{\underset{\displaystyle N}{\diagdown N \diagup}} CH_3$$

Molecular Formula; $C_5H_7N_3O_2$

Molecular Weight; 141.1

UV

Melting Point; 138-139°C

Derivatives for GCMS;

Selected ions for identification in GCMS;

Selected peaks for identification by IR;

IAC column(s) developed or available; no

<u>**FEBANTEL**</u>

RM

Reference Compound;

Merck Index No. 3879   CAS No; 58306-30-2

JECFA reference. 38th meeting

Analytical method in Section 6; Cy 4.1;

Species in which residues may occur; cattle, sheep

Parent drug; Febantel

Therapeutic category; Anthelmintic

Metabolites; Converted to fenbendazole and oxfendazole in host.

Structure;

$$S\text{—}C_6H_4\text{—}N\text{=}C\big(NHCOOCH_3\big)_2,\quad NHCOCH_2OCH_3$$

Molecular Formula; $C_{20}H_{22}N_4O_6S$

Molecular Weight; 446.5

UV

Melting Point; 129-130°C

Derivatives for GCMS;

Selected ions for identification in GCMS;

Selected peaks for identification by IR;

IAC column(s) developed or available;   no

<u>**FENBENDAZOLE**</u>

RM

Reference Compound;

Merck Index No. 3891   CAS No;   43210-67-9

JECFA reference. 38th meeting

Analytical method in Section 6; Cy 4.1;

Species in which residues may occur; cattle, sheep, horses, pigs

Parent drug; Fenbendazole

Therapeutic category; anthelmintic

Metabolites;

Structure;

Molecular Formula; $C_{15}H_{13}N_3O_2S$

Molecular Weight;   299.4

UV maximum at 297 nm

Melting Point; dec. 233°C

Derivatives for GCMS; methyl or pentafluorobenzyl

Selected ions for identification in GCMS;

Methyl-fenbendazole; EI - 327, 268, 59
Pentafluorobenzyl-fenbendazole; EI - 659, 600, 478, 181, 59
Pentafluorobenzyl-fenbendazole; PICI - 688, 660, 480, 182, 181

Selected peaks for identification by IR;

IAC column(s) developed or available; no

FLUBENDAZOLE

RM

Reference Compound.

Merck Index No. 4030   CAS No; 31430-15-6

JECFA reference.

Analytical methods in Section 6;

Species in which residues are most likely to occur; pigs and poultry

Parent drug. Flubendazole

Therapeutic category. Anthelmintic

Key Metabolites; (2-amino-1H-benzimidazol-5-yl)-4-fluorophenyl-methanone.

Structure.

$$F-C_6H_4-CO-\text{benzimidazol-2-yl}-NHCOOCH_3$$

Molecular Formula; $C_{16}H_{12}FN_3O_3$

Molecular Weight; 313.3

UV;

Melting Point;   260°C

Derivatives for GCMS;

Selected ions for identification in GCMS;

Selected peaks and relative intensity for identification by IR.

Source of compound for IR;

IAC column(s) developed or available .

HALOPERIDOL

RM

Reference Compound;

Merck Index No. 4480   CAS No; 52-86-8

JECFA reference.

Analytical method in Section 6; Cy 4.5; Cy 4.6.; Sg 4.1.

Species in which residues may occur; pigs

Parent drug; Haloperidol

Therapeutic category; tranquillizer

Metabolites;

Structure;

$$F-\!\!\bigcirc\!\!-COCH_2CH_2CH_2-N\!\!\bigcirc\!\!\overset{OH}{\underset{Cl}{\bigcirc}}$$

Molecular Formula; $C_{21}H_{23}ClFNO_2$

Molecular Weight; 375.9

UV maximum at 247nm & 241 nm in 0.1M HCl : MeOH (9:1, v/v)

Melting Point; 148-149.4°C

Derivatives for GCMS;

Selected ions for identification in GCMS;
     EI   224. Ions 237, 123 and 206 do not meet criteria (EEC 93/256)
Selected peaks for identification by IR;

IAC column(s) developed or available; no

IPRONIDAZOLE

RM

Reference Compound;

Merck Index No. 4934   CAS No;   14885-29-1

JECFA reference.   34th meeting

Analytical method in Section 6;

Species in which residues may occur; pigs and poultry

Parent drug; Ipronidazole

Therapeutic category; Antiprotozoal; Control of histomoniasis in poultry
and swine dysentery caused by *Treponema hyodysenteriae*

Metabolites;   Extensive metabolism including 2-hydroxy-ipronidazole

Structure;

$$O_2N \overset{\displaystyle CH_3}{\underset{\displaystyle N}{\diagdown N \diagup}} CH(CH_3)_2$$

Molecular Formula; $C_7H_{11}N_3O_2$

Molecular Weight;   169.2

UV

Melting Point;   60°C

Derivatives for GCMS;

Selected ions for identification in GCMS;

Selected peaks for identification by IR;

IAC column(s) developed or available;   no

<u>**ISOMETAMIDIUM CHLORIDE**</u>

RM

Reference Compound.

Merck Index No. 5028   CAS No; 34301-55-8

JECFA reference. 34th & 40th Meetings

Analytical methods in Section 6;

Species in which residues are most likely to occur; All ruminants

Parent drug. Isometamidium chloride

Therapeutic category. Antitrypanosomal agent

KEY Metabolites; Parent drug is main residue

Structure.

Molecular Formula; $C_{28}H_{26}N_7Cl$

Molecular Weight; 496.0

UV;

Melting Point; 244-245°C

Derivatives for GCMS;

Selected ions for identification in GCMS;

Selected peaks and relative intensity for identification by IR.

Source of compound for IR;

IAC column(s) developed or available .

<u>**IVERMECTIN**</u>

RM

Reference Compound;

Merck Index No. 5089   CAS No;   70288-86-7

JECFA reference. 36th meeting

Analytical method in Section 6; Cy 4.4;

Species in which residues may occur; all

Parent drug; Ivermectin is a chemically modified fermentation product
consisting of two compounds differing from each other by only one
methylene ($-CH_2-$) group. The two compounds are designated 22,23-
dihydroavermectin-B_1a and 22,23-dihydroavermectin-B_1b.
Ivermectin is a mixture of the 2 Avermectins, H_2B_1a & H_2B_1b
containing no less than 80% H_2B_1a and no more than 20% H_2B_1b

Therapeutic category; Antiparasitic

Metabolites;24-hydroxy methyl ivermectin in sheep, cattle and rats;
 3"-O-desmethyl derivatives in pigs

Molecular Formula; H_2B_1a; $C_{48}H_{74}O_{14}$: H_2B_1b; $C_{47}H_{72}O_{14}$

Molecular Weight; H_2B_1a 875.1, H_2B_1b 861.1

UV maximum in methanol   238, 245 nm

Melting Point; H_2B_1a 155-157°C

Derivatives for GCMS;

Selected ions for identification in GCMS;

Selected peaks for identification by IR;

IAC column(s) developed or available;   no

<u>**LASALOCID**</u>

RM

Reference Compound;

Merck Index No. 5204   CAS No; 25999-31-9

JECFA reference.

Analytical method in Section 6; Cy 4.2;

Species in which residues may occur;

Parent drug; Lasalocid

Therapeutic category; Coccidiostat in poultry, Ionophore, Feed additive, growth promoter

Metabolites;

Structure;

Molecular Formula; $C_{34}H_{54}O_8$

Molecular Weight; 590.8

UV maximum in 50% isopranol 248, 348 nm

Melting Point; 110-114°C

Derivatives for GCMS;

Selected ions for identification in GCMS;

Selected peaks for identification by IR;

IAC column(s) developed or available;   no

<u>**LEVAMISOLE (TETRAMISOLE)**</u>

RM

Reference Compound;

Merck Index No. 9055   CAS No; 5036-02-2

JECFA reference. 36th and 44th meetings.

Analytical method in Section 6; Sg 4.5

Species in which residues may occur; cattle, sheep, goats, pigs & poultry

Parent drug; Levamisole hydrochloride

Therapeutic category; anthelmintic, immunopotentiater

Metabolites;   Extensive

Structure;

$$C_6H_5 \diagup\diagdown N \diagdown S$$

Molecular Formula; $C_{11}H_{12}N_2S$

Molecular Weight; 204.3

UV

Melting Point; 87-89°C, hydrochloride; 264-265°C

Derivatives for GCMS; parent

Selected ions for identification in GCMS;

    EI-PI   148, 121, 203, 204

Selected peaks for identification by IR;

IAC column(s) developed or available; no

METRONIDAZOLE

RM

Reference Compound;

Merck Index No. 6033   CAS No; 443-48-1

JECFA reference. 34th meeting

Analytical method in Section 6;

Species in which residues may occur; pigs, poultry

Parent drug; Metronidazole

Therapeutic category; Antiprotozoal; Control of histomoniasis in poultry
and swine dysentery caused by *Treponema hyodysenteriae*

Metabolites; Extensive metabolism

Structure;

Molecular Formula; $C_6H_9N_3O_3$

Molecular Weight; 171.2

UV

Melting Point; 158-160°C

Derivatives for GCMS;

Selected ions for identification in GCMS;

Selected peaks for identification by IR;

IAC column(s) developed or available;   no

<u>**MONENSIN**</u>

RM

Reference Compound;

Merck Index No. 6100   CAS No; 17090-79-8

JECFA reference.

Analytical method in Section 6; Sg 4.4.

Species in which residues may occur; Poultry, cattle,

Parent drug; Monensin, or sodium salt

Therapeutic category; Ionophore, antibacterial, antifungal, antiprotozoal, coccidiostat in poultry, feed additive, growth promoter

Metabolites;

Structure;

CH3
CH3
H3C
HO CH2OH
O
O
CH3
CH3
O
CH3
O
O
OH
CH3
CH3O
CH3
HC—CH3
COOH

Molecular Formula; $C_{36}H_{62}O_{11}$

Molecular Weight; 670.9

UV no major absorbance

Melting Point; Na salt - 267-269°C

Derivatives for GCMS;

Selected ions for identification in GCMS;

Selected peaks for identification by IR;

IAC column(s) developed or available;   no

<u>**NARASIN**</u>

RM

Reference Compound;

Merck Index No. 6271   CAS No;   55134-13-9

JECFA reference.

Analytical method in Section 6; Sg 4.4

Species in which residues may occur; poultry, cattle, sheep

Parent drug; Narasin

Therapeutic category; Coccidiostat in poultry, Ionophore, Feed additive, growth promoter

Metabolites;

Structure;

(4-Me-salinomycin)

Molecular Formula; $C_{43}H_{72}O_{11}$

Molecular Weight;   765.1

UV maximum in Ethanol 285 nm

Melting Point;   98-100°C

Derivatives for GCMS;

Selected ions for identification in GCMS;

Selected peaks for identification by IR;

IAC column(s) developed or available;   no

<u>**NITROXYNIL**</u>

RM

Reference Compound;

Merck Index No.6504   CAS No; 1689-89-0

JECFA reference.

Analytical method in Section 6;

Species in which residues may occur; cattle, sheep

Parent drug; Nitroxynil

Therapeutic category; anthelmintic (fasciliocide)

Metabolites;

Structure;

$$\text{I} - \underset{\underset{\text{CN}}{|}}{\overset{\overset{\text{OH}}{|}}{\bigcirc}} - NO_2$$

Molecular Formula; $C_7H_3IN_2O_3$

Molecular Weight; 290.03

UV maximum at   ? nm, (HPLC used at 273 nm.)

Melting Point; 137-138°C

Derivatives for GCMS;

Selected ions for identification in GCMS; parent drug

     EI - 290, 273, 244, 117, 88

Selected peaks for identification by IR;

IAC column(s) developed or available; no

<u>**OXFENDAZOLE**</u>

RM

Reference Compound;

Merck Index No.6808   CAS No; 53716-50-0

JECFA reference. 38th meeting

Analytical method in Section 6; Cy 4.1;

Species in which residues may occur; cattle, sheep, pigs?

Parent drug; Oxfendazole

Therapeutic category; anthelmintic

Metabolites;

Structure;

Molecular Formula; $C_{15}H_{13}N_3O_3S$

Molecular Weight;   315.4

UV maximum at 295 nm

Melting Point; dec. 253°C

Derivatives for GCMS; Methyl or pentafluorobenzyl,

Selected ions for identification in GCMS;

 Methyl oxfendazole; EI - 343, 327, 295, 266, 250, 236, 159, 72, 59
 Pentafluorobenzyl-oxfendazole; EI - 675, 659, 627, 600, 181, 59
 Pentafluorobenzyl-oxfendazole; PICI - 701, 676, 660, 85, 71, 57

Selected peaks for identification by IR;

IAC column(s) developed or available; no

<u>**PROPIONYLPROMAZINE**</u>

RM

Reference Compound;

Merck Index No.   7730   CAS No;   3568-24-9

JECFA reference.   38th meeting

Analytical method in Section 6; Cy 4.5; Cy 4.6; Sg 4.1.

Species in which residues may occur; pigs

Parent drug; Propionylpromazine and as hydrochloride

Therapeutic category; Tranquillizer

Metabolites; none identified

Structure;

Molecular Formula; $C_{20}H_{24}N_2OS$

Molecular Weight; 340.6

UV

Melting Point; 69-70°C

Derivatives for GCMS; parent

Selected ions for identification in GCMS;
    EI   340 (base peak), 294,255, 197
Selected peaks for identification by IR;

IAC column(s) developed or available; no

<u>**RACTOPAMINE**</u>

RM

Reference Compound.

Merck Index No.   CAS No;

JECFA reference. 40th Meeting

Analytical methods in Section 6; Cy 2.3; Sg 2.1; Sg 2.4

Species in which residues are most likely to occur; pigs

Parent drug. Ractopamine hydrochloride

Therapeutic category. ß-agonist; In-feed repartitioning agent

KEY Metabolites; Ractopamine-glucuronides

Structure.

$$HO-\!\!\!\bigcirc\!\!\!-\underset{OH}{CH}-CH_2-\overset{+}{NH}_2-\underset{CH_3}{CH}-CH_2-CH_2-\!\!\!\bigcirc\!\!\!-OH \qquad Cl^-$$

Molecular Formula; $C_{18}H_{24}O_3NCl$

Molecular Weight; 337.5

UV;

Melting Point;   -   °C

Derivatives for GCMS;

Selected ions for identification in GCMS;

Selected peaks and relative intensity for identification by IR.

Source of compound for IR;
IAC column(s) developed or available .

RONIDAZOLE

RM

Reference Compound;

Merck Index No. 8128   CAS No; 7681-76-7

JECFA reference. 34th meeting

Analytical method in Section 6;

Species in which residues may occur; pigs, poultry

Parent drug; Ronidazole

Therapeutic category; Antiprotozoal; Control of histomoniasis in poultry
and swine dysentery caused by *Treponema hyodysenteriae*

Metabolites; extensive metabolism

Structure;

$$O_2N \diagdown N \diagup CH_2OOCNH_2,\ \ CH_3,\ \ N$$

Molecular Formula; $C_6H_8N_4O_4$

Molecular Weight; 200.2

UV

Melting Point; 167-169°C

Derivatives for GCMS;

Selected ions for identification in GCMS;

Selected peaks for identification by IR;

IAC column(s) developed or available;   no

<u>**SALBUTAMOL (ALBUTEROL)**</u>

RM   In preparation - calf urine and pig muscle and liver

Reference Compound

Merck Index No. 206   CAS No;   18559-94-9

JECFA reference.

Analytical method in Section 6; Cy 2.1; Cy 2.3.
                              Sg 2.1; Sg 2.2; Sg 2.3; Sg 2.4
Species in which residues may occur; pigs, calves, poultry

Parent drug; Salbutamol

Therapeutic category;   B-agonist, bronchodilator, tocolytic effects in
parturient cattle, possible aid in embryo transfer in cattle, alters
partition of nutrients on favour of increased protein to fat ratios.

Metabolites; The sulphate conjugate is the main residue in bovine and
porcine liver.

Structure;

$$HO-\underset{}{\bigcirc}\!\!-\underset{CH_2OH}{}\;\;\underset{OH\;H}{\overset{H\;\;\;H}{C}-\overset{H}{C}}-\overset{H}{N}-\underset{CH_3}{\overset{CH_3}{C}}-CH_3$$

Molecular Formula; $C_{13}H_{21}NO_3$

Molecular Weight;   239.3

UV

Melting Point;   151°C

Derivatives for GCMS;   Tri-TMS (M.W. = 455)

Selected ions for identification in GCMS

 Tri-TMS EI   426, 370, 356, 336, 280, (86 or 72 for screening)
 Tri-TMS PI-CI   456, 440, 366, also 394, 369, 350
 Tri-TMS EI   86, 369, 455 (Method Sg 2.1, Sg 2.3)
Selected peaks for identification by IR.

IAC column(s) developed or available ;   yes

<u>**SALINOMYCIN**</u>

RM

Reference Compound;

Merck Index No. 8193   CAS No; 53003-10-4

JECFA reference.

Analytical method in Section 6; Sg 4.4.

Species in which residues may occur; Poultry, cattle, sheep

Parent drug; Salinomycin

Therapeutic category; Anticoccidial, ionophore

Metabolites;

Structure;

Molecular Formula; $C_{42}H_{70}O_{11}$

Molecular Weight; 751.0

UV maximum in ethanol;water (2/1) 284 nm

Melting Point; 112.5-113.5°C

Derivatives for GCMS;

Selected ions for identification in GCMS;

Selected peaks for identification by IR;

IAC column(s) developed or available;   no

<u>**THIABENDAZOLE**</u>

RM

Reference Compound;

Merck Index No. 9126   CAS No; 148-79-8

JECFA reference. 40th meeting

Analytical method in Section 6; Cy 4.1;

Species in which residues may occur; cattle, sheep

Parent drug; Thiabendazole

Therapeutic category; Anthelmintic, fungicide

Metabolites;

Structure;

Molecular Formula; $C_{10}H_7N_3S$

Molecular Weight; 201.3

UV maximum at 301 nm

Melting Point; 304-305°C

Derivatives for GCMS; Methyl or pentafluorobenzyl,

Selected ions for identification in GCMS;
 Methyl-thiabendazole; EI - 215, 187, 156, 155, 77
 Pentafluorbenzyl-thiabendazole; EI - 381, 362, 303, 214, 181, 90
 Pentafluorbenzyl-thiabendazole; PICI - 410, 382, 202, 182, 181

IAC column(s) developed or available; no

<u>**TRICLABENDAZOLE**</u>

RM

Reference Compound.

Merck Index No.   CAS No; 68786-66-3

JECFA reference. 40th meeting

Analytical methods in Section 6;

Species in which residues are most likely to occur; all ruminants

Parent drug. Triclabendazole

Therapeutic category. Anthelmintic

KEY Metabolites; Oxidation to sulphoxide and sulphone.

Structure.

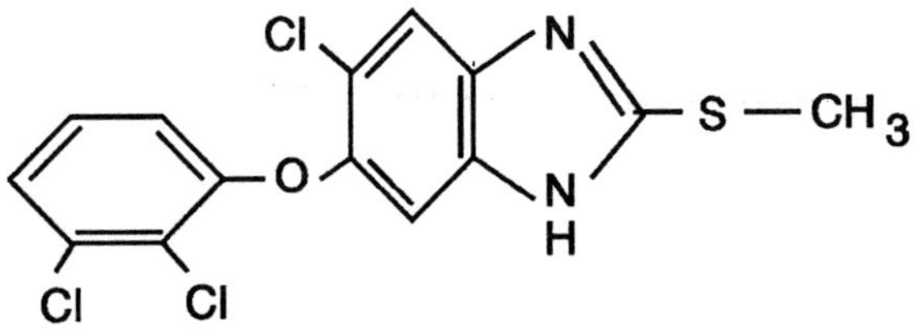

Molecular Formula; $C_{14}H_9Cl_3N_2OS$

Molecular Weight; 359.7

UV;

Melting Point;   175°C (α - modification), 162°C (β - modification)

Derivatives for GCMS;

Selected ions for identification in GCMS;

Selected peaks and relative intensity for identification by IR.

Source of compound for IR;

IAC column(s) developed or available .

<u>**XYLAZINE**</u>

RM

Reference Compound;

Merck Index No. 9889   CAS No; 7361-61-7

JECFA reference.

Analytical method in Section 6; Cy 4.5; Sg 4.1

Species in which residues may occur; pigs

Parent drug; Xylazine

Therapeutic category; tranquillizer

Metabolites;

Structure;

Molecular Formula; $C_{12}H_{16}N_2S$

Molecular Weight; 220.3

UV

Melting Point; 140-142°C

Derivatives for GCMS; parent

Selected ions for identification in GCMS;
    EI 205 (base peak), Ions 220, 177 and 145 do not meet criteria (EEC 93/256)
Selected peaks for identification by IR;

IAC column(s) developed or available; no

10.   IMPORTANT EEC LEGISLATION CONCERNING RESIDUES.

10.1 EEC PUBLISHED LIST

64/433   Council Directive on health problems affecting intra-Community trade in fresh meat. Several amendments. [OJ № L 121, 29.7.1964, pp.2012-64]

70/373   Council Directive establishing Community methods for the official control of feedingstuffs. [OJ № L 170, 3.8.1970, pp. 2-] >10 amendments.

70/524   Council Directive concerning additives in feedstuffs. c. 50 amendments. e.g. 90/167 relating to medicated feedingstuffs. [OJ № L 270, 14.12.1970, pp.1-20]

72/462   Council Directive on health and veterinary inspection problems upon importation of of bovine animals and swine and fresh meat from third countries. (several amendments). [OJ № L 302, 31.12.1972, p.28]

81/602   Council Directive concerning the prohibition of certain substances having a hormonal action and of any substances having a thyreostatic action. [OJ № L 222, 7.8.1981, pp. 32-33]

81/851   Council Directive on the approximation of the laws of Member States relating to veterinary medicinal products. [OJ № L 317, 6.11.1981, pp. 1-17]. Amended in Directives 90/676 and 90/677.

81/852   Council Directive on the approximation of the laws of the Member States relating to analytical, pharmaco-toxicological and clinical standards and protocols in respect of the testing of veterinary medicinal products. [OJ № L 317, 6.11.81, pp. 18-28]

83/90   amends 64/433 [OJ № L 59, 5.3.83, pp 10-33]

84/425   10th Commission Directive establishing Community methods for the official control of feedingstuffs. [OJ № L 238, 6.9.84, pp.34-38]

85/358   Council Directive supplementing Directive 81/602/EEC concerning the prohibition of certain substances having a hormonal action and of any substances having a thyreostatic action. [OJ № L 191, 23.7.1985, pp.46-49]

85/397   Council Directive on health and animal health problems affecting intra-Community trade in heat-treated milk. [OJ № L 226, 24.8.1985, pp. 13-18]

85/591   Concerning the introducton of Community methods of sampling and analysis for the monitoring of foodstuffs intended for human consumption. [OJ № L 372, 331.12.85, pp 50-52]

85/649   Council Directive prohibiting the use in livestock farming of certain substances having a hormonal action. [OJ № L 382, 31.12.1985, pp. 228-231]

Note; Declared invalid. Replaced by 88/146/EEC.

86/363   Council Directive on the fixing of maximum levels for pesticide
                residues of substances in and on foodstuff of animal origin.
                [OJ № L 221, 7.8.1986, pp. 43-47]

86/469   Council Directive concerning the examination of animals and
                fresh meat for the presence of residues. [OJ № L 275,
                26.9.1986, 36-46]

87/410   Commission Decision of 14th July 1987 laying down the methods
                to be used for detecting residues of substances having a
                hormonal action and of substances having a thyreostatic action.
                [OJ № L 223, 11.8.1987, pp.18-36]

88/146   Council Directive prohibiting the use in livestock farming of
                certain substances having a hormonal action. [OJ № L 70,
                16.3.1988, p.16]

88/196-206, 88/240, Commission Decisions approving the plan relating to
                the examination for hormone residues submitted by each of the
                Member States. [OJ № L 94, 12.4.1988, pp. 22-32; OJ № L 105,
                26.4.1988, p.28]

88/299   Council Directive on trade in animals treated with certain
                substances having a hormonal action and their meat, as referred
                to in article 7 of Directive 88/146/EEC. [OJ № L 128,
                21.5.1988, p.36]

89/15   Commission Decision on the importation of live animals and
                fresh meat from certain third countries. [OJ № L 8, 11.1.1989,
                pp.11-12]

89/153   Commission Decision concerning the correlation of samples taken
                for residue examination with animals and their farms of origin.
                [OJ № L 59, 2.3.89, 33-34]

89/187   Council Decision determining the powers and conditions of
                operation of Community reference laboratories provided for by
                directive 86/469 EEC concerning the examination of animals and
                fresh meat for the presence of residues. [OJ № L 66, 10.3.1989,
                pp.37-38]

89/265-276   Council Decisions approving the plan relating to the
                examination for residues other than those having a hormonal
                action submitted by each of the Member States. [OJ № L 108,
                19.4.89, pp. 20-31]

89/397   Council Directive on the official control of foodstuffs. [OJ №
                L 186, 30.6.89, pp. 23-26]

89/610   Commission Decision of 14th November 1989 laying down the
                reference methods and the list of national reference
                laboratories for detecting residues. [OJ № L 351, 2.12.1989,
                pp. 39-50]

89/662   Council Directive concerning veterinary checks in intra-
            Community trade with a view to the completion of the internal
            market. [OJ № L 395, 30.12.89. pp.13-22]

90/135   Commission Decision which deals with the plans of third
            countries for residue examination of fresh meat and animals for
            substances other than those having a hormonal action.
            Amended by Commission Decision 90/262. [OJ № L 76, 22.3.1990,
            pp.24-25]

90/167   Laying down the conditions governing the preparation, placing
            on the market and use of medicated feedingstuffs in the
            Community. [OJ № L 92, 7.4.1990, pp. 42-48]

90/424   Council Decision on expenditure in the veterinary field [OJ №
            L 224, 18.8.1990, pp. 19-28]

90/515   Commission Decision laying down the reference methods for
            detecting residues of heavy metals and arsenic. [OJ № L 286,
            18.10.1990, pp. 33-39]

90/675   Council Directive laying down the principles governing the
            organisation of veterinary checks on products entering the
            Community from third countries. [OJ № L 373, 31.12.90, pp. 1-
            14]

90/676   Amendment to Directives 81/851. (Veterinary Medicines) [OJ № L
            373, 31.12.90, pp. 15-25]

90/677   Amendment to Directives 81/851. (Veterinary Medicines) [OJ № L
            373, 31.12.90, pp. 26-28]

90/2377   Regulation laying down a Community procedure for the
            establishment of maximum residue limits of veterinary medicinal
            products in foodstuffs of animal origin. OJ № L 224,
            18.1.1990, pp.1-8]

91/61   Council Decision amending Decision 90/218/EEC [OJ № L 116,
            8.5.1990, p.27] concerning the administration of Bovine
            Somatotropin (BST). [OJ № L 37, 9.2.1991, p.39]

91/398   Commission Decision on a computerized network linking
            veterinary authorities (Animo). [OJ № L 221, 9.8.1991, p.30]

91/486   Commission Decision amending Decision 90/135/EEC relating to
            the plans of third countries concerning examination of residues
            of fresh meat for substances other than those having a hormonal
            action. [OJ № L 260, 17.9.91, pp.13-16]

91/508   Commission Directive amending the annexes to Council Directive
            70/524/EEC concerning additives in feeding stuffs. [OJ № L 271,
            27.9.1991, pp.67-69]

91/664   Council Decision designating the Community reference
            laboratories for testing certain substances for residues. [OJ №
            L 368, 31.12.1991, 17-18]

92/18   Commission Directive modifying the Annex to Council Directive
             81/852/EEC on the approximation of the laws of Member States
             relating to the analytical, pharmacotoxicological and clinical
             standards and protoco;s in respect of the testing of veterinary
             medicinal products. [O.J. № L.97., 10.4.92., pp 1-12]

92/183   Commission Decision laying down the general conditions to be
             complied with for the import of certain raw materials for the
             pharmaceutical processing industry, coming from third
             countries, which appear on the list established by Council
             Decision 79/542/EEC. [OJ № L 84, 31.3.1992, pp. 33-37]

92/675   Commission Regulation amending annexes I and III of Council
             Regulation (EEC) No. 2377/90 laying down a Community procedure
             for the establishment of maximum residue limits of veterinary
             medicinal products in foodstuffs of animal origin. [OJ № L 73,
             19.3.1992, pp. 8-14]

93/256   Commission Decision, 93/256/EEC, laying down the methods for
             detecting residues of substances having a hormonal or
             thyrostatic action. [OJ. № L.118, 14.4.93. pp 64-74]

93/257   Commission Decision, 93/257/EEC, laying down the reference
             methods and the list of national reference laboratories for
             detecting residues. [OJ. № L.118, 14.5.93, pp 75-79]

10.2. SUMMARY OF EEC LEGISLATION FOR THE CONTROL OF RESIDUES.

10.2.1. DEFINITION

The term residue is used in this context according to Directive 86/469
which says that "residue means residue of substances having a
pharmacological action and of conversion products thereof and other
substances transmitted to meat and which are likely to be dangerous to
human health".

10.2.2. LEGISLATION GIVING GENERAL RULES.

64/433 was the first Directive on health problems affecting Intra-Community
trade in fresh meat. The Directive 83/90 amended 64/433 and lays down the
ground rules as regards the examination of animals or meat for residues
that the Council shall adopt. In particular-
             - the detailed arrangements for controls.
             - the frequency of sampling.

It states that every Member State shall ensure that the following meat is
not sent from it's territory to that of another Member State
- fresh meat from animals to which stilbenes or stilbene derivatives have
been administered, and meat containing residues of these substances.
- fresh meat containing residues of other substances having a hormonal
action, antibiotics, antimony, arsenic , pesticides, or other substances
which are harmful to human health. If such residues exceed the permitted
level or, where no permitted level has been laid down, the quantity which
has been proved scientifically to be safe and on which the Scientific
Veterinary Committee (SVC) has expressed its opinion.
- fresh meat from animals to which substances likely to make the meat
dangerous or harmful to human health have been administered and on which

the SVC has expressed its opinion.

86/469 is a Directive concerning the examination of animals and fresh meat
for the presence of residues. It consists of 19 articles and 2 annexes.
The articles give definitions for the terms used, oblige Member States to
assign to a central body the coordination and implementation of the
inspections provided for and to submit plans to achieve the objectives of
the Directive. It ensures that veterinary experts from the Commission may
make on-the-spot checks. The minimum frequency of inspections is
specified. The import from third countries is allowed only in those cases,
where these countries have a legislation on the use of substances matching
the EEC legislation. The taking of samples is regulated in detail and the
procedure for treating cases of infringements.

In Annex I the residues are grouped as detailed in Section 2 of manual.
In Annex II the sampling levels and frequency and the residue testing under
reference to the grouping in Annex I are regulated.

72/462 is a Directive concerning the health and veterinary inspection
problems upon importation of bovine animals and swine and fresh meat from
third countries. It prohibits the importation to the Community of meat
containing levels of substances which are judged harmful or likely to
render consumption thereof dangerous or injurious to human health.

10.2.3. DETAILED LEGISLATION.

Following on from the basic Directives above there are many Directives and
Decisions which add detail.   Hormones were initially a major problem and
there is a specific batch of legislation for these substances (see
12.2.4.).

Other Decisions of special interest to the control of residues are
 - 87/410 which deals with the correlation of samples taken for residue
examination with animals and their farm of origin. Lays down the routine
methods to be used for the detecting of residues of substances having a
hormonal action and of substances having a thyreostatic action.
 - 89/153 which fixes the conditions of working for the Reference
laboratories.
 - 89/610 revoked and replaced by 93/257 which fixes the reference methods
and lists the National Reference Laboratories (NRL see Section 3 of manual)
for detecting residues. Council Decision 91/664 designates the four
national reference laboratories (NRL).
 - 90/135 which deals with the plans of third countries for residue
examination of fresh meat and animals for substances other than those
having a hormonal action.
 - 92/18 The Commission Directive 92/18/EEC sets out an approximation of
the laws of Member States relating to analytical, pharmacotoxicological and
clinical standards and protocols in respect of the testing of veterinary
medicinal products. Part B is on Residue Testing and requests information
on the nature and persistence of residues in order to establish practical
withdrawal times and also asks for a practical analytical method suitable
for routine use to verify compliance with the withdrawal period.

92/675 A Commission Regulation amending annexes I and III of Council
Regulation (EEC) No. 2377/90 laying down a Community procedure for the
establishment of maximum residue limits of veterinary medicinal products in
foodstuffs of animal origin.

10.2.4. LEGISLATION SPECIALLY FOR HORMONAL SUBSTANCES.

-81/602 a Directive which prohibits stilbenes and thyreostats. The
therapeutic use of other hormonal substances is regulated.

-85/358 a Directive which supplements 81/602 by introducing Community
control measures covering farm animals in their farms of origin and at the
slaughterhouses, and the meat of such animals and the meat products
obtained therefrom.

-85/649 a directive prohibiting hormonal substances for fattening purposes
whereas the use of certain substances for therapeutic purposes may be
authorised but must be strictly controlled in order to prevent any misuse
of them. The therapeutic treatment with substances having a hormonal
action is prohibited for animals intended for fattening. The import of
animals and meat to which have been administered in any way whatsoever
substances with a thyreostatic, oestrogenic, androgenic or gestagenic
action is prohibited.
A programme establishing the frequency of controls on imports from third
countries is set up.

-87/470 a Council Decision laying down the methods to be used for
detecting residues of substances having a hormonal action and of substances
having a thyreostatic action.

-88/146 a Directive on prohibiting the use in livestock of certain
substances having a hormonal action is regulating the use of these
substances further by claiming from Member States
- a list of products containing as active substances, oestradiol-17ß,
testosterone and progesterone and those derivatives which readily yield the
parent compound on hydrolysis.
- the conditions of use of these products, in particular the waiting
period necessary and detailed provisions concerning the control of these
conditions of use.
- the means of identification of use.

-88/196 & 88/200 are Commission Decisions approving the plans relating to
the examination of hormone residues submitted by Member States under
reference to Directive 86/469

-93/256 is a Commission Decision laying down the methods for detecting
residues of substances having a hormonal or thyrostatic action. However
the criteria are to be regarded as covering the analytical methods used for
all veterinary drugs and substances.

10.2.5. FUTURE LEGISLATION.

The Council is working on a Regulation laying down a Community procedure
for the establishment of residue limits of veterinary medicine products in
foodstuff of animal origin.

Directive 86/469 is being modified to cover fish and may be extended to
cover poultry.

11.   GENERAL REFERENCES.

The references listed are aimed at giving an overview of the whole subject
of residues of veterinary drugs. Specific references for each section are
included in that section.   Also each of the methods in section 6 contains
selected references.

Anabolic agents in animal production. FAO/WHO Symposium, Rome, March 1975,
EQS, (1976) Suppl V. Ed. by Lu, F.C. and Rendel, J. Georg Thieme,
Stuttgart, ISBN 3-13-536101-2

Anabolics in Animal Production. Public health aspects, analytical methods
and regulation. Symposium held at OIE, Paris Feb. 1983. Ed. by
Meissonnier, E. Soreograph, France. ISBN 92-9044-118-6

Analysis of food contaminants. Ed. by Gilbert, J. Elsevier Appl. Sc.
London and New York, (1984) ISBN 0-85334-255-5

Chemistry Quality and Assurance Hanbooks. Vol. I. Principles. Vol. II.
Specific Methods. USDA Food Safety and Quality Service. USDA and FSIS
Handbooks - continuously updated.

Drug residues in animals. Ed. by Rico, A. Academic Press Inc. (1986)

Euroresidues II. Conference on residues of veterinary drugs in food at
Veldhoven, The Netherlands, May 1993, Edited by Haagsma, N., Ruiter, A.
and Czedik-Eysenberg, P.B. ISBN 90-6159-016-7. volumes 1 & 2.

Immunoassays in food analysis. Ed. by Morris, B.A. and Clifford, M.N.
Elsevier Appl. Sc. London and New York, (1985) ISBN 0-85334-321-7

Immunoassays for Veterinary and food analysis - 1. Ed. by Morris, B.A.,
Clifford, M.N. and Jackman, R. Elsevier Appl. Sc. London and New York,
(1988) ISBN 1-85166-138-7

Manipulation of growth in farm animals. A seminar in the CEC programme of
coordination of research on beef production, Brussels, Dec., 1982. Ed. by
Roche, J.F. and O'Callaghan D. Matinus Nijhoff for the EEC, (1984), ISBN 0-
89838-617-6, EUR 8919 EN

Pharmacological basis of large animal medicine. Ed. by Bogan, J.A., Lees,
P. and Yoxall, A.T. Blackwell Scientific, Oxford, (1983), ISBN 0-632-
01055-X

Second international symposium on the analysis of anabolizing and doping
agents in biosamples. May 1990, Ghent, Belgium, Ed. by Van Peteghem, C.
J. Chromatog. (1991), $\underline{564}$, No.2, 361-583

International symposium on hormone and veterinary drug analysis, Ghent,
Belgium, May, 1992. Eds. Pardue et al. Anal. Chim. Acta. $\underline{275}$, 1-362

Van Ginkel, L.A. and Stephany, R.S. (1991) New trends in strategies for
residue analysis of growth promoting agents. Microbiol.-Ailments-
Nutrition, $\underline{9}$, 89-94

12.   ANNEXES

ANNEX I   LIST OF ABBREVIATIONS AND SYMBOLS

AA   = atomic absorption
Ac   = acetate
approx.   = approximately
B   = Belgium
b.pt. bp?   = boiling point
BCR   = Community Bureau of Reference, EEC.
Bi   = bile
B_O/T = fraction of the radioactivity of the bound fraction
B_O = radioactivity of the bound fraction of a blank sample
C   = chromatography
C-18   = CC on C-18 cartridges
C-Ac   = acetylated chromatography cartridge
C-diol   = dihydroxylated chromatography cartridges
C-Si   = silica chromatograpy cartridges
$C-SO_3H$ = sulphite chromatography cartridge
ca.   = circa, about, approximately
CC   = column C
CGE   = capillary gel electrophoresis
CI   = chemical ionization
Ci   = Curie
cm   = centimetre
conc   = concentration
CPM   = counts per minute
CSX   = ? chromatography cartridge
D   = Denmark
Dens   = densiometric
detn   = determination
Di.A   = diode array
Dial   = dialysis
DPM   = disintegrations per minute
e.g.   = for example
ECD   = electro-chemical detector
EDTA   = Ethylenediaminetetraacetic acid
EEC   = European Economic Community
Eg   = eggs
EI   = electron impact ionization
EIA   = enzyme immunoassay
equiv.   = equivalent
Et   = ethyl
EtOH   = ethyl alcohol or ethanol
F   = fat
F   = France
FAO   = Food and Agriculture Organisation
Fc   = faeces
Fig.   = figure
Fl   = fluorescence
FPT   = four plate test
G   = Germany
g   = grams
g   = gravity
GC   = gas chromatography
GIB   = growth inhibition of bacteria

Gr	=	Greece
Grav	=	gravimetric
h	=	hour
HFBA	=	heptafluorobutyric anhydride
H_2O	=	water
HPLC	=	high pressure liquid chromatography
HPTLC	=	high performance thin-layer chromatography
HRMS	=	high resolution mass spectrometry
I.S.	=	injection site - normally muscle
IA	=	immunoassay
IAC	=	immunoaffinity chromatography
IMG	=	immunogram
Ir	=	Ireland
IR	=	infrared
ISO	=	International Organisation for Standardisation
It	=	Italy
K	=	kidney
kg	=	kilogram(s)
L	=	liver
L	=	litre(s)
L	=	Luxembourg;
LC	=	liquid chromatography
LLD	=	lower limit of detection of system
LRMS	=	low resolution mass spectrometry
M	=	muscle
m	=	metre(s) or milli prefix or mass
M	=	molar
MAFF	=	Ministry of Agriculture, Fisheries and Food, United Kingdom
MAT	=	Measurements & Testing Programme, DG12.
Me	=	methyl
MeOH	=	methyl alcohol or methanol
mg	=	milligram(s)
min	=	minute(s)
Mk	=	milk
mL	=	millilitre(s)
mm	=	millimetre(s)
mp	=	melting point
MOX	=	methoxylamine hydrochloride
MS	=	mass spectrometry
MSPD	=	matrix solid-phase dispersion
MW	=	molecular weight
ng	=	nanogram(s)
NH_2	=	amino
NL	=	Netherlands (Holland)
nm	=	nanometre(s)
NMR	=	nuclear magnetic resonance
No.	=	number
NSB	=	non-specific binding = aspecific binding (ASB)
^{o}C	=	degrees Celsius (Centigrade)
P	=	Portugal
PFB	=	pentafluorobenzene-
pg	=	picogram(s)
Pl	=	plasma
ppb	=	parts per billion $(1/10^9)$
ppm	=	parts per million
ppt	=	parts per trillion $(1/10^{12})$

Pr	= propyl
ref.	= reference
R_f	= distance spot moved/distance solvent moved in TLC
RIA	= radioimmunoassay
rpm	= revolutions per minute
S	= solvent extraction
S	= Spain
Se	= Serum
sec	= second(s)
soln	= solution
SP	= spectrometry, e.g. Diode array
T	= total radioactivity (CPM OR DPM) added to a sample
Th	= Thyroid
TLC	= thin-layer chromatography
TMS(i)	= trimethylsilyl-
U	= urine
ug or μg	= microgram(s)
UK	= United Kingdom
UK-NI	= UK-Northern Ireland
uL or μL	= microlitre(s)
USDA	= United States Department of Agriculture
UV	= ultraviolet
v/v	= both components measured by volume
Vis	= visible (either by eye or in visible spectrum
w/w	= both compoents measured by weight
WHO	= World Health Organisation
wt	= weight
z	= charge

EEC Member States.

B	= Belgium
D	= Denmark
F	= France
G	= Germany
Gr	= Greece
Ir	= Ireland
It	= Italy
L	= Luxembourg
NL	= Netherlands (Holland)
P	= Portugal
S	= Spain
UK	= United Kingdom
UK-NI	= UK-Northern Ireland

Samples

Bi	= bile
Eg	= eggs
F	= fat
Fc	= faeces
I.S.	= injection site - normally muscle
K	= kidney
L	= liver
M	= muscle
Mk	= milk
Pl	= plasma

Se   = Serum
Th   = Thyroid
U   = urine
R   = retina

/   = per
%   = percentage, parts per hundred
>   = more than
<   = less than
/   = off-line hyphenated techniques
-           = on-line hyphenated techniques

E.g. HPLC/GC-MS = HPLC off-line followed by GC with on-line MS

Compounds

αE_2 = oestradiol-17α
αTB   = trenbolone-17α
Bol   = boldenone
CAP   = chloramphenicol
DE or DEN   = dienoestrol
DES   = diethylstilboestrol
E_1 = oestrone
E_3 = oestriol
EE   = ethinyloestradiol
HEX   = hexoestrol
MT   = methyltestosterone
MTU   = methylthiouracil
NT   = 19-nortestosterone
SMZ   = sulphamethazine or sulphadimidine
βE_2 = oestradiol-17β
T   = testosterone
βTB   = trenbolone-17β
TAP   = tapazole
TB or TbOH   = trenbolone
TBA   = trenbolone acetate
TU   = thiouracil
Z   = zeranol

Reference Laboratories.

RL   = Reference laboratories

BGA   = Bundesgesundamptseit, Berlin
CNEVA/LMV   = Centre National d'Etudes Veterinaires et Alimentaires,
                 Laboratoire des Medicaments Veterinaires, Fougeres
CVL   = Central Veterinary Laboratory, Weybridge
IHE   = Institut d'Hygiène et d'Épidémiologie, Brussels
ISS   = Instituto Superiore di Sanita, Rome
NFC   = National Food Centre, Dublin
RIKILT(-DLO) = Rijkskwaliteitsinstituut voor Land- en Tuinbouwprodukten,
                 Wageningen
RIVM   = Rijksinstitut voor Volksgezondheid en Milieuhygiëne,
                 Bilthoven
VRL   = Veterinary Research Laboratories, Belfast.

12.2.   ANNEX II.   CALCULATIONS OF LIMITS

12.2.1. Calculating the values for the lower limits of sensitivity,
detection, determination (quantitation or reliable measurement) and
decision (regulatory action) are a mix of statistics (at what confidence
level or how many standard deviations) and political decision. The
criteria document in section 5 and expressly covers the limit of detection
and the limit of determination.

Different values for the lower limit of decision and the lower limit of
detection were first suggested by Heitzman and Harwood (1983). They tried
to take into account the problem of non-specific interference in
immunoassays which gives rise to high values for blank materials. They
calculated the lower limit of detection as the mean value for the blank
samples plus 2 SD and suggested a lower limit of decision as an arbitrary
value higher than the lower limit of detection which took into account the
practicality of the method and the values found in animals (cattle) known
to have been treated with drug (HEX). In a later paper on residues of
monensin in cattle, Heitzman et al., (1986) suggested that the lower limit
of detection was the mean + 2 SD and the lower limit of decision was the
mean + 3 SD.

12.2.2. Lower limit of detection/determination in Section 4

As can be seen in the tables in section 4 for the routine methods used in
different Member States there are wide variations in the limits for the
measurement of residues of a particular analyte even though essentially
similar methods are used. However there is increasing agreement between
the Member States on the lower limit of decision for particular analytes.

For Reference methods the limits are more clearly defined in the Criteria
Document, EEC 93/256 (see section 5).

In the simplest situation;
  lower limit of detection is mean of 20 blank values + 3 times SD.
  lower limit of decision is mean of 20 blank values + 6 times SD.

In other situations, e.g. where peak noise has to taken into account or
identifying a spot on a TLC other approaches are outlined in section 5.

References;

Heitzman, R.J. and Harwood, D.J. (1983) The radioimmunoassay (RIA) of
hexoestrol residues in faeces, tissues and body fluids of bulls and steers.
Vet. Rec. 112, 120-123.

Heitzman, R.J., Carter, A.C. and Cottingham, J.D. (1986) An enzyme linked
immunosorbent assay (ELISA) for residues of monensin in plasma of cattle.
Br. vet. J. 142, 516-523.

12.2.3. GRAPHICAL METHOD FOR THE CALCULATION OF LIMITS USING RECOVERIES

Where spiked material is used to construct a calibration curve of added amount of spike versus the amount of spike recovered (determined from a standard curve obtained without the matrix) the limits of detection and determination can be calculated from the curve.

Matrix material is spiked in at least quadruplicate at 5 or more levels and the recovery determined by interpolation with a standard curve obtained without the matrix. The confidence limits (e.g 95%, 99% or 99.9%) for the curve are drawn. The limits are calculated from the graph as described in the schematic graph below. The individual values and the best fit linear regression line are drawn and the confidence limits. The 99% confidence limits are used in this graph and are for illustration purposes.

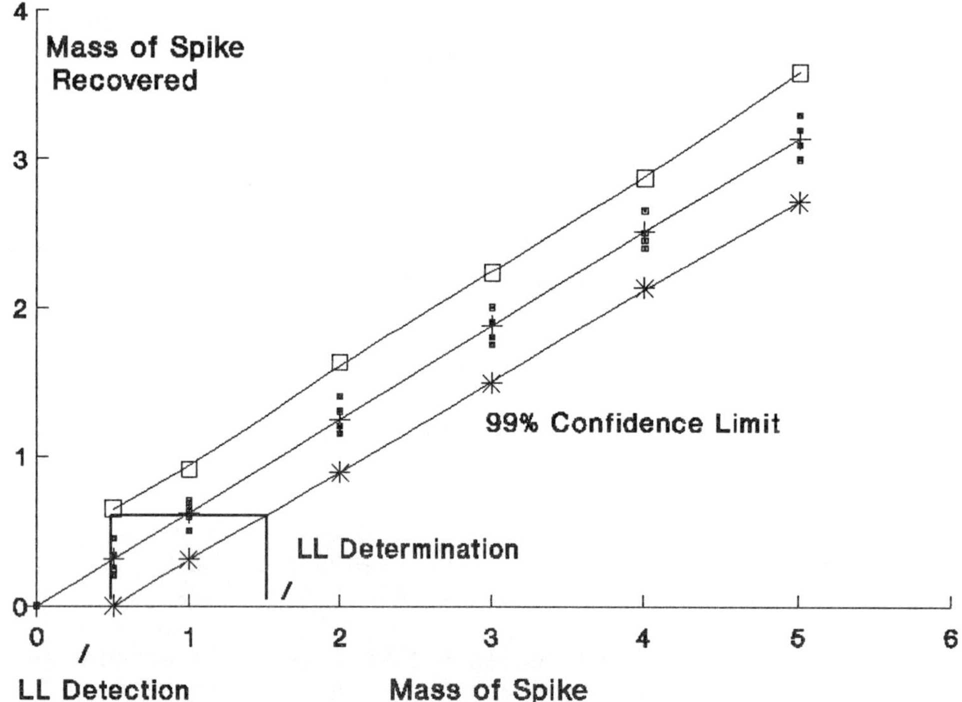

A more detailed approach to the statistical evaluation of results can be found in "Statische Methoden in der Wasseranalytik. Begriffe, Strategien, Anwendungen". Edited by Funk, W., Damman, V., Vonderheid, C. and Oehlmann, G. publ. VCH, Weinheim, D-6940. ISBN 3-527-26307-1, Chapter 4. "Nachweis- und Bestimmungsgrenze."

12.2.4. CALCULATION OF CONFIDENCE LIMITS (INTERVALS).

Data needed; mean, x;   SD, number of values, n;
            t value (see table) using degrees freedom $^{O}F = n - 1$ at
            confidence required, e.g. 95% (P<0.05);

Confidence limits = $x \pm \dfrac{SD \times t}{\sqrt{(n - 1)}}$

Table of critical t values for comparison of averages (two tailed).

| Degrees of | Confidence Interval | | |
Freedom	90%	95%	99%
1	6.31	12.71	63.66
2	2.92	4.30	9.93
3	2.35	3.18	5.84
4	2.13	2.78	4.60
5	2.02	2.57	4.03
6	1.94	2.45	3.71
7	1.90	2.37	3.50
8	1.86	2.31	3.36
9	1.83	2.26	3.25
10	1.81	2.23	3.17
11	1.80	2.20	3.11
12	1.78	2.18	3.06
13	1.77	2.16	3.01
14	1.76	2.15	2.98
15	1.73	2.09	2.95
20	1.73	2.09	2.85
25	1.71	2.06	2.79
30	1.70	2.04	2.75

13.0. INDEX

[Note: The pages are numbered separately for each section, e.g. section 3
page 5 is 3/5. The analytical methods in section 6 are numbered separately
for each method, e.g. page 3 of routine method Cy 1.2 is Cy 1.2/3.]

        Cy 1.9/1-4, Cy 2.1/1-3, Cy 2.1/10, Cy 2.2/1-6, Cy 2.3/1-7, Cy 3.1/2-
        6, Cy 3.3/1, Cy 3.5/4, Cy 3.5/6-7, Cy 3.6/3, Cy 3.6/5-6, Cy 4.1/2,
        Cy 4.3/1-2, Cy 4.3/4, Cy 4.3/6, Cy 4.6/1-6
Gel 6/7, 9/6, 9/11, 9/12, Cy 1.1/8, Cy 1.1/11-12, Cy 1.1/16, Cy 1.9/3,
        Cy 2.1/9, Cy 2.3/2, Cy 3.4/2, Cy 3.4/4, Sg 1.2/6-11, Sg 1.4/1,
        Sg 2.1/1, Sg 2.1/3, Sg 2.1/5-6, Sg 2.4/1-3, Sg 2.4/6, Sg 4.1/2,
        Sg 4.2/2, Sg 4.5/1, Sg 4.5/3-6
Growth inhibition of bacteria 4/15
Growth promoters 7/16, Cy 1.1/1, Cy 1.2/10-11, Cy 1.5/1, Cy 1.6/1,
        Cy 1.7/1, Sg 1.3/1
Haloperidol 8/9, 9/1, 9/48, Cy 4.5/3, Cy 4.5/6, Cy 4.6/3, Cy 4.6/5-6,
        Sg 4.1/3, Sg 4.1/6
Hexoestrol 2/2, 7/20, 8/4, 8/6, 8/11, 9/1, 9/7, Cy 1.1/1-2, Cy 1.2/1,
        Cy 1.2/6-7, Cy 1.2/10, Cy 1.2/12, Cy 1.2/14-15, Cy 1.7/1, Cy 1.7/8,
        Sg 1.1/1-2, Sg 1.2/6-7, Sg 1.2/12, Sg 1.3/1-3
HPLC 4/2-15, 5/20, 6/1, 6/3-7, 6/11, 7/23, 7/26-27, 7/30, 7/36, 7/38,
        8/5-7, 9/57, Cy 1.1/2-5, Cy 1.1/9-13, Cy 1.1/16, Cy 1.4/2, Cy 1.6/1-
        7, Cy 1.6/10, Cy 1.7/1-10, Cy 1.8/1-5, Cy 2.1/1, Cy 3.1/2, Cy 3.2/7-
        12, Cy 3.3/1-5, Cy 3.4/1-6, Cy 3.5/2-8, Cy 3.7/1, Cy 3.7/2-6,
        Cy 3.8/1-5, Cy 3.9/1-5, Cy 4.1/2-5, Cy 4.2/1-5, Cy 4.4/2-5, Cy 4.5/1-
        6, Cy 4.6/2, Sg 1.1/1-5, 3.4/1-5, Sg 3.5/1-6, Sg 3.6/1-6, Sg 4.1/1-6,
        Sg 4.2/1-6,   Sg 4.3/1-8, Sg 4.5/2
HPTLC 4/2-4, 4/5-9, 4/12, Cy 1.9/1-4, Cy 4.5/4, Sg 1.1/1-5, Sg 1.4/1-6,
        Sg 3.2/1-5, Sg 4.3/7-11
Hydrolysis 6/10, 7/39, 10/6, Cy 1.1/6, Cy 1.1/11, Cy 1.2/2, Cy 1.2/5,
        Cy 1.2/11-12, Cy 1.2/15, Cy 1.4/2-3, Cy 1.4/6, Cy 1.5/2-3, Cy 1.5/6,
        Cy 1.6/2, Cy 1.6/6, Cy 1.7/2, Cy 1.8/1, Cy 2.1/5, Cy 2.1/9-10,
        Cy 2.3/2-3, Cy 2.3/7, Cy 3.5/2, Cy 3.5/4, Cy 3.5/8, Sg 1.2/7-8,
        Sg 1.3/2, Sg 2.1/1-2, Sg 2.1/6, Sg 2.4/1-2, Sg 4.2/2
IAC 4/2-5, 4/7, 4/9, 4/10, 5/15, Cy 2.1/7, Cy 2.1/10
Immunoaffinity chromatography 4/15, 5/15, 6/7, 6/11, 8/10, Cy 1.1/2,
        Cy 1.1/8, Cy 1.1/11, Cy 1.1/16, Cy 2.1/5, Cy 2.1/9
Immunoassay 4/15, 5/1, 5/15, 6/4-6, 6/11, 8/10, Cy 2.1/2, Sg 2.2/1,
        Sg 2.3/1
Immunogram 5/6, 5/15
Infrared 5/15, 6/13, 8/9
Injection site 4/15, 7/17-19, 7/30, 7/32
Internal standard 5/10, 5/13, 5/21, 5/22, 6/8, 6/9, 6/12
Ipronidazole 2/3, 9/1, 9/49
Isometamidium 2/3
Ivermectin 2/3, 2/6, 4/14, 6/11, 7/1, 7/15, 7/35-36, 9/1, 9/51,
        Cy 4.4/1-5,
Kidney 2/5-6, 4/15, 6/8, 7/3-7, 7/9-10, 7/12-14, 7/16-20, 7/22, 7/25,
        7/27, 7/30, 7/34-38, 9/19, Cy 1.1/10, Cy 1.2/8, Cy 1.6/2-7,
        Cy 1.7/5,Cy 2.2/1, Cy 2.2/6, Cy 3.1/2, Cy 3.1/3, Cy 3.2/7-8,
        Cy 3.2/11, Cy 3.3/1-5, Cy 3.4/1, Cy 3.4/5-6, Cy 3.8/1, Cy 3.8/3,
        Cy 4.4/1, Cy 4.4/3, Cy 4.5/1-6, Cy 4.6/1-6, Sg 2.4/1, Sg 2.4/4-6,
        Sg 3.6/1-2, Sg 3.6/6, Sg 4.1/1-2, Sg 4.1/4, Sg 4.1/6, Sg 4.2/1-2,
        Sg 4.2/6, Sg 4.3/1-2, Sg 4.3/6-7, Sg 4.3/10
Kit(s) 6/1, 6/2, 8/10, 8/11, Cy 1.1/8, Cy 2.1/9, Cy 3.1/4, Cy 4.3/4,
        Sg 2.2/1-3, Sg 2.3/1, Sg 3.2/3
Lasalocid 2/3, 9/1, 9/52, Cy 4.2/1-5,
Levamisole 2/3, 2/6, 4/14, 9/1, 9/53, Sg 4.5/1-6
Liquid chromatography 4/15, 5/1, 5/15, 6/13, 7/2, 7/31, Cy 1.1/11-12,
        Cy 1.7/1, Cy 2.1/1, Cy 3.2/7, Cy 3.3/2, Cy 3.4/1, Cy 3.7/1-2,
        Cy 3.9/1-2, Cy 4.6/2, Sg 1.3/1, 3.4/1, Sg 4.1/2, Sg 4.3/2
Low resolution mass spectrometry 5/15

Lower limit of detection 4/15, 7/30, 8/11, Sg 2.3/1
Mass spectrometry 4/15, 5/1, 5/15, Cy 1.1/2, Cy 1.1/12, Cy 1.1/14,
        Cy 1.2/6, Cy 1.2/10-11, Cy 1.2/14, Cy 1.4/1-2, Cy 1.5/1-2, Cy 1.8/1,
        Cy 1.9/1, Cy 2.1/2, Cy 2.2/1, Cy 2.3/1, Cy 3.1/1-5, Cy 3.5/1-2,
        Cy 3.5/6, Cy 3.6/1-2, Cy 4.3/2, Cy 4.3/5, Sg 1.2/6, Sg 2.1/1,
        Sg 2.4/1, Sg 4.5/1, Sg 4.5/4
Maximum Residue Limit 5/4-7, 5/9, Cy 3.1/6, Cy 3.3/5
Measurement and Testing Programme 6/7, 8/1, Cy 1.5/6, Cy 2.3/2, Sg 3.3/6
Meat 2/5-6, 3/1, 3/3, 6/1, 6/3-4, 6/8, 6/13, 7/22, 7/24, 7/29, 7/32,
        7/37-38, 7/40, 8/10-11, 10/1-6, Cy 1.1/1-2, Cy 1.1/9, Cy 1.2/5,
        Cy 1.2/9, Cy 1.2/11-12, Cy 1.4/3, Cy 1.5/3, Cy 1.6/1, Cy 1.6/4,
        Cy 1.7/1, Cy 1.7/4, Cy 1.9/1, Cy 1.9/3-4, Cy 2.1/1, Cy 2.1/4,
        Cy 2.2/3, Cy 2.3/1, Cy 3.1/1-3, Cy 3.2/7, Cy 3.2/10, Cy 3.3/2-3,
        Cy 3.4/1, Cy 3.4/4, Cy 3.5/1-2, Cy 3.5/4, Cy 3.5/7, Cy 3.6/1,
        Cy 3.6/3-4, Cy 3.6/6, Cy 3.7/1, Cy 3.8/1, Cy 3.8/3, Cy 3.9/1-4,
        Cy 3.9/5, Cy 4.1/1, Cy 4.1/3, Cy 4.2/3, Cy 4.3/3, Cy 4.4/3, Cy 4.5/1,
        Cy 4.6/1, Cy 4.6/4, Sg 1.3/1, Sg 1.3/4-5, Sg 1.4/1-6, Sg 2.1/1-3,
        Sg 2.4/1, Sg 2.4/4-6, Sg 3.1/7-8, Sg 3.1/11, Sg 3.1/13-14, Sg 3.2/1-
        5, Sg 3.3/1-6, 3.4/1-5, Sg 3.5/4,   Sg 3.6/4, Sg 4.1/1, Sg 4.1/4,
        Sg 4.2/4, Sg 4.3/1-7, Sg 4.3/10, Sg 4.5/3
Medroxyprogesterone acetate 2/2, 8/10, 9/1, 9/8, Cy 1.1/1, Cy 1.1/8,
        Sg 1.1/1-5
Megestrol acetate 2/7, 4/6, 9/1, 9/9, Cy 1.1/1, Sg 1.1/1-5
Melengestrol 2/7, 4/6, 9/1, 9/10, Sg 1.1/1-5
Member States 2/1, 2/3, 4/1, 4/15, 5/1, 6/1, 6/4, 6/6, 7/24, 7/37, 10/1,
        10/2, 10/4, 10/5, 10/6
Methyltestosterone 2/2, 8/9-10, 9/1, 9/11, Cy 1.1/1, Cy 1.1/8, Cy 1.1/16,
        Cy 1.2/1, Cy 1.2/7-8, Sg 1.1/1-2, Sg 1.1/4, Sg 1.2/6-7, Sg 1.2/12
Metronidazole 2/3, 8/9, 9/1, 9/54
Milk 2/5-6, 4/15, 6/3-4, 6/8, 6/10, 7/3-4, 7/7-8, 7/11, 7/14, 7/24-26,
        7/28-29, 7/31-33, 7/35, 9/20, 9/22, 9/24, 10/1, Cy 1.9/3-4, Cy
        3.2/7, Cy 3.3/2, Cy 3.4/1, Cy 3.5/1-7, Cy 3.6/1, Cy 3.6/6, Cy 3.7/1-
        6, Cy 3.8/1-5, Cy 3.9/1-5, Cy 4.1/1-5, Cy 4.2/3, Cy 4.4/1, Cy 4.4/3,
        Sg 1.4/4-6, Sg 2.2/1, Sg 2.2/3, Sg 3.3/1-6, 3.4/4, Sg 4.5/3
Monensin 2/3, 9/1, 9/55, Sg 4.3/7-8
Monitoring 7/8, 7/18, 7/23, 7/36, 10/1, Cy 1.2/11, Cy 2.2/5, Cy 2.3/3,
        Cy 3.1/1, Cy 3.1/2, Cy 3.2/7, Cy 3.3/2, Cy 3.4/1, Cy 3.9/1, Cy 4.1/1,
        Cy 4.3/2, Sg 1.2/10, Sg 2.1/3, Sg 2.1/5, Sg 2.4/3, Sg 2.4/6,
        Sg 3.1/11, 3.4/1, Sg 4.5/1
MRL 2/2-5, 5/21, 7/24, 7/35, 8/1, Cy 1.1/1, Cy 1.2/1, Cy 1.6/1, Cy 1.7/1,
        Cy 1.9/1, Cy 3.1/6, Cy 3.3/5, Cy 4.1/1, Cy 4.4/1, Sg 1.4/1, Sg 3.2/1,
        Sg 3.4/1, Sg 4.5/1-3
Multiresidue 6/1, 6/7, 6/12, 7/40, Cy 1.2/1, Sg 4.1/1
Muscle 2/5-6, 4/15, 6/4, 6/8, 7/3-7, 7/9-10, 7/12-14, 7/16-19, 7/22,
        7/24-25, 7/27, 7/30-32, 7/34-38, 8/2, 9/4-5, 9/7, 9/12-16, 9/20,
        9/22, 9/32, 9/41, 9/62, Cy 1.1/1-2, Cy 1.1/4, Cy 1.1/10, Cy 1.4/1-2,
        Cy 1.6/2-9, Cy 1.7/2-3, Cy 1.7/5, Cy 1.7/7-9, Cy 1.9/1, Cy 2.1/6,
        Cy 2.2/1, Cy 3.1/3, Cy 3.2/7, Cy 3.2/11, Cy 3.4/1, Cy 3.4/6,
        Cy 3.5/2, Cy 3.5/5, Cy 3.5/8, Cy 3.6/4, Cy 3.6/6, Cy 3.8/1, Cy 3.8/3,
        Cy 4.2/1, Cy 4.2/3, Cy 4.4/1, Cy 4.4/3, Sg 1.1/1, Sg 1.4/1, Sg 3.3/1,
        Sg 3.3/4, Sg 3.3/6, Sg 3.5/1-2, Sg 3.5/6, Sg 3.6/1-2, Sg 3.6/6
Narasin 2/3, 9/1, 9/56, Sg 4.3/7-8
Neomycin 7/29, 8/4, 9/1, 9/27, Sg 3.6/1-5
Nitrofurans 2/2, 2/6, 3/2, 4/13, 5/20, 6/3, 6/4, Cy 3.9/1-2, Cy 3.9/5,
        Sg 3.4/1-2, 3.4/5
Nitrofurazone 2/2, 9/1, 9/28, Cy 3.9/1-2, Cy 3.9/5, Sg 3.4/2
Nitroxynil 4/14, 9/1, 9/57

Nortestosterone 2/2, 2/7, 3/2, 4/3, 6/2, 7/1, 7/15-16, 7/20-23, 8/4, 8/10,
     8/11, 9/1, 9/12, Cy 1.1/1-2, Cy 1.1/8, Cy 1.1/10, Cy 1.1/16,
     Cy 1.2/1, Cy 1.2/7, Sg 1.1/1-2, Sg 1.1/4, Sg 1.2/6-7, Sg 1.2/12
NRL 3/1, 5/17, 10/5
Oestradiol 2/2, 2/7, 6/2, 7/1, 7/2-5, 7/7, 7/12, 7/14, 7/17, 7/22, 8/9-11,
     9/1, 9/17, 10/6, Cy 1.1/1, Cy 1.1/5, Cy 1.1/8, Cy 1.1/13, Cy 1.2/1,
     Cy 1.2/7-8, Sg 1.1/1-2, Sg 1.1/4, Sg 1.2/6-7, Sg 1.2/12
Oxfendazole 2/3, 2/6, 4/14, 7/1, 7/15, 7/34, 7/35, 9/1, 9/45, 9/58,
     Cy 4.1/1-2, Cy 4.1/5
Oxytetracyline 2/2, 9/1, 9/30, Cy 3.8/4-5
Penicillin 6/2, 7/1, 7/15, 7/28-31, 8/10, 9/21, Sg 3.1/8-9, Sg 3.1/13
Pharmacokinetics 7/28
Plasma 2/7, 4/15, 6/8, 6/10, 7/5, 7/17, 7/30, 7/37-38, 7/40, 8/11,
     Cy 1.1/1, Cy 1.1/16, Cy 1.6/1, Cy 1.6/10, Cy 1.7/10, Cy 1.9/3-4,
     Cy 2.1/2, Cy 2.1/10, Cy 2.2/1-6, Sg 1.1/1, Sg 1.4/4-6
Precision 5/3-7, 5/20, 6/5, Cy 1.1/4, Cy 1.1/15, Cy 1.6/9, Cy 1.9/4,
     Cy 2.2/5, Cy 3.5/7, Cy 3.6/6, Cy 3.7/5, Cy 3.9/5, Cy 4.1/5, Cy 4.2/5,
     Cy 4.4/5, Sg 1.3/5, Sg 1.4/6, Sg 2.2/3, Sg 3.3/6, Sg 3.5/5, Sg 3.6/6,
     Sg 4.5/6
Pregnant 2/7, 7/3-9, 7/10, 7/12, 7/13, 7/21, 7/34, 9/12
Progesterone 2/2, 6/2, 7/1-3, 7/5, 7/6, 7/8, 7/10-11, 8/9-11, 9/1, 9/18,
     10/6, Cy 1.1/8, Cy 1.2/1, Cy 1.2/7
Propionylpromazine 2/3, 9/1, 9/59, Cy 4.6/3, Cy 4.6/5-6, Sg 4.1/3,
     Sg 4.1/6
Quality control 5/8, 5/10, 5/17, 5/21, 6/12, 8/1, 8/12, Sg 3.5/6
Ractopamine 2/3, 9/1, 9/60, Cy 2.3/1-6, Sg 2.1/1-5, Sg 2.4/1-5
Radioimmunoassay 4/15, 6/13, 7/8, 7/17, 7/18, 7/20, 7/23, 7/40, Cy 1.2/10,
     Cy 1.5/1, Cy 1.6/1, Cy 1.6/7, Cy 1.7/1, Cy 1.7/8, Cy 3.5/2, Cy 3.6/1,
     Sg 1.3/1, Sg 1.3/4, Sg 3.3/1, Sg 3.3/5
Reference Laboratories 3/1, 4/1, 5/17, 6/1, 10/2-5, Cy 1.7/10, Sg 1.3/6
Reference Material 5/2, 5/3, 5/10, 8/8, Cy 3.4/1, Cy 3.4/5-6, Cy 3.6/6
RIA 4/2-7, 4/9, 4/10, 4/15, 6/2, 6/6, 6/10-11, 7/20, 8/5-7, 8/10,
     Cy 1.6/1-10, Cy 1.7/1-10, Cy 3.6/6, Sg 1.3/1-6, Sg 2.2/2, Sg 2.3/1,
     Sg 3.3/1-2, Sg 3.3/5-6
RIKILT 3/4, 5/1, 6/6, 8/4, 8/8, 9/1, 9/12, Cy 2.1/9, Cy 2.3/2, Cy 3.9/1,
     Cy 3.9/4-5, Sg 3.2/5, 3.4/1-2, Sg 4.3/1, Sg 4.3/6-7
RIVM 3/1, 3/3-4, 4/15, 5/1, 6/6-7, 6/12, 8/4-8, 8/12, 9/4-5, 9/7, 9/42,
     Cy 1.1/3, Cy 1.1/5, Cy 1.1/8-16, Cy 2.1/4, Cy 2.1/6, Cy 2.1/9,
     Cy 3.5/2, Cy 3.5/7, Cy 3.6/6, Cy 4.6/3, Sg 4.1/3
RMs 5/23, 6/7, 6/12, 7/32, 8/1-8, 9/1, Cy 1.1/3, Cy 1.7/10, Cy 1.9/4,
     Cy 2.3/7, Cy 3.4/6, Cy 3.5/7, Cy 3.6/6, Sg 1.1/5, Sg 1.2/11,
     Sg 1.3/6, Sg 1.4/6, Sg 2.1/6, Sg 2.2/3, Sg 2.3/5, Sg 2.4/6
Ronidazole 2/3, 2/6, 9/1, 9/61, 3.4/1-2, 3.4/5
Routine method 2/7, Sg 1.1/1, Sg 1.2/6, Sg 4.3/7
Salbutamol 2/3, 4/9, 6/3, 7/15, 7/37, 7/39, 8/4, 8/10-11, 9/1, 9/62,
     Cy 1.1/8, Cy 2.1/1-2, Cy 2.1/6-9, Cy 2.3/1-2, Cy 2.3/6, Sg 2.1/1-2,
     Sg 2.1/5, Sg 2.2/1-3, Sg 2.3/1-5, Sg 2.4/1-4
Salinomycin 2/3, 9/1, 9/56, 9/63, Sg 4.3/7-8
Serum 4/15, 6/8, 6/10, 7/30, 8/11, Cy 1.1/16, Cy 1.6/10, Cy 1.7/10,
     Cy 2.1/2,Cy 2.1/10, Cy 4.4/1, Sg 2.2/1, Sg 2.3/1-2
Spiramycin 2/3, 2/5, 9/31, Sg 3.1/7
Standard 5/2, 5/4, 5/6, 5/9, 5/10, 5/11, 5/12, 5/13, 5/14, 5/18, 5/20,
     5/21, 5/22, 5/23, 6/3, 6/8, 6/9, 6/12, 7/5, 7/28, 8/1, 8/5, 8/6, 8/7
Stilbenes 2/1, 2/7, 3/2, 4/2, 6/2, 6/6, 7/1, 7/15, 7/19, 8/5-7, 8/10,
     10/4, 10/6, Cy 1.1/2, Cy 1.2/10-14, Cy 1.7/1-5, Cy 1.7/10, Sg 1.2/10,
     Sg 1.3/1-6
Sulphadimidine 2/2, 6/2, 7/1, 7/15, 7/24-27, 8/10-11, 9/1, 9/32,

        Cy 3.1/2-6, Cy 3.2/7-8, Cy 3.2/10-12, Cy 3.3/1-5, Cy 3.4/1-6,
        Sg 3.1/8-9, Sg 3.1/13, Sg 3.2/5
Sulphaquinoxaline 2/2, 9/1, 9/33, Cy 3.1/3, Cy 3.2/12, Sg 3.2/5
Tapazole 2/2, 9/1, 9/13, Cy 1.9/1, Sg 1.4/1
Testosterone 2/2, 2/7, 6/2, 7/1-3, 7/5-6, 7/7, 7/9-10, 7/20, 8/9, 8/10-11,
        9/1, 9/3, 9/19, 10/6, Cy 1.1/1-2, Cy 1.1/5, Cy 1.1/8, Cy 1.2/1-2,
        Cy 1.2/6-7, Sg 1.1/1-2, Sg 1.1/4, Sg 1.2/6-7, Sg 1.2/12
Thiabendazole 2/3-4, 4/14, 7/1, 7/15, 7/34-35, 9/1, 9/64, Cy 4.1/1-2,
        Cy 4.1/5
Thiouracil 2/2, 9/1, 9/14, Cy 1.9/1, Sg 1.4/1-2
Trenbolone 2/2, 2/7, 3/2, 4/4, 6/2, 7/1, 7/15-18, 8/4, 8/10-11, 9/1, 9/15,
        Cy 1.1/1-2, Cy 1.1/8, Cy 1.1/11, Cy 1.1/13, Cy 1.1/16, Cy 1.2/7,
        Cy 1.2/9, Cy 1.4/1-6, Cy 1.5/5, Cy 2.1/1, Sg 1.1/1-2, Sg 1.1/4,
        Sg 1.2/6-7, Sg 1.2/12
Triclabendazole 2/3, 7/1, 7/15, 7/35, 9/1, 9/65
Trimethoprim 2/3, 2/5, 6/4, 7/26, 8/9, 9/1, 9/34
Tylosin 2/3, 8/11, 9/1, 9/35, Sg 3.1/7
Urine 2/7, 4/15, 6/8, 6/10, 6/12-13, 7/8, 7/15-23, 7/27, 7/30, 7/36-40,
        8/2, 8/5-7, 8/10-11, 9/4-5, 9/7-8, 9/12-16, 9/19, 9/32, 9/41-42,
        9/62, Cy 1.1/1-2, Cy 1.1/10, Cy 1.1/12, Cy 1.1/14, Cy 1.1/16,
        Cy 1.4/1, Cy 1.6/1-2, Cy 1.6/4-5, Cy 1.6/7, Cy 1.6/9-10, Cy 1.7/1-2,
        Cy 1.7/5, Cy 1.7/8 Cy 1.7/10, Cy 1.8/1, Cy 1.8/3, Cy 1.8/5, Cy 1.9/3,
        Cy 2.1/1-2, Cy 2.1/4-5, Cy 2.1/7-8, Cy 2.1/10, Cy 2.2/1, Cy 2.3/1-4,
        Cy 2.3/7, Cy 3.5/1-8, Sg 1.1/1, Sg 1.2/6-7, Sg 1.2/9-11, Sg 1.3/1,
        Sg 1.3/4, Sg 1.3/6, Sg 1.4/4, Sg 2.1/1, Sg 2.1/3, Sg 2.1/6, Sg 2.2/1-
        3, Sg 2.3/1-6, Sg 2.4/1, Sg 3.2/1, Sg 4.1/1
USDA 5/17, 5/21, 5/23, 7/25, 7/28, 11/1, Sg 3.2/1
VRL 3/4, 8/4, Cy 3.2/12
Withdrawal time 7/24, 7/27, 7/34, 7/36, 7/38
Xenobiotic 2/7, 7/1, 7/15-16, Cy 1.1/1, Cy 1.2/1, Cy 1.8/1, Sg 1.1/1,
        Sg 1.2/6, Sg 1.2/11
Xylazine 9/1, 9/66, Cy 4.5/3, Cy 4.5/6, Cy 4.6/3, Cy 4.6/5-6, Sg 4.1/3,
        Sg 4.1/6
Zeranol 2/2, 4/5, 7/18, 8/4, 8/8, 9/1, 9/16, Cy 1.1/13, Cy 1.5/1-2,
        Cy 1.6/1, Cy 1.6/8, Sg 1.2/12

EDITORS ACKNOWLEDGEMENTS

The Editor thanks sincerely all those who have assisted and contributed to this edition of the "manual". Special thanks are extended to Achim Boenke of DG12 for his management and encouragement in the project and to Claire Gaudot of DG6 for help with sections 4 and 5. Thanks are also extended to the staff of both the Community Reference Laboratories and National Reference Laboratories for their much needed advice and contributions.

For up-to-date information on European Community research

consult

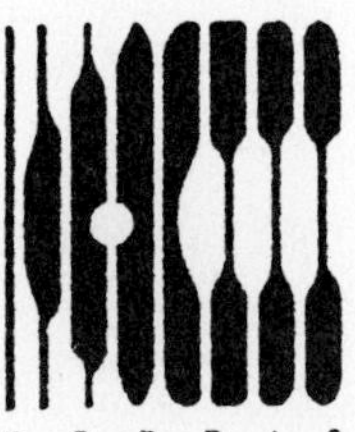

CORDIS
The Community Research and Development Information Service

CORDIS is an on-line service set up under the VALUE programme to give quick and easy access to information on European Community research programmes.

The CORDIS service is at present offered free-of-charge by the European Commission Host Organisation (ECHO). A menu-based interface makes CORDIS simple to use even if you are not familiar with on-line information services. For experienced users, the standard Common Command Language (CCL) method of extracting data is also available.

CORDIS comprises eight databases:

- RTD-News: short announcements of Calls for Proposals, publications and events in the R&D field

- RTD-Programmes: details of all EC programmes in R&D and related areas

- RTD-Projects: containing 14,000 entries on individual activities within the programmes

- RTD-Publications: bibliographic details and summaries of more than 50,000 scientific and technical publications arising from EC activities

- RTD-Results: provides valuable leads and hot tips on prototypes ready for industrial exploitation and areas of research ripe for collaboration

- RTD-Comdocuments: details of Commission communications to the Council of Ministers and the European Parliament on research topics

- RTD-Acronyms: explains the thousands of acronyms and abbreviations current in the Community research area

- RTD-Partners: helps bring organisations and research centres together for collaboration on project proposals, exploitation of results, or marketing agreements.

For more information and CORDIS registration forms, contact
ECHO Customer Service
CORDIS Operations
BP 2373
L-1023 Luxembourg
Tel.: (+352) 34 98 11   Fax: (+352) 34 98 12 34

If you are already an ECHO user, please indicate your customer number.

European Communities – Commission

EUR 15127 – Residues in food-producing animals and their
                products:
                Reference materials and methods – 2nd edition

R. J. Heitzman

Luxembourg: Office for Official Publications of the European Communities
1994 – Nos, 512 pp, num. tab., fig – 21.0 × 29.7 cm

ISBN 0-632-03786-5

Food quality, especially public concern about residues in meat, is one of
the important issues in Europe. This is the first revision of a book whose
purpose is to bring together and update the activities in residues of
veterinary drugs within the Community. The increasing vigilance and
control of residues of veterinary drugs in farm animals and their primary
products relies on effective control of residues. This is only made
possible by having adequate technical resources to carry out relevant
legislation. The analytical methodology used must have an acceptable
quality assurance supported by good quality control criteria, sufficient
reference materials and technical data.

This book addresses each of these needs in detail. There is a summary of
relevant EEC legislation including a selection of Maximum Residue Limits
(MRLs). The methods used in each Member State for the examination of
residues of a large number of drugs is summarised and a selection of the
methods are described in detail. There is supporting information on
residues and chemical/physical data of the most important veterinary drugs.
Also one section of the book covers quality assurance and gives the
criteria for the methods to be used in routine analysis of residues.